HEAD, NECK, and OROFACIAL
INFECTIONS

Second Edition

James R. Hupp, DMD, MD, JD, MBA, FACS
Founding Dean and Professor Emeritus
School of Dental Medicine
East Carolina University
Greenville, North Carolina
Retired
Hollis, New Hampshire

Elie M. Ferneini, DMD, MD, MHS, MBA, FACS
Medical Director
Beau Visage Med Spa
Private Practice
Ferneini Maxillofacial Surgical Institute
Cheshire, Connecticut;
Associate Clinical Professor
Division of Oral and Maxillofacial Surgery
University of Connecticut
Farmington, Connecticut;
Associate Clinical Professor
Department of Surgery
Frank H Netter MD School of Medicine
Quinnipiac University
North Haven, Connecticut

ELSEVIER

Elsevier
3251 Riverport Lane
St. Louis, Missouri 63043

HEAD, NECK, AND OROFACIAL INFECTIONS, SECOND EDITION   ISBN: 978-0-443-11245-4

Previous edition copyrighted 2016.

Publishing Director, Education Content: Kristin Wilhelm
Senior Content Development Manager: Ranjana Sharma
Senior Content Strategist: Kelly Skelton
Senior Content Development Specialist: Rishabh Gupta
Publishing Services Manager: Deepthi Unni
Project Manager: Nayagi Anandan
Design Direction: Patrick Ferguson

Printed in India

Last digit is the print number: 9 8 7 6 5 4 3 2 1

To my beloved wife, Moniek, whose love, devotion, and unwavering support have been the bedrock of my journey to complete this work. Her grace has been my lighthouse, guiding me through the tempests toward realization.

To my children, Michael, Isabella, and Anthony: my greatest inspiration. Their zest for life fuels my ambition and challenges me to exceed my boundaries, striving for excellence in all I undertake.

I extend a heartfelt gratitude to my parents and elder brothers, the architects of my values. They have imbued me with the ethos of education and perseverance, nurturing my growth and fostering my aspirations.

This book is a tribute to my family, whose collective spirit and encouragement have been indispensable. To them, I dedicate this endeavor, a reflection of our shared journey and the love that binds us.

EMF

To Carmen, my true love and best friend, whose wisdom and loving support of me and our kids has made the world a far better place; our accomplished children Jamie, Justin, Joelle, and Jordan, and the amazing individuals they married, Ted, Natacha, Joe, and Jordan; and our marvelous grandkids, Peyton, Morgan, Owen, and Elliot.

JRH

Contributors

Shelly Abramowicz, DMD, MPH, FACS
Professor in Surgery and Pediatrics
Department of Oral and Maxillofacial Surgery
Emory University School of Medicine
Chief, Section of Oral and Maxillofacial Surgery
Children's Healthcare of Atlanta
Atlanta, Georgia

Odai Abushanab, DMD
Resident
Department of Oral and Maxillofacial Surgery
Rutgers University
Newark, New Jersey

Davis Aasen, MD
Resident Physician
Department of Surgery, Division of Otolaryngology-Head
    and Neck Surgery
University of Connecticut Medical School
Farmington, Connecticut

Amir Azari, DMD, MD
Surgeon
Private Practice
Facial and Oral Surgery Center, Bend;
Maxillofacial Surgeon
Shriners Cleft Lip and Palate Program
Shriners Hospital, Portland
Oregon

Ali Banki, DO, FAAD, FAOCD
Assistant Clinical Professor
Department of Medicine
University of New England College of Osteopathic
    Medicine
Biddeford, Maine
Clinical Associate
Department of Dermatology
University of Connecticut School of Medicine
Farmington, Connecticut
Medical Director
Banki Dermatology and Cosmetic Center
Glastonbury, Connecticut

Mohammad Banki, MD, DMD, FACS
Clinical Associate Professor of Surgery
Department of Surgery
Warren Alpert Medical School of Brown University
Providence, Rhode Island
Surgical Director
Artistic Contours
Warwick, Rhode Island

R. Bryan Bell, MD, DDS, FACS, FRCS(Ed)
Physician Executive and Director
Division of Surgical Oncology, Radiation Oncology and
    Clinical Programs
Providence Cancer Institute
Medical Director
Providence Head and Neck Cancer Program
Providence Cancer Institute
Member
Earle A. Chiles Research Institute
Providence Cancer Institute
Portland, Oregon

Tyler T. Boynton, DMD
Private Practice
Department of Oral and Maxillofacial Surgery
Napa Sonoma Oral Surgery and Dental Implants
Sonoma, California

Joseph V. Califano, DDS, PhD
Professor and Co-Director of Predoctoral Periodontics
    Division of Periodontology/Department of Regenerative
and Reconstructive Sciences
Oregon Health and Science University
Portland, Oregon

Daniel P. Caruso, DDS, MD
Fellow
Department of Oral and Maxillofacial Surgery
University of Florida College of Medicine
Jacksonville, Florida

Charles L. Castiglione, MD MBA FACS
Clinical Professor of Surgery
UCONN School of Medicine
Clinical Professor of Oral and Maxillofacial Surgery
UCONN School of Dental Medicine
Hartford Hospital
Hartford, Connecticut

Frank M. Castiglione Jr, MD
Associate Clinical Professor
Department of Dermatology
Yale University
New Haven, Connecticut

Kaylie Catlin, MD, DDS
Resident
Department of Oral and Maxillofacial Surgery
University of Alabama at Birmingham
Birmingham, Alabama

William Chung, DDS, MD
Clinical Professor and Residency Program Director
Department of Oral and Maxillofacial Surgery
Indiana University
Indianapolis, Indiana

Christopher W. Cutler, DDS, PhD
Professor and Chair
Department of Periodontics
Augusta University
Augusta, Georgia

Chad Dammling, DDS, MD
Oral & Maxillofacial Surgeon- Private Practice
Carolina Centers for Oral and Facial Surgery
Raleigh, North Carolina

Fionna Feller, MD
Assistant Professor
Department of Infectious Disease
Vanderbilt University Medical Center;
Section of Infectious Diseases
Veteran Affairs Tennessee Valley Healthcare
Nashville, Tennessee

Antoine M. Ferneini, MD, FACS
Section Chief
Division of Vascular Surgery
Midstate Medical Center
Meriden, Connecticut
Private Practice
Connecticut Vascular Center, PC
North Haven, Connecticut

Elie M. Ferneini, DMD, MD, MHS, MBA, FACS
Medical Director
Beau Visage Med Spa
Private Practice
Ferneini Maxillofacial Surgical Institute
Cheshire, Connecticut;
Associate Clinical Professor
Division of Oral and Maxillofacial Surgery
University of Connecticut
Farmington, Connecticut;
Associate Clinical Professor
Department of Surgery
Frank H Netter MD School of Medicine
Quinnipiac University
North Haven, Connecticut

Susan L. Fink, MD, PhD
Associate Professor
Department of Laboratory Medicine and Pathology
University of Washington
Seattle, Washington

Thomas R. Flynn, DMD
Oral and Maxillofacial Surgeon
Retired
Reno, Nevada

Jacob Gady, DMD, MD
Private Practice
Department of Oral and Maxillofacial Surgery
Connecticut Center for Oral, Facial, and Implant Surgery
West Hartford, Connecticut

Morton Goldberg, DMD, MD
Clinical Professor Emeritus
Division of Oral and Maxillofacial Surgery
School of Dental Medicine, University of Connecticut,
    Farmington
Connecticut

Michael T. Goupil, DDS, MEd, MBA
Emeritus Faculty
University of Connecticut
Farmington, Connecticut

Steven Halepas, DMD, MD
Resident,
Department of Oral and Maxillofacial Surgery
Columbia University
New York, New York

Neil Haycocks, MD, PhD
Assistant Medical Examiner
Utah Office of the Medical Examiner
Utah Department of Health & Human Services
Adjunct Instructor
Department of Pathology
University of Utah School of Medicine
Salt Lake City, Utah

Gabriel M. Hayek, DMD, MD
Private Practice
Department of Oral and Maxillofacial Surgery
Avon Oral, Facial, and Dental Implant Surgery
Avon, Connecticut
Pediatric Cleft and Craniofacial Surgeon
Connecticut Children's Medical Center
Hartford, Connecticut

Cindy Hoffman, DO, FAOCD, FAAD, MBA
Department of Dermatology
St. Barnabas Hospital
Bronx, New York

James R. Hupp, DMD, MD, JD, MBA, FACS
Founding Dean and Professor Emeritus
School of Dental Medicine
East Carolina University
Greenville, North Carolina
Retired
Hollis, New Hampshire

Kyle Johnson, MD
Private Practice
Plains Ear, Nose, Throat, and Facial Plastic Surgery
West Fargo, North Dakota

Walter M. Jongbloed, MD
Resident
Division of Otolaryngology, Department of Surgery
University of Connecticut
Farmington, Connecticut

Alexa J. Kacin, MD
Resident
Department of Otolaryngology–Head and Neck Surgery
Beth Israel Deaconess Medical Center
Harvard Medical School
Boston, Massachusetts

Hilal A. Kanaan, MD, MS
Neurosurgeon
Department of Neurosurgery
East Carolina University Health
Greenville, North Carolina

James A. Katancik, DDS, PhD
Professor and Chair
Regenerative and Reconstructive Sciences
Oregon Health and Science University, Portland, Oregon

Baber N. Khatib, MD, DDS, FACS, FRCD(C)
Oral and Maxillofacial Surgeon
Head and Neck Microvascular Reconstructive Surgeon
OMFS/Microvascular Reconstructive Surgery
Head and Neck Surgical Associates
Providence Franz Cancer Center
Director
Portland 3D Printing Lab
Portland, Oregon

Brian Kinard, DMD, MD
Associate Professor
Department of Oral and Maxillofacial Surgery
University of Alabama at Birmingham
Birmingham, Alabama

Antonia Kolokythas, DDS, MSc, MSed, FACS
Professor and Department Chair
Department of Oral and Maxillofacial Surgery
Augusta University
OMFS Chair and Program Director
Department of Oral and Maxillofacial Surgery and
    Hospital Dentistry
Augusta University
Augusta, Georgia

Kevin C. Lee, DDS, MD
Fellow
Department of Head and Neck Surgery
Roswell Park Comprehensive Cancer Center
Buffalo, New York

Stuart E. Lieblich, DMD
Clinical Professor
Department of Oral and Maxillofacial Surgery
University of Connecticut
Private Practice
Avon Oral and Maxillofacial Surgery
Avon, Connecticut

Maricar Malinis, MD
Associate Professor
Section of Infectious Diseases
Department of Internal Medicine
Yale School of Medicine
New Haven, Connecticut

Regan C. Manayan, MD
Resident
Division of Otolaryngology–Head and Neck Surgery
Beth Israel Deaconess Medical Center
Clinical Fellow
Department of Otolaryngology–Head and Neck Surgery
Harvard Medical School
Boston, Massachusetts

Nishant D. Merchant, MD, FACS
Assistant Professor of Surgery
UConn Health/ Hartford Hospital;
Associate Program Director
Acute Care Surgery Fellowship
UConn Health/ Hartford Hospital
Acute Care Surgeon
Department of Surgery
Hartford, Connecticut

Michael Miloro, DMD, MD, FACS
Professor and Head
Department of Oral and Maxillofacial Surgery
University of Illinois
Chicago, Illinois
Division Chief
Department of Oral and Maxillofacial Surgery
UI Health Hospital
Chicago, Illinois

Thomas S. Murray, MD, PhD
Professor
Department of Pediatrics
Section Infectious Diseases and Global Health
Yale University School of Medicine
New Haven, Connecticut

Keyur Y. Naik, MD, DDS
Fellow
Department of Head and Neck Surgery
High Desert Oral and Facial Surgery
University Medical Center of El Paso
El Paso, Texas

James G. Naples, MD
Assistant Professor of Otolaryngology
Department of Otolaryngology–Head and Neck Surgery
Beth Israel Deaconess Medical Center
Harvard Medical School
Boston, Massachusetts

Timothy John O'Brien, MD
Ear, Nose, and Throat Surgeon
Department of Otolaryngology
Hartford Hospital
Hartford, Connecticut

Kourosh Parham, MD, PhD, FACS
Professor
Department of Surgery, Otolaryngology–Head and
Neck Surgery
University of Connecticut Health
Farmington, Connecticut

Zachary S. Peacock, DMD, MD, FACS
Walter C. Guralnick Chair
Department of Oral and Maxillofacial Surgery
Massachusetts General Hospital;
Department of Oral and Maxillofacial Surgery, Harvard
School of Dental Medicine
Boston, Massachusetts

Robert Piorkowski, MD, FACS
Emeritus Surgeon
Division of Surgical Oncology
Department of Surgery
Hartford Hospital
Hartford, Connecticut

**Philip M. Preshaw, BDS, FDS RCSEd, FDS (Rest Dent)
RCSEd, PhD**
Dean and Professor of Periodontology
Department of Periodontology
School of Dentistry
University of Dundee
Dundee, United Kingdom

Elizabeth Roderick, MD
Acute Care Surgeon
Department of Surgery
Hospital of Central Connecticut
New Britain, Connecticut

Daniel P. Russo, MD
Resident Physician
Department of Surgery, Division of Otolaryngology–Head
and Neck Surgery
University of Connecticut Medical School
Farmington, Connecticut

Thomas Schlieve, DDS, MD
Associate Professor
Department of Surgery, Division of Oral and Maxillofacial
Surgery
UT Southwestern Medical Center
Dallas, Texas

David Shafer, DMD
Chief and Associate Professor
Division of Oral and Maxillofacial Surgery
School of Dental Medicine
University of Connecticut
Farmington, Connecticut

Rabie M. Shanti, DMD, MD
Director, Oral and Maxillofacial Surgery Residency
Training Program
Department of Oral and Maxillofacial Surgery
Rutgers School of Dental Medicine
Newark, New Jersey

Anthony M. Spina, MD, DDS
Director and Vice Chair
Board of Directors
OMS National Insurance Company
Schaumburg, Illinois

Sarah M. Stano, DO
Resident
Department of Dermatology
St. Barnabas Hospital
Bronx, New York

Lance Davis Thompson, MD, DDS
Oral and Maxillofacial Surgeon
Department of Surgery
Head and Neck Surgical Associates
Portland, Oregon

Patrick Clyne Thompson
Medical doctor
Vascular surgeon
Vascular surgery
Connecticut vascular center
North haven, Connecticut

Stevan H. Thompson, BS, DDS, ABOMS, ABOMP
Associate Professor
Surgical Sciences and OMS
East Carolina University SoDM
Greenville, North Carolina

Kiley Trott, MD
Assistant Professor
Department of Otolaryngology
Yale University
New Haven, Connecticut

Katherine Zamecki-Vedder, MD, FACS, FAAO
Attending Physician
Department of Ophthalmology
Connecticut Eye Consultants, PC
Danbury, Connecticut

Vincent B. Ziccardi, DDS, MD
Professor, Chair, and Associate Dean for
    Hospital Affairs
Oral and Maxillofacial Surgery
Rutgers University
Chief of Service
Dental Medicine
University Hospital
Newark, New Jersey

Preface

Infections located in the head, neck, and orofacial regions are commonly seen by healthcare providers in their offices, clinics, and emergency units. Due to the complex nature of the anatomy in this region and large number of vital structures, such as the brain, eyes, and mediastinum, infections in this area of the body must be quickly recognized, diagnosed, and managed to protect patients from serious morbidity or loss of life.

Head, Neck, and Orofacial Infections: An Interdisciplinary Approach was, in its initial edition, the first book to present in-depth, up-to-date information needed by those faced with patients with infections of the head and neck and orofacial complex. This second edition updates the first particularly in the areas of diagnosis and antibiotic management. Many new expert authors were recruited to help ensure the book's contents are authoritative.

Like the first edition, this book is designed to be of value to a large range of health professionals, including:

Physicians—family physicians, infectious disease specialists, internists, hospitalists, pediatricians, critical care physicians, anesthesiologists, clinical pathologists, and radiologists.

Surgeons—general surgeons, head and neck surgeons, otolaryngologists, neurosurgeons, plastic surgeons, pediatric surgeons, oral-maxillofacial surgeons, dermatologists, ophthalmologists, and trauma surgeons.

Nursing professionals—nurse practitioners, nurse anesthetists, hospital-based nurses, nurses responsible for hospital and clinic infection control, and nurses helping manage emergency facilities and operating room suites.

Dental professionals—general dentists, pediatric dentists, periodontists, endodontists, anesthesiologists, oral-maxillofacial radiologists, and pathologists.

Acknowledgments

I wish to thank and acknowledge the many individuals whose expertise has resulted in this outstanding contribution to the medical literature. This first includes my co-editor Dr. Elie M. Ferneini, a tireless talented surgeon, writer, and all-round gracious individual. I also appreciate the entire Elsevier staff involved in producing this work, in particular Rishabh Gupta, Lauren Boyle, Nayagi Anandan, Patrick Ferguson, and Deepthi Unni. It is also important to recognize my faculty during residency, Dr. Morton Goldberg and the late Dr. Richard Topazian. Their original concept for a book dedicated to infections in orofacial region was titled *Oral and Maxillofacial Infections*. It served as the impetus and basis for the first edition of this book, which we have greatly expanded to cover the entire head, neck, and orofacial region.

JRH

I would like to express my deepest gratitude to the mentors, colleagues, residents, and students who have contributed to and inspired the creation of this significant textbook. Their unwavering support and belief in my abilities have been instrumental in bringing this project to fruition.

I would like to extend a special acknowledgment to my esteemed co-editor, Dr. James R. Hupp, whose expertise and visionary leadership within our specialty have played a pivotal role in shaping the content and ensuring the accuracy and relevance of the information presented within this text. Additionally, I am profoundly grateful to Dr. Morton Goldberg and the late Dr. Richard Topazian for their visionary foresight in envisioning a textbook dedicated to head and neck infection. Their seminal contributions to the field have paved the way for this groundbreaking work.

Furthermore, I would like to express my heartfelt appreciation to the entire publishing team at Elsevier for their unwavering commitment to excellence, meticulous attention to detail, and tireless efforts in bringing this project to fruition. Their expertise and support have been indispensable throughout the entire process.

In closing, I would like to extend my deepest gratitude to all those who have contributed to the creation of this significant textbook. Your collective efforts, unwavering support, and invaluable insights have transformed mere words into a comprehensive body of knowledge that will undoubtedly shape the academic discourse within our field for years to come.

EMF

Contents

Appendices

PART 1

General Topics Related to Head, Neck, and Orofacial Infections

1

Immunobiology of Infectious Disease

JOSEPH V. CALIFANO, CHRISTOPHER W. CUTLER, AND PHILIP M. PRESHAW

The human immune system is a biologic marvel designed to identify and destroy or alter pathogens, foreign material, and abnormal cells that threaten an individual. This chapter presents a detailed discussion of the immune system as it relates to infectious pathogens.

Throughout our lives we are constantly encountering microorganisms capable of causing infectious disease. We have, through the evolutionary processes of natural selection, developed a complex and highly organized immune system comprising molecules, cells, and tissues that protect us from agents of infection. Although infections clearly do occur, most interactions with potentially pathogenic bacteria, viruses, or fungi do not result in a productive infection. For infection to occur, the inoculum and virulence of the organism must be of a magnitude sufficient to overwhelm the immune system.

Our immune system is generally divided into two major branches, innate immunity and adaptive immunity (Figure 1-1). It is important to note that these two branches must coordinate closely to ensure that early sentinel innate function translates into pathogen destruction.[1] Innate immunity provides the first line of defense against infection. It includes physical barriers such as the skin and mucosa, phagocytic cells (e.g., neutrophils, macrophages, dendritic cells), specialized pattern recognition receptors (PRRs) that bind and detect classes of macromolecules on pathogens not found in eukaryotic cells (e.g., lipopolysaccharide, lipoteichoic acid, single-stranded DNA, double-stranded RNA [dsRNA]), and molecules that promote inflammation, chemotaxis, and opsonization (e.g., cytokines, complement, acute phase proteins, arachidonic acid metabolites). Infectious agents are often eliminated by innate immunity, thereby preserving health. However, when a pathogen is encountered, the innate immune system can be overwhelmed or circumvented, leading to successful replication of the pathogen within the host, that is, a productive infection. Dendritic cells are the bridge cells of the immune response, serving to sense danger and alert the adaptive immune system to action, shaping the resultant effector responses.[2] Effector responses may be dominated by B cells, differentiating into plasma cells, which secrete antibody (i.e., a humoral response). Opsonizing antibodies specific to the pathogen facilitate its phagocytosis and clearance. It also

may be dominated by a T cell response consisting of helper T cells that assist macrophage clearance or cytotoxic T cells that clear intracellular pathogens like viruses and some bacteria, such as *Mycobacterium tuberculosis*. Innate immunity is the most rapid, not requiring prior exposure to the microorganism to respond to it. Adaptive immunity, on initial exposure to a pathogen, requires 3 to 7 days for a response to occur. With multiple exposures to the pathogen over time, either naturally or through immunization, there is a decrease in the lag time and an increase in the magnitude and efficacy of the adaptive immune response.

Cells of the Immune System

The cells of the immune system are derived from pluripotent stem cells in the bone marrow. The stem cells then differentiate into lymphoid and myeloid progenitors.

The lymphoid progenitor ultimately differentiates into B lymphocytes (produced in the bone marrow), T lymphocytes (produced in the thymus), and natural killer (NK) cells. NK cells are innate immune cells that recognize virally infected cells and neoplastic cells. B lymphocytes, when activated further, differentiate into memory B cells and antibody-secreting plasma cells. T lymphocytes can differentiate into helper T cells, cytotoxic T cells, and regulatory T cells. These different subpopulations of T cells are distinguished from each other by the types of cytokines they produce and by the surface molecules that they display (Figure 1-2).

The myeloid precursor further differentiates into neutrophils (polymorphonuclear leukocytes), macrophage–monocytes, basophils, eosinophils, mast cells, and dendritic cells. It also can differentiate into an erythroblast from which red blood cells are derived, and a megakaryocyte from which platelets are derived (see Figure 1-2).

Polymorphonuclear leukocytes comprise the majority of the granulocytes circulating in the blood. Macrophages are also phagocytic cells, are derived from circulating monocytes, and are located in the tissues in readiness to encounter pathogens. Polymorphonuclear leukocytes and macrophages are the primary phagocytic cells of the body; they kill pathogens by ingesting them and exposing them to an array of enzymes, reactive oxygen species, and antimicrobial peptides contained within lysosomes.

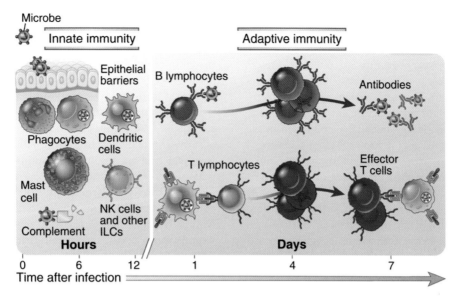

• **Figure 1-1** Components and Kinetics of Innate and Adaptive Immunity. The mechanisms of innate immunity provide the initial defense against infections. Adaptive immune responses develop later and require the activation of lymphocytes. The kinetics of the innate and adaptive immune responses are approximations and vary in different infections. *ILCs,* innate lymphoid cells; *NK,* natural killer. (From Abbas AK, Lichtman AH, Pillai SP. *Cellular and Molecular Immunology.* 10th ed. Philadelphia: Elsevier; 2022.)

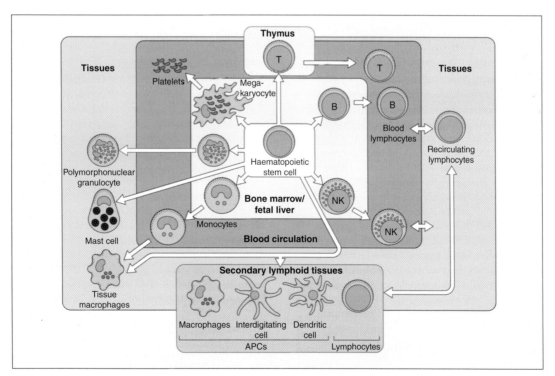

• **Figure 1-2** Origin of Cells of the Immune System. All cells shown here arise from the hemopoietic stem cell. Platelets are released into the circulation. Polymorphonuclear granulocytes and monocytes pass from the circulation into the tissues. Mast cells can be found in all tissues. B cells mature in the fetal liver and bone marrow in mammals, whereas T cells mature in the thymus. The origin of large granular lymphocytes with natural killer *(NK)* activity is probably the bone marrow. Lymphocytes recirculate through the secondary lymphoid tissues. Interdigitating cells and dendritic cells act as antigen-presenting cells *(APCs)* in secondary lymphoid tissues. (From Male D, Stokes R, Male V. *Immunology.* 9th ed. Philadelphia: Elsevier; 2021.)

Mast cells are granulocytes that contain granules containing histamine and heparin. They are located throughout the body, being particularly present in tissues surrounding blood vessels and in close proximity to epithelial surfaces (skin and mucosa). They play a key role in allergic responses and anaphylaxis and in immune responses to pathogens. Mast cells and basophils are functionally similar to each other, the difference being that mast cells are located in the tissues, whereas basophils are found in the circulation. Activation, and subsequent release of histamine by degranulation, results from binding with immunoglobulin E (IgE) and with complement proteins.

DCs are antigen-presenting cells (APCs) that are located in the tissues. These phagocytic cells when immature express a large array of C-type lectin receptors to recognize a broad spectrum of microbes. Upon uptake, immature DCs process the antigens and undergo a maturation program, required to successfully present the antigen to naïve T cells bearing the cognate T cell receptor (TCR) to stimulate their clonal expansion.

Primary and Secondary Lymphoid Tissues

The cells described in the previous section can be found in many locations throughout the body. Among these are the primary and secondary lymphoid tissues (Figure 1-3). The primary lymphoid tissues are the bone marrow and thymus. All cells involved in immunity are derived from the bone marrow. In addition, T lymphocyte development is completed in the thymus, where positive and negative selection allow T cells to be selected that can recognize antigen presented to them in association with self-major histocompatibility molecules with high affinity, but not recognize self-major histocompatibility molecules alone with high affinity. This allows them to be functional but not autoreactive, which could result in autoimmune disease. The secondary lymphoid tissues include lymph nodes in many locations throughout the body; spleen, tonsils, adenoids, and Peyer's patches in the small intestine. All the secondary lymphoid tissues have T cell–rich zones where antigen presentation can occur and B cell–rich zones where B cells are part of lymphoid follicles. B cells in lymphoid follicles exhibit rapid proliferation and differentiation into antibody-secreting plasma cells in response to antigen and T cell–derived growth factors.

Sites in the body that are likely to encounter pathogenic organisms through ingestion or respiration have a higher concentration of secondary lymphoid tissue. Also present at sites of chronic exposure to microbes (e.g., periodontal lamina propria in periodontitis patients),[3] is the formation of tertiary lymphoid tissues, consisting of DC-CD4+ T cell conjugates. The head and neck have a substantial system of

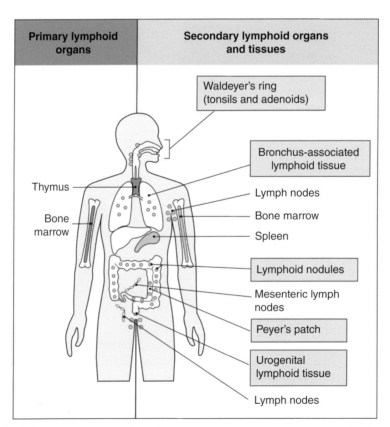

• **Figure 1-3** Primary and Secondary Lymphoid Tissue. Primary lymphoid tissues are the bone marrow and thymus. Secondary lymphoid tissues include lymph nodes in many locations throughout the body; spleen, tonsils, adenoids, and Peyer's patches in the small intestine.

lymph drainage from the oral cavity, pharynx, nose, nasal cavity, paranasal sinuses, nasal pharynx, and pharynx to help prevent infection as a result of exposure through ingestion of food, mastication, and respiration. Secondary lymphoid tissues in the head and neck include many lymph nodes, palatine tonsils, lingual tonsils, and adenoids. It is interesting to note that surgery in the oral cavity performed under aseptic but nonsterile conditions typically does not result in a postsurgical infection. Surgery under the same conditions in sterile tissue sites would likely result in such an infection. The relative resistance to postsurgical infection may result from the greater proportion of lymphoid tissue in this anatomic region.

Innate Immunity

Innate immunity includes barriers to infection (see Figure 1-1). Examples are skin, mucosa, saliva, mucus, tears, acid pH in the stomach, and ciliated respiratory epithelium. The importance of innate immunity becomes clear when one considers the risk of infection that follows severe burns in which the connective tissue is directly exposed to the environment. Infection is a significant cause of morbidity and mortality in patients with severe burns involving large areas of the body. Intact skin and mucosa thus are physical barriers to infection. The epithelium of skin and mucosa is constantly sloughing or exfoliating. This impedes the attachment of pathogenic organisms as they are shed along with the dead cells to which they are attached. Secretions in the respiratory tract, gastrointestinal tract, and eyes serve to flush the epithelial surfaces and further cleanse them. In the respiratory tract, this action is enhanced as ciliated respiratory epithelial cells "sweep" mucus and any potential pathogens out of the lungs, nasal cavity, and paranasal sinuses, and from there into the esophagus to be swallowed and join the gastric contents in conditions of very low pH. Acidity of the stomach acts to inactivate and kill pathogens that enter the gastrointestinal tract.

Antimicrobial molecules are additional barriers to infection; among them are lysozyme, phospholipase A_2, antimicrobial peptides, and acute phase proteins. Lysozyme is secreted by neutrophils and macrophages; it is present in tissues and most secretions, including saliva, and catalyzes hydrolysis of peptidoglycan. Breakdown of bacterial peptidoglycan disrupts the cell wall, especially in gram-positive bacteria. Phospholipase A_2 is produced by neutrophils and epithelial cells. It digests fatty acids in the cell wall and leads to bacterial lysis. Phagocytes, epithelial cells, and salivary glands are all sources of antimicrobial peptides (e.g., defensins, cathelicidins). These molecules form pores or otherwise affect the permeability of the cell membrane, resulting in cellular lysis. Acute phase proteins (e.g., C-reactive protein [CRP], mannose-binding protein [MBP; also known as mannose-binding lectin]) are produced by the liver. They bind to surface carbohydrates of dead or dying host cells (i.e., CRP) or microbial carbohydrate (CRP and MBP) and in turn activate complement through the lectin pathway.

Once complement is activated, the pathogen is opsonized by C3b.[4]

If the barriers and antimicrobial molecules fail to eliminate the pathogen, it will gain access to the subcutaneous tissues. As this occurs, cells of the immune system such as fibroblasts, epithelial cells, and endothelial cells begin to recognize broad classes of macromolecules associated with pathogenic organisms that are not found in humans (e.g., lipopolysaccharide, lipoteichoic acid, flagellin, hypomethylated CpG-rich DNA, dsRNA, N-formylmethionyl-leucyl-phenylalanine [FMLP]). These macromolecules are termed *pathogen-associated molecular patterns* (PAMPs). Similarly, the same cells recognize molecules from damaged host tissues that are elaborated as a result of infection. The receptors that recognize these pathogen-derived molecules are termed *pattern recognition receptors* (PRRs). Examples of PRRs include Toll-like receptors (TLRs) and nucleotide-binding oligomerization domain–like receptors (NLRs), retinoic acid-inducible gene 1–like receptors (RLRs), and the FMLP receptor (Table 1-1).[4]

There are as many as 13 different TLRs. Each recognizes particular macromolecules and molecular patterns. The patterns recognized by some of the key TLRs are summarized in Figure 1-4. TLRs are found on macrophage–monocytes, neutrophils, fibroblasts, epithelial cells, endothelial cells, and DCs. TLRs are transmembrane proteins, some of which are located on the surfaces of cells (e.g., TLR1, TLR2, TLR4, TLR5, TLR6, TLR11), whereas others are located within cells at the endosomal-lysosomal compartment (TLR3, TLR7, TLR8, TLR9). When a pathogen-derived molecule engages the TLR, intracellular second messengers in turn activate expression of genes for proinflammatory cytokines.[5,6]

The process by which interactions between PAMPs and TLRs lead to activation of expression of genes for proinflammatory cytokines is highly complex, and it is referred to as *intracellular signaling*. The process of signal transduction results from recruitment of adaptor proteins that are present within the cytoplasm as the means by which to transfer the signal from the surface-bound TLR to the nucleus, where gene expression will occur.[7,8] Adaptor proteins include myeloid differentiation primary response protein 88 (MYD88), TIR domain-containing adaptor protein inducing interferon-β (IFN-β) (TRIF), TRIF-related adaptor molecule (TRAM), and TIR domain-containing adaptor protein (TIRAP). The adaptor proteins associate (by structural or conformational changes) with the cytoplasmic domains of TLRs by interactions between the Toll/IL-1 (TIR) domains present in each TLR and each adaptor. The MYD88 adaptor is used by all TLR family members except TLR3, which signals via the TRIF adaptor. TLR4 signals via both MYD88 and TRIF (Figure 1-5).[6]

The recruitment of adaptor proteins leads to a cascade of downstream signaling events that differ according to the adaptor molecule concerned. However, in broad terms, the outcome of each signaling pathway results in activation of transcription factors such as nuclear factor-κB (NF-κB) and

TABLE 1-1   Pattern Recognition Molecules of the Innate Immune System

Pattern Recognition Receptors	Location	Specific Examples	Ligands (PAMPs or DAMPs)
Cell-Associated			
TLRs	Plasma membrane and endosomal membranes of DCs, phagocytes, B cells, endothelial cells, and many other cell types	TLRs 1-9	Various microbial molecules including bacterial LPS, peptidoglycans, viral nucleic acids
NLRs	Cytosol of phagocytes, epithelial cells, and other cells	NOD1/2	Bacterial cell wall peptidoglycans
		NLRP family (inflammasomes)	Intracellular crystals (urate, silica); changes in cytosolic ATP and ion concentrations; lysosomal damage
RLRs	Cytosol of phagocytes and other cells.	RIG-1, MDA-5	Viral RNA
CDSs	Cytosol of many cell types	AIM2; STING-associated CDSs	Bacterial and viral DNA
CLRs	Plasma membranes of phagocytes	Mannose receptor, DC-SIGN	Microbial surface carbohydrates with terminal mannose and fucose
		Dectin-1, Dectin-2	Glucans present in fungal and bacterial cell walls
Scavenger receptors	Plasma membranes of phagocytes	CD36	Microbial diacylglycerides
N-Formyl met-leu-phe receptors	Plasma membranes of phagocytes	FPR and FPRL1	Peptides containing N-formylmethionyl residues

TABLE 1-1	Pattern Recognition Molecules of the Innate Immune System—cont'd		
Pattern Recognition Receptors	**Location**	**Specific Examples**	**Ligands (PAMPs or DAMPs)**
Soluble			
Pentraxins	Plasma	C-reactive protein	Microbial phosphorylcholine and phosphatidylethanolamine
Collectins	Plasma	Mannose-binding lectin	Carbohydrates with terminal mannose and fucose
	Alveoli	Surfactant proteins SP-A and SP-D	Various microbial structures
Ficolins	Plasma	Ficolin	N-Acetylglucosamine and lipoteichoic acid components of the cell walls of gram-positive bacteria
Complement	Plasma	Various complement proteins	Microbial surfaces

TLR, toll-like receptor; *NOD*, nucleotide-binding oligomerization domain; *NLRP*, nucleotide-binding oligomerization domain leucine-rich repeat and pyrin domain; *RIG*, retinoic acid-inducible gene; *MDA*, anti-melanoma differentiation associated gene; *AIM*, absent in melanoma; *STING*, stimulator of interferon genes associated cytosolic *DNA* sensor; *CLR*, C-type lectin receptors; *FPR*, formyl peptide receptors; *FPRL*, formylpeptide receptor-like; *DC-SIGN*, dendritic cell-specific intercellular adhesion molecule grabbing non-integrin.

From Abbas AK, Lichtman AH, Pillai SP. *Cellular and Molecular Immunology*. 10th ed. Philadelphia: Elsevier; 2022.

IFN regulatory factors that control the transcription of DNA. TLR signaling leads to expression of proinflammatory cytokines, including tumor necrosis factor-α (TNF-α), type I IFNs, interleukin-1 (IL-1), IL-6, IL-8, and IL-12. These cytokines activate phagocytes, recruit phagocytes to sites of infection, promote maturation of DCs, increase the resistance of cells to viral infection, activate NK cells, and support the development of adaptive immunity for the pathogen (see Figure 1-5).

NLRs are another family of PRRs. They are located intracellularly and, like TLRs, recognize the presence of molecular patterns uniquely associated with pathogens. Once engaged, they also result in the expression of genes for proinflammatory cytokines.

RLRs recognize dsRNA, which is unique to some RNA viruses and when present is indicative of a viral infection. Engagement of RLR by viral dsRNA also increases the expression of proinflammatory cytokines.

Neutrophils also have a receptor for the *N*-formylated tripeptide, FMLP. Every bacterial protein is synthesized, beginning with these three amino acids, the first of which is unique to prokaryotes. Once protein synthesis is complete,

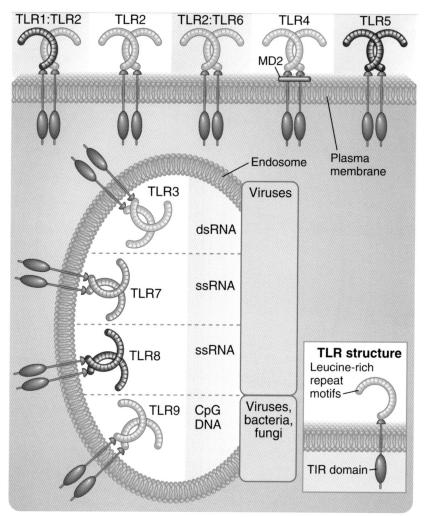

• **Figure 1-4** Toll-like Receptors 1 to 9 and Their Specificity. *dsRNA*, double-stranded RNA; *LPS*, lipopolysaccharide; *ssRNA*, single-stranded RNA; *TLR*, toll-like receptor. (From Abbas AK, Lichtman AH, Pillai SP. *Cellular and Molecular Immunology*. 10th ed. Philadelphia: Elsevier; 2022.)

this tripeptide is cleaved off. Where bacteria are present, so is FMLP; therefore, FMLP is a potent chemotactic factor and induces neutrophil chemotaxis toward increasing concentrations of this molecule.

As cells begin to encounter a pathogen and their PRRs are engaged, they will secrete proinflammatory cytokines. These proinflammatory molecules play a significant role in innate immunity. They help in activating phagocytes (neutrophils, macrophages), NK cells, and DCs and in recruitment of these cells to sites of infection. In addition, complement and cellular adhesion molecules participate in innate immunity and the inflammatory process.

As mentioned previously, some of the key proinflammatory cytokines that are released when PRRs (i.e., TLRs and NLRs) are engaged include TNF-α, type I interferons, IL-1, IL-6, IL-8, IL-12, and lipid mediators. The source of TNF-α in innate immunity is principally the macrophage. It stimulates endothelial cells to express intercellular adhesion molecule 1 (ICAM-1). Immune cells, especially neutrophils and monocytes, express leukocyte function–associated antigen 1 (LFA-1) on their surface that binds to ICAM-1 and

allows these cells to exit the circulation at sites of inflammation, trauma, and infection. Neutrophils and macrophages are also activated by TNF-α. This cytokine also stimulates the liver to release acute phase proteins that activate complement, thereby promoting chemotaxis, opsonization, bacterial lysis, vasodilation, and increased vascular permeability.

Macrophages and fibroblasts release type I IFNs, which activate NK cells and increase cellular resistance to viral infection. NK cells are important in the initial defense against viral infection. They recognize cells infected with a wide variety of viruses and then kill the infected cell. Macrophages and endothelial cells release IL-1, IL-6, and IL-8. The effects of IL-1 in innate immunity are similar to those of TNF-α. IL-6 stimulates the production of acute phase proteins in the liver and supports proliferation of B cells as an adaptive immunity is developing. Chemokines, including IL-8, are chemotactic for immune cells, especially neutrophils. They help direct these cells to sites of infection. Macrophages and DCs secrete IL-12. This cytokine stimulates NK cells to produce high levels of IFN-γ, which in turn stimulates many cells, especially macrophages. When activated, macrophages also release lipid

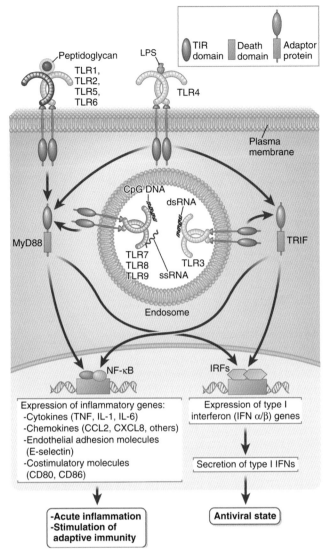

• **Figure 1-5** Toll-Like Receptors *(TLRs)* Signal Transduction and Inflammatory Gene Expression. TLRs 1, 2, 5, and 6 use adaptor protein MYD88 and activate transcription factors NK-κB and AP-1. TLR3 uses adaptor protein TRIFF and activates IRF transcription. TLR 4 can activate both pathways. TLR 7 and 9 in the endosome use MYD88 and activate both NK-κB and IRFs. *dsRNA,* double -stranded RNA; *IFN,* interferon; *IRFs,* interferon regulatory factors; *NF-kB,* nuclear factor kappa B; *ssRNA,* single -stranded RNA; *TIR,* Toll IL-1 receptor; *TLR,* toll-like receptor; *TRIF,* TIR-domain containing adapter-inducing interferon beta. (From Abbas AK, Lichtman AH, Pillai SP. *Cellular and Molecular Immunology.* 10th ed. Philadelphia: Elsevier; 2022.)

mediators that have proinflammatory activity, including the metabolites of arachidonic acid, prostaglandins, and leukotrienes. Prostaglandins (e.g., prostaglandin E_2 [PGE_2]) increase vascular permeability and result in vasodilation, as well as having positive feedback effects on cytokine and prostaglandin secretion, and activating osteoclastic bone resorption. Leukotrienes are chemotactic for neutrophils and support the vascular effects of prostaglandins.

In addition to the proinflammatory cytokines, complement proteins are also an important component of innate immunity (Figure 1-6). As indicated previously, acute phase proteins can activate complement through the lectin

pathway. In addition, many bacterially derived molecules (especially lipopolysaccharide) can activate complement through the alternate pathway. Once activated, several important complement proteins are generated. Among them are C3a, C3b, and C5a. Phagocytes have receptors for C3b on their surface. As the complement cascade is activated, C3b is deposited on the surface of the pathogen, and it serves as an opsonin and facilitates phagocytosis. The complement protein C3a increases vascular permeability and results in vasodilation. A gradient of C5a emanating from sites of infection serves as a potent chemotactic agent, particularly for neutrophils and monocytes. Finally, the terminal sequence of the complement cascade forms the membrane attack complex that creates a pore in the pathogen, disturbs osmotic balance, and thus results in cell lysis.[4]

Adaptive Immunity

Once the barriers (e.g., epithelium, mucosa) are breached, the pathogenic organism gains access to subcutaneous tissues. Immune cells release proinflammatory cytokines as part of innate immunity, and these molecules, as well as antigen from the pathogen, stimulate development of an adaptive immune response. If innate immunity quickly clears the pathogen locally, a strong adaptive immune response may not be necessary. However, if the pathogen is successful in replicating within the host tissues and disseminates more widely throughout the body, there is grave danger to the host, necessitating a strong adaptive immune response.

Antigens, Epitopes, and Antigen Receptors

The adaptive immune response differs from innate immunity in that it recognizes specific antigens from a pathogen. Rather than responding through receptors with the ability to recognize broad classes of pathogen-associated macromolecules (i.e., PAMPs), the receptors in adaptive immunity recognize macromolecules (i.e., proteins, carbohydrates, lipids, nucleic acids) that derive from the particular invading organism at the species and strain level. In fact, if we examine a particular protein derived from the infecting pathogen, several receptors will recognize different sites or epitopes on the protein (an epitope is that part of an antigen that is recognized by the immune system, and typically constitutes five to seven amino acids of a protein). The receptors (antibody molecules and the TCR) recognize epitopes in a specific "lock-and-key" manner (Table 1-2, Figure 1-7). Therefore, if the secondary or tertiary conformation of the protein is affected by denaturing the protein (e.g., after heat denaturation), then the epitope may no longer be present because the three-dimensional configuration of the epitope's amino acids may have been lost (see Figure 1-7).

Adaptive immunity can be thought of as having two general types: (1) cellular, which is primarily focused on defense from intracellular pathogens (e.g., viruses, certain bacteria such as *M. tuberculosis,* malignant tumor cells), and

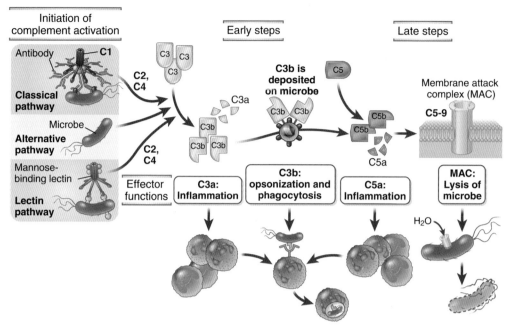

• **Figure 1-6** Complement Activation. The activation of the complement system may be initiated by three distinct pathways, all of which lead to the production of C3b (the early steps). C3b initiates the late steps of complement activation, culminating in the production of peptides that stimulate inflammation (C5a) and polymerized C9, which forms the membrane attack complex, so called because it creates holes in plasma membranes. The principal functions of major proteins produced at different steps are shown. (From Abbas AK, Lichtman AH, Pillai SP. *Cellular and Molecular Immunology*. 10th ed. Philadelphia: Elsevier; 2022.)

TABLE 1-2	Antigen Receptors *Antibody and the T Cell Receptor*	
Feature	**Immunoglobulin (Ig)**	**T Cell Receptor (TCR)**
Antigen-binding site	Made up of three CDRs in V_H and three CDRs in V_L domains	Made up of three CDRs in $V\alpha$ and three CDRs in $V\beta$ domains (in the most common form of TCR)
Nature of antigen that may be bound	Macromolecules (proteins, lipids, polysaccharides) and small chemicals	Peptide-MHC complexes
Nature of antigenic determinants recognized	Linear and conformational determinants of various macromolecules and chemicals	Linear determinants of peptides; only few amino acid residues of a peptide bound to an MHC molecule
Affinity of antigen binding	K_d 10^{-7}–10^{-11} M; average affinity of Igs increases during immune response	K_d 10^{-5}–10^{-7} M
On-rate and off-rate	Rapid on-rate, variable off-rate	Slow on-rate, slow off-rate

CDR, complementarity-determining region; K_d, dissociation constant; *MHC*, major histocompatibility complex V_H, variable domain of the heavy chain immunoglobulin; V_L, variable domain of the light chain immunoglobulin; $V\alpha$ and $V\beta$, variable domains of the T cell receptor alpha and beta chains.
From Abbas AK, Lichtman AH, Pillai SP. *Cellular and Molecular Immunology*. 10th ed. Philadelphia: Elsevier; 2022.

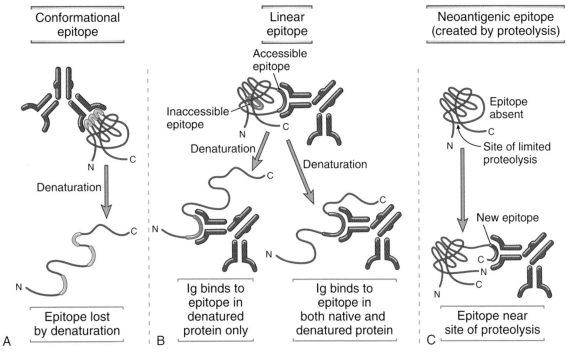

• **Figure 1-7** Antibody, Antigen, Epitope. A protein antigen has an epitope of 5 to 7 amino acids that is recognized by the antibody's antigen combining site. The amino acids are often not adjacent (i.e., not a linear epitope) on the protein polypeptide chain but rather are located near each other by virtue of the secondary structure and form a conformational epitope. A conformational epitope is lost by denaturation. (From Abbas AK, Lichtman AH, Pilla SP. *Cellular and Molecular Immunology*. 10th ed. Philadelphia: Elsevier; 2022.)

(2) humoral, which is primarily focused on defense from extracellular pathogens (e.g., bacteria, fungi, parasites). The former involves cytokines from T helper (T$_h$) cells and effector cells, such as cytolytic T (T$_{CTL}$) cells, macrophage–monocytes, and NK cells. The latter involves B lymphocytes that differentiate into antibody-secreting plasma cells and B memory cells. They do so with the help of cytokines from Th cells.

The antigen receptor for the B cell is the surface antibody molecule. It recognizes soluble or free native antigen (i.e., not denatured or processed). The antigen-combining sites on the antibody molecule recognize the epitope in a specific lock-and-key fashion. The antigen receptor for the T cell is the TCR (see Table 1-2). The TCR recognizes only processed antigen that must be presented to the T cell (i.e., it is not a native antigen and is not free or soluble antigen). Antigen presentation involves internalizing of the native molecule by an APC (e.g., a DC), processing of the molecule into small pieces, association of the fragments with a special cleft on the major histocompatibility complex (MHC) molecules, and expression of the same on the cell surface. The T cell and its TCR then recognize the processed antigen in association with self-MHC molecules in a specific lock-and-key fashion (see Table 1-2).

The T cell and B cell antigen receptors and, in particular, their antigen-combining sites are unique to the particular cell clone and relate to its antigen specificity. Immature lymphocytes have germline DNA sequences in the genes responsible for their antigen receptors. Once the cell is mature, these genes eventually encode for two glycoprotein transmembrane proteins that compose the α and β chains of the TCR or the two heavy-chain transmembrane glycoproteins and two associated light chains that constitute the surface antibody molecule that is the B cell receptor. These genes are composed of a large number of DNA segments separated by noncoding DNA (Figures 1-8 and 1-9). There are constant region gene segments that do not vary among different cell clones and are present for each chain (four for antibody and two for the TCR). There are also variable region (V), diversity (D), and joining (J) gene segments. There are many different V, D, and J segments. For antibody molecules, the variable portions of the heavy chains are composed of V, D, and J gene segments and the light chains only V and J. For the TCR, the variable region of the α chain is composed of V and J gene segments, and the β chain is composed of V, D, and J segments. As the lymphocyte develops into a mature B or T cell, the germline DNA is subjected to recombination and mutation among the gene segments and deletion of many of the V, D, and J genes, so that a particular set of V and J or V, D, and J genes are directly joined to one another. This process occurs on each of the heavy and light chains of the antibody genes and the α and β chains of the TCR. There are also some inaccuracies in the splicing of these gene segments and insertions of a small number of nucleotides at the joints, resulting in additional diversity. This genetic recombination

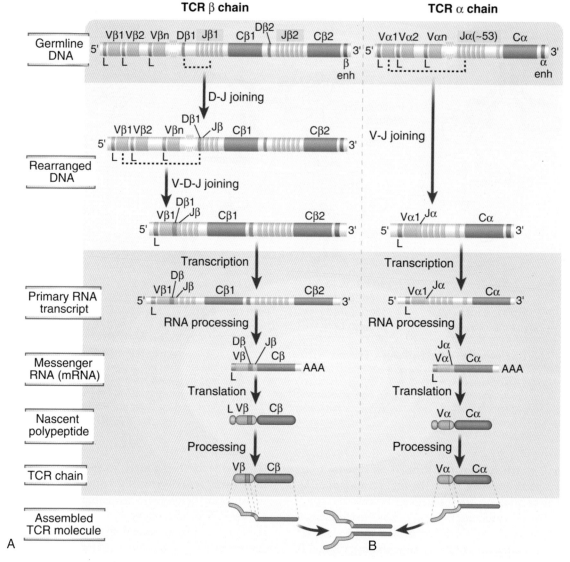

• Figure 1-8 Generation of Diversity T Cell Receptor. As the lymphocyte develops into a mature T cell, the germline DNA is subjected to recombination and mutation among the gene segments and deletion of many of the V, D, and J genes, so that a particular set of V and J or V, D, and J genes are directly joined to one another. This process occurs on each of the α and β chains of the T cell receptor. This genetic recombination and rearrangement in the germline DNA allows for an extremely high level of variation in the final DNA sequence in the antigen-combining sites of the antigen receptors. (From Abbas AK, Lichtman AH, Pillai SP. *Cellular and Molecular Immunology.* 10th ed. Philadelphia: Elsevier; 2022.)

and rearrangement in the germline DNA allows for an extremely high level of variation in the final DNA sequence in the antigen-combining sites of the antigen receptors; this is referred to as *generation of diversity*. It allows, through this random process, the production of unique antigen-combining sites in the B cell surface antibody or TCR that allows an immune response to essentially any possible antigen in the environment.

Antigen Presentation and the Major Histocompatibility Complex

T lymphocytes have several subsets: T_h cells, which can be further subdivided into T_{h1}, T_{h2}, T_{h17}, T follicular helper (T_{fH}) cells; T_{CTL} cells, which are the primary effector cells in cellular immunity; and regulatory T (T_{reg}) cells, which help in regulation of immunity. They encounter and recognize antigen that is processed and presented to them. T cells require that antigen be processed and presented, rather than responding directly to antigen, to limit incidence of autoimmune diseases. T_h and T_{reg} cells are CD4$^+$, which indicates that they recognize antigen presented in association with MHC class II molecules (i.e., they recognize antigen together with components of self that are involved in the presentation of pieces of the antigen). Not all cells possess class II MHC; therefore, only certain cells can present antigen to CD4$^+$ cells. APCs with high levels of MHC class II molecules on their surface include DCs,

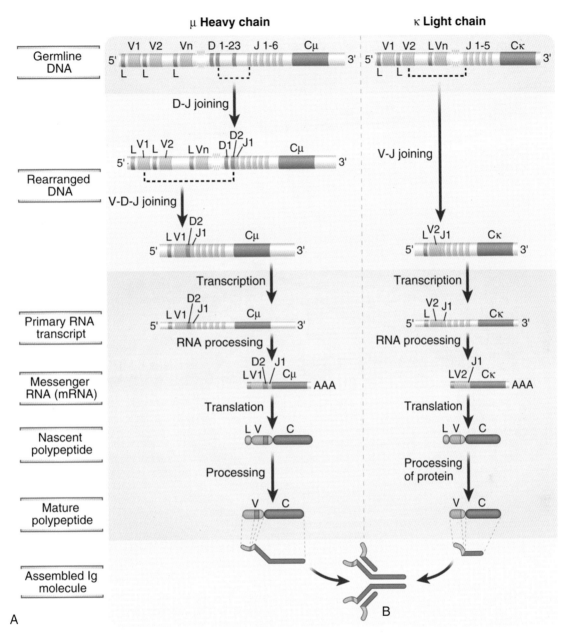

• Figure 1-9 Generation of Diversity B cell Receptor/Antibody. As the lymphocyte develops into a mature B cell, the germline DNA is subjected to recombination and mutation among the gene segments and deletion of many of the V, D, and J genes, so that a particular set of V and J or V, D, and J genes are directly joined to one another. This process occurs on each of the heavy and light chains of the antibody genes. There are also some inaccuracies in the splicing of these gene segments and insertions of a small number of nucleotides at the joints, resulting in additional diversity. This genetic recombination and rearrangement in the germline DNA allows for an extremely high level of variation in the final DNA sequence in the antigen-combining sites of the antigen receptors. (From Abbas AK, Lichtman AH, Pillai SP. *Cellular and Molecular Immunology*. 10th ed. Philadelphia: Elsevier; 2022.)

macrophage–monocytes, Langerhans cells, and B cells. They all have the ability to present antigen to $CD4^+$ T_h and T_{reg} cells. T_{CTL} cells are $CD8^+$, which indicates that they recognize antigen in the context of MHC class I. MHC class I molecules are expressed on all nucleated cells. When a cell is infected with a virus, the T_{CTL} cells can then recognize viral antigens that are presented by the infected cell in association with class I MHC molecules (Figure 1-10). The

TCRs in each case recognize the combination of the fragment of the foreign antigen and the self-MHC molecule. It is important to note that T cells can only recognize antigen that is processed and presented to them in association with self-MHC molecules. Therefore, APCs from one person cannot present antigen to another person's T cells, unless they are monozygotic twins, because they will not share the same MHC molecules. As an aside, MHC molecules are also the

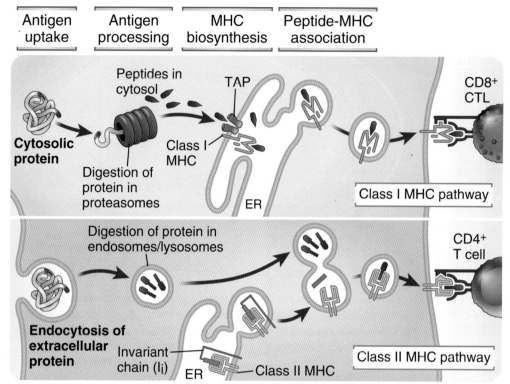

• **Figure 1-10** Antigen Processing and Presentation. Antigen presentation to CD8⁺ T cells: Protein antigens for viral or tumor specific antigens present in the cytosol of any nucleated cell are broken up into peptides by a proteasome. They are then associated with class I MHC molecules on the surface of the cell and recognized by the T cell receptor on the CD8⁺ cell. Antigen presentation to CD4⁺ T cells: Protein antigens are taken up by endocytosis or phagocytosis and are then within a lysosome of an antigen-presenting cell. Once in the lysosome they are broken up into peptides by hydrolytic enzymes, associated with class II MHC molecules on the surface of the cell, and recognized by the T cell receptor on the CD4⁺ cell. MHC, major histocompatibility complex; CTL, cytotoxic T lymphocyte; ER, endoplasmic reticulum; TAP, transporter associated with antigen processing. (From Abbas AK, Lichtman AH, Pillai SP. *Cellular and Molecular Immunology*. 10th ed. Philadelphia: Elsevier; 2022.)

transmembrane glycoproteins involved with tissue typing and responsible for graft rejection in tissue transplantation.

Clonal Selection

At any given time, the large numbers of T and B lymphocytes we have are composed of many clones, with each clone comprising only a small number of cells, all of which share the same receptor and specificity (Figures 1-11 and 1-12). When we have an infection (or are immunized with a vaccine), almost all the lymphocytes lack reactivity with the antigens from the pathogen. Lymphocytes that have receptors with affinity for specific antigen of the invading organism will be activated by engagement of their receptor by the antigen along with costimulatory signals. When this occurs, these cells will undergo rapid cell division and, through the resulting proliferation, temporarily represent a large proportion of the circulating T and B cells in the body. This situation will remain until the pathogen is cleared by the resulting immune response. It usually takes 3 to 7 days of lag time for this response to occur after initial exposure. Once that pathogen is cleared, the number of lymphocytes will return to normal. Some of the cells that are reactive with the pathogen will persist as B and T memory cells in

secondary lymphoid tissues. If the same pathogen is encountered again in the future, the lag time will be shorter (Figure 1-13). In addition, each time there is an exposure to antigens of a particular pathogen, there is competition for antigen among the memory cells. As a result, the cells with higher affinity (i.e., antigen receptors that bind the antigen more tightly and effectively) will be more likely to be stimulated. This process of "natural selection" of cells with the most avid and effective receptors results in the phenomenon of affinity maturation. Thus, multiple exposures not only decrease the lag time, but also increase the efficacy and efficiency of the adaptive immune response.

T Cell Maturation In the Thymus

B cells mature in the bone marrow, and essentially all B cells that effectively rearrange their germline DNA to a functional surface antibody receptor become part of the B cell repertoire. This can result in B cells that generate antibody molecules that recognize self-antigens (i.e., autoantibody), and this sets up the potential for autoimmune disease. For most people, autoimmunity is prevented by the T cell maturation process that occurs in the thymus. Immature T cells generated in the bone marrow mature and rearrange

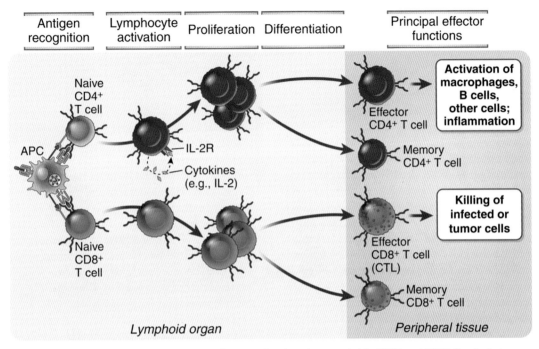

• **Figure 1-11** Clonal Selection T cells. Processed antigen is presented to CD4⁺ and CD8⁺ T cells that have receptors specific for the antigen (i.e., there is clonal selection of these particular T cells). There is then activation and clonal expansion followed by effector helper and cytolytic function. *APC*, antigen presenting cell; *CTL*, cytotoxic T lymphocyte. (From Abbas AK, Lichtman AH, Pillai SP. *Cellular and Molecular Immunology*. 10th ed. Philadelphia: Elsevier; 2022.)

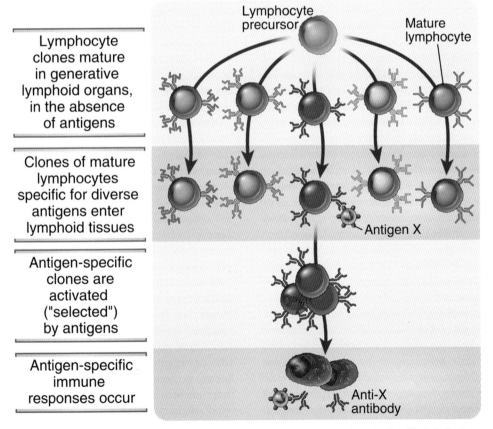

• **Figure 1-12** Clonal Selection B cells. B cells recognize native antigen and receive T cell help in the form of cytokine growth factors. They are then activated and clonal expansion occurs. During this process the B cells further differentiate into antibody secreting plasma cells and B memory cells. (From Abbas AK, Lichtman AH, Pillai SP. *Cellular and Molecular Immunology*. 10th ed. Philadelphia: Elsevier; 2022.)

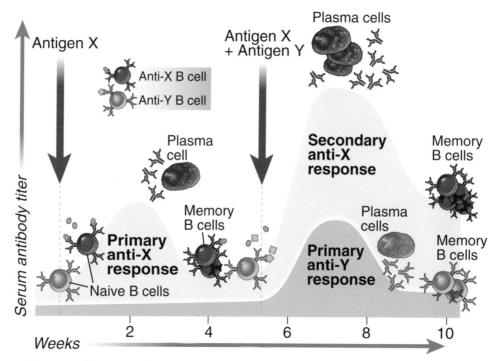

• **Figure 1-13** Primary and Secondary Response. When B cells encounter antigen in the primary response, there is a long lag time before the B cell differentiates into a plasma cell and secretes antibody. This antibody is mostly IgM and of lower affinity. With subsequent exposure in the secondary response, B memory cells compete for antigen. Cells with surface antibody receptors with the highest affinity will more readily bind antigen and become stimulated. This natural selection process increases the affinity of the antibody with each exposure to antigen. During the secondary response class switch usually occurs and the lag time is shorter. (From Abbas AK, Lichtman AH, Pillai SP. *Cellular and Molecular Immunology*. 10th ed. Philadelphia: Elsevier; 2022.)

their germline DNA and express TCRs in the thymus. As the T cells mature, thymic stromal cells assess the level of affinity of the TCR for the self-MHC molecules on their surface. T cells with receptors that have low affinity for self-MHC are positively selected because they have good potential to recognize processed foreign antigen in association with self-MHC with high affinity. Those without affinity for self-MHC are not selected. T cells that have high affinity for self-MHC are deleted because they would likely be autoreactive and promote autoimmune disease. This process evolved to prevent cell-mediated autoimmune disease and prevent autoimmune disease mediated by autoantibody, because autoreactive B cells will not have T cells reactive with autoantigens to provide the required T cell help in the form of cytokine growth factors.

Cellular Immunity

Once CD4$^+$ T$_h$ cells leave the thymus, they circulate throughout the body. As they move through T cell–rich zones in the secondary lymphoid tissue, they sample foreign antigen presented by DCs. If they encounter antigen that their TCR recognizes, they are stimulated. They exchange stimulatory signals in the form of cytokines and reciprocal receptor engagement. The T cell then proliferates and expands so that many clones of the pathogen- or antigen-specific T cell are produced and circulate throughout all the secondary lymphoid tissues to help eliminate the pathogenic organism.

Depending on the type of interaction and signals received from the APC, the T$_h$ cell is further differentiated into one of several T$_h$ subsets.[9] Each produces a different set of growth factors that support an immune response that is tailored to the particular pathogen (e.g., bacteria/extracellular versus virus/intracellular). The T cell subsets are T$_{h1}$, T$_{h2}$, Th$_{17}$, and T$_{fH}$ cells. T$_{h1}$ cells secrete IL-2, IFN-γ, and TNF-α and especially support cellular immune responses to viral infections. These cytokines are important in stimulating macrophage–monocytes, T$_{CTL}$ cells, and NK cells. T$_{h2}$ cells secrete IL-4, IL-5, IL-10, and transforming growth factor (TGF)-β, which support B cell growth and differentiation and, therefore, antibody responses important for extracellular bacterial infections. Th$_{17}$ cells secrete IL-6, IL-17, IL-22, and TNF-α, which support innate immunity and antibody responses (Figure 1-14).[10] T$_{fH}$ cells (fH = follicular helper) are unique helper cells that reside in the B cell–rich zone of secondary lymphoid tissue where lymphoid follicles are located. They help support and regulate B cell growth and maturation within the lymphoid follicle (see Figure 1-14).[11,12] T$_{reg}$ cells secrete IL-10 and TGF-β, which regulate and dampen the adaptive immune response. These cytokines especially inhibit T$_{h1}$ cytokines. It is important to

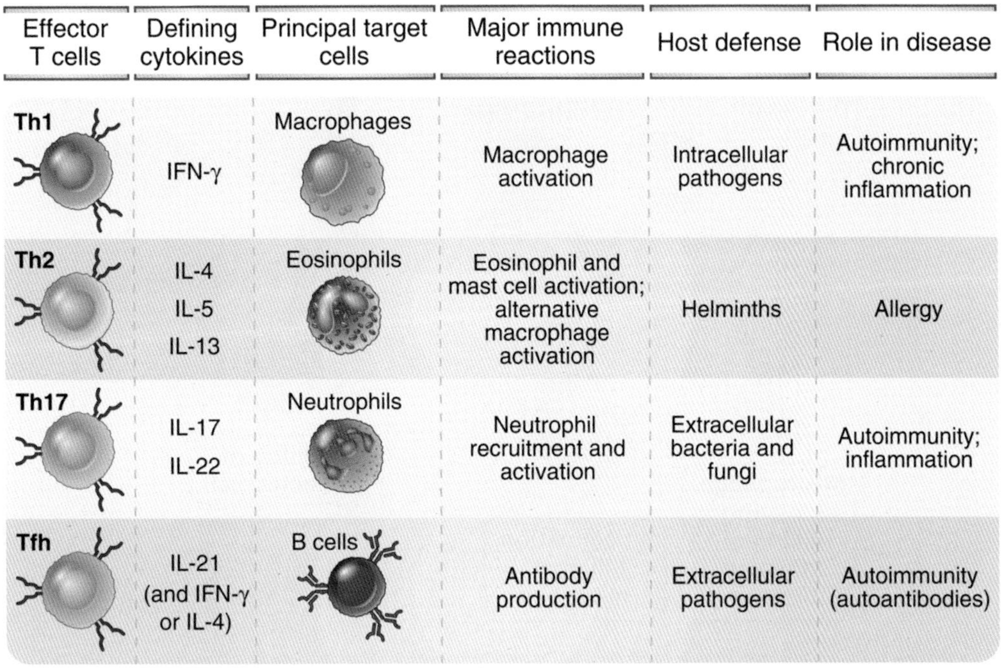

Effector T cells	Defining cytokines	Principal target cells	Major immune reactions	Host defense	Role in disease
Th1	IFN-γ	Macrophages	Macrophage activation	Intracellular pathogens	Autoimmunity; chronic inflammation
Th2	IL-4 IL-5 IL-13	Eosinophils	Eosinophil and mast cell activation; alternative macrophage activation	Helminths	Allergy
Th17	IL-17 IL-22	Neutrophils	Neutrophil recruitment and activation	Extracellular bacteria and fungi	Autoimmunity; inflammation
Tfh	IL-21 (and IFN-γ or IL-4)	B cells	Antibody production	Extracellular pathogens	Autoimmunity (autoantibodies)

• **Figure 1-14** T Helper Cell Subtypes and Their Function. Naïve CD4$^+$ T cells may differentiate into distinct subsets of effector cells in response to antigen, costimulators, and cytokines. The columns to the right list the major differences between the best-defined subsets. *Th*, T helper cell; *Tfh*, T follicular helper cell; *IL*, interleukin. (From Abbas AK, Lichtman AH, Pillai SP. *Cellular and Molecular Immunology*. 10th ed. Philadelphia: Elsevier; 2022.)

note that during an adaptive immune response to an infection, no one particular T helper subset is exclusively active. Rather, all or many are active, and some predominate as appropriate to the particular type of infection. For example, one may have both T_{h1} and T_{h2} helper cells supporting antibody production in response to a bacterial infection. The T helper cell functions to provide growth factors to stimulate and support the proliferation and differentiation of the appropriate effector cells to control the infection (Figures 1-15 and 1-16).

When the infection is intracellular, a cellular immune response, involving T_{h1} cytokines (IL-2, IFN-γ, TNF-α) predominates. Phagocytes, T_{CTL} cells, and NK cells are activated and kill virally infected cells to clear the pathogen. In the case of T_{CTL}, viral antigens expressed on the surface of infected cells are presented in the context of MHC class I molecules. The cytolytic T cell then kills the infected cell by releasing perforin (cytolytic proteins located in the granules of T_{CTL} that, on degranulation, insert into the plasma membrane of the target cell, forming a pore) to assist in delivering granzymes that are also released to the cytoplasm, where they induce apoptosis or programmed cell death. NK cells also kill virally infected cells. Rather than the specific way in which T_{CTL} cells recognize viral antigen, NK cells can recognize a wide variety of virally infected cells and kill them by inducing apoptosis similarly to T_{CTL} cells. In addition, NK cells have Fc receptors that can bind the constant region of opsonizing antibody. If antibody is produced that binds to viral antigens on the surface of a virally infected cell, the NK cell can use antibody-dependent cellular cytotoxicity to identify and then kill the cell (see Figures 1-15 and 1-16).

Humoral Immunity

When an infection involves an extracellular pathogen such as a bacterial species, antibody production becomes important for antigen-specific opsonization and toxin neutralization and clearance (Figure 1-17). T_{h2} (and sometimes T_{h1} and Th_{17}) cells provide the cytokine growth factors that support proliferation and differentiation of antigen-specific B cells. B cells express antibodies, all with the same specificity (i.e., the same hypervariable region) on a particular B cell, on their cell surface to function as their antigen receptors. Upon activation, these B cells then further differentiate into B memory cells and antibody-secreting plasma cells that produce the same antibody that bound to the antigen.[13] Antibody then binds to the surface of the pathogen, opsonizing it. The antibody may also fix complement through the classical pathway that can further opsonize the bacterium by depositing C3b on its surface. Phagocytes have Fc receptors that bind the constant region of antibody molecules that have bound to the surface of a pathogen or toxin. They also have C3 receptors that allow them to use the opsonin C3b. Furthermore, the bacteria can be lysed by the complement membrane attack complex (see Figure 1-17).

Antibody molecules have a characteristic Y-shaped structure comprising two heavy and two light polypeptide chains, each containing hypervariable regions [fraction

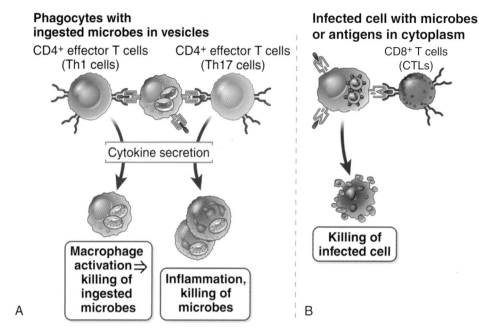

• **Figure 1-15** T Cells and Killing of Extracellular and Intracellular Pathogens. T_{h1} and T_{h17} cells secrete cytokines that support clearance of extracellular pathogens **(A)**; T_{CTL} cells that are stimulated by cytokines identify host cells with intracellular infection and kill those cells **(B)**. *CTLs*, cytotoxic T lymphocytes; *Th*, T helper cell; *CD*, cluster of differentiation. (From Abbas AK, Lichtman AH, Pillai SP. *Cellular and Molecular Immunology.* 10th ed. Philadelphia: Elsevier; 2022.)

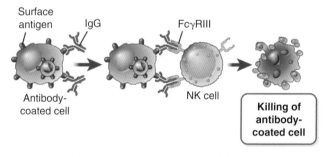

• **Figure 1-16** Antibody Dependent Cell-Mediated Cytotoxicity. Virally infected host cell expresses viral antigens on its surface. These antigens can be recognized by viral antigen -specific antibody secreted by the plasma cell. The NK cell can recognize the virally infected cell by engaging the antibody through its Fc receptor and then kill the infected cell. $Fc_\gamma R$, immunoglobulin G constant region receptor on the NK cell; *NK*, natural killer; *IgG*, immunoglobulin G. (From Abbas AK, Lichtman AH, Pillai, SP. *Cellular and Molecular Immunology.* ed 10, Philadelphia: Elsevier; 2022.

antibody binding, F(ab)$_2$], which account for the specificity of the molecule in binding to antigen, and constant regions (fraction crystallizable [Fc]), which result in biologic activity such as binding to Fc receptors on phagocytic cells. Antibody can be of different functional classes (IgM, IgG, IgA, IgE, and IgD) and subclasses (IgG$_1$, IgG$_2$, IgG$_3$, IgG$_4$, IgA$_1$, and IgA$_2$). Functions of antibodies include activation of complement, prevention of attachment of microbes, opsonization, and agglutination and immobilization of pathogens.

In the primary antibody response, IgM is usually produced. It forms a structure of five basic IgM units (a pentamer) bound together by small polypeptide chains, resulting in a large molecule in the circulation that is highly effective in activating complement and in immobilizing bacteria by binding to flagella. Monomeric IgM (single unit) is found on the surface of B cells, where it functions as an antigen receptor. With continued exposure to antigen or infection, class switching can occur and is under the control of T$_h$ cells based on the cytokines being produced. Antibodies of the IgM and IgG classes are typically found circulating in serum. Similar to IgM, IgG also activates complement, and being a smaller molecule existing as a single unit (a monomer), it can leave the circulation and enter the tissues of the body. IgG performs a unique role in pregnancy, crossing the placenta to enter the fetal circulation and thus providing immune protection to the fetus while its immune system is still developing.

Antibody of the IgA class is typically found in secretions, including saliva, tears, and mucus. It is found as a monomer and a dimer, and the dimeric form is transported across mucosal surfaces to enter the lumen of the gastrointestinal, genitourinary, and respiratory tracts. This secreted form of IgA (S-IgA) provides the main form of antibody protection for mucosal surfaces. S-IgA therefore plays a key role in defense against infection by blocking the attachment of microorganisms to the mucosa.

IgD is mainly located on the surface of B cells and, along with monomeric IgM, functions as an antigen receptor.

Antibody of the IgE class is typically found free in only minute amounts, and it has an important role in anaphylaxis. Almost all the IgE produced by plasma cells is rapidly

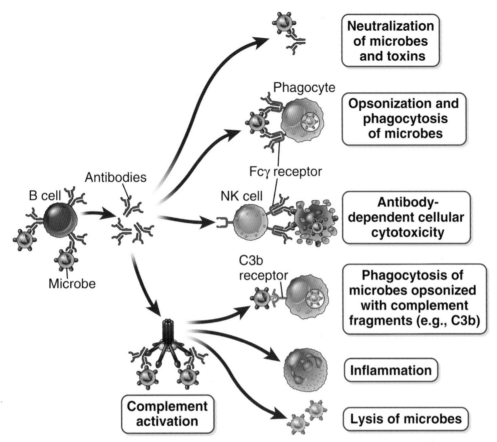

• **Figure 1-17** Antibody and the Response to Infection. Antibody molecules function in the defense against infection in several ways. They neutralize toxins, opsonize microbes to facilitate phagocytosis (either directly or indirectly through complement fixation), can facilitate NK cell antibody dependent cyto-toxicity, and can potentiate inflammation and cell lysis through complement activation. *FcγR*, immunoglobulin G constant region receptor; *NK*, natural killer. (From Abbas AK, Lichtman AH, Pillai SP. *Cellular and Molecular Immunology*. 10th ed. Philadelphia: Elsevier; 2022.)

bound by mast cells, basophils, and eosinophils that have very high affinity Fcε receptors on their surface that bind IgE. When multiple IgE molecules bound by Fcε receptors on the cell surface bind antigen and are therefore cross-linked, mast cell, basophil, or eosinophil degranulation occurs. This can result in immediate type I hypersensitivity. These cells appear to be important in the immune response to parasitic infections.

Regulation of the Immune Response

The immune response is heavily regulated at every level. Every cell and cytokine feeds back in some fashion to prevent an excessive response to the invading pathogen. An inflammatory response that is excessive, especially if it is not directed specifically toward the pathogen, has the potential to cause tissue damage and harm the host (which can be recognized as the signs and symptoms of specific chronic diseases). This text does not allow for a comprehensive and complete review of every regulatory process in the immune response. What follows are some examples of immunoregulation.

One such example involves the pathogenic condition *Papillon-Lefèvre syndrome*. In this condition, a defective enzyme prevents normal immunoregulation and results in a systemic disease that includes severe periodontitis. Affected individuals have a defective cathepsin C gene. As bacterial dental plaque (biofilm) accumulates on the teeth, bacterial macromolecules induce cells of the periodontal tissues to release the chemokine macrophage inflammatory protein-1α (MIP-1α). This chemokine (also known as chemokine [C-C motif] ligand 3 [CCL3]) is then chemotactic for phagocytes, especially neutrophils. As neutrophils accumulate at the site, they release inactive serine proteases. In systemically healthy individuals, the serine proteases are activated when they are cleaved by the protease cathepsin C. When activated, the serine proteases digest the MIP-1α and thus prevent excessive accumulation of neutrophils. In patients with Papillon-Lefèvre syndrome, the cathepsin C gene has a mutation rendering the enzyme inactive. The serine proteases from the neutrophils are therefore also inactive and unable to digest and limit the local concentration of MIP-1α. As a result, neutrophils accumulate at high levels in the periodontal tissues and are activated by bacteria-specific macromolecules and inflammatory cytokines present in the local environment. The resulting high numbers of activated neutrophils in the connective tissues release hydrolytic enzymes that destroy the connective tissue and bone that normally support the teeth. This typically results in rapidly progressing periodontitis at a young age (grade C periodontitis, with rapid rate of progression), typically leading eventually to loss of teeth. An additional symptom of this disease is palmar-plantar keratosis.

T_h cells, especially $CD4^+$ cells, are central to regulation of immunity. In a T_{h1}-dominated response to an intracellular pathogen, high levels of IL-2 and IFN-γ are released. This promotes the activation of macrophage–monocytes and the release of additional cytokines that support cellular immunity, including TNF-α, IL-1, IL-12, and IL-18. In addition to supporting cellular immunity, IFN-γ downregulates the activity of T_{h2} cells and their cytokines, which would dampen B cell activation and the production of antibody. Conversely, when there is an infection with an extracellular pathogen, T_{h2} cells and their cytokines predominate; these include IL-4, IL-5, IL-6, IL-10, and IL-13, which support the development of B cells that eventually differentiate into antibody-secreting plasma cells. In addition, IL-10 limits the release of IFN-γ by T_{h1} cells. The T_{h2} cytokines IL-4, IL-5, IL-6, and IL-13 also limit the release of cytokines by the macrophage–monocytes.

T_{reg} cells (also $CD4^+$) are important cells in immunoregulation. They recognize antigen presented to them and, as they are activated, release IL-4, IL-10, and TGF-β. These cytokines reduce the activity of DCs so that antigen presentation is dampened. These cytokines also directly inhibit the release of IL-2, IL-5, and TNF-α, thereby reducing the activity of T_h and T_{CTL} cells.

The activity of the immune system is also subject to the effects of the emotional state of the individual. Psychological stress, especially if chronic, induces the release of cortisol and catecholamines. Cells involved with immunity have receptors for circulating cortisol and catecholamines, both of which are immunosuppressive. In fact, chronic stress can lead to an increased susceptibility to infection.

References

1. Shanker A, Marincola FM. Cooperativity of adaptive and innate immunity: implications for cancer therapy. *Cancer Immunol Immunother.* 2011;60(8):1061-1074.
2. Litman GW, Rast JP, Fugmann SD. The origins of vertebrate adaptive immunity. *Nat Rev Immunol.* 2010;10(8):543-553.
3. Jotwani R, Cutler CW. Multiple dendritic cell (DC) subpopulations in human gingiva and association of mature DCs with CD4+ T-cells in situ. *J Dent Res.* 2003;82:736-741.
4. Abbas A. *Cellular and Molecular Immunology.* 10th ed. Philadelphia: Elsevier; 2021.
5. Abdelsadik A, Trad A. Toll-like receptors on the fork roads between innate and adaptive immunity. *Hum Immunol.* 2011; 72:1188-1193.
6. Barton GM, Kagan JC. A cell biological view of Toll-like receptor function: regulation through compartmentalization. *Nat Rev Immunol.* 2009;8:535-542.
7. Kenny EF, O'Neill LAJ. Signaling adaptors used by Toll-like receptors: an update. *Cytokine.* 2008;43(3):342-349.
8. Hennessy EJ, Parker AE, O'Neill LA. Targeting Toll-like receptors: emerging therapeutics? *Nat Rev Drug Discov.* 2010;9:293-307.
9. Murphy KM, Stockinger B. Effector T cell plasticity: flexibility in the face of changing circumstances. *Nat Immunol.* 2010; 11(8):674-680.
10. Steinman L. A brief history of T(H)17, the first major revision in the T(H)1/T(H)2 hypothesis of T cell-mediated tissue damage. *Nature Med.* 2007;13:139-145.
11. Ramiscal RR, Vinuesa CG. T-cell subsets in the germinal center. *Immunol Rev.* 2013;252:146-155.
12. Tangye SG, Ma CS, Brink R, et al. The good, the bad and the ugly: TFH cells in human health and disease. *Nat Rev Immunol.* 2013;13(6):412-426.
13. Goodnow CC, Vinuesa CG, Randall KL, et al. Control systems and decision making for antibody production. *Nat Immunol.* 2010;11(8):681-688.

Bibliography

Abbas A. *Cellular and Molecular Immunology.* 10th ed. Philadelphia: Elsevier; 2022.
Murphy K. *Janeway's Immunobiology.* 10th ed. New York: Norton & Company; 2022.

2

Bacteriology of the Head and Neck Regions

THOMAS S. MURRAY AND KILEY TROTT

The head and neck regions of the human body are home to a wide variety of bacteria that inhabit both the skin and mucosal surfaces. Traditionally, the clinical microbiology laboratory has used various nutrient-rich culture media to grow and identify bacteria from patient specimens. Phenotypic and biochemical properties of the isolated bacteria distinguish pathogens from commensal organisms. More recently many clinical microbiology laboratories rely on matrix assisted laser desorption/ionization time of flight (MALDI-TOF) mass spectrometry to rapidly identify pathogenic organisms.[1] Outside of the clinical laboratory, the introduction of large-scale, high-throughput DNA sequencing to identify bacterial populations that both colonize and infect the human body is changing our understanding of the important role bacteria play in both causing disease and maintaining health.

The human microbiome is the genomic composition of the microbial population (the microbiota), numbering in the trillions, that inhabits the human body.[2] The vast majority of these bacteria are not recovered with standard growth techniques and identified as a result of deep sequencing DNA technology that has expanded our knowledge of the microbes that constitute this diverse, complex population.[2] This technology allows for the sequencing of hundreds of thousands of bacterial DNA sequences from a single specimen to identify all bacteria present in the sample. Generally, samples from a specific location or niche of the human body (e.g., oral cavity, sinuses, skin, adenoids) are collected and microbial DNA from the sample is extracted, amplified, and sequenced with comparison to a reference database for bacterial identification. Major advantages of this technology are the ability to identify organisms that are not readily recovered by bacterial culture and gather information on large numbers of different bacteria from a single specimen.[3] The final result is a detailed population profile of commensal bacteria for specific regions of the body, including different anatomic sites of the head and neck (Table 2-1).[4-13]

Infectious processes are likely due to the complex interactions among the host immune system, pathogenic bacteria, and the resident commensal microbes. This is especially important when considering the microbial population of the head and neck. Dysbiosis of healthy oral microbiota can lead to infection, and emerging evidence also suggests relationships to a variety of cancers.[14]

Commensal Flora of the Head, Neck, and Oral Cavity

The application of deep DNA sequencing to the human microbiota early in life confirms the importance of the neonatal microbiome, although controversy remains as to when colonization commences. Although some have suggested the fetus is colonized in utero, other data support the uterus as sterile with neonatal microbial colonization by maternal flora beginning at delivery.[6] Multiple factors influence the evolution and development of the bacterial populations that colonize the skin, oral cavity, and gut. These factors include, but are not limited to, the type of delivery (vaginal versus cesarean section), breast feeding or formula, length of time in the hospital, exposure to antibiotics, transition to solid food, and the presence or absence of teeth.[6,7] The local environment also plays an important role in the kinds of bacteria present in a given location of the body. Environmental factors that will determine the bacterial population include, but are not limited to, the available nutrients, pH, moisture levels, other competitive bacteria occupying the same niche, and exposure to the host immune system. The neonate is initially colonized by pioneering organisms that transitions to a more mature, stable bacterial population that resembles the climax microbial community of adults by 3 to 6 years of age.[6]

However, for a given individual, the microbiome can change over time with changes in overall health. In addition, there is significant variation across different individuals on examining bacterial populations at the same anatomic site. Different physiologic states and behaviors have profound effects on the commensal flora of the individual presumably by altering the microenvironment for bacterial growth in favor of certain organisms at the expense of others.[6] The emergence of teeth during infancy

TABLE 2-1	Common Microbiota of the Head and Neck
Location (Reference)	**Bacteria***
Outer ear[10]	Alloiococcus Corynebacterium Staphylococcus non-aureus
Inner ear[11]	Carnobacteria Comamonada Corynebacteria Flavobacterium Moraxella Pasteurella Staphylococcus Viridans group Streptococcus
Sinuses-[17,18]	Corynebacteria Cyanobacteria Propionibacterium Staphylococcus aureus and non-aureus
Esophagus[13]	Fusobacterium Haemophilus Neisseria Prevotella Viridans group Streptococcus
Larynx[16]	Fusobacterium Gemella Neisserria Parvimonas Prevotella Viridans group Streptococcus
Tonsils/adenoids[12,19,20]	Fusobacterium Gemella Haemophilus Moraxella Neisseria Prevotella Porphyromonas Staphylococcus Streptococcus pyogenes Viridans group Streptococcus
Nose[9]	Haemophilus Neisseria Moraxella Staphylococcus aureus Streptococcus pneumoniae Viridans group Streptococcus
Oral cavity-saliva and plaques[4,5,8,15]	Actinomyces Cornybacterium Haemophilus Fusobacterium Neisseria Porphyromonas Prevotella Rothia Veillonella Viridans group Streptococcus

*More common genera of bacteria have been selected. Bacteria have been isolated from both healthy and diseased individuals of all ages. Note many bacterial genera are present in most locations of the head and neck. (Reviewed in reference 7.)

profoundly changes the oral flora by changing the microenvironment. As another example, smoking alters the microflora of the oral cavity, with increased numbers of potentially pathogenic bacteria present compared with the oral flora of nonsmokers.[15] In one study, patients with squamous cell carcinoma of the larynx had vastly different microbial populations than control patients with vocal cord polyps.[16] Changes to the mucosal surfaces because of chemotherapy can alter the microbial population. Many studies have now characterized bacterial communities of different regions of the head and neck for both healthy and diseased populations of various ages (see Table 2-1).[7]

Given that laboratory cultivation techniques recover a limited number of organisms, it is not surprising that culture-independent techniques have identified previously unrecognized commensal flora, especially among the anaerobic bacteria. The increased sensitivity of these molecular techniques compared with culture-based approaches has also revealed large numbers of bacterial populations in healthy subjects at sites not previously thought to be colonized. For example, DNA-based studies of healthy adults have identified bacterial populations in the middle meatus of the sinus that include *Staphylococcus aureus, Staphylococcus epidermidis, Propionibacterium acnes,* and anaerobic *Cyanobacterium* species.[17,18] Although the diversity and populations of bacteria vary among individuals and studies, the common conclusion is that the sinuses of healthy asymptomatic individuals are colonized with bacterial populations, including potential pathogens such as *S. aureus*. It also raises the possibility that there are as yet unrecognized organisms contributing to clinical disease that do not grow under routine laboratory growth conditions.

In many cases bacterial infections of the head and neck are caused by bacterial flora that often colonize the skin, oral cavity, or respiratory tract and contiguous spaces without causing disease. When there is disruption of this homeostasis between host and microbes because of a change in the host or bacterial population, certain bacteria (e.g., *S. aureus, Streptococcus pneumoniae*) behave as pathogens that cause invasive infection and clinical symptoms. Surgically removed adenoids and tonsils contain common pathogens that cause acute otitis media, and these organisms can migrate from the posterior airway to the inner ear to cause infection when homeostasis is disrupted.[19,20]

Pathogenesis of Acute and Chronic Bacterial Infections

Acute Infection

Acute infections occur when a change in the host environment or the bacterial population in a region permits invasion of a pathogenic bacteria, resulting in clinical signs and symptoms consistent with infection. Acute infection initially requires bacteria express surface molecules that facilitate adhesion to an epithelial, mucosal, or artificial surface. Attached bacteria then secrete a variety of virulence factors that interact with host tissue and the immune response to produce inflammation consistent with symptomatic infection. If the bacteria are able to penetrate the host surface into a previously sterile site and replicate, effectively dealing with host defenses, then invasive disease occurs. These general principles of acute infection are applicable to multiple pathogens discussed later.

Surface Adhesion

The first step in acute infection is adhesion to a surface, typically a mucosal surface for head and neck infections. Bacteria may possess one or more multiple surface structures or surface-exposed proteins that facilitate adhesion to the epithelial cell layer. For example, both *S. pneumoniae* and *Haemophilus influenzae,* pathogens of the upper respiratory tract and contiguous spaces, express the surface phosphorylcholine ChoP, which in pneumococcus binds the platelet-activating factor receptor found on epithelial cells of the nasopharynx. Multiple pathogens, including *Pseudomonas aeruginosa,* a common cause of otitis externa, display fimbriae on the cell surface, thin structures that extend and retract, attaching the bacteria to surfaces such as epithelial cells. *P. aeruginosa* also expresses a single flagellum used for motility to get the bacterium to the host surface and attach once it makes contact (Figure 2-1).

Virulence Factor Production

In many cases, bacteria successfully colonize the mucosal cell layer without causing clinical symptoms and disease. However, when bacteria invade a sterile space or secrete virulence factors, the ensuing tissue damage and inflammatory response results in clinical signs and symptoms. Bacteria have evolved an incredible variety of surface-associated and secreted virulence factors to cause cellular damage and inactivate host defenses. For example, gram-negative pathogens have lipopolysaccharide on the cell surface that interacts with Toll-like receptor (TLR) 4 of the innate immune system to generate a robust proinflammatory response.

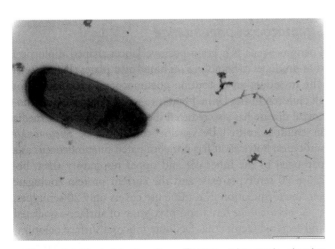

• **Figure 2-1 Bacterial Flagellum.** Flectron micrograph showing *Pseudomonas aeruginosa* with a single, unipolar flagellum important for interaction with the host innate immune system (via Toll-like receptor-5) as well as bacterial adhesion to host surfaces.

Although this response can lead to bacterial death and resolution of infection, it can also cause tissue damage that facilitates bacterial invasion across surfaces into sterile sites. Several different pathogens of the head and neck secrete proteins that form pores in host cell membranes, disrupting the host cell and resulting in lysis. Common examples discussed later in more detail include streptolysin produced by *S. pneumoniae* and the *S. aureus* Panton-Valentine leukocidin (PVL) toxin. In addition to secreting virulence factors directly into the environment, several bacteria possess needle-like structures that insert into host cell membranes. These structures allow bacteria to pump virulence factors directly into the cytosol of host cells, resulting in cell death and facilitating bacterial invasion. *P. aeruginosa* has a type III secretion system that injects molecules into host cells, including ExoU, a phospholipase expressed by some strains that causes rapid cell necrosis.

Surviving the Host Response to Infection

Given the vast array of defenses the body possesses to protect against infection, bacteria are armed with multiple mechanisms to survive within a dangerous host environment. Pathogenic bacteria avoid phagocytosis by neutrophils and macrophages through a variety of means. Many gram-negative and gram-positive bacteria possess a polysaccharide capsule that is antiphagocytic and offers a competitive advantage compared with unencapsulated strains. In addition to the exopolysaccharide capsule, surface proteins such as the M-protein of *Streptococcus pyogenes* (group A *Streptococcus*) also prevent engulfment by host cells. A variety of secreted proteins disrupt opsonization by averting deposition of complement on the bacterial surface. Another important immune defense mechanism that bacteria must deal with is the neutrophil extracellular trap (NET), extracellular fibrils that engulf and destroy bacteria. Respiratory pathogens have developed numerous ways to protect themselves from NETs. Some secrete enzymes that degrade the DNA component of NETs (e.g., the DNAse of *S. pyogenes*), whereas others exhibit surface molecules that allow for survival within the NET after engulfment. In addition, many of the cytolytic pore-forming toxins described previously target immune cells. For example, PVL and pneumolysin can both lyse white blood cells recruited to the site of infection. Additional secreted proteins cleave antibody or complement or inactivate host defensin molecules to survive the host response.

Chronic Infection and Biofilm Formation

Under certain circumstances, an acute infection is not completely resolved despite an aggressive immune response with or without antimicrobial therapy and chronic infection results. A number of chronic infections of the head and neck, such as chronic otitis media and chronic rhinosinusitis, are challenging to treat with antibiotic therapy alone. The bacterial strategy for long-term survival in the host now known to be an important component of most chronic infections is the formation of bacterial biofilms. These organized communities of bacteria often colonize a surface but may also exist as aggregates in liquid such as mucus and saliva and are more resistant to antibiotic therapy.[21] Importantly they may be polymicrobial, with multiple types of microbes coexisting in the same community.[21,22] Virtually all of the pathogens of the head and neck described in this chapter form biofilms that contribute to persistence in the hostile host environment.

There is an inverse relationship comparing the bacterial lifestyle of tissue destruction, invasion, and acute infection with that of host colonization, biofilm formation, and chronic disease. When genes encoding proteins required for biofilm formation are upregulated, genes encoding proteins that are virulence factors during acute infection are downregulated. Alternatively, during acute infection when virulence factors for invasion are upregulated, genes encoding proteins present in biofilms are turned off. This paradigm argues that the same bacterial strain may display an acute or chronic phenotype, depending on the environment and host response, and may serve to explain how initial acute infections become chronic and more difficult to treat over time with the same strain of bacteria.

Surface-associated biofilm formation is initiated with contact and adhesion (Figure 2-2). The presence of a foreign body provides an ideal surface for bacterial colonization, chronic infection, and biofilm formation. Biofilms form on teeth and contribute to dental caries, and they allow for bacterial colonization of mucosal and epithelial surfaces.[22] Attachment to a foreign or host surface requires many of the same factors mentioned for acute infection, such as flagella, fimbriae, or surface adhesins. Next, the bacteria aggregate into microcolonies followed by cell division and the formation of a mature biofilm with channels that allow for gas exchange and nutrient acquisition. Bacteria at the base of the biofilm exhibit decreased metabolism compared with bacteria closer to the surface; therefore, antibiotics that require metabolic activity, such as protein or cell wall synthesis, are less active even if the drugs do penetrate the biofilm.

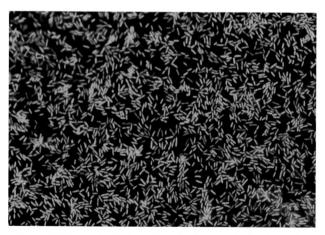

• **Figure 2-2** Bacterial Surface Colonization. The initial step in both colonization and surface-associated biofilm formation is attachment. In this example, *Pseudomonas aeruginosa* expressing green fluorescent protein adhere to the surface, "colonizing" a glass slide.

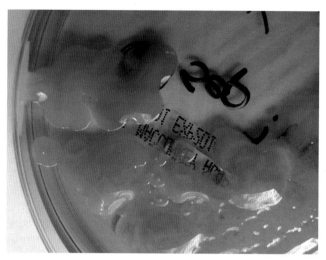

• **Figure 2-3** Exopolysaccharide, a bacterial virulence factor. Mucoid *Klebsiella pneumoniae* grown on MacConkey agar plates secrete an abundance of exopolysaccharide that in vivo prevents phagocytosis and antibiotic penetration.

The biofilm is protected by an extracellular matrix consisting of both bacterial and host material that inhibits both phagocytosis and antibiotic penetration. Some bacterial strains produce a mucoid phenotype because of increased production of exopolysaccharide (Figure 2-3). These mucoid strains are particularly difficult to eradicate and commonly cause chronic infection. Importantly, biofilms are not static, and bacteria released from the biofilm are capable of colonizing nearby surfaces, spreading infection within the host.

The list of potential pathogens of the head and neck region is extensive (Table 2-2). Several pathogens that more commonly cause invasive disease in multiple locations of the head and neck and those that cause disease in the oral cavity are discussed here in more detail.

Common Bacterial Pathogens of the Ear, Sinuses, and Contiguous Regions

Streptococcus pneumoniae

Pneumococcus is a gram-positive lancet-shaped diplococci that produces α-hemolysis on blood agar plates (Figure 2-4). The introduction of routine pneumococcal vaccination for all children in the United States to reduce invasive pneumococcal disease has also reduced the rates of acute otitis media in children caused by vaccine containing *S. pneumoniae* serotypes; however, it has not eliminated pneumococcus as a pathogen of the inner ear and upper respiratory tract, because 90 serotypes exist and the current protein conjugate vaccine formulation in routine use covers only 20 serotypes.

S. pneumoniae has a complex array of surface-associated and secreted factors that facilitate mucosal surface colonization, mitigate the host immune response, and promote invasion of the host.[23] The negatively charged polysaccharide capsule is required for virulence and protects against upper respiratory secretions and phagocytosis. However, the

TABLE 2-2 Infections Caused by Bacteria Commonly Found in the Head and Neck

Bacteria	Common Infections of Head and Neck	Systemic Infectious Complications
Actinomyces species	Dental plaque/caries	Actinomycosis
Aggregatibacter actinomycetemcomitans	Periodontitis	Association with increased risk for coronary artery disease
Capnocytophaga species	Periodontitis (particularly juvenile periodontitis)	Endocarditis, fulminant sepsis in asplenic patients
Fusobacterium species	Periodontitis, pharyngitis, tonsillitis, peritonsillar abscess	Lemierre syndrome (septic thrombophlebitis of the internal jugular vein), sepsis
Haemophilus influenzae	Epiglottitis, rhinosinusitis, otitis media	Meningitis, septic arthritis, osteomyelitis, cellulitis, pneumonia, bronchitis
Moraxella catarrhalis	Otitis media, rhinosinusitis	COPD exacerbation, pneumonia
Prevotella intermedia	Dental plaque/caries, periodontitis	Brain or lung abscess
Staphylococcus aureus	Peritonsillar abscess, cervical lymphadenitis, rhinosinusitis	Pneumonia, endocarditis, skin and soft tissue infection, sepsis, toxic shock syndrome, osteomyelitis, septic arthritis, pneumonia
Streptococcus pneumoniae	Otitis media, rhinosinusitis	Pneumonia, sepsis, meningitis
Streptococcus pyogenes	Pharyngitis, peritonsillar abscess, cervical lymphadenitis	Rheumatic fever, poststreptococcal glomerulonephritis, skin and soft tissue infection, toxic shock syndrome
Viridans group streptococci	Dental plaque/caries	Endocarditis, sepsis

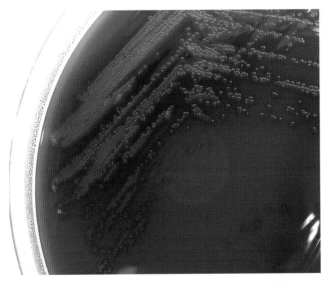

• **Figure 2-4** α-Hemolysis of *Streptococcus pneumoniae.* The *green* around each pneumococcal colony is due to the conversion of hemoglobin to methemoglobin in the blood agar plate. Viridans streptococci colonies are similar in appearance and distinguished from pneumococcus by optochin susceptibility.

capsule does not promote binding to epithelial cells, and its size is decreased when the bacteria interacts with host epithelial cells. Additional surface adhesions bind components of the extracellular matrix, such as fibronectin and epithelial cell receptors. *S. pneumoniae* strains secrete antimicrobial peptides, including those that target other pneumococcal serotypes to colonize a mucosal surface already crowded with other commensal flora.[23]

The immune system is also the target of several secreted virulence factors. Pneumolysin is a cytotoxic protein that targets the cholesterol-containing membranes of host membranes for pore formation and cell lysis. Pneumolysin is important for pneumococcal respiratory infections and invasion into the bloodstream. In addition to lysing cells, it also activates the immune response with proinflammatory cytokines leading to the recruitment of CD4± T cells.[23] Examples of pneumococcal mitigation of the host immune response include a secreted metalloprotease that cleaves immunoglobulin A1 (IgA1) to degrade antibody in the respiratory tract and surface expression of PsPA, a protein that prevents C3 complement fixation on the bacterial surface.[23]

Currently, many circulating strains of *S. pneumoniae* are resistant to many commonly used antipneumococcal antimicrobial agents. For example, resistance to penicillin results from mutations in penicillin-binding proteins required for cell wall synthesis. Resistance to other drugs such as the macrolides and quinolones is also increasing. Thus, when pneumococcus is isolated from an invasive head and neck infection, antibiotic susceptibility testing is recommended to guide therapy.

Moraxella catarrhalis

Moraxella catarrhalis is an oxidase-positive, gram-negative diplococci that does not exhibit hemolysis on blood agar plates (Figure 2-5). *M. catarrhalis* specifically binds the respiratory epithelium and the extracellular matrix of the

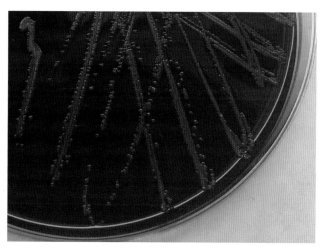

• **Figure 2-5** *Haemophilus influenzae* growth on chocolate agar plate. *H. influenzae* is fastidious and requires factor V and factor X for growth. These factors are available to the bacteria in chocolate agar composed of lysed erythrocytes.

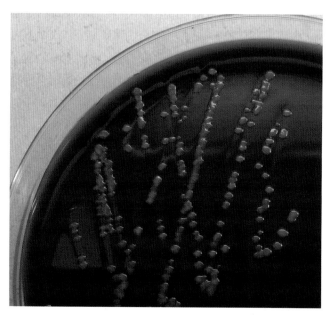

• **Figure 2-6** *Moraxella catarrhalis* growth on blood agar plate. Note the complete absence of hemolysis (γ-hemolysis) around the colonies.

human upper respiratory tract and has been recovered from the biofilms of children with chronic otitis media.[24,25] Although *M. catarrhalis* does not possess a polysaccharide capsule, it does have a number of surface adhesins. Examples of important adhesins include the outer membrane proteins, lipooligosaccharide, and ubiquitous surface protein A (UspA). UspA1 binds both epithelial cells and extracellular matrix to facilitate colonization and biofilm formation.[26] UspA2 functions to bind and inactivate complement and lipooligosaccharide, and outer membrane proteins function to reduce serum-dependent bacterial killing.[25] Variable alleles on the UspA2 locus, such as UspA2H and Usp2V, also have been identified that play a role in adherence, serum resistance, and biofilm formation. Isolates from respiratory tract infections in children exhibit increased Usp2 levels compared with UspA2H, suggesting a role for Usp2 in childhood disease.[26] Similar to *P. aeruginosa*, *M. catarrhalis* also possesses surface fimbriae, called *type IV pili*, that are important for epithelial cell binding and biofilm formation. After mucosal colonization, *M. catarrhalis* is capable of invading epithelial cells, although the exact mechanisms remain to be elucidated.[24] This also has been observed in vivo, because *M. catarrhalis* has been identified in adenoid and tonsillar specimens from patients.[19] The vast majority of *M. catarrhalis* secrete a β-lactamase that confers resistance to therapy with ampicillin alone. Successful treatment requires either the addition of a β-lactamase inhibitor to a penicillin, a cephalosporin if a β-lactam antibiotic is preferred, or an antibiotic from an alternative class.

Haemophilus influenzae

H. influenzae is a fastidious, thin, gram-negative rod that is oxidase positive and requires chocolate agar plates that contain partially lysed red blood cells (Figure 2-6). Six encapsulated serotypes (a to f) exist, and historically *H. influenzae* type B (Hib) was the cause of most invasive disease. The introduction of routine childhood vaccination

against Hib has virtually eliminated invasive disease with this strain in the United States. The majority of infections caused by *H. influenzae*, such as acute otitis media, are due to unencapsulated, nontypeable strains.[27] Nontypeable *H. influenzae* has a number of virulence factors that are similar to those of *M. catarrhalis*, a competitor for mucosal colonization of the upper airway. Surface pili bind both host cells and extracellular matrix components. The outer membrane protein P2 displays antigenic variation to avoid recognition by antibody, allowing for the persistence of chronic infection despite the host immune response.[28] Another well-studied group of adhesins are the autotransporters.[29] An example is HapA, a protein that promotes bacterial aggregation and adherence to respiratory epithelial cells.[29] Another is *H. influenzae* adhesin (Hia), which is upregulated during human bronchial epithelial cell infection models.[30]

H. influenzae invasion of epithelial cells is postulated to occur by multiple endocytic pathways and requires actin. In addition, mechanisms may exist that promote intracellular survival, such as the IgA1 protease IgaB, which can cleave lysosomal proteins.[30] *H. influenzae* also can penetrate epithelial cell layers between cells, disrupting tight junctions without causing cell death. In addition to causing invasive disease, strong evidence from animal models and human patients demonstrate that certain nontypeable strains of *H. influenzae* exist in biofilms, often coexisting with other bacteria.[31] The aggregation of bacteria promoted by HapA on the epithelial cell surface contributes to the initial stages of biofilm formation. These biofilms are stabilized by extracellular DNA and can even survive within NETs produced by activated neutrophils.[31] Nontypeable *H. influenzae* has been recovered from surgically removed human tonsils, demonstrating the long-term viability of these strains in vivo.[20] Interestingly, low concentrations of antibiotics promote

H. influenzae biofilm formation, and the clinical implications of this observation require careful consideration.

Streptococcus pyogenes

Group A streptococcus is a catalase-negative, gram-positive coccus that is seen in long chains when visualized using Gram stain. *S. pyogenes* is a human pathogen that causes pharyngitis and invasive soft tissue disease, and can both colonize and invade the skin and throat (see Table 2-2). The capacity of *S. pyogenes* to cause infection has been well studied, and just a few of the best-known virulence factors will be described.

Among the most recognized virulence factors that determine the serotype is the surface M protein. M1 is among the most prevalent serotypes and a frequent cause of invasive disease. M protein has multiple functions: It acts as an adhesin, binds fibrinogen to prevent phagocytosis and, along with the DNase SDA1 and a hyaluronidase capsule, prevents killing by NETS, enhancing survival during the initial neutrophil response.[32] The neutrophil response is also muted by SpyCEP, a protease that cleaves interleukin-8, a potent chemokine that attracts neutrophils to the infection site.[33] Phagocytosis is also inhibited by the IgG peptidase IdeS, which cleaves the heavy chain of *S. pyogenes'* surface-associated IgG, disrupting opsonization.[32] Streptolysin O is a pore-forming cytolysin familiar to clinicians because antibodies to it are used to document recent *S. pyogenes* infection. Streptolysin O also induces apoptosis in immune cells and facilitates invasion into sterile sites. Strains of *S. pyogenes* also produce a variety of superantigens, which are molecules that bind T cells outside of the major histocompatibility complex pocket, eliciting a profound immune response that can lead to clinical syndromes such as toxic shock syndrome.[32]

S. pyogenes has been a model system to understand the regulation of virulence factors that promote acute infection and those that favor biofilm formation.[32,33] The major regulator of *S. pyogenes* virulence is the CovS/CovR two-component response regulator system. Two-component systems used by most pathogenic bacteria have one protein—a sensor kinase that senses signals from the environment and responds by phosphorylating a paired response regulator that alters the transcription of a specific set of genes. The CovS/CovR proteins control the majority of *S. pyogenes* virulence factors discussed previously, and they serve as a switch regulating genes encoding proteins that favor either colonization and biofilm formation or virulence factor production and acute invasive infection.

As an example, CovS/CovR upregulates the cysteine protease SpeB, which degrades both host immune factors such as antibody, antimicrobial peptides, and precytokines while also degrading bacterial virulence factors. The activity of SpeB dampens both the immune response and bacterial invasiveness, favoring colonization of the upper airway. When SpeB activity is decreased, bacterial virulence factor production and the host inflammatory response are upregulated, promoting invasive disease. This inverse relationship has held up when comparing SpeB activity from clinical isolates that caused more severe disease (low SpeB, increased virulence factors) with those causing less severe disease (high SpeB, decreased virulence factor production).[32] It follows that CovR/CovS mutants should express less SpeB and demonstrate increased virulence, but with more difficulty colonizing the mucosal surface. In fact, this is true of clinical isolates. CovR also suppresses capsule production so that CovR mutants have larger capsules and demonstrate increased capacity for invasive disease. These large capsules do not bind the mucosal surface well such that upper airway colonization and biofilm formation are diminished and the bacteria are cleared more easily from the surface.[32] This example highlights how bacteria can tightly regulate gene expression to survive changing environments. The bacterial proteins required for initial surface adhesion are often of little value later in the infectious process when invasion requires tissue destruction.

Staphylococcus aureus

S. aureus is a gram-positive catalase- and coagulase-positive organism that classically forms clusters when visualized with Gram stain. Importantly, when recovered from primary clinical specimens such as abscesses, *S. aureus* may appear as pairs of cocci or as a single bacterium. It is β-hemolytic (complete hemolysis) on blood agar, and many colonies have a gold or tan appearance (Figure 2-7), in contrast to coagulase-negative staphylococci, which generally exhibit no hemolysis (γ-hemolysis).

Both methicillin-susceptible *S. aureus* (MSSA) and methicillin-resistant *S. aureus* (MRSA) can colonize the skin and nasal mucosa and cause invasive disease. Methicillin resistance occurs when *S. aureus* expresses the *mecA* gene encoding penicillin-binding protein PBP2a that is not present in MSSA strains. *MecA* is found on a chromosomal cassette, often with other antimicrobial resistance genes, that can

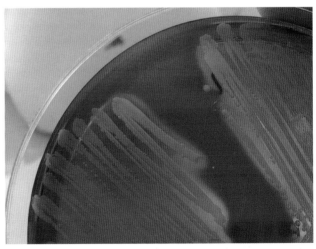

• **Figure 2-7** β-Hemolysis of *Staphylococcus aureus*. *S. aureus* produces hemolysins that lyse red blood cells and produce complete clearing (β-hemolysis) around the bacterial colonies when grown on blood agar plates.

move to other *S. aureus* strains by horizontal gene transfer. MRSA and MSSA have large numbers of virulence factors that contribute to both colonization and disease, and a selection of these are highlighted in this chapter.

S. aureus has a number of microbial surface components recognizing adhesive matrix molecules (MSCRAMMs) that bind extracellular matrix components such as fibronectin and collagen to enable adhesion to the host. Protein A is an MSCRAMM that is intimately involved in interactions with the immune response, binding IgG to prevent opsonization, C3 of the complement pathway, and a receptor for tumor necrosis factor-α. A variety of superantigens function to impair neutrophil migration to the site of infection, and several molecules inactivate complement by inhibiting convertases.[34]

In addition to adhesins, *S. aureus* also expresses multiple toxins that contribute to pathogenesis. One of the best studied is the PVL toxin, a pore-forming toxin consisting of the LukS and LukF proteins that requires interaction with a host receptor for the lysis of white blood cells. Although many studies associate PVL-positive *S. aureus* with more severe and invasive disease, other studies reach different conclusions.[35-37] The results may depend on the animal model being studied, the location of infection, and the presence or absence of other virulence factors in the strain.[37] *S. aureus* also expresses α and δ hemolysins that lyse red blood cells. δ-Toxin is a phenol-soluble modulin peptide, one of a family of phenol-soluble modulin peptides with cytolytic properties secreted by *S. aureus*.[35] The coagulase activity of *S. aureus* is due to two enzymes that promote fibrin clots, binding prothrombin and converting fibrinogen to fibrin. These fibrin clots enhance abscess formation and promote biofilm formation when bacteria are attached to surfaces such as catheters. This activity is counterbalanced by staphylokinase, which converts plasminogen to plasmin, resulting in the breakdown of fibrin clots. This allows the escape of the bacteria from the clot.[35]

In addition to MRSA, *S. aureus* can be resistant to a variety of other commonly used antistaphylococcal agents such as clindamycin and trimethoprim–sulfamethoxazole. Fortunately, high-level resistance to vancomycin has been described only rarely for *S. aureus*. When *S. aureus* infection is suspected, knowledge of the local antimicrobial resistance patterns is critical in choosing empiric therapy. The initial antibiotic choice can be adjusted once the organism is confirmed and antimicrobial susceptibilities are known.

Common Bacterial Pathogens of the Teeth, Mouth, and Pharynx

Viridans Group Streptococci

These streptococcal species are Gram positive and display α-hemolysis, resulting in a green color around the colonies that gives rise to the name (*viridis* is Latin for "green"). Rarely, these species can be nonhemolytic (γ-hemolysis), or β-hemolytic in the case of *Streptococcus anginosus*. Common viridans streptococci include *S. mitis, S. anginosus, S. mutans* group, *S. salivarius*, and *S. bovis*. Viridans streptococci

are prevalent colonizers of the healthy human mouth (see Table 2-1). Viridans streptococci are implicated in the formation of dental caries and are pathogenic when introduced into fascial planes of the head and neck forming abscesses. In addition, viridans streptococci bacteremia is a known cause of subacute native and prosthetic valve endocarditis.

Virulence factors of the viridans streptococci are not fully elucidated, but several of the known factors are included here. For initial colonization of oral mucosal surfaces, viridans streptococci produce a series of adhesins similar to those found in pneumococcus. Interestingly, IgA antibodies appear to be strain specific, and as one strain is cleared, another strain takes its place through clonal and antigenic diversity via genetic recombination among different streptococcal species.[38] In addition, several species within this group also possess IgA1 protease.[39] Viridans streptococci are fierce competitors in the colonization of the mucosal surface of the mouth, producing bacteriocidins that have bactericidal activity against other organisms, killing more virulent species of streptococci and staphylococci. Additionally it has been identified that *Streptococcus intermedius* produces a sialidase, allowing for tissue sugar modification, thought to play a role in biofilm formation and colonization.[40]

Current literature has not fully elucidated the features that enable viridans streptococcus to behave as a commensal pathogen in some hosts and host locations (mouth) and as a pathogen in other hosts or locations. However, the different virulence factors of *S. mutans* help to explain its diversity as a pathogen. In the mouth, the polysaccharides produced by exoenzymes from *S. mutans* are the main constituents of the insoluble matrix on which plaque biofilms form and dental caries develop.[41] In the bloodstream, *S. mutans* expresses two bacteriophage-encoded proteins (PblA and PblB) that bind directly to platelets and contribute to the pathogenesis of subacute endocarditis.[39] Type k *S. mutans* produces a collagen-binding protein that interacts with damaged cerebral blood vessels to convert ischemic to hemorrhagic stroke.[42] There are differing levels of other factors when comparing commensal and pathogenic states. One example is intermedilysin, a cholesterol-dependent cytolysis, found at high levels in abscesses and lower levels in dental plaques.[38]

Actinomyces Species

Actinomyces species are facultative, anaerobic, non–spore-forming, filamentous, gram-positive rods that commonly inhabit the oropharynx. Although individual bacteria are filamentous, colonies form fungus-like branched networks of hyphae. *Actinomyces* species grow slowly in culture and are not acid-fast, distinguishing them from *Nocardia* species. *Actinomyces* species are pathogenic locally in the oral cavity or through direct extension into fascial planes as abscesses. Of the myriad species of *Actinomyces* identified, the most common pathogens include *A. israelii, A. viscosus, A. naeslundii, A. turicensis,* and *A. radingae*. Systemic disease can also result through exposure of *Actinomyces* species to the bloodstream or through aspiration of organisms into pulmonary tissue. Local infection with *Actinomyces* species occurs at the level of the teeth and gingiva. *Actinomyces* species isolated from supragingival plaques and root surface caries are implicated in the development of gingivitis.[43]

Infection can spread when normal mucosal barriers are disrupted, leading to abscesses with connecting sinus tracts. These abscesses are most commonly found in the face and neck as cervicofacial actinomycosis, but they can also occur throughout the thorax, abdomen, pelvis, and central nervous system. Understanding of the virulence factors used by *Actinomyces* species is limited. One hypothesis is that cell wall lipoproteins induce an overzealous immune response through TLR-2, leading to extension of disease beyond mucosal surfaces.[43] In addition, cell wall peptidoglycan induces alveolar bone resorption and osteoclastogenesis, in addition to recruitment of inflammatory cytokines.[44] *Actinomyces* species form biofilms, and *Actinomycosis* infections can be polymicrobial and involve 5 to 10 other bacterial species that may contribute to pathogenesis.[45] Certain species also have fimbriae that can bind to collagen and teeth, which may contribute to the development of osteomyelitis.[45]

Prevotella Species

Prevotella species are small anaerobic gram-negative rods frequently identified when the microbiome of different regions of the head and neck are determined with deep sequencing (see Table 2-1). The species of *Prevotella* most linked with human disease are *P. intermedia, P. melaninogenica, P. bivia, P. nigrescens,* and *P. disiens. P. intermedia* is implicated in periodontal disease, usually in association with *Porphyromonas gingivalis* and *Aggregatibacter actinomycetemcomitans.*[46] *Prevotella* species are also implicated in chronic sinusitis, middle ear infections, brain abscesses, and intraabdominal abscesses. Virulence mechanisms for *Prevotella* species include attachment to the mucosa, immune system evasion, and increased production of virulence factors when the organism transitions from commensal to pathogen. *P. intermedia* uses proteases to interfere with complement-mediated bacterial killing.[46] Interestingly, one study demonstrated an increased level of proteolytic activity in pathologic *P. intermedia* clinical isolates compared with those recovered from healthy mouths.[47]

Another important virulence factor in *Prevotella* species is the extracellular polymetric substance (EPS). EPS provides scaffolding for biofilm formation, a critical step in the development of dental caries and periodontal disease. In addition, EPS serves as a capsule that facilitates mucosal adherence and resistance to phagocytosis.[48] Interestingly, *P. intermedia* disables and kills neutrophils, a characteristic not found in other endodontic pathogens such as *Fusobacterium nucleatum, S. intermedius, Parvimonas micra,* and *P. intermedia.*[49] Enzyme secretion systems, such as the type VI secretion and type IX/Por secretion systems secrete proteases and hemolysins that can contribute to virulence.[50]

Fusobacterium Species

Fusobacterium species are anaerobic, elongated, gram-negative rods. There are multiple species of *Fusobacterium,* but the one most associated with human disease is *F. necrophorum,* a cause of periodontal disease, tonsillitis, peritonsillar abscess, and thrombophlebitis of the jugular vein (Lemierre syndrome). Although many *Fusobacterium* species are included in normal human oral flora, it remains unclear whether *F. necrophorum* is a commensal organism or is present only as a pathogen.[51] Virulence factors for *F. necrophorum* are well known as they relate to zoonotic infections, but their relationship to human disease is not clear. Adhesins and fimbriae play a critical role in host cell attachment.[51] Leukotoxin is a known virulence factor of *F. necrophorum* that likely facilitates abscess formation.[51] Endotoxin and hemolysin also appear to be important virulence factors in the formation of abscesses and for increased necrosis of locally infected tissue.[51] Novel genome-based studies of *F. necrophorum* attempting to identify virulence factors found genes encoding fibrinolysin that may indicate a mechanism to prevent fibrin barriers.[52] Hemagglutinin and a not yet identified factor leading to platelet aggregation are most associated with the thrombotic consequences found in Lemierre syndrome.

Capnocytophaga Species

Capnocytophaga species are filamentous, thin, gram-negative rods with a tapered end (fusiform) that are capnophilic. *Capnocytophaga* species colonize the human oropharynx and are associated with periodontitis, septicemia in patients with splenic or liver dysfunction, and, rarely, endocarditis. There is an association with dog bites, and *Capnocytophaga* species are a prominent cause of post–dog bite infections.[53] Virulence mechanisms are not well understood; however, some species produce EPS that suppresses host complement. In addition, some strains produce β-lactamases; therefore, empiric therapy for *Capnocytophaga* species should include a β-lactamase inhibitor if a β-lactam antibiotic is considered.[54]

Conclusions

It is increasingly apparent that the commensal bacteria of the head, neck, and oral cavity play a critical role in maintaining human health. New DNA sequencing techniques have shown commensal organisms to be ubiquitous throughout the oral cavity and contiguous spaces. These commensals can become infective when host defenses, including the protective epithelial barrier of the surface, are damaged. Pathogenic bacteria have evolved similar strategies to successfully colonize mucosal surfaces, evade the host immune response, and invade soft tissue. For bacteria of the head and neck, the virulence factors expressed during colonization differ from those expressed during acute infection. This tight regulation, along with interaction with the host immune system and inflammatory response, tip the balance in favor of either colonization or infection with signs and symptoms of disease.

The most common infections of this region are dental caries and periodontal disease that develop after a proliferation of bacterial commensals and subsequent upregulation of virulence factors or exchange of genetic information between more pathogenic species and these commensals. Local oral cavity infections, such as caries, gingivitis, periodontitis, or abscess (periapical or periodontal), wreak havoc in the mouth, potentially affecting patient comfort and socialization. These infections can extend to surrounding structures, leading to life-threatening necrotizing infections, severe abscess formation, or local vascular complications, such as Lemierre syndrome, resulting in significant morbidity and occasional mortality.

However, the emerging literature on this topic strongly suggests that there are additional consequences of dental caries and periodontal disease beyond the oral cavity with profound implications for human health. Examples include cardiovascular disease, diabetes mellitus, preterm birth, and low birth weight. These links are currently poorly understood, with many studies demonstrating an association between specific bacteria in the oral cavity and pathogenic lesions outside the head, neck, and mouth. For example, periodontal pathogen burden in subgingival biofilm samples is associated with carotid intima-media thickness and risk for nonfatal myocardial infarction.[55] In addition, both the DNA of periodontal pathogens and the culture-viable bacteria have been isolated from atherosclerotic plaques. In one of the most convincing association studies, *A. actinomycetemcomitans* identified in high concentrations in saliva increased the risk of coronary artery disease compared with hosts with lower concentrations of *A. actinomycetemcomitans*.[55]

The coronavirus disease of 2019 (COVID-19) pandemic caused by severe acute respiratory syndrome coronavirus-2 (SARS-CoV-2) produced a renewed focus on illness of the upper respiratory tract and its accompanying microbiome. Research focused both on comparative differences within the microbiome in those with COVID-19 and uninfected controls, as well as the associations between the upper respiratory tract microbiome and COVID-19 severity.[56] In patients with COVID-19, overall upper respiratory tract bacterial load may increase and the relative abundance of certain microbial species may correlate with COVID-19 severity.[56]

Additionally, members of the oral microbiome may act synergistically with SARS-CoV-2 and aid progression of infection. *F. nucleatum,* discussed earlier, has been implicated in multiple diseases such as decreased lung function in chronic obstructive pulmonary disease, the development of inflammatory bowel disease, colorectal cancer, and potentially oral squamous cell carcinoma.[57,58] Higher numbers of *F. nucleatum* have been recovered in patients with COVID-19. Interestingly, *F. nucleatum* can induce the upregulation of the SARS-CoV-2 receptor angiotensin-converting enzyme 2 in human respiratory epithelial cells and the release of proinflammatory cytokines, thus aiding SARS-CoV-2 infection.[59]

There is a history of connecting an organism associated with the head and neck region to a systemic disorder, *S. pyogenes* (group A streptococcus), and rheumatic heart disease. In the case of rheumatic fever, investigators in the early 1900s identified a link between *S. pyogenes* pharyngitis and the subsequent development of rheumatic fever. Despite a century of understanding of this important link, uncovering the pathogenesis of rheumatic fever evolved, moving from direct bacterial invasion of affected systemic organs, to toxin-mediated disease, and to the currently favored theory of an autoimmune process brought on by molecular mimicry in genetically susceptible individuals.[60] Similar links associating head and neck bacteria with systemic diseases are intriguing and also evolving. Future work, with the help of deep sequencing technology, will aim to elucidate these relationships. It may turn out that therapies that alter the bacterial population of the oral cavity modify the risk for common systemic diseases, such as cancer and coronary artery disease and possibly even modify the risk of viral infections.

Acknowledgments

We would like to acknowledge the contribution of the author from the previous edition, Dr. Todd Cassesse.

References

1. Tsuchida S, Umemura H, Nakayama T. Current status of matrix-assisted laser desorption/ionization-time-of-flight mass spectrometry (MALDI-TOF MS) in clinical diagnostic microbiology. *Molecules.* 2020;25(20):4775.
2. Cho I, Blaser MJ. The human microbiome: at the interface of health and disease. *Nat Rev Genet.* 2012;13(4):260-270.
3. Weinstock GM. Genomic approaches to studying the human microbiota. *Nature.* 2012;489(7415):250-256.
4. D'Agostino S, Ferrara E, Valentini G, Stoica SA, Dolci M. Exploring oral microbiome in healthy infants and children: a systematic review. *Int J Environ Res Public Health.* 2022;19(18):11403.
5. Lamont RJ, Koo H, Hajishengallis G. The oral microbiota: dynamic communities and host interactions. *Nat Rev Microbiol.* 2018;16(12):745-759.
6. Martino C, Dilmore AH, Burcham ZM, Metcalf JL, Jeste D, Knight R. Microbiota succession throughout life from the cradle to the grave. *Nat Rev Microbiol.* 2022;20(12):707-720.
7. Samarrai R, Frank S, Lum A, Woodis K, Weinstock G, Roberts D. Defining the microbiome of the head and neck: a contemporary review. *Am J Otolaryngol.* 2022;43(1):103224.
8. Sedghi L, DiMassa V, Harrington A, Lynch SV, Kapila YL. The oral microbiome: role of key organisms and complex networks in oral health and disease. *Periodontology 2000.* 2021;87(1):107-131.
9. Allen EK, Pitkaranta A, Maki M, et al. Bacteria in the nose of young adults during wellness and rhinovirus colds: detection by culture and microarray methods in 100 nasal lavage specimens. *Int Forum Allergy Rhinol.* 2013;3(9):731-739.
10. Frank DN, Spiegelman GB, Davis W, Wagner E, Lyons E, Pace NR. Culture-independent molecular analysis of microbial constituents of the healthy human outer ear. *J Clin Microbiol.* 2003;41(1):295-303.
11. Hilty M, Qi W, Brugger SD, et al. Nasopharyngeal microbiota in infants with acute otitis media. *J Infect Dis.* 2012;205(7):1048-1055.

12. Jensen A, Fago-Olsen H, Sorensen CH, Kilian M. Molecular mapping to species level of the tonsillar crypt microbiota associated with health and recurrent tonsillitis. *PLoS One.* 2013; 8(2):e56418.

13. Norder Grusell E, Dahlen G, Ruth M, et al. Bacterial flora of the human oral cavity, and the upper and lower esophagus. *Dis Esophagus.* 2013;26(1):84-90.

14. Irfan M, Delgado RZR, Frias-Lopez J. The oral microbiome and cancer. *Front Immunol.* 2020;11:591088.

15. Brook I. The impact of smoking on oral and nasopharyngeal bacterial flora. *J Dent Res.* 2011;90(6):704-710.

16. Gong HL, Shi Y, Zhou L, et al. The composition of microbiome in larynx and the throat biodiversity between laryngeal squamous cell carcinoma patients and control population. *PLoS One.* 2013;8(6):e66476.

17. Aurora R, Chatterjee D, Hentzleman J, Prasad G, Sindwani R, Sanford T. Contrasting the microbiomes from healthy volunteers and patients with chronic rhinosinusitis. *JAMA Otolaryngol Head Neck Surg.* 2013;139(12):1328-1338.

18. Ramakrishnan VR, Feazel LM, Gitomer SA, Ir D, Robertson CE, Frank DN. The microbiome of the middle meatus in healthy adults. *PLoS One.* 2013;8(12):e85507.

19. Ren T, Glatt DU, Nguyen TN, et al. 16S rRNA survey revealed complex bacterial communities and evidence of bacterial interference on human adenoids. *Environ Microbiol.* 2013;15(2): 535-547.

20. Singh K, Nordstrom T, Morgelin M, Brant M, Cardell LO, Riesbeck K. *Haemophilus influenzae* resides in tonsils and uses immunoglobulin D binding as an evasion strategy. *J Infect Dis.* 2014;209(9):1418-1428.

21. Sauer K, Stoodley P, Goeres DM, et al. The biofilm life cycle: expanding the conceptual model of biofilm formation. *Nat Rev Microbiol.* 2022;20(10):608-620.

22. Bowen WH, Burne RA, Wu H, Koo H. Oral biofilms: pathogens, matrix, and polymicrobial interactions in microenvironments. *Trends Microbiol.* 2018;26(3):229-242.

23. Kadioglu A, Weiser JN, Paton JC, Andrew PW. The role of Streptococcus pneumoniae virulence factors in host respiratory colonization and disease. *Nat Rev Microbiol.* 2008;6(4):288-301.

24. Murphy TF, Parameswaran GI. *Moraxella catarrhalis*, a human respiratory tract pathogen. *Clin Infect Dis.* 2009;49(1):124-131.

25. de Vries SP, Bootsma HJ, Hays JP, Hermans PW. Molecular aspects of *Moraxella catarrhalis* pathogenesis. *Microbiol Mol Biol Rev.* 2009;73(3):389-406.

26. Blakeway LV, Tan A, Peak IRA, Seib KL. Virulence determinants of *Moraxella catarrhalis*: distribution and considerations for vaccine development. *Microbiology (Reading).* 2017;163(10):1371-1384.

27. Van Eldere J, Slack MP, Ladhani S, Cripps AW. Non-typeable *Haemophilus influenzae*, an under-recognised pathogen. *Lancet Infect Dis.* 2014;14(12):1281-1292.

28. St Geme JW III. Molecular and cellular determinants of nontypeable *Haemophilus influenzae* adherence and invasion. *Cell Microbiol.* 2002;4(4):191-200.

29. Spahich NA, St Geme JW III. Structure and function of the *Haemophilus influenzae* autotransporters. *Front Cell Infect Microbiol.* 2011;1:5.

30. Duell BL, Su YC, Riesbeck K. Host-pathogen interactions of nontypeable *Haemophilus influenzae*: from commensal to pathogen. *FEBS Lett.* 2016;590(21):3840-3853.

31. Swords WE. Nontypeable *Haemophilus influenzae* biofilms: role in chronic airway infections. *Front Cell Infect Microbiol.* 2012;2:97.

32. Cole JN, Barnett TC, Nizet V, Walker MJ. Molecular insight into invasive group A streptococcal disease. *Nat Rev Microbiol.* 2011;9(10):724-736.

33. Lynskey NN, Lawrenson RA, Sriskandan S. New understandings in *Streptococcus pyogenes*. *Curr Opin Infect Dis.* 2011;24(3): 196-202.

34. Zecconi A, Scali F. *Staphylococcus aureus* virulence factors in evasion from innate immune defenses in human and animal diseases. *Immunol Lett.* 2013;150(1-2):12-22.

35. Otto M. *Staphylococcus aureus* toxins. *Curr Opin Microbiol.* 2014;17:32-37.

36. Tong SY, Davis JS, Eichenberger E, Holland TL, Fowler Jr VG. *Staphylococcus aureus* infections: epidemiology, pathophysiology, clinical manifestations, and management. *Clin Microbiol Rev.* 2015;28(3):603-661.

37. Watkins RR, David MZ, Salata RA. Current concepts on the virulence mechanisms of methicillin-resistant *Staphylococcus aureus*. *J Med Microbiol.* 2012;61(Pt 9):1179-1193.

38. Sitkiewicz I. How to become a killer, or is it all accidental? Virulence strategies in oral streptococci. *Mol Oral Microbiol.* 2018;33(1):1-12.

39. Mitchell J. *Streptococcus mitis*: walking the line between commensalism and pathogenesis. *Mol Oral Microbiol.* 2011;26(2):89-98.

40. Takao A, Nagamune H, Maeda N. Sialidase of *Streptococcus intermedius*: a putative virulence factor modifying sugar chains. *Microbiol Immunol.* 2010;54(10):584-595.

41. Bowen WH, Koo H. Biology of *Streptococcus mutans*-derived glucosyltransferases: role in extracellular matrix formation of cariogenic biofilms. *Caries Res.* 2011;45(1):69-86.

42. Nakano K, Hokamura K, Taniguchi N, et al. The collagen-binding protein of *Streptococcus mutans* is involved in haemorrhagic stroke. *Nat Commun.* 2011;2:485.

43. Shimada E, Kataoka H, Miyazawa Y, Yamamoto M, Igarashi T. Lipoproteins of *Actinomyces viscosus* induce inflammatory responses through TLR2 in human gingival epithelial cells and macrophages. *Microbes Infect.* 2012;14(11):916-921.

44. Sato T, Watanabe K, Kumada H, Toyama T, Tani-Ishii N, Hamada N. Peptidoglycan of *Actinomyces naeslundii* induces inflammatory cytokine production and stimulates osteoclastogenesis in alveolar bone resorption. *Arch Oral Biol.* 2012;57 (11):1522-1528.

45. Gajdács M, Urbán E, Terhes G. Microbiological and clinical aspects of cervicofacial *Actinomyces* infections: an overview. *Dent J (Basel).* 2019;7(3):85.

46. Potempa M, Potempa J, Kantyka T, et al. Interpain A, a cysteine proteinase from *Prevotella intermedia*, inhibits complement by degrading complement factor C3. *PLoS Pathog.* 2009;5(2): e1000316.

47. Yanagisawa M, Kuriyama T, Williams DW, Nakagawa K, Karasawa T. Proteinase activity of *Prevotella* species associated with oral purulent infection. *Curr Microbiol.* 2006;52(5):375-378.

48. Yamanaka T, Yamane K, Furukawa T, et al. Comparison of the virulence of exopolysaccharide-producing *Prevotella intermedia* to exopolysaccharide non-producing periodontopathic organisms. *BMC Infect Dis.* 2011;11:228.

49. Matsui A, Jin JO, Johnston CD, Yamazaki H, Houri-Haddad Y, Rittling SR. Pathogenic bacterial species associated with endodontic infection evade innate immune control by disabling neutrophils. *Infect Immun.* 2014;82(10):4068-4079.

50. Sharma G, Garg N, Hasan S, Shirodkar S. *Prevotella*: an insight into its characteristics and associated virulence factors. *Microb Pathog.* 2022;169:105673.

51. Riordan T. Human infection with *Fusobacterium necrophorum* (necrobacillosis), with a focus on Lemierre's syndrome. *Clin Microbiol Rev.* 2007;20(4):622-659.

52. Thapa G, Jayal A, Sikazwe E, Perry T, Mohammed Al Balushi A, Livingstone P. A genome-led study on the pathogenesis of *Fusobacterium necrophorum* infections. *Gene.* 2022;840:146770.

53. Butler T. *Capnocytophaga canimorsus*: an emerging cause of sepsis, meningitis, and post-splenectomy infection after dog bites. *Eur J Clin Microbiol Infect Dis.* 2015;34(7):1271-1280.

54. Ehrmann E, Handal T, Tamanai-Shacoori Z, Bonnaure-Mallet M, Fosse T. High prevalence of beta-lactam and macrolide resistance genes in human oral *Capnocytophaga species. J Antimicrob Chemother.* 2014;69(2):381-384.

55. Hyvarinen K, Mantyla P, Buhlin K, et al. A common periodontal pathogen has an adverse association with both acute and stable coronary artery disease. *Atherosclerosis.* 2012;223(2):478-484.

56. Shilts MH, Rosas-Salazar C, Strickland BA, et al. Severe COVID-19 is associated with an altered upper respiratory tract microbiome. *Front Cell Infect Microbiol.* 2021;11:781968.

57. Bao L, Zhang C, Lyu J, et al. Beware of pharyngeal *Fusobacterium nucleatum* in COVID-19. *BMC Microbiol.* 2021;21(1):277.

58. Torralba MG, Aleti G, Li W, et al. Oral microbial species and virulence factors associated with oral squamous cell carcinoma. *Microb Ecol.* 2021;82(4):1030-1046.

59. Takahashi Y, Watanabe N, Kamio N, et al. Expression of the SARS-CoV-2 receptor ACE2 and proinflammatory cytokines induced by the periodontopathic bacterium *Fusobacterium nucleatum* in human respiratory epithelial cells. *Int J Mol Sci.* 2021;22(3):1352.

60. Benedek TG. The history of bacteriologic concepts of rheumatic fever and rheumatoid arthritis. *Semin Arthritis Rheum.* 2006; 36(2):109-123.

3

Nonbacterial Microbiology of the Head, Neck, and Orofacial Region

MARICAR MALINIS AND FIONNA FELLER

Various infectious diseases can involve the head and neck. Nonbacterial causes include viruses, fungi, and parasites. This chapter describes the clinical manifestation, diagnosis, and treatment of a variety of nonbacterial infections of the head and neck.

Viral Infections

Viral and virally related diseases have a variety of head and neck manifestations that can range from an inflammatory presentation to malignancy.

Herpesviruses

Herpesviruses are double-stranded DNA viruses that can establish latency and reactivate during a net state of immunosuppression. Five herpesviruses that have significant clinical and pathologic head and neck presentations are herpes simplex viruses (HSV-1 and HSV-2), varicella-zoster virus (VZV), Epstein-Barr virus (EBV), cytomegalovirus (CMV), and the Kaposi's sarcoma (KS)–associated virus, human herpesvirus-8 (HHV-8).

Herpes Simplex Virus

Humans are the natural host for HSV-1 and -2. HSV-1 is more commonly associated with oral, labial, and ocular infections, whereas HSV-2 is more closely associated with genital infections. There is a frequent overlap in the presentation of both viruses.

Transmission is by person-to-person contact through infected secretions or mucocutaneous surfaces. After the primary infection, HSV becomes latent in neural tissue, particularly the dorsal root ganglion. Disease manifestations are more likely from reactivation secondary to stress, trauma, and immunosuppression. Cell-mediated immunity contains infection in their lytic state or active replication, whereas humoral immunity modulates latent HSV infection at the neurons. Disseminated disease can occur in patients with cell-mediated immunosuppression (e.g., AIDS, solid organ or hematopoietic stem cell transplant recipients).

Clinical Manifestations

Primary HSV-1 infection manifests as gingivostomatitis, characterized by painful ulceration and vesicular lesion involving the tongue, buccal, and sublingual mucosa and palate (Figure 3-1). Infrequently, pharyngitis can occur. Primary HSV infection is more often associated with constitutional symptoms, prolonged symptom duration, and prolonged viral shedding compared with disease reactivation.

HSV-1 reactivation manifests as cutaneous and mucocutaneous disease. Herpes labialis (i.e., cold sore) is a vesicle or ulceration limited to the lips. Cutaneous lesions may be limited to a dermatome, like herpes zoster (shingles). Herpes gladiatorum is a cutaneous HSV-1 manifestation involving the face, neck, and arms seen more commonly in wrestlers and rugby players.[1]

HSV-1 and, infrequently, HSV-2 (in neonates) can inoculate the eye and result in conjunctivitis, blepharitis, or keratitis (corneal ulceration). Blepharitis can occur as a result of vesicles along the lid margin and periorbital skin. Corneal ulceration and scarring may cause vision loss. Although rare, acute retinal necrosis can occur with HSV infection.

Diagnosis

Diagnostic tests include Tzanck smear, viral culture, serology, immunofluorescence staining, and polymerase chain reaction (PCR).[2] A Tzanck smear can be performed on a scraped sample to assess for cytopathic effect. However, it is unable to differentiate HSV-1, HSV-2, and VZV because of similar cytologic changes. Viral cultures can differentiate the herpesviruses. Scrapings can be examined for herpes antigen via immunofluorescence. Serology is helpful in distinguishing HSV-1 and HSV-2. Real-time HSV PCR can confirm HSV infection in clinical specimens.

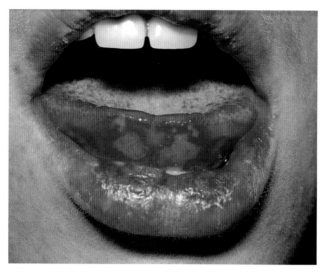

• **Figure 3-1** Herpes Simplex Involving the Lips and Tongue. (From Regezi JA, Sciubba JJ, Jordan RCK. *Oral Pathology: Clinical Pathologic Correlations.* 6th ed. St Louis: Saunders; 2012.)

Treatment

Antiviral treatment includes acyclovir, valacyclovir, and famciclovir. These antivirals interfere with DNA viral synthesis. Valacyclovir and famciclovir have better bioavailability and less frequent dosing compared to acyclovir. Chronic suppression to reduce frequency of HSV reactivation can be offered to patients with recurrent episodes. Resistance to acyclovir and its analogues infrequently occurs. Resistance testing to acyclovir and consideration of alternative therapy such as foscarnet and cidofovir are recommended if there is lack of clinical improvement with standard therapy. A novel antiviral, pritelivir which is a nucleoside analog that has activity against acyclovir-resistant HSV and can reduce genital viral shedding, is currently studied through a randomized controlled trial in immunocompromised hosts.[3,4]

Varicella-Zoster Virus

VZV has two distinct clinical presentations: varicella (chickenpox) and herpes zoster (shingles). Varicella is the primary infection and can be acquired by inhalation of infectious respiratory secretion or direct contact with a mucocutaneous lesion. Herpes zoster is the recurrent infection in individuals with prior primary infection. After the primary varicella infection, VZV enters the dorsal root ganglia and spinal cord, where it remains latent until it reactivates akin to HSV.

Clinical Manifestations

Primary infection appears as an erythematous papule that evolves into vesicles or bullae. Lesions become pustular in 3 to 4 days and crusted in 7 to 10 days. Scarring can persist for months to years after primary infection. Reactivation of the disease is often limited to dermatomal distribution. Reactivation of latent virus in the geniculate ganglion can

manifest as Ramsay Hunt syndrome, which is characterized by facial palsy, ear and facial pain, and ear canal vesicular lesions. Reactivation of the latent virus involving the trigeminal nerve's ophthalmic division can result in herpes ophthalmicus, described as conjunctivitis or a corneal ulcer causing vision loss. VZV can manifest as acute retinal necrosis. The ophthalmic manifestation requires urgent evaluation and treatment because of potential vision loss. Postherpetic neuralgia is a complication of herpes zoster in 10 to 15% of all patients and manifests with pain, numbness, dysesthesia, and allodynia along the affected dermatome (Figure 3-2) persisting months after the initial onset of the rash.

Diagnosis

The diagnosis is based solely on clinical presentation. Laboratory tests, such as direct immunofluorescence testing and PCR of swabbed unroofed vesicles, are helpful to establish diagnosis.

Treatment and Prevention

Supportive care is the cornerstone of management of primary infection. Antiviral treatment with acyclovir, valacyclovir, or famciclovir should be considered in those who developed herpes zoster within 72 hours of symptoms to reduce symptom duration and risk of postherpetic neuralgia. Recombinant zoster vaccine reduces the risks for herpes zoster and postherpetic neuralgia by approximately 90%.[5] The vaccine should be offered to immunocompetent adults 50 years and older and immunocompromised adults older than 19 years. Two doses of the vaccine are required 2 to 6 months apart.[6]

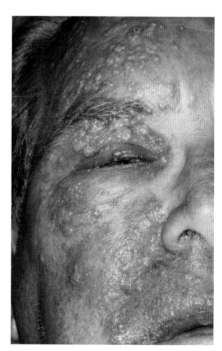

• **Figure 3-2** Herpes Zoster Involving the Face. (From Neville BW, Damm DD, Allen CM, et al. *Oral and Maxillofacial Pathology.* 4th ed. St Louis: Saunders; 2016.)

Epstein-Barr Virus

The Epstein-Barr virus (EBV) is a ubiquitous herpesvirus with approximately 90% seroprevalence in adults. EBV acquired during childhood is largely subclinical. Transmission is by direct contact with salivary secretion. After primary infection, the virus achieves latency in B cells.

Clinical Manifestation

Infectious mononucleosis is most associated with EBV primary infection. It is a self-limiting syndrome characterized by fever, fatigue, tonsillopharyngitis, lymphadenopathy, and the presence of atypical lymphocytes in a peripheral smear. Lymphadenopathy often involves the posterior cervical chain and is frequently symmetric in presentation. A generalized maculopapular rash can occur with antibiotic exposure, more commonly with amoxicillin or ampicillin. The presence of heterophile antibodies (immunoglobulin [Ig] M reacting with sheep or horse red blood cells) and symptoms compatible with infectious mononucleosis establishes the diagnosis of EBV. If the heterophile antibody is negative, a serologic assay can confirm the diagnosis of acute infection with presence of IgM viral capsid antigen antibody.

Oral hairy leukoplakia is a result of EBV infection of oral squamous epithelial cells and can be seen in immunosuppressed patients, including those with HIV infection (Figure 3-3). It appears as white, shaggy plaque and painless lesions commonly seen on the tongue's lateral border but can also involve the buccal mucosa and gingiva. It cannot be scraped, in contrast to oral thrush caused by *Candida*. The diagnosis is made clinically, but biopsy is helpful to rule out other causes of leukoplakia. EBV has been associated with malignancies such as Burkitt lymphoma, Hodgkin lymphoma, T cell lymphoma, and nasopharyngeal carcinoma.

Treatment

The treatment of mononucleosis is primarily supportive care. There is no proven benefit of antiviral treatment. The incidence of oral hairy leukoplakia can been reduced in people living with HIV by taking antiretroviral treatment.

Cytomegalovirus

The seroprevalence of CMV is 60% by 6 years of age, and it increases with age, approaching 90% by the age of 80 years.[7] Primary infection can occur with exposure to saliva, genital secretions, blood, or tissue and perinatally. After primary infection, CMV establishes latency in the host's cells or tissues, including polymorphonuclear cells, T-lymphocytes, endothelial vascular tissue, fibroblasts, salivary glands, and renal epithelial cells. Reactivation from latent infection can occur in the setting of immunosuppression or acute illness.

Clinical Manifestations and Diagnosis

Primary infection with CMV in immunocompetent individuals may manifest as asymptomatic illness or mononucleosis-like. The latter is characterized by fever, malaise, lymphadenopathy, and laboratory findings of lymphocytosis and atypical lymphocytes. The heterophil agglutinin test is negative in CMV mononucleosis and positive in EBV mononucleosis. In contrast with EBV, CMV mononucleosis is not typically associated with exudative tonsillopharyngitis. A maculopapular rash can similarly occur after antibiotic exposure.

CMV esophagitis can manifest as odynophagia and dysphagia. The diagnosis is confirmed by detection of intranuclear inclusion bodies in biopsied tissue (Figure 3-4).

CMV retinitis is more commonly seen in patients with advanced immunosuppression, such as with HIV/AIDS. People living with HIV and have CD4 less than 50 cells/mm^3 are at risk for CMV retinitis. Retinal disease rarely occurs in solid organ or bone marrow transplant recipients. The diagnosis is made by fundoscopic examination demonstrating white fluffy retinal infiltrate with hemorrhage (Figure 3-5). Elevated CMV viral load in blood or plasma detected by PCR assay correlates with disease activity in patients with AIDS.[8]

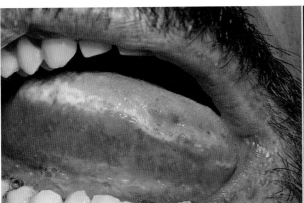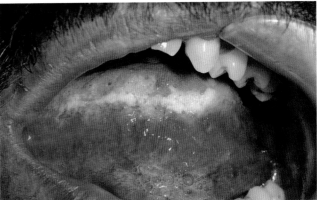

• **Figure 3-3** Oral Hairy Leukoplakia Associated With Epstein-Barr Virus. (From Regezi JA, Sciubba JJ, Jordan RCK. *Oral Pathology: Clinical Pathologic Correlations.* 6th ed. St Louis: Saunders; 2012.)

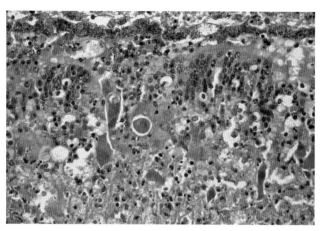

• **Figure 3-4** Cytomegalovirus Inclusion Bodies in Esophageal Tissue Biopsy. (From Gilbert-Barnes E. *Potter's Pathology of the Fetus, Infant and Child.* 2nd ed. St Louis: Mosby; 2007.)

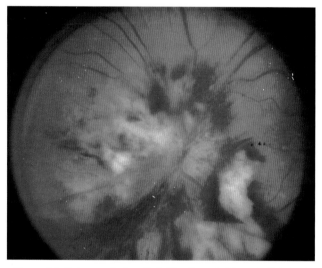

• **Figure 3-5** Cytomegalovirus Retinitis. (From Goldman L, Schafer AI. *Goldman's Cecil Medicine.* 24th ed. Philadelphia: Saunders; 2012.)

Treatment

CMV mononucleosis is self-limited and managed by supportive care. On the other hand, CMV disease (i.e., esophagitis and retinitis) requires either intravenous ganciclovir or oral valganciclovir. An induction dose is given for 21 days followed by a maintenance regimen. In patients with HIV/AIDS, antiretroviral treatment facilitates recovery of CMV-specific T cell–mediated immunity. In the setting of ganciclovir-resistant CMV, foscarnet, cidofovir, and maribavir can be given. Foscarnet and cidofovir are given intravenously and causes nephrotoxicity. Maribavir was recently approved by the U.S. Food and Drug Administration (FDA) for treatment of CMV resistant or refractory to ganciclovir. It has better tolerability and safety profile with lower rates of myelosuppression and renal impairment than other anti-CMV agents. However, it cannot be used for CMV retinitis or meningoencephalitis.[9]

Human Herpesvirus-8

Human herpesvirus-8 (HHV-8), or KS–associated herpesvirus, is a γ herpesvirus associated with malignancies, including KS, primary effusion lymphoma, and Castleman's disease. HHV-8 infects various cell types, including B cells, macrophages, endothelial cells, and epithelial cells. After primary infection, it establishes latency in B cells and glandular epithelial cells. Seroprevalence rates differ among different geographic regions. Prevalence appears to be higher among homosexual males, and it correlates with number of homosexual partners. Transmission of HHV-8 by saliva was suggested by studies.

Clinical Manifestations

The primary infection in immunocompetent children can be characterized by a febrile maculopapular skin rash.[10] Otherwise, it can be asymptomatic. In an immunocompromised state, reactivation of disease can lead to malignancy such as KS.

KS is a vascular neoplasm that is classified into four types: classic (occurs in middle or old age), endemic (described in sub-Saharan Africa before AIDS), iatrogenic (associated with immunosuppressive drug therapy, including transplant recipients), and AIDS associated (epidemic).

KS occurred more commonly in patients with AIDS before the era of highly active antiretroviral treatment.[11] KS may manifest with cutaneous and visceral involvement. Cutaneous lesions of KS involves the face, oral mucosa, lower extremity, and genitalia. It is a nonpainful, nonpruritic papule or plaque-like lesion. The color varies depending on vascularity and can be pink, red, violet, and brown. Oral cavity lesions was observed in one third of patients with KS (Figure 3-6) and commonly involves the palate and gingiva.

Diagnosis

Biopsy of the lesion confirms the diagnosis.

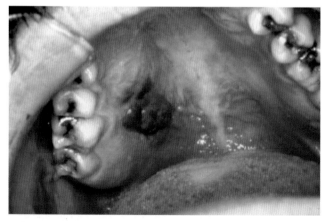

• **Figure 3-6** Kaposi Sarcoma of the Hard Palate. (From Daniel SJ, Harfst SA, Wilder R. *Mosby's Dental Hygiene: Concepts, Cases, and Competencies.* 2nd ed. St Louis: Mosby; 2008.)

Treatment

The treatment of AIDS-related KS involves reversal of immunosuppression by highly active antiretroviral treatment initiation.[12] On rare occasions, local or systemic chemotherapy is indicated.

Human Immunodeficiency Virus

HIV is a retrovirus infecting T helper cells (CD4$^+$), macrophages, and dendritic cells. CD4$^+$ count declines as a result of direct viral killing and cytotoxic-mediated cell (CD8+) killing of infected cells.

HIV can be transmitted by sexual contact, blood exposure, needle-stick injuries, and maternal to fetal transmission. Acute retroviral syndrome or acute HIV infection manifests with fever, malaise, cervical lymphadenopathy, and pharyngitis similar to mononucleosis.

Diagnosis

Patients with symptoms suggestive of acute retroviral syndrome should be screened for HIV. The Centers for Disease Control and Prevention (CDC) guidelines recommend screening with a fourth-generation combined antigen–antibody immunoassay with confirmatory HIV-1/HIV-2 antibody differentiation assay and an RNA test to resolve reactive immunoassay with a negative confirmatory test result (Figure 3-7).[13]

With low CD4$^+$, infected patients can develop opportunistic infections such as oral candidiasis, KS, and hairy leukoplakia. Other common head and neck lesions include aphthous stomatitis, periodontal disease, non-Hodgkin lymphoma, and lymphadenopathy. Reactivation of herpesviruses (e.g., CMV, HSV) can occur depending on the degree of immunosuppression.

Treatment

The mainstay of HIV treatment is antiretroviral therapy. Current guidelines from the U.S. Department of Health and Human Services (DHHS) and the International Antiviral Society–USA Panel recommend treatment in all patients with HIV infection, regardless of CD4 cell count. Guidelines for selection of medication, laboratory monitoring, and patient evaluation is beyond the scope of this book, but resources are found at http://www.iasusa.org and https://hivinfo.nih.gov/home-page.

Human Papilloma Virus

Human papilloma virus (HPV) is a double-stranded DNA virus that infects squamous stratified epithelia of the body and can cause benign or malignant tumors. At least 184 types have been identified to date. Certain HPV types have a predilection for skin or mucosa.

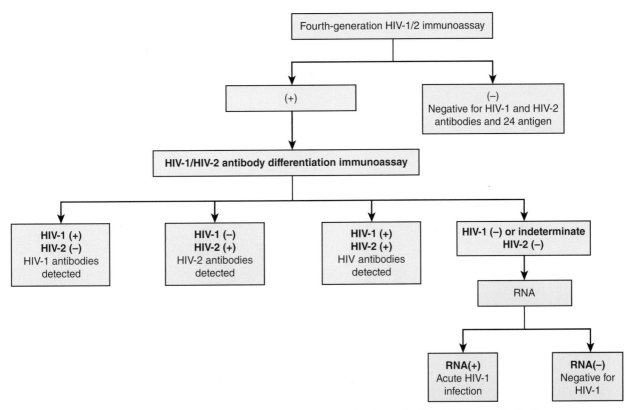

• **Figure 3-7** Detection of Acute HIV Infection in Two Evaluations of a New HIV Diagnostic Testing Algorithm – United States, 2011-2013. (Reproduced from Centers for Disease Control and Prevention. Detection of acute HIV infection in two evaluations of a new HIV diagnostic testing algorithm – United States, 2011-2013. *MMWR Morb Mortal Wkly Rep.* 2013;62:489.)

Clinical Manifestation, Diagnosis, and Treatment

Cutaneous HPV infection, more commonly known as *warts*, is the most common manifestation. Close personal contact is likely the mode of transmission in cutaneous warts. Verrucae plana (Figure 3-8) is the type most found in distribution of face, neck, and hands. It can appear as multiple, slightly elevated papules with irregular contours and smooth surfaces. The diagnosis of warts is essentially based on physical examination. Treatment includes the use of keratolytic agents (e.g., salicylic acid), cryotherapy, or laser surgery.

Mucosal HPV can cause oral lesions of several types. HPV types 6, 11, and 16 infections cause squamous papilloma; HPV types 2, 4, and 57 cause verrucae vulgaris; and HPV types 3 and 13 cause focal epithelial hyperplasia.[14,15]

Recurrent respiratory papillomatosis is an HPV infection of the upper aerodigestive tract, but more commonly has laryngeal involvement during early childhood or early adult life. In young children, acquisition is likely via the passage through an infected birth canal, because HPV types are similar to those of anogenital warts.[16] Among adults, the risk of recurrent respiratory papillomatosis is associated with an increased number of sexual partners and oral-genital contact.

HPV virus has been strongly associated with malignancy. HPV types 16, 18, 31, 33, 35, 39, 45, 51, 52, 56, 58, 59, and 66 are considered high risk for oncogenesis.[17] Oropharyngeal cancer has been associated with HPV among the younger population and those with high-risk sexual behavior. There are currently 3 HPV vaccines available: 9-valent (Gardasil 9), quadrivalent (Gardasil), and bivalent (Cervarix) vaccines. The CDC recommends initiating HPV vaccine series before age 15 to improve immunogenicity compared to 3-dose series started after age 15. Catch-up vaccination should be offered for all adults through age 26 years.[18]

Coxsackie Virus

Coxsackie viruses belong to the *Enterovirus* genus and further divided into Coxsackie A and Coxsackie B. These viruses can be transmitted easily by direct contact or oral route. Infection can occur all year in temperate climates, but peaks during summer and fall. Coxsackie A virus is an important head and neck pathogen as it commonly causes herpangina and hand, foot, and mouth disease (HFMD).

Clinical Manifestation

Herpangina (Figure 3-9) is a clinical syndrome characterized by fever, sore throat, painful swallowing, and a papulovesicular enanthem with surrounding erythema involving the fauces and soft palate.[2] The lesions can progress to ulcerations. Enanthems persist 5 to 7 days and resolve spontaneously. Herpangina is commonly caused by Coxsackie A serotypes 1 to 10, 16, and 22, and Coxsackie B serotypes 1 to 5.[19,20]

HFMD is a clinical syndrome characterized by fever, enanthem (mucosal membrane lesion), and exanthem. The enanthem has a vesiculoulcerative appearance with surrounding erythema involving the tongue, palate, and buccal and gingival mucosa, but sparing the oropharynx (Figure 3-10).[2] Exanthem typically appears 1 or 2 days after the enanthem and is characterized by nonpainful, nonpruritic, and macular, maculopapular, or vesicular rash involving the hands, feet, buttocks, upper thighs and arms, or feet (Figure 3-11).[21] Spontaneous resolution can occur within 7 to 10 days. Several enteroviruses are associated with HFMD,

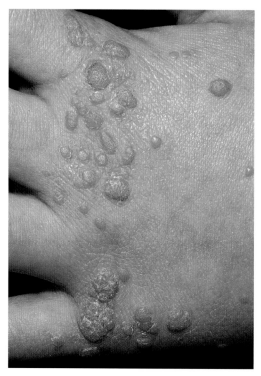

• **Figure 3-8** Verruca Plana on Hand. (From Habif T. *Clinical Dermatology: A Color Guide to Diagnosis and Therapy*. 6th ed. Philadelphia: Saunders; 2016.)

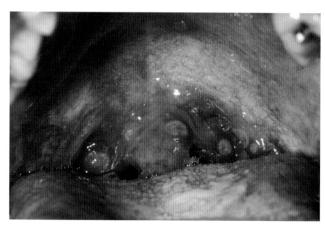

• **Figure 3-9** Herpangina. (From Neville BW, Damm DD, Allen CM, et al. *Oral and Maxillofacial Pathology*. 4th ed. St Louis: Saunders; 2016.)

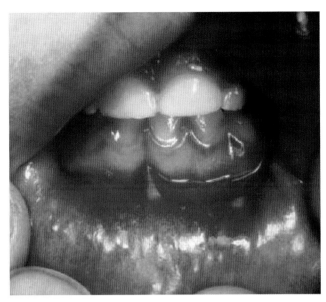

• **Figure 3-10** Oral Lesions in a Patient With Hand, Foot, and Mouth Disease. (From Ferri FF. *Ferri's Color Atlas and Text of Clinical Medicine.* Philadelphia: Saunders; 2009.)

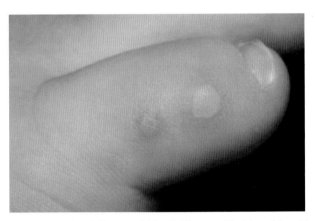

• **Figure 3-11** Hand, Foot, and Mouth Disease. Vesicles of the skin of the toe. (From Neville BW, Damm DD, Allen CM, et al. *Oral and Maxillofacial Pathology.* 4th ed. St Louis: Saunders; 2016.)

but Coxsackie A serotype 16 has been more frequently associated with large outbreaks.[22,23]

Diagnosis

The diagnosis for herpangina and HFMD is made clinically based on the typical appearance of the lesions. Confirmation by cell culture or nucleic acid amplification (e.g., PCR) may be warranted if diagnosis is uncertain or in patients with complications that can include rhombencephalitis, acute flaccid paralysis, aseptic meningitis, or myocarditis.[24] Samples from the throat, stool, or vesicular fluid of an exanthema or enanthem are appropriate for testing.

Treatment

HFMD and herpangina are self-limiting diseases, and therapeutic options are limited to symptomatic relief and

supportive care. Children who are unable to tolerate solid food and liquids by mouth because of painful oral lesions will require hospitalization for hydration with intravenous fluids. Infection spread can be prevented by hand hygiene. In a hospital setting, contact precautions in addition to standard precautions is implemented for the duration of the illness.

Mumps

Mumps virus is a single-stranded RNA virus belonging to the genus *Paramyxovirus*. Only one serotype exists, but there are 13 genotypes.[25] Humans are the natural host of this virus. Mumps is highly infectious, inoculates through nose or mouth, and is transmitted by direct contact, respiratory droplets, or fomites. Incubation period is between 16 and 18 days from exposure to onset of symptoms. An infected patient is typically contagious 1 to 2 days before the onset of symptoms, which continue for a few more days.

Clinical Manifestation

Prodromal symptoms include low-grade fever, malaise, anorexia, and headache. Within 48 to 72 hours, parotid gland enlargement and tenderness could be appreciated. Occasional earache can precede the parotid enlargement. On examination, the enlarged parotid gland obscures the angle of the mandible. Contralateral parotid gland enlargement occurs in 90% of patients, but this may be delayed by several days.[25] Patients may experience trismus and difficulty with mastication. The parotid gland returns to normal size within 7 days. Complications are rare, but meningitis, encephalitis, orchitis, and pancreatitis can occur.

Diagnosis and Treatment

Clinical diagnosis is made by exposure history and physical findings. Diagnosis is confirmed by detection of one of the following: mumps-specific IgM antibodies, a fourfold rise in IgG mumps-specific antibody in serum or detection of mumps virus, or viral nucleic acid in clinical specimen (saliva, urine, seminal fluid, or cerebrospinal fluid).[26] The disease is self-limited, and therapy is mainly symptomatic and supportive.

Mumps can be prevented by administration of measles, mumps, and rubella (MMR) vaccine. Per the Advisory Committee on Immunization Practices guidelines, the first dose of the MMR vaccine is recommended at 12 to 15 months old and a second dose is given at 4 to 6 years old.

Mpox

Mpox is an orthopoxvirus infection that can be transmitted from animal-to-human by contact of infected body fluids, bite, or consumption of infected raw meat. Person-to-person transmission most commonly occurs through direct close contact, usually through contact of affected skin lesions or mucous membranes, including respiratory secretions and genital contact. The most common transmission in the 2022 mpox outbreak was sexual contact, with most cases identified in men who have sex with men. Transmission through fomites has been reported with low incidence.[27]

Clinical Manifestation

Infected persons may be asymptomatic during the mpox incubation period, which lasts approximately 3 to 17 days, then develop a characteristic rash that can involve various parts of the body, including the head and neck. The rash usually begins as small, deep-seated painful macules that evolve to well-circumscribed papules, pustules, and vesicles, often with central umbilication, followed by scabbing and crusting in 1 to 2 weeks (Figure 3-12). In the 2022 mpox outbreak, proctitis was a common manifestation especially in those practicing anal-receptive sex. Systemic symptoms such as fever, chills, lymphadenopathy, fatigue, headache, and myalgias can also be present.[28]

Diagnosis and Treatment

Patients with compatible rash and relevant epidemiologic exposures should be tested for mpox.

Diagnosis is established by isolating mpox virus DNA on PCR testing or next-generation sequencing from samples of the rash. The mpox virus also can be isolated in culture. Clinical specimens can be obtained by swabbing the rash using a dry synthetic swab vigorously without de-roofing the lesion. Antigen and antibody testing are not recommended because they do not distinguish between orthopoxviruses.[27]

Treatment is mainly supportive, and antivirals can be offered for severe disease. Although there is no specific antiviral available against mpox, select patients can be offered antivirals that have been studied to be effective against other orthopoxviruses. These include tecovirimat and brincidofovir, both of which are approved by the FDA for treatment of human smallpox disease. Clinical trial assessing the efficacy of tecovirimat in treating mpox is ongoing. Tecovirimat can be offered as postexposure prophylaxis for immunocompromised hosts for which mpox vaccination is contraindicated. Brincidofovir is used for patients with severe disease who do not improve on tecovirimat or have contraindications to receiving tecovirimat.[29,30]

Individuals who have been exposed to mpox or are at high risk for mpox infection can be offered vaccination for both preexposure and postexposure prophylaxis. Postexposure prophylaxis (PEP) should be administered as soon as possible, ideally within 4 days, but can be given up to 14 days after exposure. Currently, there are two smallpox vaccines approved by the FDA to curb the mpox outbreak: live-attenuated Modified Vaccinia Ankara (MVA) vaccine (JYNNEOS) and live vaccinia vaccine (ACAM2000). The MVA vaccine is FDA-approved for preexposure and postexposure prophylaxis for mpox. The MVA is a live attenuated viral vaccine that does not replicate well in humans; therefore, it can be safely administered to immunocompromised hosts. In contrast, the live vaccinia vaccine replicates in human cells and is contraindicated in those with immunocompromising conditions. To date, there are no published data on the safety and efficacy of both vaccines. Vaccinia immune globulin intravenous (VIGIV) can be considered as PEP in patients with severe immunodeficiency, though data are lacking on its efficacy for mpox treatment.[29,30]

SARS-CoV-2

Coronavirus disease (COVID-19) is a respiratory disease caused by the novel severe acute respiratory syndrome coronavirus 2, or SARS-CoV-2 discovered in 2019 and is responsible for the current pandemic. The virus is transmitted person-to-person through aerosolization of infected respiratory droplets. Asymptomatic patients can transmit infection through viral shedding. SARS-CoV-2 has evolved over time, with many variants discovered to date. Current variants of concern include Delta (B.1.617.2 lineage) and Omicron (XBB 1.5 lineage).[31]

Clinical Manifestation

Symptoms of COVID-19 can include fever, chills, cough, dyspnea, sore throat, anosmia, dysgeusia, congestion, and rhinorrhea. Individuals may present with headache, fatigue, myalgia, diarrhea, nausea, and vomiting. Although the severity of illness varies among each SARS-CoV-2 variant, it is established that presence of multiple comorbidities is associated with severe disease. The incubation period is around 14 days after exposure, with most patients becoming symptomatic within 5 days.[32] However, the median incubation period differs slightly with each SARS-CoV-2 variant as well. Chest imaging may show ground-glass

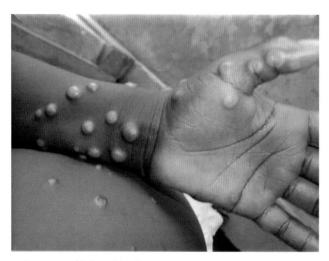

• **Figure 3-12** Various Manifestations of Mpox Rash. Lesions range from single versus many and macules, pustules, nodules, and vesicles involving any body part. Examples: https://www.cdc.gov/poxvirus/monkeypox/clinicians/clinical-recognition.html; https://www.who.int/health-topics/monkeypox#tab=tab_1.

opacities with mixed consolidation, pleural or septal thickening, or air bronchograms, though some individuals can present with normal chest radiograph findings.[33] Supporting laboratory findings can include lymphopenia, elevated inflammatory markers (C-reactive protein, erythrocyte sedimentation rate, ferritin), and elevated lactate dehydrogenase levels.

Diagnosis and Treatment

Diagnosis is established through molecular testing via nucleic acid amplification test (NAAT) or antigen test. NAAT is the recommended initial test due to higher sensitivity in both symptomatic and asymptomatic individuals. Respiratory tract specimens for NAAT can be obtained from nasopharyngeal swabs, saliva, or lower respiratory tract. Antigen tests, which are obtained through nasopharyngeal swabs only, are more convenient and rapid but have lower sensitivity especially in asymptomatic individuals. The CDC recommends that a negative test in symptomatic patients or those with recent exposure be followed by repeat testing with either a second antigen test after 48 hours or NAAT. Antibody tests for nucleocapsid protein (N), spike protein (S), or receptor-binding domain of S protein (RBD) are available. Detection of S protein and RBD antibodies is associated with either prior immunization or prior SARS-CoV-2 infection. Meanwhile, presence of N protein antibody usually indicates prior infection.[34]

Available COVID-19–directed therapies have changed over time according to variants of concern. Available therapies approved by the FDA at the time of this writing include nirmatrelvir/ritonavir, remdesivir, and molnupiravir.[35] Molnuporavir and nirmatrelvir/ritonavir are oral antivirals that can be given for mild to moderate COVID-19 in individuals considered at high risk to develop severe disease. Before prescribing nirmatrelvir/ritonavir, the patient's medication list should be reviewed carefully for potential drug-drug interaction with ritonavir. Both medications should be taken within 5 days of symptom onset. Remdesivir is an intravenous antiviral that can be offered to hospitalized patients (for 5 to 10 days' duration) and nonhospitalized patients (for 3 days' duration) who are at risk of progressing to severe disease. Monoclonal antibodies' emergency use authorization was withdrawn by the FDA because they are not effective against circulating Omicron variants. High-titer COVID-19 convalescent plasma can be considered an adjunctive treatment for COVID-19 in immunocompromised hosts. Other supportive treatments for hospitalized patients with severe COVID-19 include immunomodulators such as corticosteroids and interleukin-6 inhibitors, and antithrombotic therapy. COVID-19 treatment guidelines by the National Institutes of Health and Infectious Diseases Society of America are available on their respective websites.

There are currently four SARS-CoV2 vaccines approved by the FDA: BNT162b2 (mRNA), mRNA-1273 (mRNA), NVX-CoV2373 (protein subunit), and AD26.COV2.S (viral vector) vaccines. These vaccines have been shown to be safe and effective. There is a small risk of myocarditis and pericarditis associated with the mRNA vaccine among young males. AD26.COV2.S is the least preferred because of the rare occurrence thrombosis with thrombocytopenia syndrome, occurring in four cases per million vaccine doses.[36]

Fungal Infections

Mycoses represent infection by fungal organisms. With rare exception, mycoses are not transmissible from patient to patient, and contact isolation in the health care setting is not indicated. Mycoses are divided into yeast or yeast-like and molds. Table 3-1 summarizes the most common mycoses involving the orofacial region.

Yeast

Candida Species

Candida organisms are yeast because they are fungi that are present in a unicellular form. They are small (4 to 6 μm), thin-walled, ovoid cells that reproduce by budding. They are recovered from soil, animals, the hospital environment, and food. They are normal commensals of humans and are commonly found on the skin, in the gastrointestinal and female genital tracts, and in the urine of patients with indwelling Foley catheters.

Clinical Manifestations

The most common candida involving the head and neck is *Candida albicans*. The defense mechanism of intact integument is of importance in maintaining resistance to cutaneous candidiasis.

Oral thrush was first described at the time of Hippocrates and Galen. Berg in 1841 established the fungal cause of thrush in newborns (Figure 3-13). *Candida* species form smooth, creamy white patches on the tongue and soft or hard palate. The patches are a pseudomembrane consisting of *Candida,* epithelial cells, leukocytes, bacteria, and focal debris. The patches are removable by scraping and leaving a raw, bleeding, and painful surface. Patients with chronic mucocutaneous candidiasis commonly have a dysfunction of the lymphocytic system that places the patient at risk of *Candida* infection. Patients with AIDS are also highly susceptible to oral thrush because of lymphopenia and the role of T helper cells, which are essential for regulation of phagocytosis.[37] Other risk factors are diabetes, steroid use, antibiotic use, neutropenia, and other immunosuppressive conditions.

Other oral manifestations of *Candida* infection are the following:
- *Angular cheilitis,* which represents a nonspecific inflammatory reaction to the corners of the mouth because of candida (Figure 3-14).
- *Candida leukoplakia,* which consists of a raised firm white plaque of the oral mucosa that cannot be removed

TABLE 3-1	Summary of Common Fungal Infections Involving the Head and Neck			
Fungal	**Type**	**Infection Site**	**Diagnosis**	**Treatment**
Candida	Budding yeast	Pseudomembranous angular cheilitis Leukoplakia Atrophic candidiasis	KOH, routine culture	Topical, systemic azole
Histoplasma capsulatum	Yeast	Ulcerative lesions on the tongue	GMS stain on biopsy, histoplasma antigen	Itraconazole, IV amphotericin
Cryptococcus neoformans	Yeast	Gingivitis Sinusitis Salivary gland	GMS stain on biopsy, culture, cryptococcal antigen	Fluconazole, IV amphotericin ± flucytosine
Coccidioides immitis	Yeast	Cervical lymphadenopathy Nodular lesion of the nasolabial fold	GMS stain of tissue, anticoccidioidal antibodies	Self-limited, fluconazole, IV amphotericin
Paracoccidioides brasiliensis	Yeast	Ulcerative/granulomatous lesions of the mouth, larynx, and pharynx	GMS stain of tissue	Sulfonamide, IV amphotericin, ketoconazole, itraconazole, posaconazole
Penicillium marneffei	Yeast	Ulcerative or nodular lesions on skin, larynx, and pharynx	Identification of organism	IV amphotericin ± flucytosine
Fusarium species	Yeast	Sinusitis	GMS stain of tissue, culture of tissue	IV amphotericin, caspofungin, voriconazole, posaconazole
Aspergillus species	Mold	Allergic sinusitis Fungus ball Mycetoma Invasive sinusitis Otitis Oral	GMS stain of tissue, culture of tissue	Supportive, surgery, voriconazole, IV amphotericin, echinocandin
Mucor species	Mold	Rhinocerebral Oral	GMS stain of tissue, culture of tissue	Surgery, IV amphotericin, posaconazole

GMS, Gomori methenamine silver; *IV*, intravenous; *KOH*, potassium hydroxide.

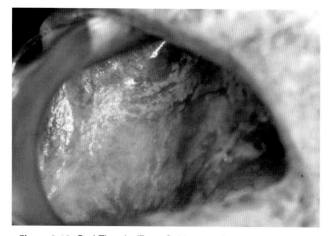

• **Figure 3-13** Oral Thrush. (From Goldman L, Schafer AI. *Goldman's Cecil Medicine.* 24th ed. Philadelphia: Saunders; 2012.)

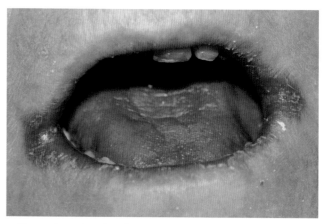

• **Figure 3-14** Angular Cheilitis. (From Neville BW, Damm DD, Allen CM, et al. *Oral and Maxillofacial Pathology.* 4th ed. St Louis: Saunders; 2016.)

by scraping, is usually found on the side of the tongue, and can affect the cheeks (Figure 3-15).
- *Acute atrophic candidiasis, chronic atrophic candidiasis,* or *"denture sore mouth,"* which is described as erythematous tongue, or thinning of the mucous membrane.

Diagnosis

The yeast form, pseudohyphae, and hyphae stain positive with a Gram stain. Identification is also facilitated by 10% potassium hydroxide. *Candida* grows well in routine blood culture bottles and on agar plates, and they do not require special fungal media for cultivation (Figure 3-16).

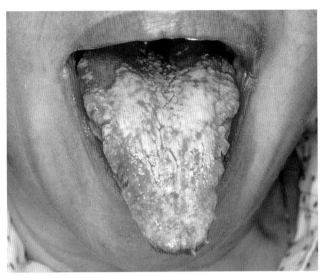

• **Figure 3-15** Candidal Leukoplakia. (From Ibsen O, Phelan J. *Oral Pathology for the Dental Hygienist.* 6th ed. St Louis: Saunders; 2014.)

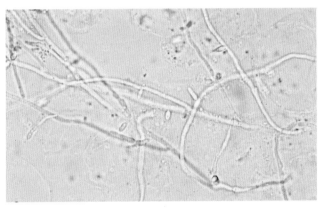

• **Figure 3-16** *Candida* in Yeast Form and Pseudohyphae. (From Zitelli BJ, McIntire SC, Nowalk AJ. *Zitelli and Davis' Atlas of Pediatric Physical Diagnosis.* 6th ed. Philadelphia: Saunders; 2012.)

Treatment

The treatment of oral candidiasis includes topical agents, such as mycostatin or clotrimazole, or systemic azole agents, such as fluconazole, ketoconazole, or itraconazole. If there is no response to treatment in an immunocompromised host, the possibility of *Candida glabrata* infection should be considered because it may not be susceptible to fluconazole. Echinocandin given intravenously may be considered for such cases. Currently there are two FDA-approved treatments for recurrent fluconazole-resistant *Candida* (i.e., ibrexafungerp and oteseconazole), but both are restricted to vulvovaginal candidiasis.[38]

Histoplasma capsulatum

Histoplasma capsulatum is a dimorphic fungus, first identified by Darling in 1905 in Panama.[39] It exists as a mold in soil and as a yeast in humans (Figure 3-17). It causes infections commonly in the Midwestern and Southeastern United States, specifically from the Ohio and Mississippi rivers into the Canadian provinces of Québec and Ontario.

Histoplasmosis is acquired by inhalation of mycelial fragments and microconidia from the soil. It remains a frequent cause of opportunistic infection in immunocompromised hosts.

Clinical Manifestations

Most oral lesions are ulcerative (Figure 3-18) or nodular and can involve the skin, tongue, palate, or buccal mucosa. They can mimic squamous oral cancer. Disseminated disease can occur in immunocompromised hosts.

Diagnosis

The diagnosis of histoplasmosis requires isolation of the organism from body fluid or tissue. The antigen detection and PCR analysis assay, which detects polysaccharide antigen in the serum or the urine by enzyme-linked immunosorbent assay, are the mainstays of the diagnosis of histoplasmosis.

Histopathology demonstrates macrophages with budding yeast organisms. Special stains include periodic acid–Schiff stain, Gomori methenamine silver (GMS) stain, or Grocott's silver stain.

Treatment

Infections caused by *Histoplasma capsulatum* are usually self-limited and do not require treatment. Individuals with mild to moderate symptoms lasting longer than 4 weeks can be offered itraconazole. Recommended treatment for disseminated/severe histoplasmosis is liposomal amphotericin-B for 1 to 2 weeks, followed by itraconazole for total of at least 12 weeks. Adjunctive corticosteroids can be considered in cases of severe respiratory disease.[40]

Cryptococcus neoformans

Cryptococcus neoformans is an encapsulated oval yeast (4 to 6 μm) surrounded by a capsule that can measure up to 30 μm. It is a common opportunistic pathogen worldwide in the immunosuppressed host. *C. neoformans* serotype A is the most common serotype infecting patients with AIDS. It is mainly found in the southwest United States and Central and South America. The mode of transmission is from inhalation of the yeast from the environment, mainly from soil contaminated by guano from birds; it is also associated with trees and rotting wood.

Clinical Manifestations

Cryptococcus species can rarely cause gingivitis, sinusitis, and salivary gland enlargement. The oral lesions are craterlike, nonhealing ulcers that are tender to palpation or are friable plaques.

Diagnosis

C. neoformans appears as spherical budding yeast and the organism capsule on India ink stain (Figure 3-19). It grows on laboratory agar media within 48 to 72 hours. Cryptococcal antigen in the serum is elevated in cases of disseminated infection. Despite localized presentation of cryptococcosis, cryptococcal meningitis should be ruled out

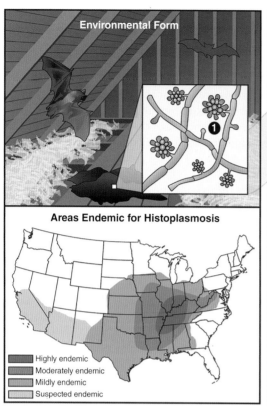
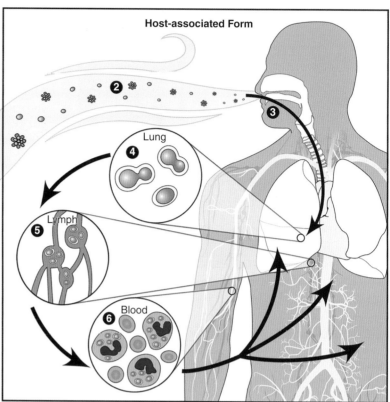
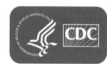

In the environment, *Histoplasm capsulatum* exists as a mold (1) with aerial hyphae. The hyphae produce macroconidia and microconidia (2) spores that are aerosolized and dispersed. Microconidia are inhaled into the lungs by a susceptible host (3). The warmer temperature inside the host signals a transformation to an oval, budding yeast (4). The yeast are phagocytized by immune cells and transported to regional lymph nodes (5). From there they travel in the blood to other parts of the body (6).

• **Figure 3-17** Biology of Histoplasmosis. (From Centers for Disease Control and Prevention, Atlanta, Ga.)

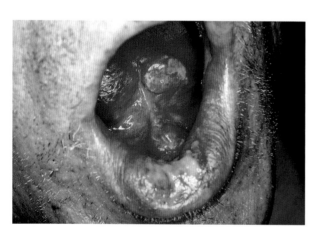

• **Figure 3-18** Oral Lesions of Histoplasmosis. (From Regezi JA, Sciubba JJ, Jordan RCK. *Oral Pathology: Clinical Pathologic Correlations*. 6th ed. St Louis: Saunders; 2012.)

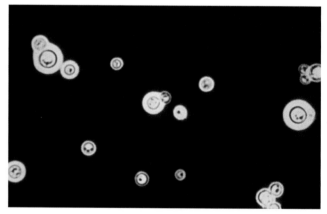

• **Figure 3-19** India Ink Demonstrating *Cryptococcus neoformans*. (From Murray P. *Medical Microbiology.* 5th ed. Philadelphia: Mosby; 2005.)

by obtaining cerebrospinal fluid for fungal culture or cryptococcal antigen testing.

Treatment

Localized disease can be treated with fluconazole. Disseminated disease should be treated with amphotericin B with or without flucytosine.

Coccidioides immitis

Coccidioides immitis is endemic to the soils of certain regions of the western United States. It is a dimorphic fungus that appears as either a mycelium or a spherule.[41] Both forms of growth are asexual. Infection occurs after inhalation of arthroconidia (Figure 3-20).

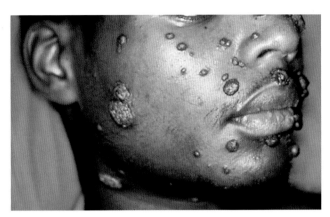

• **Figure 3-20** Skin Lesions of Coccidiomycosis. (From Fitzpatrick JE. *Dermatology Secrets plus.* 4th ed. Philadelphia: Mosby; 2011. Courtesy James E. Fitzpatrick.)

Clinical Manifestations

Extrapulmonary dissemination occurs in immunocompromised patients by hematogenous spread and can result in cervical lymphadenopathy or ulcerative nodular skin lesions of the face with predilection to the nasolabial fold.[42]

Diagnosis

Identifying spherules in clinical specimen (Figure 3-21) or detecting serum-specific anticoccidioidal antibodies supports the diagnosis of coccidioidomycosis.

Treatment

The disease is usually self-limited. Treatment option includes fluconazole or amphotericin B.

Paracoccidioides brasiliensis

Paracoccidioidomycosis is the most important endemic fungal disease; it is reported only in Latin America from Mexico to Argentina. Brazil constitutes the center of the endemic area. *Paracoccidioides brasiliensis* is a thermally dimorphic fungus. It appears as an oval-to-round yeast with a size of 4 to 40 μm surrounded by a translucent double-contoured cell wall resembling a mariner's wheel.

Clinical Manifestations

Paracoccidioidomycosis is a polymorphic, progressive disease. Extrapulmonary manifestations involve the skin, mucosa, and lymph nodes (mainly cervical nodes). Painful, mulberry-like ulcerations and granulomatous lesions with raised border are seen in the mouth, lips, gingiva, tongue, and palate. On occasion, lesions can be seen in the nose (Figure 3-22), larynx, and pharynx.[43,44]

Diagnosis

Direct microscopy of specimen can identify the fungus on a wet mount. GMS stain is used to identify fungus on a tissue biopsy specimen (Figure 3-23). PCR also can be used on both exudate and tissue. Serology detection is helpful for diagnosis and follow-up. Skin testing has not been clinically reliable for diagnosis.

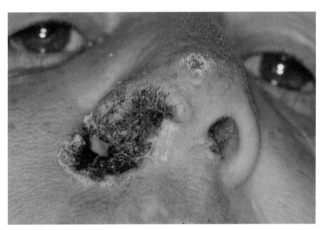

• **Figure 3-22** Paracoccidioidomycosis Involving the Nose. (From Marques SA. Paracoccidioidomycosis. *Clin Dermatol.* 2012;30[6]: 610-615.)

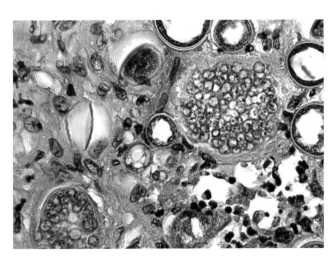

• **Figure 3-21** Spherules With Thick Capsule and Filled With Endospores of *Coccidioides* Species. Demonstrated by hematoxylin-eosin stain seen in tissue. (From Kradin RL. *Diagnostic Pathology of Infectious Disease.* Philadelphia: Saunders; 2010.)

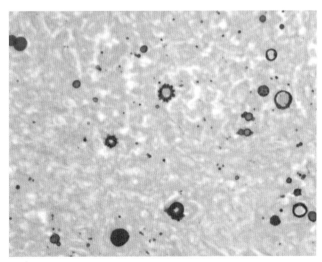

• **Figure 3-23** Paracoccidioides Seen in Tissue by Gomori Methenamine Silver Stain. (From Kradin RL. *Diagnostic Pathology of Infectious Disease.* Philadelphia: Saunders; 2010.)

Treatment

Treatment with sulfonamides, amphotericin B, or both is not always successful. Other treatment options include ketoconazole, itraconazole, or posaconazole.

Talaromyces marneffei

Talaromyces marneffei is a thermally dimorphic fungus that causes life-threatening disseminated infection. The rapid expansion of the AIDS epidemic in Thailand has led to a marked increase in the rate of talaromycosis but the disease has been described in both HIV-infected and uninfected individuals. The mode of transmission is inhalation of the conidia.

Clinical Manifestations

Skin lesions, such as papules, pustules, nodules, ulcers, or abscess, can occur on the face (Figure 3-24). In patients with AIDS, lesions also can be seen on the palate and pharynx. It can be associated with purulent discharge, granuloma, or necrosis.

Diagnosis

Clinical suspicion is raised based on presentation and epidemiologic exposure. The diagnosis is based on identification of the organism on smear, histopathology, or culture of tissue (Figure 3-25). Microscopic examination reveals yeast forms measuring 2 to 3 × 2 to 6 μm, both within phagocyte and extracellular. The extracellular forms may appear "sausage-like" consisting of three cells divided by two transverse septa.

Treatment

The recommended treatment is intravenous amphotericin B, with or without flucytosine, followed by itraconazole.[45]

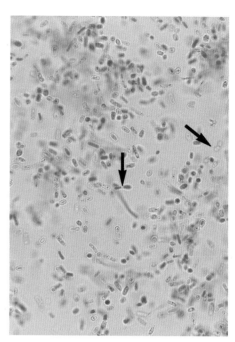

• **Figure 3-25** *Penicillium marneffei* in Yeast Form by Gomori Methenamine Silver Stain. (From Tille P. *Bailey and Scott's Diagnostic Microbiology.* 13th ed. St Louis: Mosby; 2014.)

Molds

Fusarium Species

Fusarium species is common in soil. The modes of entry are inhalation, ingestion, or following a traumatic inoculation of the organism. Fusariosis occurs mostly in immunocompromised hosts, particularly bone marrow transplant patients or those with prolonged neutropenia, and it is associated with a high mortality rate. Sinusitis can precede dissemination.[46]

Diagnosis

The diagnosis is made by either blood or tissue culture growth or demonstration of characteristic fungal hyphae in tissue. Histopathologic examination should demonstrate septated hyphae of *Fusarium* species with GMS stain or periodic acid–Schiff stains (Figure 3-26).

Treatment

Treatment options include amphotericin B, caspofungin, voriconazole, or posaconazole. Susceptibility testing may assist in choice of appropriate antifungal therapy.

Aspergillus Species

The genus *Aspergillus* was first recognized in 1729 by Micheli, who associated the shape of the sporulating head of the mold with an aspergillum used to sprinkle holy water. *Aspergillus* species are widespread in nature and ubiquitous, found in soil, in decaying vegetation, in the air, and in the water supply. There are more than 180 *Aspergillus* species,

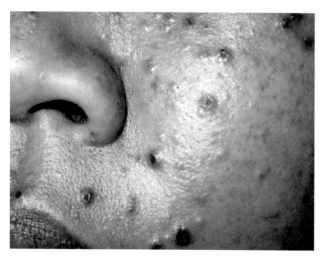

• **Figure 3-24** Skin Lesions on the Face Caused by *Penicillium marneffei.* (From Guerrant RL, Walker DH, Weller PF. *Tropical Infectious Diseases.* 3rd ed. Edinburgh: Saunders; 2011.)

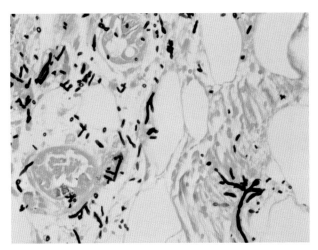

• **Figure 3-26** *Fusarium* Species Shown by Gomori Methenamine Silver Stain *(arrows)*. (From Kradin RL. *Diagnostic Pathology of Infectious Disease.* Philadelphia: Saunders; 2010. Courtesy Mirian Sotto, Department of Dermatology, Hospital das Clinicas, University of São Paulo, São Paulo, Brazil.)

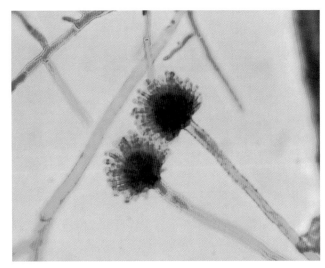

• **Figure 3-27** Conidial Head of *Aspergillus fumigatus* by Gomori Methenamine Silver Stain. (From Murray PR. *Medical Microbiology.* 7th ed. Philadelphia: Saunders; 2013.)

most of which reproduce asexually. The most common species causing invasive disease are *Aspergillus fumigatus* (66%). *Aspergillus flavus* (14%), *Aspergillus terreus* (5%), and *Aspergillus niger* (5%) are less common.[47] The usual route of infection for invasive aspergillosis is inhalation of *Aspergillus conidia.* On occasion, infection follows local tissue invasion after surgery or contaminated devices.[48]

Clinical Manifestations

The variety of clinical syndromes associated with aspergillosis range from colonization, to allergic response to the fungus, to invasive disease.

Aspergillus species can be a colonizer of the sinuses and the ear canal. *Aspergillus* species occasionally cause allergic fungal sinusitis in patients with chronic allergic sinusitis and nasal polyps. In all mycetoma cases, the active agent was an *Aspergillus* organism.[49]

Aspergillus species also can be accompanied by fungus ball of the sinuses without tissue invasion. Maxillary sinuses are the most involved in sinus aspergilloma because of *A. fumigatus* or *A. flavus.*[50]

Otomycosis is a condition of otitis externa with evidence of mold growth clinically. It is usually caused by *A. niger* forming black tuft or *A. fumigatus* with a greenish mold.[51]

Prolonged and profound neutropenia, solid organ or bone marrow transplant, and steroid and tumor necrosis factor-α medications increase the risk for invasive aspergillosis.[52] It commonly manifests as acute invasive rhinosinusitis. The presence of epistaxis and an ulcer or eschar should be the clue to invasive fungal disease. The infection can spread to the paranasal sinuses, palate, orbit, or brain with a high mortality rate.

Other presentations can manifest as an oral aspergillosis after an endodontic procedure, especially in the maxillary segment. It manifests as swelling, pain, and violaceous discoloration of the oral mucosa that can progress to a necrotic ulcer.

Diagnosis

Aspergillus species are easily cultured. A distinguishing characteristic is their ability to grow at 37°C. Most strains of *A. fumigatus* grow at a temperature of 45°C and above, which can be used to identify the species.

A. fumigatus hyphae are hyaline, septated, and usually branched at an acute angle. The conidial head (Figure 3-27) is columnar with conidiophores that are smooth-walled and uncolored, or darkened in the upper portion near the vesicle. Conidia can appear smooth to rough, measuring 2 to 3.5 μm in diameter.

Computed tomographic (CT) scanning of the sinuses can be used to confirm a fungus ball (Figure 3-28) and assess the extent of the infection in invasive disease. Demonstration of characteristic fungal hyphae on histopathologic examination confirms the diagnosis.

Treatment

The treatment consists of voriconazole, isavuconazole, or amphotericin B. Surgical debridement might be required.

Mucorales

The Mucorales order is a subset of the Zygomycetes (formerly Phycomycetes) class and contains the order Mucorales, the family Mucoraceae, and the genera *Absidia, Mucor,* and *Rhizopus.*[53] Mucormycosis refers to infection with fungi in the order of Mucorales. *Rhizopus* species are the most common causative organisms (Figure 3-29).

Clinical Manifestations

Rhinocerebral manifestation is the most common presentation and can manifest in two distinct patterns: a rapidly

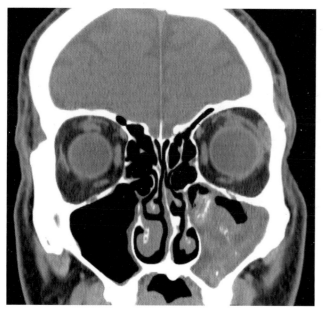

• **Figure 3-28** Fungus Ball on Computed Tomographic Scan of the Sinuses. (From Flint PW, Haughey BH, Robbins KT, et al. *Cummings Otolaryngology: Head and Neck Surgery.* 6th ed. Philadelphia: Saunders; 2015.)

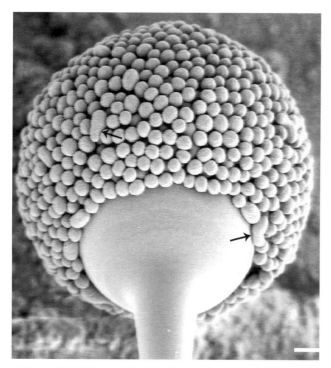

• **Figure 3-29** *Rhizopus* Species Sporangiospores *(arrow).* (From Jennessen J, Schnürer J, Olsson J, et al. Morphological characteristics of sporangiospores of the tempe fungus *Rhizopus oligosporus* differentiate it from other taxa of the *R. microsporus* group. *Mycol Res.* 2008;112[Pt 5]:547-563.)

progressive form with a high mortality rate[54,55] or the rarer slowly progressive chronic form of the disease.

Acute rhinocerebral mucormycosis (ARM) manifests in a rapidly fulminant manner with fever, headache, lethargy, mucosal necrosis, and ophthalmologic findings such as

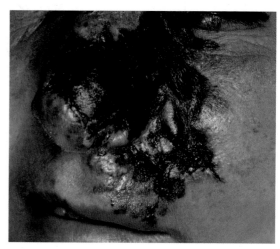

• **Figure 3-30** Fungal Sinusitis Caused by *Mucor* Species. (From Requena L, Sitthinamsuwan P, Santonia C, et al. Cutaneous and mucosal mucormycosis mimicking pancreatic panniculitis and gouty panniculitis. *J Am Acad Dermatol.* 2011;66:975-984.)

proptosis, ptosis, ophthalmoplegia, and visual changes (Figure 3-30). Cranial nerve involvement is often present. Maxillary sinusitis and oral involvement have been described. Oral lesions are ulcerative with a black necrotic surface. Massive tissue destruction can occur if there is a delay in treatment. ARM usually develops in critically ill patients with diabetic ketoacidosis or immunodeficiency. The incidence of ARM has risen in the past several decades, possibly because of the increased use of steroids, cytotoxic drugs, and other immunosuppressive medical therapies (e.g., bone marrow transplant) or simply because of increased recognition of the disease. The prognosis of the disease has not been thoroughly evaluated in the relevant literature, overshadowed by the more aggressive acute form of the disease. The largest series available reports an overall survival rate of 83%.[56,57]

Chronic rhinocerebral mucormycosis is a rare representation of the mucormycoses group of infections. The disease can manifest with atypical symptoms that can result in delayed diagnosis. It should be considered in individuals with predisposing conditions listed in the previous paragraph.

Diagnosis

Histopathologic finding of broad nonseptate hyphae confirms the clinical diagnosis (Figure 3-31).[58]

Treatment

The treatment involves surgical debridement and intravenous amphotericin B followed by oral posaconazole or isavuconazole.[55]

Parasitic Infections

Myiasis

Myiasis is an infestation of fly larvae that grows inside the host while feeding on its tissue. The most common human

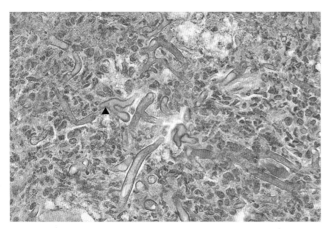

• **Figure 3-31** Broad, Nonseptate Hyphae *(arrow)* Seen on Tissue is Characteristic of *Mucor* Species. (From Klatt EC. *Robbins and Cotran Atlas of Pathology.* 3rd ed. Philadelphia: Saunders; 2015.)

botfly is *Dermatobia hominis.* The infection most commonly occurs in tropical areas like Mexico, South America, Central America, and the Caribbean.

Eggs are laid in the soil or on sand floors. When the larvae hatch at night, they seek a blood meal from sleeping human hosts (Figure 3-32).[59] The bite may be slightly painful and can cause local edema. Cutaneous myiasis is the most common, but nasopharyngeal myiasis causing infestation of the nose, mouth, sinuses, and ear has been reported (Figure 3-33). Treatment consists of manual or surgical removal of the larvae.

Encephalitozoon hellem

Encephalitozoon hellem is a microsporidium and intracellular parasite mainly in mammals and birds. It has been associated with sinusitis and disseminated disease, specifically in an immunocompromised host and in patients with AIDS.

Clinical Manifestations

E. hellem can cause rhinitis, sinusitis, and nasal polyposis.

Diagnosis

Visualization of the organism is accomplished using Chromotrope 2R, Giemsa, Brow-Hopps Gram stain, acid-fast staining, in aspirate, with epithelial cells on tissue biopsy.

Treatment

Albendazole and fumagillin can be effective treatment options.

Trypanosoma cruzi

Trypanosoma cruzi is a protozoan flagellate that causes the American trypanosomiasis or Chagas disease. It is transmitted by various species of bloodsucking insects or kissing bugs.[60] *T. cruzi* are found in the southern Americas from the southern half of the United States to Argentina (Figure 3-34).

Illness occurs 1 week after skin infiltration. An indurated lesion of the skin (called a *chagoma*) occurs with erythema

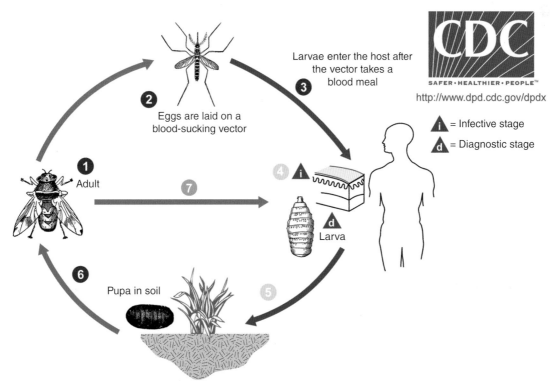

• **Figure 3-32** Biology of Myiasis. (Courtesy Centers for Disease Control and Prevention, Atlanta, Ga.)

and swelling accompanied by local lymph node involvement. Both hypersalivation and salivary gland hypertrophy have been described.

Diagnosis

Serologic tests for *T. cruzi* infection include enzyme-linked immunosorbent assay (ELISA), immunoblot, and

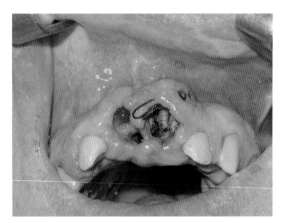

• **Figure 3-33** Myiasis Involving the Oral Cavity. (From Gealh WC, Ferreira GM, Farah GJ, et al. Treatment of oral myiasis caused by *Cochliomyia hominivorax*: two cases treated with ivermectin. *Br J Oral Maxillofac Surg.* 2009;47:23-26.)

immunofluorescent assay. Patient with suspected chronic *T. cruzi* infection should undergo two different serologic tests. If results are discordant, further testing with PCR or blood culture can be pursued. For acute infection, diagnosis can be made by observation of parasites in blood smear by microscopic inspection. Serologic findings can be obtained in 8 months in suspected cases of congenital infection to confirm seroconversion.[61]

Treatment

Treatment is recommended by the CDC for people with acute infection, infants with congenital infection, and for those with immunocompromising condition. Certain patients with chronic infection may benefit from treatment. Benznidazole is approved by the FDA for treatment of Chagas disease in pediatric patients aged 2 to 12 years of age.

Toxoplasma gondii

Toxoplasma gondii is an intracellular protozoan parasite that can infect most warm-blooded animals, including humans. It is estimated that 22.5% of the U.S. population 12 years and older are infected with *T. gondii*. Infection can occur through ingestion of undercooked

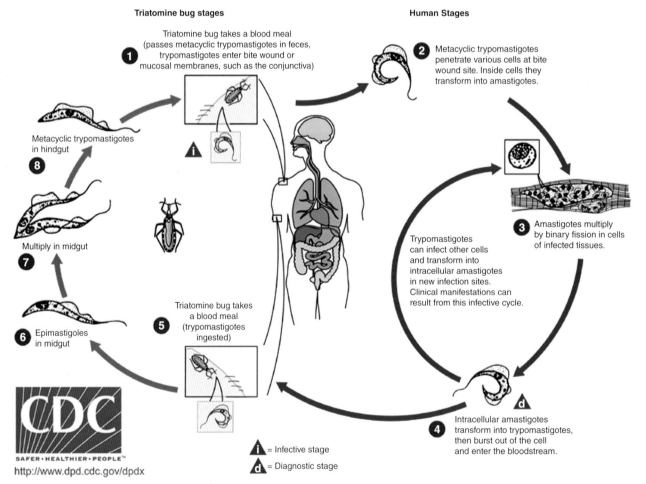

• **Figure 3-34** Life Cycle of *Trypanosoma cruzi*. (Courtesy Centers for Disease Control and Prevention, Atlanta, Ga.)

or contaminated meat with tissue cysts, consumption of food or water contaminated with cat feces, mother to child (congenital), and rarely by organ transplant or blood transfusion. Domestic cats belonging to the family Felidae are considered definitive hosts for toxoplasma. The life cycle of toxoplasma is illustrated in Figure 3-35.[62]

Clinical Presentation

Acute infection in 80 to 90% of immunocompetent individuals is usually asymptomatic.[63] When symptomatic, the most common manifestation is bilateral, symmetric, nontender, and nonfluctuant cervical lymphadenopathy, but generalized lymphadenopathy can occur. Fever, chills, sweats, myalgias, pharyngitis, and diffuse maculopapular rash may be present.

Chorioretinitis can occur congenitally or postnatally (Figure 3-36). Symptoms include eye pain, photophobia, tearing, and blurred vision.

Diagnosis

The diagnosis can be made by direct detection of the parasite or serologic testing.[64] The demonstration of positive IgM and negative IgG during acute infection and both positive IgM and IgG 2 weeks later makes diagnosis more likely. IgG antibody avidity testing can help to determine whether infection is acute or chronic.[65] IgG antibody early during infection binds to antigen less avidly compared with antibodies of prior infection.

Diagnosis of chorioretinitis involves demonstration of characteristic eye lesions and serologic testing.

Treatment

Acute infection is often self-limited and does not require treatment unless symptoms are severe. First-line regimens include pyrimethamine plus sulfadiazine and pyrimethamine plus clindamycin. Leucovorin (folinic acid) should be given when taking pyrimethamine.

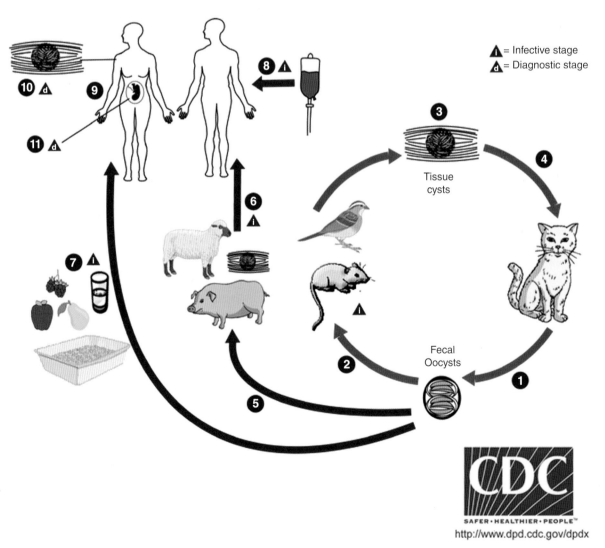

• **Figure 3-35** Life Cycle of *Toxoplasmosis* Species. (From Centers for Disease Control and Prevention, Atlanta, Ga.)

For chorioretinitis, an ophthalmologist should be involved with the treatment. Treatment duration is 4 to 6 weeks or longer depending on the patient's response.

Leishmania

Leishmaniasis is a tropical disease caused by a heterogeneous group of protozoa belonging to the genus *Leishmania,*

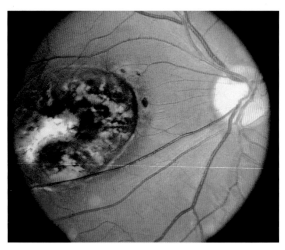

• **Figure 3-36** Toxoplasmic Chorioretinitis. (From Swartz MH. *Textbook of Physical Diagnosis.* 7th ed. Philadelphia: Saunders; 2014.)

is transmitted by sand fly vector, and is found on every continent except for Australia and Antarctica. The life cycle of *Leishmania* species is illustrated in Figure 3-37.[66]

Clinical Manifestations

In the Old World (Eastern Hemisphere), leishmaniasis is found in parts of Asia, the Middle East, Africa, and southern Europe. In the New World (Western Hemisphere), it is found in parts of Mexico, Central America, and South America except Chile and Uruguay. It can be asymptomatic or have cutaneous, mucocutaneous, or visceral involvement depending on the species involved. Discussion in this chapter will be limited to cutaneous manifestation and its complications relevant to head and neck infection.

Cutaneous leishmaniasis can have a range of clinical manifestations depending on the parasite virulence and host immune response. Manifestations include localized cutaneous leishmaniasis, diffuse cutaneous leishmaniasis, or mucosal leishmaniasis.

Localized cutaneous leishmaniasis occurs on exposed areas of the skin, including the face. It begins as a pink-colored papule that enlarges into a nodule or plaque-like lesion and progresses to a painless ulcer with an indurated border. Manifestations can differ depending on the species, as listed in Table 3-2.

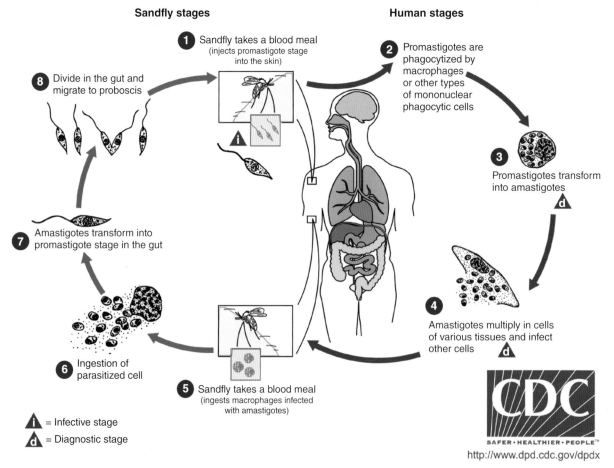

• **Figure 3-37** Life Cycle of *Leishmania* Species. (Courtesy Centers for Disease Control and Prevention, Atlanta, Ga.)

Diffuse cutaneous leishmaniasis caused by *L. aethiopica,* *L. mexicana,* and *L. amazonensis* is uncommon. This infection occurs mainly in individuals with cell-mediated immune deficiency (e.g., AIDS). The disease begins as a nonulcerating localized lesion (nodule or plaque) and then disseminates into other skin areas.

Mucosal leishmaniasis is caused primarily by the *Viannia* subgenus including *L. (Viannia) braziliensis, L. (Viannia) guyanensis,* and *L. (Viannia) panamensis.* Mucosal involvement occurs from hematogenous or lymphatic spread from cutaneous lesions and can manifest any time from a few months to decades after infection. Mucosal destruction and erosion usually involve the nose, mouth, or nasal septum. Cheek, palate, pharynx, epiglottis, larynx, and trachea also can be affected. Facial or upper airway destruction can lead to aspiration, respiratory compromise, even death. Vocal cord and pharyngeal examination is required if the patient is infected with New World cutaneous leishmaniasis or if symptoms suggestive of nasal, oral, or hypopharyngeal involvement are present.[67-69]

Diagnosis

The diagnosis of cutaneous leishmaniasis should be considered in any patient with skin lesions with exposure to an endemic area. The definitive diagnosis involves visualization of parasite in the specimen, positive culture, or molecular analysis by PCR. A reference laboratory, such as the CDC, should be contacted to obtain appropriate instructions before biopsy and handling of the specimen.

Treatment

The treatment of cutaneous leishmaniasis requires expert consultation with an infectious disease specialist. Treatment should be individualized because certain regimens can be effective only against particular *Leishmania* species. Typical agents that have been used in the United States for treatment include pentavalent antimonial compound, liposomal amphotericin, and miltefosine.[66] Amphotericin B deoxycholate, pentamidine, and azoles (ketoconazole, itraconazole, fluconazole) have been used in select cases of leishmaniasis (Figures 3-38 and 3-39).

Echinococcus granulosus

Echinococcus granulosus is a tapeworm (Figure 3-40) that is endemic in Mediterranean countries, South America, Australia, New Zealand, and East Africa. Infections in humans occur after direct contact with infected dogs or ingestion of food contaminated by stool containing ova. The life cycle is illustrated in Figure 3-41.[70]

Hydatid cyst in the neck region has been reported but is rare.[71] Cysts are typically slow growing, fluctuant, and painless. The diagnosis of hydatid cyst depends on history of exposure, clinical presentation, laboratory evaluation, and radiographic findings. The value of serologic testing is controversial because of false-positive and false-negative results. Ultrasonography is considered the most sensitive

TABLE 3-2	Summary of Leishmania Species With Localized Cutaneous Leishmaniasis	
Subgenus	Complex	Cutaneous Manifestation
Old World (Eastern Hemisphere)		
Leishmania species	*L.L. major* (moist or rural oriental sore)	Multiple lesions Has thick crust Size can expand to ≥6 cm in diameter Resolve within 2-4 mo[71]
	L.L. tropica (dry or urban oriental sore)	Few lesions typically 1-2 cm, but facial lesions can be larger Dry and crusted May persist from 6-15 mo[72]
	L.L. aethiopica	Solitary lesion with or without satellite papules May involve mucocutaneous margins excluding oral or nasal mucosa
	L.L. infantum-chagasi	Slow-growing nodules May or may not have visceral involvement
New World		
Leishmania spp.	*L.L. mexicana* (Chiclero ulcer)	Chronic small ulcers Limited to one or few lesions Spontaneously heal ~14 wk[73]
Viannia spp.	*L.V. braziliensis*	Multiple ulcers or nodules Lymphocutaneous involvement Fever, malaise, or lymphadenopathy may be present prior to skin lesion[74] Can last 6-12 mo May be associated with mucosal leishmaniasis

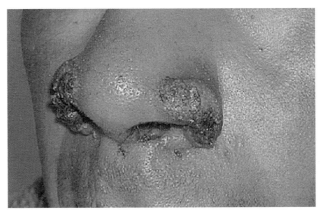

• **Figure 3-38** Mucosal Leishmaniasis Affecting the Nares. (From Virgilio GR, Hale BR. A case of mucocutaneous leishmaniasis. *Otolaryngol Head Neck Surg.* 2005;132:800-801.)

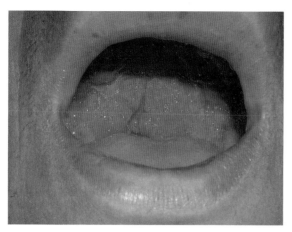

• **Figure 3-39** Mucosal Leishmaniasis Involving the Palate. (From Virgilio GR, Hale BR. A case of mucocutaneous leishmaniasis. *Otolaryngol Head Neck Surg.* 2005;132:800-801.)

radiographic modality in detecting membrane, septa, and hydatid sand within the cyst. Other modalities also include CT and magnetic resonance imaging. Evaluation for simultaneous extracervical involvement should be performed. Fine-needle aspiration should be considered carefully because of the risk of cyst content spillage, which can induce anaphylactic reaction and dissemination. Treatment of hydatid cyst involves surgical removal with the goal of total removal of cyst. More recently, puncture, aspiration, injection of protoscolicidal agent (95% ethanol or hypertonic saline), and reaspiration have been used more increasingly as the preferred treatment.[72] Medical management with albendazole should be offered in only select cases when surgery is not an option. Treatment duration is uncertain.

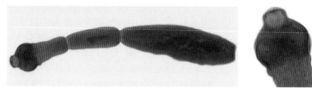

• **Figure 3-40** *Echinococcus granulosus.* (Courtesy Centers for Disease Control and Prevention, Atlanta, Ga.)

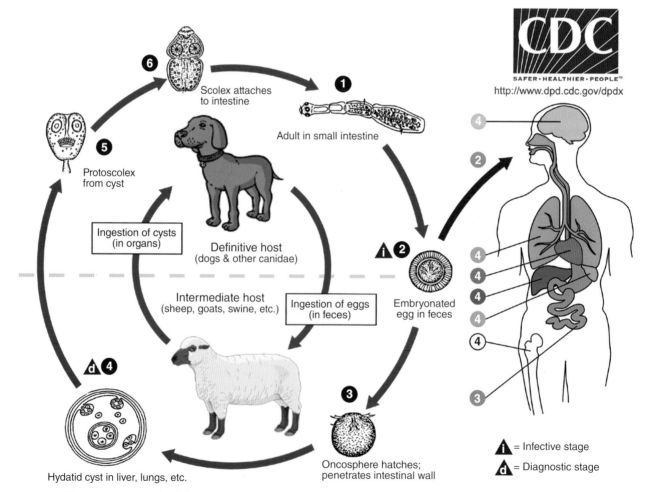

• **Figure 3-41** Life Cycle of *Echinococcus* Species. (Courtesy Centers for Disease Control and Prevention, Atlanta, Ga.)

References

1. Turbeville SD, Cowan LD, Greenfield RA. Infectious disease outbreaks in competitive sports: a review of the literature. *Am J Sports Med.* 2006;34:1860-1865.

2. Mandell GL, Bennett JE, Dolin R. *Mandell, Douglas, and Bennett's principles and practice of infectious diseases.* 8th ed. Philadelphia: Elsevier Saunders; 2014.

3. Wald A, Timmler B, Magaret A, et al. Effect of pritelivir compared with valacyclovir on genital HSV-2 shedding in patients with frequent recurrences: a randomized clinical trial. *JAMA.* 2016;316(23):2495-2503.

4. AiCuris Anti-infective Cures AG, Mespace, Inc. *Trial on Efficacy and Safety of Pritelivir Tablets for Treatment of Acyclovir-Resistant Mucocutaneous HSV (herpes simplex virus) Infections in Immunocompromised Subjects (PRIOH-1).* USA: NIH U.S. National Library of Medicine, Clinicaltrials.gov; 2017.

5. Cunningham AL, Lal H, Kovac M, et al. Efficacy of the herpes zoster subunit vaccine in adults 70 years of age or older. *N Engl J Med.* 2016;375:1019-1032.

6. Centers for Disease Control and Prevention. *Shingrix Recommendations.* Updated on January 24, 2022. Available at: https://www.cdc.gov/vaccines/vpd/shingles/hcp/shingrix/recommendations.html.

7. Staras SA, Dollard SC, Radford KW, et al. Seroprevalence of cytomegalovirus infection in the United States, 1988-1994. *Clin Infect Dis.* 2006;43:1143-1151.

8. Spector SA, Wong R, Hsia K, et al. Plasma cytomegalovirus (CMV) DNA load predicts CMV disease and survival in AIDS patients. *J Clin Invest.* 1998;101:497-502.

9. Avery RK, Alain S, Alexander BD, et al. Maribavir for refractory cytomegalovirus infections with or without resistance post-transplant: results from a phase 3 randomized clinical trial. *Clin Inf Dis.* 2022;75:690-701.

10. Andreoni M, Sarmati L, Nicastri E, et al. Primary human herpesvirus 8 infection in immunocompetent children. *JAMA.* 2002;287:1295-1300.

11. Beral V, Peterman TA, Berkelman RL, et al. Kaposi's sarcoma among persons with AIDS: a sexually transmitted infection? *Lancet.* 1990;335:123-128.

12. International Collaboration on HIV. Cancer: highly active antiretroviral therapy and incidence of cancer in human immunodeficiency virus-infected adults. *J Natl Cancer Inst.* 2000;92:1823-1830.

13. Centers for Disease Control and Prevention. Detection of acute HIV infection in two evaluations of a new HIV diagnostic testing algorithm—United States, 2011-2013. *MMWR Morb Mortal Wkly Rep.* 2013;62:489-494.

14. Miller CS, White DK, Royse DD. In situ hybridization analysis of human papillomavirus in orofacial lesions using a consensus biotinylated probe. *Am J Dermatopathol.* 1993;15:256-259.

15. Neville BW. *Oral and Maxillofacial Pathology.* 3rd ed. St Louis: Elsevier Saunders; 2008.

16. Derkay CS, Wiatrak B. Recurrent respiratory papillomatosis: a review. *Laryngoscope.* 2008;118:1236-1247.

17. Shah JP, Patel SG, Singh B, et al. *Jatin Shah's Head and Neck Surgery and Oncology.* 5th ed. Philadelphia: Elsevier Mosby; 2019.

18. Centers for Disease Control and Prevention. *HPV Vaccination Recommendation.* Updated on November 16, 2021. Available at: https://www.cdc.gov/vaccines/vpd/hpv/hcp/recommendations.html.

19. Puenpa J, Mauleekoonphairoj J, Linsuwanon P, et al. Prevalence and characterization of enterovirus infections among pediatric patients with hand foot mouth disease, herpangina and influenza like illness in Thailand. *PLoS One.* 2014:9:e98888.

20. Mirand A, Henquell C, Archimbaud C, et al. Outbreak of hand, foot and mouth disease/herpangina associated with coxsackievirus A6 and A10 infections in 2010, France: a large citywide, prospective observational study. *Clin Microbiol Infect.* 2012;18:E110-E118.

21. Hubiche T, Schuffenecker I, Boralevi F, et al. Dermatological spectrum of hand, foot and mouth disease from classical to generalized exanthema. *Pediatr Infect Dis J.* 2014;33:e92-e98.

22. Wu PC, Huang LM, Kao CL, et al. An outbreak of coxsackievirus A16 infection: comparison with other enteroviruses in a preschool in Taipei. *J Microbiol Immunol Infect.* 2010;43:271-277.

23. Chang LY, Lin TY, Huang YC, et al. Comparison of enterovirus 71 and coxsackie-virus A16 clinical illnesses during the Taiwan enterovirus epidemic, 1998. *Pediatr Infect Dis J.* 1999;8:1092-1096.

24. Jiang M, Wei D, Ou WL, et al. Autopsy findings in children with hand, foot, and mouth disease. *N Engl J Med.* 2012;367:91-92.

25. Hviid A, Rubin S, Muhlemann K. Mumps. *Lancet.* 2008;371:932-944.

26. Centers for Disease Control and Prevention. *Questions and Answers about Lab Testing.* Updated December 20, 2012. Available at: https://www.cdc.gov/mumps/lab/specimen-collect.html#:~:text=If%20it%20has%20been%20%3C3,serum%20specimen%20for%20IgM%20detection.

27. World Health Organization. *Monkeypox.* Updated May 19, 2022. Available at: https://www.who.int/news-room/fact-sheets/detail/monkeypox.

28. Centers for Disease Control and Prevention. *Clinical Recognition of Mpox.* Updated August 23, 2022. Available at: https://www.cdc.gov/poxvirus/monkeypox/clinicians/clinical-recognition.html#:~:text=Lesions%20often%20occur%20in%20the,appear%20on%20palms%20and%20soles.

29. Centers for Disease Control and Prevention. *Treatment Information for Healthcare Professionals.* Updated February 23, 2023. Available at: https://www.cdc.gov/poxvirus/monkeypox/clinicians/treatment.html#:~:text=Vaccinia%20Immune%20Globulin%20Intravenous%20(VIGIV),-VIGIV%20is%20licensed&text=Data%20are%20not%20available%20on%20the%20effectiveness%20of%20VIGIV%20in,benefit%20from%20treatment%20with%20VIGIV.

30. American Society of Transplantation. *Monkeypox FAQ for Transplant Community.* August 4, 2022. Available at: https://www.myast.org/monkeypox-faqs-transplant-community.

31. Centers for Disease Control and Prevention. *Monitoring Variant Proportions.* Updated February 23, 2023. Available at: https://covid.cdc.gov/covid-data-tracker/#variant-proportions.

32. Wiersinga WJ, Rhodes A, Cheng AC, et al. Pathophysiology, transmission, diagnosis, and treatment of coronavirus disease 2019 (COVID-19): a review. *JAMA.* 2020;324:782-793.

33. Carotti M, Salaffi F, Sarzi-Puttini P, et al. Chest CT features of coronavirus disease 2019 (COVID-19) pneumonia: key points for radiologists. *Radiol Med.* 2020;125:636-646.

34. Centers for Disease Control and Prevention. *Overview of Testing for SARS-CoV-2.* Updated on September 28, 2022. Available at: https://www.cdc.gov/coronavirus/2019-ncov/hcp/testing-overview.html.

35. National Institutes of Health. *COVID-19 Treatment Guidelines: Antiviral Agents, Including Antibody Products.* Last updated December 28, 2022. Available at: https://www.covid19treatment guidelines.nih.gov/therapies/antivirals-including-antibody-products/summary-recommendations/.

36. Centers for Disease Control and Prevention. *Interim Clinical Considerations for Use of COVID-19 Vaccines Currently Approved or Authorized in the United States.* Updated on January 23, 2023. Available at: https://www.cdc.gov/vaccines/covid-19/clinical-considerations/interim-considerations-us.html.

37. Lilic D, Gravenor I. Immunology of chronic mucocutaneous candidiasis. *J Clin Pathol.* 2001;54:81-83.

38. Sobel JD. New antifungals for vulvovaginal candidiasis: what is their role? *Clin Infect Dis.* 2023;76(5):783-785.

39. Darling S. A protozoal general infection producing pseudotubercles in the lung and focal necrosis in the liver, spleen and lymph nodes. *JAMA.* 1906;46:1283-1285.

40. Wheat LJ, Freifeld AG, Kleiman MB, et al. Clinical practice guidelines for the management of patients with histoplasmosis: 2007 update by the Infectious Diseases Society of America. *Clin Infect Dis.* 2007;45:807-825.

41. Abuodeh RO, Orbach MJ, Mandel MA, et al. Genetic transformation of Coccidioides immitis facilitated by Agrobacterium tumefaciens. *J Infect Dis.* 2000;181:2106-2110.

42. Galgiani JN. Coccidioidomycosis. *Western J Med.* 1993;159:153-171.

43. Bicalho RN, Santo MF, de Aguiar MC, et al. Oral paracoccidioidomycosis: a retrospective study of 62 Brazilian patients. *Oral Dis.* 2001;7:56-60.

44. Sant'Anna GD, Mauri M, Arrarte JL, et al. Laryngeal manifestations of paracoccidioidomycosis (South American blastomycosis). *Arch Otolaryngol Head Neck Surg.* 1999;125:1375-1378.

45. Sirisanthana T, Supparatpinyo K, Perriens J, et al. Amphotericin B and itraconazole for treatment of disseminated Penicillium marneffei infection in human immunodeficiency virus-infected patients. *Clin Infect Dis.* 1998;26:1107-1110.

46. Anaissie E, Kantarjian H, Ro J, et al. The emerging role of Fusarium infections in patients with cancer. *Medicine (Baltimore).* 1988;67:77-83.

47. Patterson TF, Kirkpatrick WR, White M, et al. Invasive aspergillosis: disease spectrum, treatment practices, and outcomes. I3 Aspergillus Study Group. *Medicine (Baltimore).* 2000;79:250-260.

48. Gettleman LK, Shetty AK, Prober CG. Posttraumatic invasive Aspergillus fumigatus wound infection. *Pediatr Infect Dis J.* 1999;18:745-747.

49. Thompson GR, Patterson TF. Fungal disease of the nose and paranasal sinuses. *J Allergy Clin Immunol.* 2012;129:321-326.

50. Ferguson BJ. Fungus balls of the paranasal sinuses. *Otolaryngol Clin North Am.* 2000;33:389-398.

51. Kaur R, Mittal N, Kakkar M, et al. Otomycosis: a clinicomycologic study. *Ear Nose Throat J.* 2000;79:606-609.

52. Marr KA, Carter RA, Crippa F, et al. Epidemiology and outcome of mould infections in hematopoietic stem cell transplant recipients. *Clin Infect Dis.* 2002;34:909-917.

53. Roden MM, Zaoutis TE, Buchanan WL, et al. Epidemiology and outcome of zygomycosis: a review of 929 reported cases. *Clin Infect Dis.* 2005;41:634-653.

54. Kwon-Chung KJ. Taxonomy of fungi causing mucormycosis and entomophthoramycosis (zygomycosis) and nomenclature of the disease: molecular mycologic perspectives. *Clin Infect Dis.* 2012;54(suppl 1):S8-S15.

55. Spellberg B, Edwards Jr J, Ibrahim A. Novel perspectives on mucormycosis: pathophysiology, presentation, and management. *Clin Microbiol Rev.* 2005;18:556-569.

56. Turner JH, Soudry E, Nayak JV, et al. Survival outcomes in acute invasive fungal sinusitis: a systematic review and quantitative synthesis of published evidence. *Laryngoscope.* 2013;123:1112-1118.

57. Teixeira CA, Medeiros PB, Leushner P, et al. Rhinocerebral mucormycosis: literature review apropos of a rare entity. *BMJ Case Rep.* 2013;2013:bcr2012008552.

58. Mohindra S, Mohindra S, Gupta R, et al. Rhinocerebral mucormycosis: the disease spectrum in 27 patients. *Mycoses.* 2007;50:290-296.

59. Centers for Disease Control and Prevention. *Parasites—Myiasis Biology.* Updated July 19, 2013. Available at: https://www.cdc.gov/parasites/myiasis/index.html.

60. Centers for Disease Control and Prevention. *Parasites—American Trypanosomiasis Biology.* Updated November 2, 2010. Available at: https://www.cdc.gov/dpdx/trypanosomiasisamerican/index.html.

61. Suarez C, Nolder D, Garcia-Mingo A, et al. Diagnosis and clinical management of Chagas disease: an increasing challenge in non-endemic areas. *Res Rep Trop Med.* 2022;13:25-40.

62. Centers for Disease Control and Prevention. *Parasites—Toxoplasmosis Biology.* Updated January 10, 2013. Available at: https://www.cdc.gov/dpdx/toxoplasmosis/index.html.

63. Remington JS. Toxoplasmosis in the adult. *Bull N Y Acad Med.* 1974;50:211-227.

64. Montoya JG, Liesenfeld O. Toxoplasmosis. *Lancet.* 2004;363:1965-1976.

65. Hedman K, Lappalainen M, Seppaia I, et al. Recent primary toxoplasma infection indicated by a low avidity of specific IgG. *J Infect Dis.* 1989;159:736-740.

66. Centers for Disease Control and Prevention. *Parasites—Leishmaniasis Biology.* Updated January 10, 2013. Available at: https://www.cdc.gov/dpdx/leishmaniasis/index.html.

67. Minodier P, Parola P. Cutaneous leishmaniasis treatment. *Travel Med Infect Dis.* 2007;5:150-158.

68. Herwaldt BL, Arana BA, Navin TR. The natural history of cutaneous leishmaniasis in Guatemala. *J Infect Dis.* 1992;165:518-527.

69. Barral A, Guerreiro J, Bomfim G, et al. Lymphadenopathy as the first sign of human cutaneous infection by Leishmania braziliensis. *Am J Trop Med Hyg.* 1995;53:256-259.

70. Centers for Disease Control and Prevention. *Parasites—Echinococcosis Biology.* Updated December 12, 2012. Available at: https://www.cdc.gov/dpdx/echinococcosis/index.html.

71. Ustundag E, Yayla B, Muezzinoglu B, et al. Pathology quiz case: cervical hydatid cyst. *Arch Otolaryngol Head Neck Surg.* 2006;132:695-696.

72. Moro P, Schantz PM. Echinococcosis: a review. *Int J Infect Dis.* 2009;13:125-133.

73. Aronson N, Herwaldt BL, Libman M, et al. Diagnosis and treatment of leishmaniasis: clinical practice guidelines by the Infectious Diseases Society of America (IDSA) and the American Society of Tropical Medicine and Hygiene (ASTMH). *Clin Infect Dis.* 2016;63(12):1539-1557. doi:10.1093/cid/ciw742.

74. Barral A, Guerreiro J, Bomfim G, Correia D, Barral-Netto M, Carvalho EM. Lymphadenopathy as the first sign of human cutaneous infection by Leishmania braziliensis. *Am J Trop Med Hyg.* 1995;53(3):256-259. doi:10.4269/ajtmh.1995.53.256.

4

Anatomy Relevant to Head, Neck, and Orofacial Infections

STEVAN H. THOMPSON

The anatomy of the head and neck is complex because it is composed of varied tissues and anatomic structures, as well as being contained in a compact space. This chapter is a succinct overview to be used in concert with the remaining chapters of this text to assist in the visualization of important aspects related to clinical assessment and surgical interventions concerning head, neck, and orofacial infections. In the 1930s, Grodinsky and Holyoke described the fascial layers and the concepts related to the spread of infection through contiguous potential anatomic spaces. Knowledge of these compartments and interfascial spaces is fundamental to understanding the spread of head and neck space infections. Because of the compactness of the anatomic structures, once an infection violates its initial immunologic barriers, the potential to involve a much larger number of important anatomic structures becomes imminent in the clinical timeline.

A thorough knowledge of the anatomy and the most common scenarios related to the varied infections that can occur allows the clinician to treat a patient more effectively. This knowledge, harnessed with the patient's clinical information and contemporary imaging modalities, has the ability to more clearly define the anatomic extent of a patient's pathologic condition.

Epithelial Surfaces

Scalp

The scalp is composed of five layers consisting of the overlying skin, dense connective tissue, the fibrous sheet of aponeurosis epicranialis (galea aponeurotica), the subaponeurotic space, and the pericranium.

Anatomic boundaries affect the spread of infection in the scalp because of various muscle attachments to the cranial bones. The occipitofrontalis muscle attaches to the occiput and mastoid part of the temporal bone, the epicranial aponeurosis, and the temporal fascia attachment to the zygomatic arch. These attachments limit potential posterior and lateral spread of infections from the scalp. However, the frontalis muscle attaches to the skin and subcutaneous tissue anteriorly, and not the frontal bone or nasal root. As a result, there is no muscle attachment limiting the anterior spread of infection.

The subaponeurotic space is considered the "danger space" because it is composed of loose connective tissue and the emissary veins (Figure 4-1). Localized infection within this layer can spread through the calvaria via the emissary veins to the intracranial dural venous sinuses. These emissary veins provide a connection to intracranial structures, such as the superior sagittal sinus, sigmoid sinus, and suboccipital venous plexus. Involvement of these vascular structures can result in severe systemic disease or neurologic dysfunction.

Skin

The skin is composed of the epidermis, the dermis, and the hypodermis (Figure 4-2). The dermis contains adnexal skin structures, such as hair follicles and sebaceous glands, which can succumb to infections that can spread to the adjacent structures. Subcutaneous nerves, vessels, and lymphatics travel in the hypodermis, which is a fatty layer of loose connective tissue. In the head and neck, the hypodermis can contain muscle, such as the platysma. The platysma is a remnant of more extensive mammalian skin-associated musculature. A deep subdermal plexus of vessels exists in the hypodermis. Infections can involve the epidermis, dermis, or hypodermal tissues; however, rapid spread occurs most readily within the loose connective tissue layer that composes the hypodermis.

Internal Lining Mucosa

The internal lining mucosa is composed of an epithelial layer that is keratinized or nonkeratinized (Figure 4-3). In some areas, the lining epithelial layer may consist of

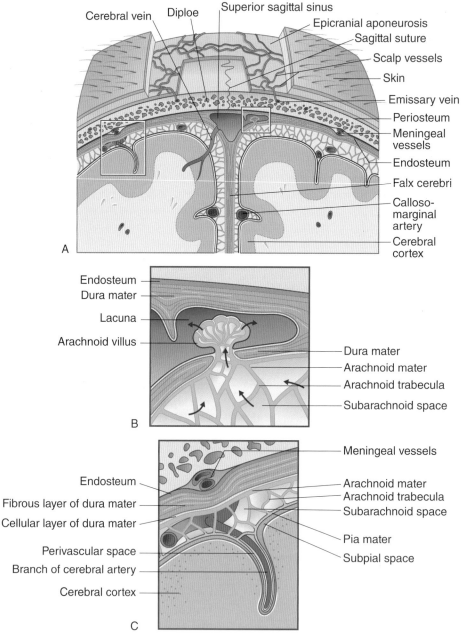

• **Figure 4-1** Depiction of the Scalp, Skull, and an Emissary Vein. (From FitzGerald MJT, Gruener G, Mtui E. *Clinical Neuroanatomy and Neuroscience*. 6th ed. Edinburgh: Saunders; 2012.)

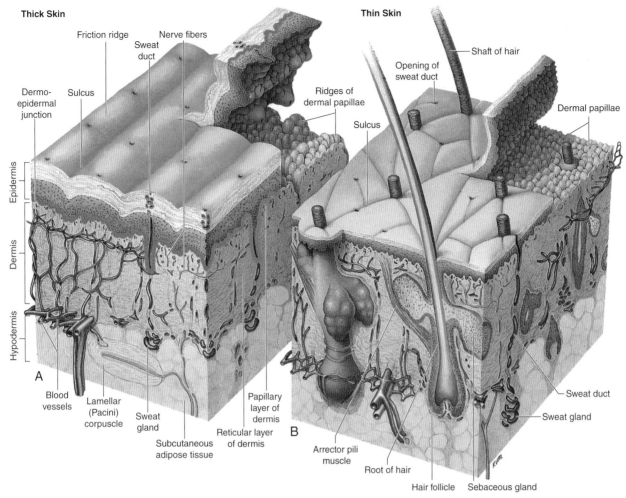

Thick Skin

Friction ridge
Nerve fibers
Sweat duct
Dermo-epidermal junction
Sulcus
Epidermis
Dermis
Hypodermis
A
Blood vessels
Lamellar (Pacini) corpuscle
Sweat gland
Subcutaneous adipose tissue
Reticular layer of dermis
Papillary layer of dermis

Thin Skin

Shaft of hair
Opening of sweat duct
Ridges of dermal papillae
Sulcus
Dermal papillae
B
Arrector pili muscle
Root of hair
Hair follicle
Sebaceous gland
Sweat gland
Sweat duct

• **Figure 4-2 A** and **B,** Microscopic anatomy of the skin. (From Patton KT, Thibodeau GA. *Anatomy and Physiology*. 8th ed. St Louis: Mosby; 2013.)

specialized structures such as olfactory, respiratory, or taste (Figure 4-4).

The underlying layer is composed of the lamina propria. Specialized tissues such as minor salivary glands, mucous glands, or taste buds may be present in this layer (Figure 4-5). Infections can involve the surface epithelial or lamina propria layers of the lining mucosa. Differing pathologic conditions can cause distinct tissue changes with specific clinical appearances and differing propensities to affect the deeper contiguous structures.

Spatial Boundaries and Fascial and Clinical Anatomic Considerations

Fascial Layers, Boundaries, and Anatomic Compartments and Spaces

Fascia is an enveloping sheet of dense fibrous connective tissue beneath the skin (Figures 4-6 and 4-7). Separate layers invest deeper muscle tissue. The superficial fascia is a loose connective tissue layer immediately deep to the skin. It contains fat, blood vessels, lymphatics, glands, and

nerves. The deep fascia, also known as the investing fascia, envelops muscles and supports the tissues like an elastic sheath. It can provide fibrous sheaths for tendons, muscle origins and insertions, and the formation of retinacula (Figure 4-8).

The superficial cervical fascia is contiguous with the superficial musculoaponeurotic system and the temporoparietal fascia. It invests the platysma, cutaneous nerves, vessels, and fat.

The deep cervical fascia (DCF; Box 4-1) is composed of three layers: superficial, middle, and deep (Figure 4-9).

The superficial (investing) layer of the DCF envelops the trapezius muscle, sternocleidomastoid muscle, submandibular gland, and parotid gland. Superiorly, this layer is contiguous with the deep temporal fascia and parotideomasseteric fascia. The temporal space is between the temporalis fascia and the temporal bone periosteum. It contains the internal maxillary artery and mandibular nerve. The temporalis muscle divides the temporal space into superficial and deep compartments. A suprasternal split allows encasement of the anterior and posterior borders of the manubrium, and the inferior suprasternal space of Burns.

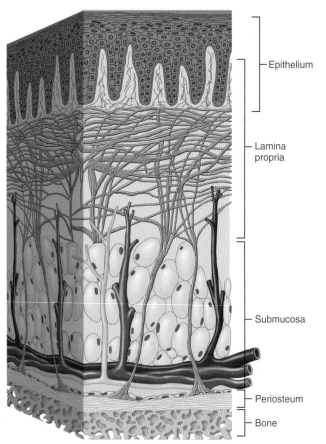

• **Figure 4-3** Microscopic Anatomy of the Oral Mucosa. (From Nanci A. *Ten Cate's Oral Histology.* 8th ed. St Louis: Mosby; 2013.)

Epithelium

Lamina propria

Submucosa

Periosteum

Bone

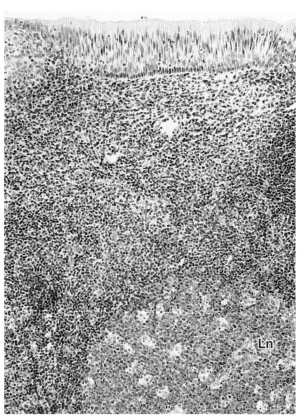

• **Figure 4-4** Histology Showing Normal Ciliated Respiratory Mucosa. *Ln,* Lymph node. (From Gartner LP. *Color Textbook of Histology.* 3rd ed. Philadelphia: Saunders; 2007.)

Ln

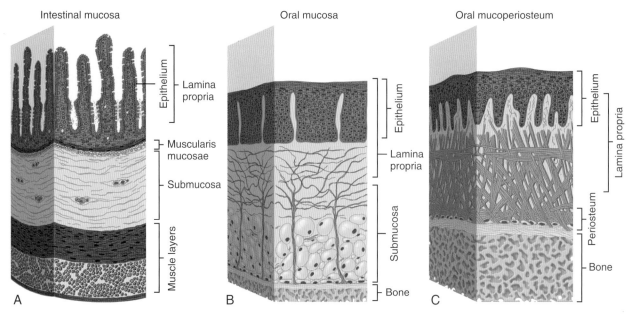

Intestinal mucosa

Oral mucosa

Oral mucoperiosteum

Epithelium

Lamina propria

Muscularis mucosae

Submucosa

Muscle layers

Epithelium

Lamina propria

Submucosa

Bone

Epithelium

Lamina propria

Periosteum

Bone

A   B   C

• **Figure 4-5** **A** to **C,** Example of the microscopic variability in several types of lining mucosa. (From Nanci A. *Ten Cate's Oral Histology.* 8th ed. St Louis: Mosby; 2013.)

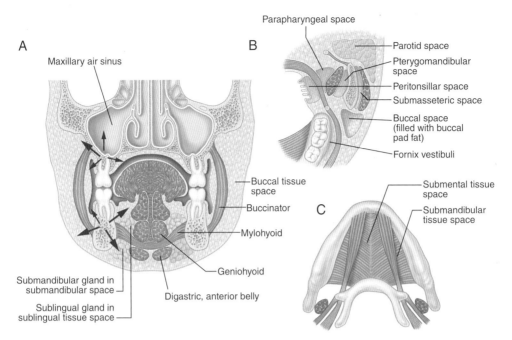

• **Figure 4-6** Depiction of Primary Odontogenic Periapical Infection Routes and Adjacent Anatomic Spaces. (**A,** From Standring S. *Gray's Anatomy: The Anatomical Basis of Clinical Practice*. 41st ed. Philadelphia: Churchill Livingstone; 2016. **B** and **C,** Redrawn from Berkovitz BKB, Holland GR, Moxham BJ. *Oral Anatomy, Histology, and Embryology*. 4th ed. Edinburgh: Mosby; 2009.)

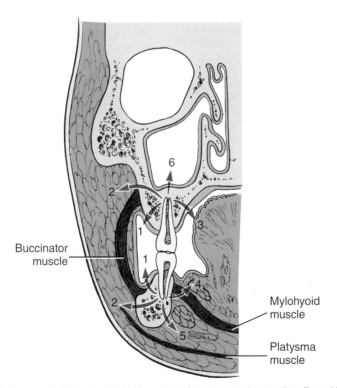

• **Figure 4-7** *Red arrows* indicate the contiguous anatomic structures that can be affected by an odontogenic periapical infection. *1,* Vestibule; *2,* buccal space; *3,* palate; *4,* floor of mouth/sublingual; *5,* submandibular; *6,* maxillary sinus. (Adapted from Flint PW, Haughey BH, Lund VJ, et al., eds. *Cummings Otolaryngology: Head and Neck Surgery*. 5th ed. Philadelphia: Mosby; 2010.)

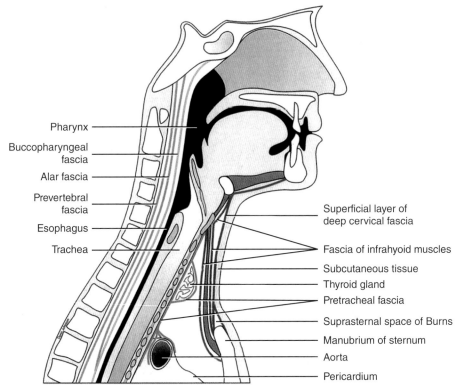

Pharynx
Buccopharyngeal fascia
Alar fascia
Prevertebral fascia
Esophagus
Trachea

Superficial layer of deep cervical fascia
Fascia of infrahyoid muscles
Subcutaneous tissue
Thyroid gland
Pretracheal fascia
Suprasternal space of Burns
Manubrium of sternum
Aorta
Pericardium

• **Figure 4-8** Axial Plane Depiction of the Cervical Fascia. (From Bagheri SC, Bell RB, Khan HA. *Current Therapy in Oral and Maxillofacial Surgery*. St Louis: Saunders; 2012. Copyright Donn Johnson at Atlanta VA Medical Center Art Department.)

• BOX 4-1   Deep Cervical Fascia Components

A. Investing/superficial/anterior
   1. Investing layer
   2. Temporal
   3. Parotideomasseteric
B. Middle layer divisions
   1. Sterno-omohyoid
   2. Sternothyroid-thyrohyoid
   3. Visceral
      a. Buccopharyngeal
      b. Pretracheal
      c. Retropharyngeal
C. Posterior/deep divisions
   1. Alar
   2. Prevertebral

It folds to become the stylomandibular ligament. Within or deep to the superficial layer of the DCF, superficial to the facial artery and vein, the marginal mandibular branch of the facial nerve can be found. Severe infections of this layer can result in decreased function of the marginal mandibular branch, resulting in an asymmetry of the ipsilateral lower lip commissure on smiling or pursing of the lips.

The middle layer consists of fascia surrounding the infrahyoid muscles, and has two layers that envelop the sternohyoid/omohyoid and sternothyroid/thyrohyoid structures. The visceral fascia envelops the thyroid, trachea, larynx,

esophagus, and pharynx. The buccopharyngeal fascia covers the buccinator muscle and the pharynx to blend with the pretracheal fascia. The pretracheal fascia invests the thyroid gland, trachea, and larynx and fuses inferiorly with the fibrous pericardium. There is no deep fascia in the face. The pharyngobasilar fascia at the skull base is the tissue that connects and suspends the pharyngeal musculature and ensures that the nasopharynx does not collapse.

The deep layer consists of the alar and prevertebral fascia. The alar fascia splits from the prevertebral fascia to run between the vertebral transverse processes, and joins the carotid sheath laterally. The prevertebral fascia is a sheath that encloses the vertebral column and its muscles. It contains axillary vessels, the brachial plexus, and sympathetic trunks. The soft tissue width in the adult at C2-C3 is 3 to 7 mm and at C6-C7 is less than 20 mm. Lateral plain film radiography can show infection-related abnormalities within these anatomic measurements. The prevertebral fascia extends laterally as the axillary sheath, and fuses with the anterior longitudinal ligament at the T3 vertebral level. Between the alar and prevertebral fascia lies the "danger space" that extends from the skull base to the diaphragm and is contiguous with the posterior mediastinum (Figure 4-10). Infections have the ability to involve the mediastinum structures from the retropharyngeal, pretracheal, and prevertebral spaces (Figure 4-11).

The carotid sheath is a tubular structure composed of all three layers of the DCF; it contains the vagus nerve, internal

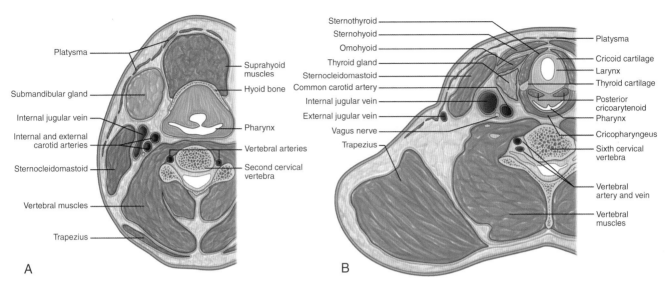

• **Figure 4-9** **A** and **B,** Axial plane depiction of the deep cervical fascial layers *(blue)* at two different levels of the neck. (From Ellis H, Mahadevan V. The anterior triangle of the neck. *Surgery [Oxford].* 2014;32 [suppl 2]:e28-e40.)

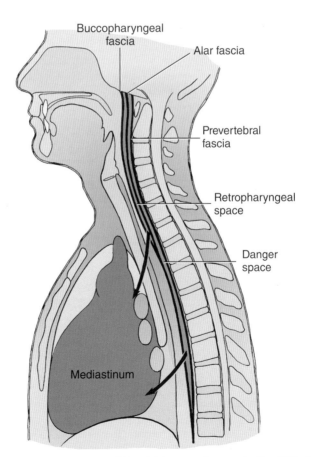

• **Figure 4-10** Sagittal Plane Depiction of Fascial Spaces Communication With the Mediastinum. (From Hupp JR, Ellis E, Tucker MR. *Contemporary Oral and Maxillofacial Surgery.* 6th ed. St Louis: Mosby; 2014.)

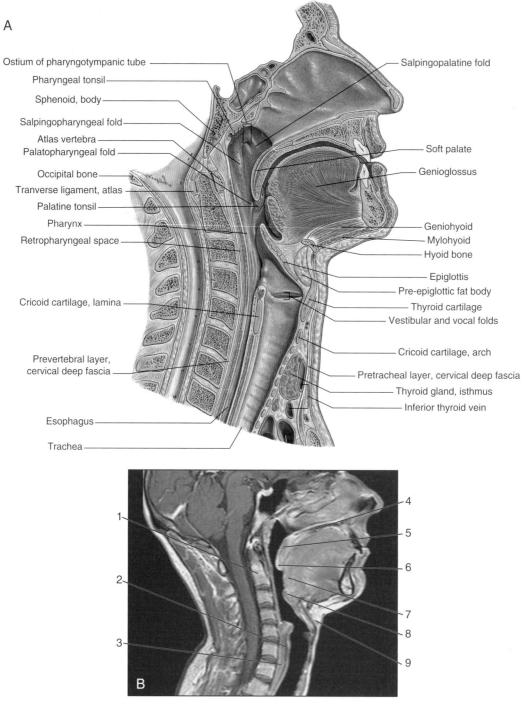

A

Ostium of pharyngotympanic tube

Pharyngeal tonsil

Sphenoid, body

Salpingopharyngeal fold

Atlas vertebra

Palatopharyngeal fold

Occipital bone

Tranverse ligament, atlas

Palatine tonsil

Pharynx

Retropharyngeal space

Cricoid cartilage, lamina

Prevertebral layer, cervical deep fascia

Esophagus

Trachea

Salpingopalatine fold

Soft palate

Genioglossus

Geniohyoid

Mylohyoid

Hyoid bone

Epiglottis

Pre-epiglottic fat body

Thyroid cartilage

Vestibular and vocal folds

Cricoid cartilage, arch

Pretracheal layer, cervical deep fascia

Thyroid gland, isthmus

Inferior thyroid vein

• **Figure 4-11 A,** Sagittal plane depiction of fascial spaces. **B,** Corresponding MRI also includes the posterior cranial fossa, cerebellum, and cervical spinal cord. *1,* Dens of axis. *2,* Lamina of cricoid cartilage. *3,* Esophagus. *4,* Hard palate. *5,* Soft palate. *6,* Uvula. *7,* Pharyngeal part of tongue. *8,* Epiglottis. *9,* Hyoid bone. (From Standring S. *Gray's Anatomy: the Anatomical Basis of Clinical Practice.* 41st ed. Philadelphia: Churchill Livingstone; 2016. Courtesy Dr. Roger JS Chinn.)

jugular vein, and common and internal carotid arteries. Eleven "spaces" created by the fascial layers are present in the deep neck. They should be considered both real and potential spaces.

The hyoid bone is an important anatomic structure that limits the spread of infection. Spaces can be described in relation to the hyoid bone as suprahyoid, infrahyoid, or traversing the length of the neck, to potentially extend from the skull base and involve the mediastinum as the caudal extension.

Dentition and Dentoalveolar Complex: Primary Odontogenic Space Infections

The primary odontogenic space infections involve fascial spaces that are in direct association with the dentoalveolar complex (see Figure 4-7). The dentoalveolar complex is composed of the teeth and surrounding gingival and bony tissues.

Dentoalveolar infections that increase in the inoculum volume and propagate from the dentition generally travel through the alveolar medullary bone that exhibits the least amount of structural resistance (Figure 4-12). Three important factors for resistance to the spread of infection are root apex proximity to the cortical plate, medullary bone volume and density, and cortical bone thickness and density. Cone-beam computed tomography (CBCT) imaging displays this three-dimensional architecture. There are predictable patterns of extension of these infections based on the anatomy and architecture of the surrounding bone and associated muscle attachments to the facial bones (Figure 4-13). The

extragnathic soft tissue clinical presentation depends on how the pathogenic inoculum spreads in relation to the position of the muscle attachments.

The mandibular incisors and canines often show labial extension in the vestibule. Lingual extension involving the incisors can occur (Figure 4-14). The mandibular premolars and molars often show buccal extension. The maxillary incisors, canines, and buccal root of the first premolars often show labial extension. Infections of the premolar palatal root more often spread to the palate.

The maxillary second premolar and molars frequently show a buccal extension, with the exception of infections involving the palatal root of the molars. The attachments of the buccinator, mylohyoid, and other facial muscles can affect the extension of infection from the apical regions of the root systems. For example, in the maxilla if the apex of the root is superior to the attachment of the buccinator muscle, the infection will occupy the buccal space. If the apex of the root is inferior to the attachment of the buccinator muscle, the infection will occupy the vestibular space. A similar association exists in the mandible based on the location of the root apex to the muscle attachment. If it is superior to the buccinator muscle attachment, the infection will occupy the vestibular space; if it is inferior to the attachment, it will occupy the buccal space. Plain film intraoral (Figure 4-15) and panoramic radiography of the tooth root system apex region are frequently used as part of the initial diagnostic assessment of a tooth-related infection (pulpal, periodontal, or both).

The palatine tonsils and peritonsillar area in children (Figure 4-16), and odontogenic structures (see Figure 4-12) in adults are the most prevalent initial anatomic origins of deep neck space infections for these two age groups.

The deep spaces associated with infections arising from the dentition (odontogenic) can be divided based on their association with an initial occurrence in the maxilla or mandible. A primary odontogenic fascial space is directly contiguous with the source of the dentoalveolar odontogenic infection (see Figure 4-6). A secondary odontogenic fascial space is in close proximity to a primary space, and can become involved because of the anatomic association (see Figure 4-7 and Box 4-2).

Table 4-1 lists the various spaces with identifying borders. Table 4-2 is a synopsis of the predominant clinical findings when certain fascial spaces are involved with a bacterial infection.

Masticator Space

The masticator space is a secondary odontogenic fascial space, and it encompasses the submasseteric, pterygomandibular, temporal, and deep temporal (infratemporal) fascial spaces. Given the contents of this space, and the proximity to the airway, infections within the masticator space are important to recognize and treat early in the clinical timeline (Figure 4-17). Various muscles of mastication, including the medial pterygoid, lateral pterygoid, masseter, and temporalis muscles, can be involved, resulting

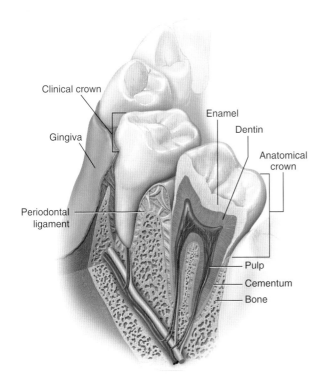

• **Figure 4-12** Depiction of the Dentition and Dentoalveolar Complex. (From Nanci A. *Ten Cate's Oral Histology: Development, Structure, and Function*. 8th ed. St Louis: Mosby; 2013.)

Labels in figure:
Clinical crown
Gingiva
Periodontal ligament
Enamel
Dentin
Anatomical crown
Pulp
Cementum
Bone

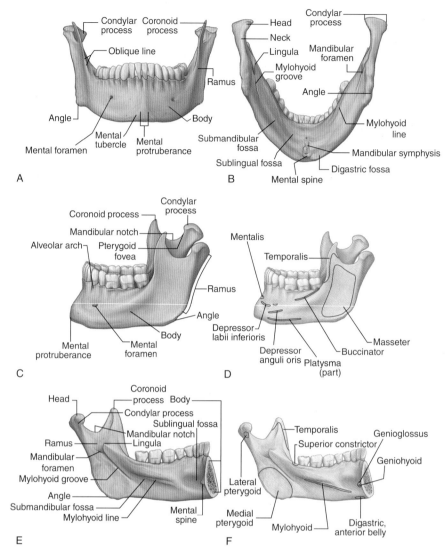

• **Figure 4-13** Mandible Bony Muscle Attachments. The soft tissue extension of a periapical infection is guided by the apical root system–bone muscle attachment relationship. (Redrawn with permission from Putz R, Pabst R. *Sobotta Atlas of Human Anatomy: Head, Neck, Upper Limb*. 14th ed. Vol. 1. Munich: Elsevier GmbH; 2008.)

in difficulty opening the mouth (trismus). With significant trismus, adequate intraoral evaluation becomes difficult, as does airway management. For this reason, early signs of trismus should immediately raise concern. Rapid spread to contiguous areas, including the parapharyngeal, parotid, and retropharyngeal spaces, can occur, posing imminent risk to airway patency. For this reason, aggressive surgical drainage is required with maintenance of a protected airway in the immediate postoperative setting. Surgical drainage is best achieved from combined intraoral and extraoral approaches.

Vestibular Space

The vestibule is an oral mucosa–lined trough immediately adjacent to the alveolar bone of the mandible both lingually and buccally, and lateral to the maxillary alveolar bone. The attachment of musculature to the lateral aspects of both the maxilla and mandible determine the relative depth of

the vestibular mucosal fold. The lingual mandibular vestibule is contiguous with the floor of the mouth. The major structures forming the boundaries of the floor of the mouth are the mylohyoid and genioglossus muscles. The attachments of the buccinator muscle bilaterally onto the lateral aspects of the maxilla and mandible form the major boundary for the buccal vestibular spaces. Posteriorly, the buccinator muscle connects with the pterygomandibular raphe and superior constrictor muscle. Isolated vestibular space infections can be treated locally with removal of the source.

Buccal Space

The buccal space occupies the area between the buccinator muscle medially and overlying facial skin. The anterior boundary is the modiolus, which is composed of the intersection of the following muscles: orbicularis oris, buccinator, levator anguli oris, depressor anguli oris, zygomaticus

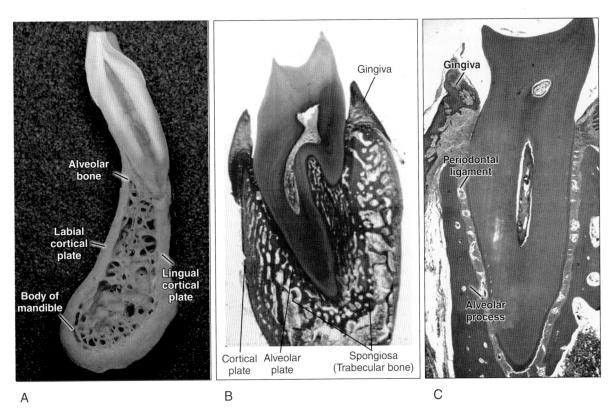

• **Figure 4-14** **A** to **C,** Dentoalveolar complex showing the relationship of the root system structure and the alveolar bone support. The root system morphology, three-dimensional intraosseous root system position, and medullary cortical bone architecture and density all contribute to how a periapical infectious process can involve the buccal or lingual cortex. Muscle bony attachment position affects further soft tissue extension. Plain film radiography requires approximately 60% bone mineral loss before pathology changes become evident. (From Nanci A. *Ten Cate's Oral Histology: Development, Structure, and Function.* 8th ed. St Louis: Mosby; 2013. **A,** Courtesy T. Tambasco de Oliveira.)

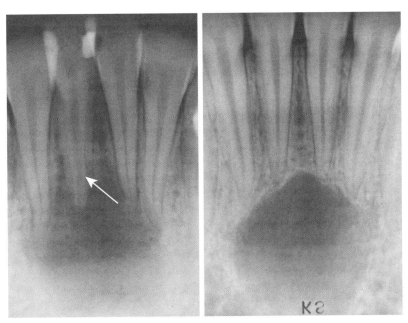

• **Figure 4-15** *Left side,* Periapical inflammation and infection of pulpal etiology. The *arrow* indicates the nonvital tooth pulpal etiology. *Right side,* Solitary bone cavity. Not related to pathology of the dentition pulp tissue or periodontium. (From Neville BW, Damm DD, Allen CM, et al., eds. *Oral and Maxillofacial Pathology.* 4th ed. St Louis: Elsevier; 2016.)

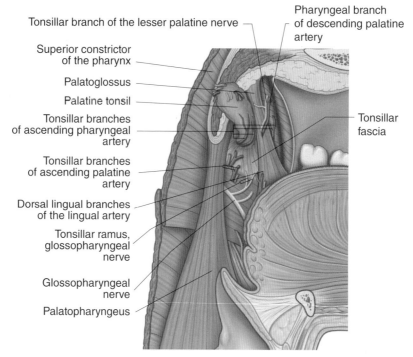

• **Figure 4-16** Palatine Tonsil Region of the Pharynx. (From Standring S. *Gray's Anatomy: The Anatomical Basis of Clinical Practice.* 41st ed. Philadelphia: Churchill Livingstone; 2016.)

major, risorius, platysma, and levator labii superioris. These structures together form the commissure of the mouth. The buccinator muscle separates the vestibular space from the buccal space. Entry of infections into the buccal space depends on their relationship to the attachment of the buccinator muscle. Infections confined to the buccal space are limited by the attachments of the investing fascia to the zygomatic arch and inferior border of the mandible. Therefore, these bony landmarks should remain easily palpable on clinical examination. If these structures are not readily palpable, there must be concern for involvement of adjacent fascial spaces. The approach for surgical drainage is best achieved intraorally.

Palatal Space

The palatal space is composed of the soft tissue lingual to the maxillary dentition, including the hard palate, and extending to the soft palate tissue border. It forms the roof of the oral cavity together with the soft palate–uvula structures. Infections entering the palatal space are commonly associated with pathologic conditions of the palatal roots of maxillary multi-rooted teeth. Effective surgical drainage can be obtained intraorally.

Canine Space

The canine space is the area at the apex of the maxillary canine root system (canine fossa), bordered by the zygomaticus minor, orbicularis oris, levator labii superioris, levator labii superioris alaeque nasi, and levator anguli oris muscles. Infections in this space will obliterate the nasolabial fold on

TABLE 4-1   Borders of the Fascial Spaces of the Head and Neck

Space	Anterior	Posterior	Superior	Inferior	Superficial or Medial*	Deep or Lateral†
Buccal	Modiolus	Pterygomandibular raphe, pterygomandibular space	Zygomatic arch Maxilla	Mandible	Subcutaneous tissue and skin	Buccinator muscle
Infratemporal space	Posterior surface of the maxilla	Styloid process	Greater wing of the sphenoid bone Infratemporal crest	Lateral pterygoid muscle Pterygomandibular space	Lateral pterygoid plate*	Mandibular ramus Coronoid process†
Infraorbital	Nasal cartilages	Buccal space	Quadratus labii superioris muscle	Oral mucosa	Quadratus labii superioris muscle	Levator anguli oris Maxilla
Submandibular	Anterior belly digastric muscle	Posterior belly digastric muscle Stylohyoid muscle Stylopharyngeus muscle	Inferior and medial surfaces of the mandible Mylohyoid muscle	Digastric tendon	Platysma Investing fascia	Mylohyoid muscle Hyoglossus muscle Superior constrictor muscle
Submental	Inferior mandibular border	Hyoid bone	Mylohyoid muscle	Investing fascia	Investing fascia	Anterior bellies of digastric muscle†
Sublingual	Lingual mandible	Submandibular space Tongue base	Oral mucosa	Mylohyoid muscle	Muscles of the tongue*	Lingual mandible†
Pterygomandibular space	Buccal space	Parotid gland	Lateral pterygoid muscle	Inferior border of the mandible	Medial pterygoid muscle*	Ascending ramus Medial mandible†
Submasseteric	Buccal space	Parotid gland	Zygomatic arch	Inferior border of the mandible	Lateral ascending ramus*	Masseter muscle†
Lateral pharyngeal	Superior and middle constrictor muscles	Carotid sheath Scalene muscle fascia	Superior skull base	Hyoid bone	Pharyngeal constrictor muscles and retropharyngeal space*	Medial pterygoid muscle†
Retropharyngeal	Superior and middle constrictor muscles	Alar fascia	Skull base	Fusion of alar and prevertebral fasciae at C6-T4		Carotid sheath and lateral pharyngeal space†
Pretracheal	Fasciae of the sternothyroid-thyrohyoid muscles	Retropharyngeal space	Thyroid cartilage	Superior mediastinum	Fasciae of the sternothyroid-thyrohyoid muscles	Visceral fascia (DCF) over trachea and thyroid gland
Parotid‡	Mandibular ramus	Mastoid process and sternocleidomastoid muscle	Parotideomasseteric fascia	Stylomandibular ligament and submandibular space	Stylomandibular ligament and lateral pharyngeal space*	Parotideomasseteric fascia
Carotid sheath	Sternocleidomastoid muscle and lateral pharyngeal space	Lateral extension of the retropharyngeal space	Skull base	Connective tissue of the aortic arch		
Peritonsillar space	Palatoglossus muscle	Palatopharyngeus muscle	Soft palate	Base of the tongue	Oropharyngeal mucosa and palatine tonsil*	Superior constrictor muscle and buccopharyngeal fascia†

*Medial border.
†Lateral border.
‡The parotid space is partially encased by the parotideomasseteric fascia and can encroach upon the other adjacent fascial spaces.
Modified from Hupp JR, Ellis E, Tucker MR. *Contemporary Oral and Maxillofacial Surgery.* 6th ed. St Louis: Mosby; 2014.

TABLE 4-2 Clinical Findings Relevant to Fascial Space Anatomy

Space	Probable Originating Site	Contents	Signs and Symptoms (in Addition to Pain, Swelling, Erythema)	Surgical Approach for I&D
Buccal	Maxillary molars and premolars Mandibular premolars	Facial A/V/N, deep facial A/V, buccal A/V, parotid duct, buccal fat pad, transverse facial A/V	Zygomatic arch and inferior border of the mandible readily palpable, trismus	Intraoral or extraoral
Infraorbital	Maxillary canine	Infraorbital nerve and vessels	May see lower eyelid involvement	Intraoral or extraoral
Submandibular	Mandibular molars	Submandibular gland, facial A/V, lymph nodes	Odynophagia or dysphagia, inferior border of the mandible difficult to palpate, concern for airway obstruction	Extraoral
Submental	Mandibular anterior teeth Fracture of the symphysis	Anterior jugular vein, lymphatics	Floor of mouth elevation	Extraoral
Sublingual	Mandibular premolars and molars Direct trauma	Hypoglossal nerve, lingual A/V/N, sublingual gland and ducts, submandibular ducts	Floor of mouth elevation, odynophagia/dysphagia, altered tongue mobility, concern for airway obstruction	Extraoral
Pterygomandibular	Mandibular third molars Fracture of the angle of the mandible	Mandibular nerve, inferior alveolar A/V, sphenomandibular ligament	Trismus, concern for airway obstruction, odynophagia/dysphagia	Intraoral and extraoral
Submasseteric	Mandibular third molars, fracture of the angle of the mandible	Masseteric A/V	Trismus	Intraoral
Lateral pharyngeal	Mandibular third molars Tonsils Infection of adjacent fascial spaces	Maxillary A; ascending pharyngeal A; internal carotid A; internal jugular V; cranial nerves IX; X, XI, XII; sympathetic trunk; superior cervical ganglion; deep cervical lymph nodes	Concern for airway obstruction, odynophagia, dysphagia, trismus, soft palate and uvula displacement/deviation	Intraoral
Retropharyngeal	Adjacent fascial spaces	Lymphatics	Dysphagia, odynophagia, concern for airway obstruction	Intraoral
Pretracheal	Adjacent fascial spaces	Trachea and esophagus	Dysphagia, odynophagia, stridor, hoarseness	Extraoral
Parotid	Parotid gland	Parotid gland and duct, cranial VII, facial nerve V, external carotid A	Trismus	Extraoral
Carotid sheath	Adjacent fascial spaces	Carotid artery, internal jugular vein, vagus nerve, sympathetic post-ganglionic fibers	Pharyngitis, Horner syndrome (possible late event)	Extraoral
Infratemporal space	Maxillary molars	Pterygoid muscles, pterygoid venous plexus, branch of the mandibular nerve, otic ganglion, chorda tympani, br. of maxillary artery	Trismus	Intraoral or extraoral
Peritonsillar	Tonsils	Palatine tonsils, glossopharyngeal nerve, tonsillar and palatine branch of ascending pharyngeal and maxillary arteries, peritonsillar veins	Trismus, odynophagia, dysphagia, uvular deviation, "hot potato voice"	Intraoral

A/V, Artery/vein; A/V/N, artery/vein/nerve; I&D, incision and drainage.
Adapted and modified from Flynn TR. Anatomy of oral and maxillofacial infections. In Topazian RG, Goldberg MH, Hupp JR, eds. Oral and Maxillofacial Infections. 4th ed. Philadelphia: WB Saunders; 2002. With permission.

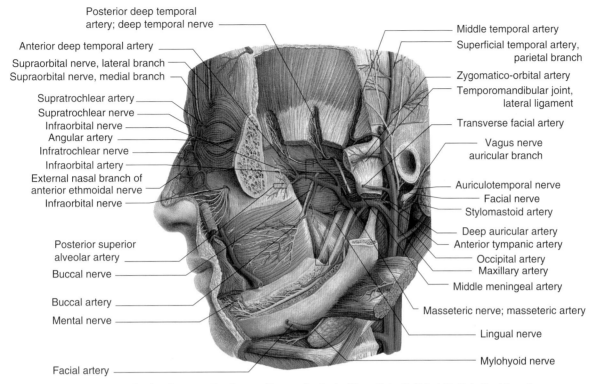

Posterior deep temporal artery; deep temporal nerve

Anterior deep temporal artery

Supraorbital nerve, lateral branch

Supraorbital nerve, medial branch

Supratrochlear artery

Supratrochlear nerve

Infraorbital nerve

Angular artery

Infratrochlear nerve

Infraorbital artery

External nasal branch of anterior ethmoidal nerve

Infraorbital nerve

Posterior superior alveolar artery

Buccal nerve

Buccal artery

Mental nerve

Facial artery

Middle temporal artery

Superficial temporal artery, parietal branch

Zygomatico-orbital artery

Temporomandibular joint, lateral ligament

Transverse facial artery

Vagus nerve auricular branch

Auriculotemporal nerve

Facial nerve

Stylomastoid artery

Deep auricular artery

Anterior tympanic artery

Occipital artery

Maxillary artery

Middle meningeal artery

Masseteric nerve; masseteric artery

Lingual nerve

Mylohyoid nerve

• **Figure 4-17** Region Deep to the Ramus–Zygomatic Arch. (From Putz R, Pabst R. *Sobotta Atlas of Human Anatomy*: *Head, Neck, Upper Limb*. 14th ed. Vol. 1. Munich: Elsevier GmbH; 2006.)

clinical examination. The canine space lies inferior to the infraorbital space, which allows for local anesthesia to be given at the site of the infraorbital foramen before surgical drainage. Effective surgical drainage can be achieved using an intraoral approach.

Mental Space

The mental space occupies the soft tissue region anterior to the mandibular symphysis and is limited by the attachments of the mentalis muscle. It lies inferior to the mandibular labial vestibule.

Submandibular Space

The submandibular space is of particular anatomic interest because the progression of infections into this space can readily spread to contiguous areas. Clinically, once an infection has progressed from the buccal space to the submandibular space, the inferior border of the mandible becomes obscured. Posteriorly, the submandibular space freely communicates with the pterygomandibular, sublingual, lateral pharyngeal, and retropharyngeal spaces; therefore, treatment should occur as early as possible to prevent airway compromise. In the setting of pan-space infections, Ludwig's angina is commonly described. This infection has been described classically as bilateral involvement of the sublingual, submental, and submandibular spaces. Because the location of these spaces is inferior to the tongue base, infections here can result in elevation of the floor of the mouth and posterior displacement of the tongue base into the airway (see Figure 4-39).

Cavernous Sinus

The cavernous sinuses are positioned on either side of the sella turcica and sphenoid bone body. They are between the meningeal and periosteal layers of the dura mater. The anterior boundary is the superior orbital fissure, and the posterior boundary is the petrous part of the temporal bone. They connect with the pterygoid venous plexus (see Figure 4-29) by the emissary veins, superior and inferior ophthalmic veins, middle cerebral vein, and sphenoparietal sinus. They are connected with each other by an intercavernous sinus (reticulated venous plexus) situated between the optic chiasm and sphenoid sinuses. The internal carotid artery and abducens nerve (VI) are medially situated within each sinus. The oculomotor (III), trochlear (IV), ophthalmic (V1), and maxillary (V2) nerves are positioned near the lateral sinus wall from a superior to inferior location (Figures 4-18 and 4-19).

The superior ophthalmic vein receives blood from the orbital roof and scalp, and the inferior ophthalmic vein receives blood from the orbital floor. The superior and inferior ophthalmic veins drain into the pterygoid venous plexus and cavernous sinus. The cavernous sinus drains posteriorly into the petrosal sinuses (superior and inferior). The superior petrosal sinus connects to the transverse and sigmoid sinus. The inferior petrosal sinus connects to the sigmoid sinus–internal jugular vein, and basilar plexus–internal vertebral venous plexus. Signs and symptoms of infection can include papilledema, exophthalmos-proptosis, diplopia, ophthalmoplegia, eyelid edema, chemosis, sluggish pupillary response (autonomic nervous system damage), upper

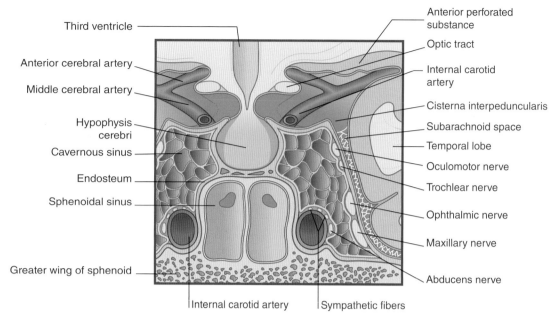

• **Figure 4-18** Coronal Depiction of the Cavernous Sinus Anatomy and Contents. (From FitzGerald MJT, Gruener G, Mtui E. *Clinical Neuroanatomy and Neuroscience*. 6th ed. Edinburgh: Saunders; 2012.)

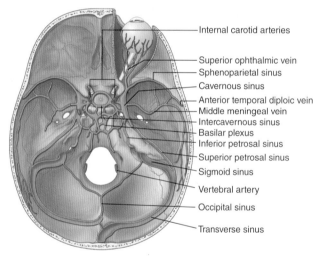

• **Figure 4-19** Axial Depiction of the Intracranial Cavernous Sinus Structures and Venous Connections. (From Standring S. *Gray's Anatomy: The Anatomical Basis of Clinical Practice*. 41st ed. Philadelphia: Churchill Livingstone; 2016.)

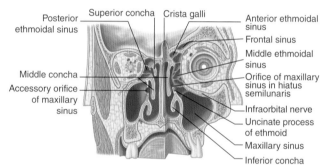

• **Figure 4-20** Coronal Depiction of the Nasal Cavity, Paranasal Sinuses, and Orbit Regions. (From Standring S. *Gray's Anatomy: The Anatomical Basis of Clinical Practice*. 41st ed. Philadelphia: Churchill Livingstone; 2016.)

eyelid ptosis (cranial nerve III damage and sympathetic plexus damage on the internal carotid artery), and vision loss (optic nerve and central retinal artery and vein damage). Spread of infection or emboli can occur from the upper lip or paranasal face area (e.g., anterior facial vein, ophthalmic veins) and from the pterygoid space via the pterygoid venous plexus that connects directly via the foramen ovale.

Orbit and Surrounding Spaces

The orbital space lies posterior to the orbital septum and includes the contents of the bony orbit, the globe, extraocular muscles, and fat. The bony orbit is formed by the confluence of the frontal, maxillary, zygomatic, sphenoid, lacrimal, palatine, and ethmoid bones. Within the bony orbit lie the superior and inferior orbital fissures. The structures that pass through the superior orbital fissure include the superior ophthalmic vein and the lacrimal, frontal, trochlear, oculomotor, nasociliary, and abducens nerves. The infraorbital nerve and vein, zygomatic nerve, and inferior ophthalmic vein pass through the inferior orbital fissure. The optic canal connects the orbit and the middle cranial fossa; therefore, infections within the bony orbit can spread to the brain. Communication with the nasal apparatus can occur via the nasolacrimal system, and extension to the maxillary sinus and maxilla can occur via the inferior orbital fissure (Figures 4-20 and 4-21).

The periorbital space includes the area overlying the orbicularis oculi muscle, the eyelid tissue superficial to the orbital septum and tarsal plate (preseptal), including the overlying skin of the eyelid (Figure 4-22).

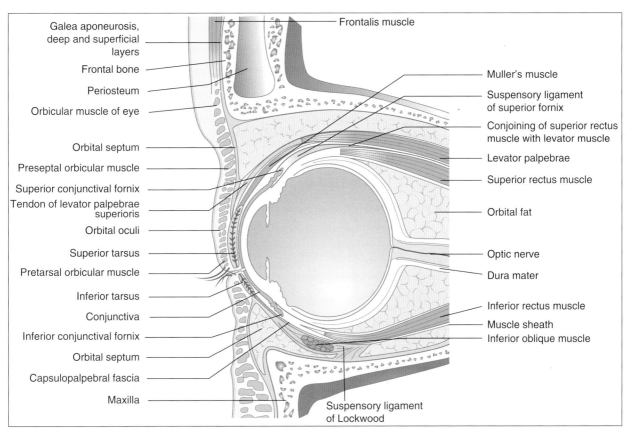

• **Figure 4-21** Sagittal Depiction of the Periorbital Anatomy and Orbital Contents. (From Moy RL, Fincher EF. *Procedures in Cosmetic Dermatology Series: Blepharoplasty*. St Louis: Mosby; 2006.)

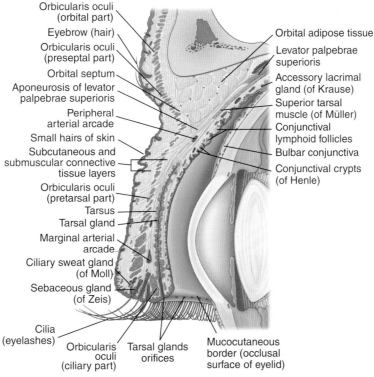

• **Figure 4-22** Sagittal Depiction of the Periorbital Upper Eyelid Anatomy. (From Standring S. *Gray's Anatomy: The Anatomical Basis of Clinical Practice*. 41st ed. Philadelphia: Churchill Livingstone; 2016.)

The infraorbital space lies below the inferior orbital rim between the canine fossa and involving the lower inferior edge of the orbicularis oculi muscle. This space contains the infraorbital nerve and vessels as they exit the infraorbital foramen on the anterior surface of the maxillary bones. Contiguous spaces include the buccal, canine, and periorbital preseptal areas.

Ear

Auricle (Pinna)

The parts of the external ear most often affected by infections are the perichondrium, ear cartilage and overlying skin (Figure 4-23), and the skin lining the external acoustic meatus (EAM). The external third of the EAM is composed of cartilage, and the remainder is bone (tympanic, squamous, and petrous part of the temporal bone). Specialized cerumen and sebaceous glands are present. The lateral and superior portions of the auricle drain to the superficial parotid lymph nodes. The medial surface drains to the mastoid and deep cervical lymph nodes. The remaining tissues of the auricle drain to the superficial cervical lymph nodes. The auricle receives its arterial blood supply from the superficial temporal, posterior auricular, deep auricular, and anterior tympanic branches of the maxillary artery. The venous drainage is as follows: the superficial temporal vein to the maxillary and retromandibular veins, the posterior auricular vein to the posterior retromandibular and external jugular veins, the maxillary vein to the superficial temporal and retromandibular vein, and draining veins (external acoustic meatus) to the pterygoid plexus.

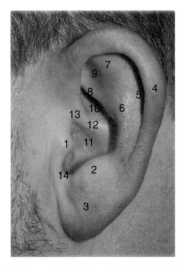

• **Figure 4-23** Photograph Depicting the Auricle Anatomic Subunits. *1,* Tragus. *2,* Antitragus. *3,* Lobe. *4,* Helix. *5,* Scapha. *6,* Antihelix. *7,* Superior crus. *8,* Anterior crus. *9,* Fossa triangularis. *10,* Cymba concha. *11,* Cavum concha. *12,* Helical radix. *13,* Helical crus. *14,* Intertragal incisure. (From Niamtu J. *Cosmetic Facial Surgery.* St Louis: Mosby; 2011.)

Middle Ear (Tympanic Cavity)

The middle ear is located in the petrous portion of the temporal bone; it has a mucous membrane lining (Figure 4-24). The boundaries are the tegmen tympani (roof), jugular fossa (floor), membranous lateral wall, labyrinthine (medial) wall, and carotid canal/internal carotid artery (anterior). The middle ear connects with the nasopharynx via the pharyngotympanic tube in an anteromedial position. It connects posteriorly with the mastoid air cells and mastoid antrum, via the aditus (inlet). Other adjacent anatomic structures include the floor of the middle cranial fossa, the temporal lobe of the brain, the superior bulb of the internal jugular vein, the posterior cranial fossa and sigmoid sinus, and the canal of the facial nerve. The arterial supply of the middle ear is from the stylomastoid branch of the posterior auricular artery, the anterior tympanic branch of the maxillary artery, the inferior tympanic branch of the ascending pharyngeal artery, and the caroticotympanic branch of the internal carotid artery. Venous drainage is to the pterygoid venous plexus and superior petrosal sinus. Lymphatic drainage is to the deep cervical lymph nodes. The pharyngotympanic tube venous drainage is to the pterygoid venous plexus. Lymphatic drainage is also to the deep cervical lymph nodes.

Inner Ear

The inner (internal) ear is contained in the petrous portion of the temporal bone. Adjacent structures are the middle ear, facial nerve, vestibulocochlear nerve, pharyngotympanic tube, chorda tympani nerve, internal carotid artery, and the contents of the cranial fossa (Figure 4-25).

Mastoid Air Cells

The mastoid air cells communicate with the middle cranial fossa via the petrosquamous fissure and the tympanic cavity (middle ear), as described previously (Figure 4-26).

Nose and Paranasal Structures

Pterygoid Venous Plexus

The pterygoid venous plexus is an extensive valveless plexus of veins that parallels the medial two thirds of the maxillary artery on the lateral aspect of the medial pterygoid muscle, within the infratemporal fossa. It communicates with the facial vein (Figure 4-27) via the deep facial vein, inferior ophthalmic vein, maxillary vein, pharyngeal venous plexus, and cavernous sinus. Given the extensive communication between the various venous structures, the spread of infection via venous drainage is readily apparent (Figures 4-28, 4-29, and 4-30).

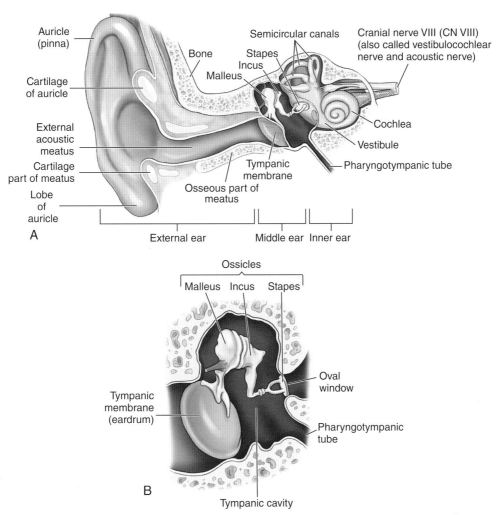

• **Figure 4-24 A** and **B,** Auditory apparatus. (From LaFleur Brooks M, LaFleur Brooks D. *Exploring Medical Language*. 9th ed. St Louis: Mosby; 2014.)

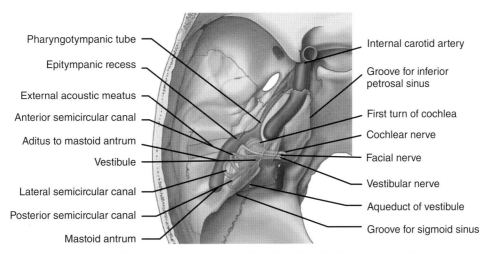

• **Figure 4-25** Temporal Bone Auditory Apparatus. (From Standring S. *Gray's Anatomy: The Anatomical Basis of Clinical Practice*. 41st ed. Philadelphia: Churchill Livingstone; 2016.)

A

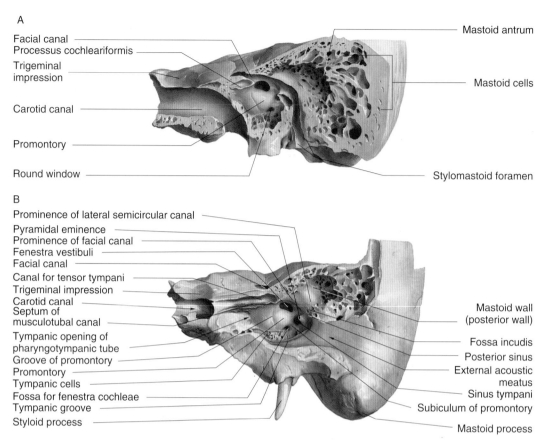

Facial canal
Processus cochleariformis
Trigeminal impression
Carotid canal
Promontory
Round window

Mastoid antrum
Mastoid cells
Stylomastoid foramen

B

Prominence of lateral semicircular canal
Pyramidal eminence
Prominence of facial canal
Fenestra vestibuli
Facial canal
Canal for tensor tympani
Trigeminal impression
Carotid canal
Septum of musculotubal canal
Tympanic opening of pharyngotympanic tube
Groove of promontory
Promontory
Tympanic cells
Fossa for fenestra cochleae
Tympanic groove
Styloid process

Mastoid wall (posterior wall)
Fossa incudis
Posterior sinus
External acoustic meatus
Sinus tympani
Subiculum of promontory
Mastoid process

• **Figure 4-26** Depiction of the Mastoid Air Cells. (From Standring S. *Gray's Anatomy: The Anatomical Basis of Clinical Practice.* 41st ed. Philadelphia: Churchill Livingstone; 2016.)

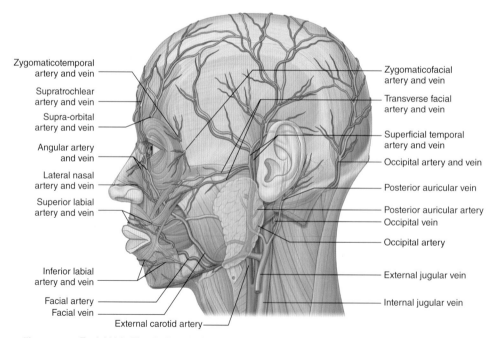

Zygomaticotemporal artery and vein
Supratrochlear artery and vein
Supra-orbital artery and vein
Angular artery and vein
Lateral nasal artery and vein
Superior labial artery and vein
Inferior labial artery and vein
Facial artery
Facial vein
External carotid artery

Zygomaticofacial artery and vein
Transverse facial artery and vein
Superficial temporal artery and vein
Occipital artery and vein
Posterior auricular vein
Posterior auricular artery
Occipital vein
Occipital artery
External jugular vein
Internal jugular vein

• **Figure 4-27** Facial Vein That Indirectly Communicates With the Cavernous Sinus. (From Standring S. *Gray's Anatomy: The Anatomical Basis of Clinical Practice.* 41st ed. Philadelphia: Churchill Livingstone; 2016.)

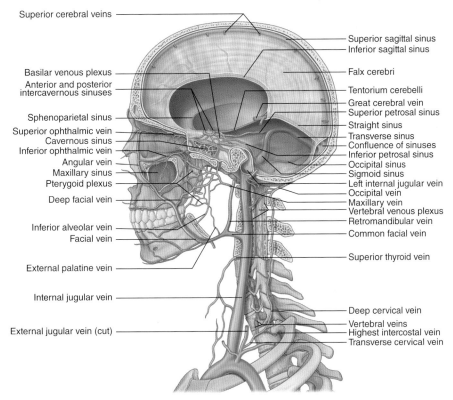

• **Figure 4-28** Pterygoid Venous Plexus and Deep Veins of the Head and Neck. (From Standring S. *Gray's Anatomy: The Anatomical Basis of Clinical Practice.* 41st ed. Philadelphia: Churchill Livingstone; 2016.)

Nasolacrimal Apparatus

The nasolacrimal apparatus is composed of the lacrimal gland and ducts, punctum, caruncle, papilla, canaliculi, sac, and nasolacrimal duct. The duct opens into the nasal cavity via the inferior meatus, which lies beneath the inferior turbinate. This relationship between the lacrimal system and the nose allows for the spread of nasal infections to the orbit, and vice versa (Figure 4-31).

Nasal Cavity and Paranasal Sinuses

The nasal cavity (Figure 4-32) is lined by mucosa attached to the underlying perichondrium and periosteum (Figures 4-33 and 4-34). The mucosa is continuous with adjacent structures, including the nasopharynx posteriorly, the superior and lateral paranasal sinuses, and the lacrimal sac and conjunctiva superiorly. The superior one third serves an olfactory function, and the lower two thirds serve a respiratory function. All the paranasal sinuses drain into the lateral walls of the nasal cavity. The nasal cavity communicates with the pterygopalatine fossa through the sphenopalatine foramen. A deviated nasal septum or inflamed and swollen mucosa may block the openings of the paranasal sinuses. A paranasal sinus infection can involve or originate in the nasal cavity and nasopharynx areas.

The anterior cranial fossa, orbits, anterior ethmoidal air cells, and nasal cavity surround the frontal sinus, which communicates with the hiatus semilunaris (middle nasal meatus) via the frontonasal duct. The posterior bony wall of the frontal sinus is thin, and infections can erode into the anterior cranial fossa.

The ethmoidal air cells or ethmoid sinuses are subdivided and surrounded by the anterior cranial fossa, nasal cavity, and orbits. The posterior cells drain directly into the superior nasal meatus, the middle cells drain into the summit of the ethmoidal bulla (middle nasal meatus), and the anterior cells drain into the anterior aspect of the hiatus semilunaris. Ethmoid sinus infections can erode through the thin medial orbital wall into the orbit and potentially extend into the cranial cavity. Lymphatic drainage of the anterior and middle cells is to the submandibular lymph nodes, and the posterior cells drain to the retropharyngeal lymph nodes.

The larger maxillary sinuses lie below the orbital floor and drain into the posterior aspect of the hiatus semilunaris (see Figure 4-33; Figures 4-35 and 4-36). They are surrounded by the orbit, infraorbital canal and its contents, maxillary teeth, nasal cavity, overlying soft tissue structures of the cheek, infratemporal fossa, and pterygopalatine fossa. Infections of the maxillary sinus may originate in the maxillary dentition or arise de novo within the sinus cavity. Because of this association, infections within the maxillary sinuses can manifest with odontogenic symptomatology and vice versa. The lymphatic drainage is to the submandibular lymph nodes.

The sphenoidal sinus is between the hypophysis and the sphenoethmoidal recess. It is surrounded by the hypophyseal fossa and hypophysis, optic chiasm, nasopharynx, pterygoid

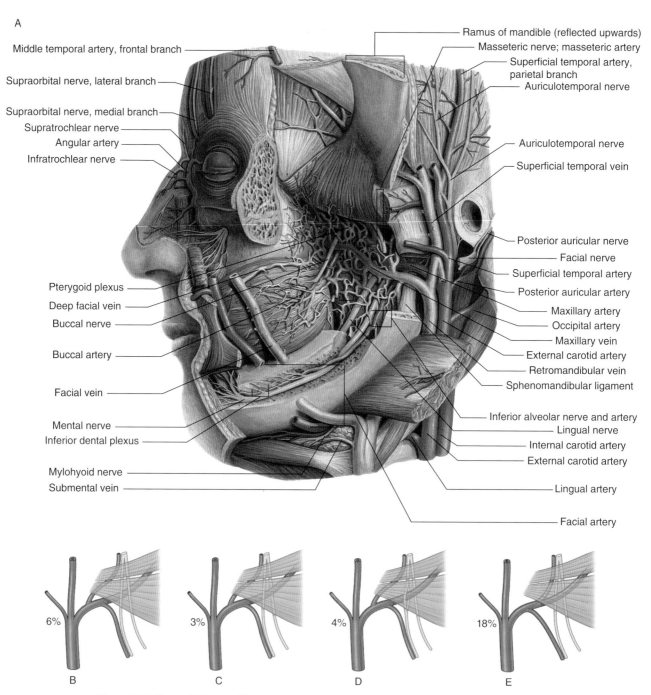

A

Middle temporal artery, frontal branch

Supraorbital nerve, lateral branch

Supraorbital nerve, medial branch

Supratrochlear nerve

Angular artery

Infratrochlear nerve

Ramus of mandible (reflected upwards)

Masseteric nerve; masseteric artery

Superficial temporal artery, parietal branch

Auriculotemporal nerve

Auriculotemporal nerve

Superficial temporal vein

Posterior auricular nerve

Facial nerve

Superficial temporal artery

Posterior auricular artery

Maxillary artery

Occipital artery

Maxillary vein

External carotid artery

Retromandibular vein

Sphenomandibular ligament

Pterygoid plexus

Deep facial vein

Buccal nerve

Buccal artery

Facial vein

Mental nerve

Inferior dental plexus

Mylohyoid nerve

Submental vein

Inferior alveolar nerve and artery

Lingual nerve

Internal carotid artery

External carotid artery

Lingual artery

Facial artery

6%   3%   4%   18%

B   C   D   E

• **Figure 4-29** Pterygoid Venous Plexus and Internal Maxillary Artery Anatomic Variability in the Infra-temporal Fossa. (From Putz R, Pabst R. *Sobotta Atlas of Human Anatomy: Head, Neck, Upper Limb*. 14th ed. Vol. 1. Munich: Elsevier GmbH; 2008.)

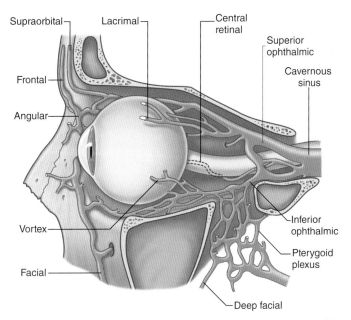

• **Figure 4-30** Depiction of the Pterygoid Venous Plexus With Venous Connections. (From Standring S. *Gray's Anatomy: The Anatomical Basis of Clinical Practice*. 41st ed. Philadelphia: Churchill Livingstone; 2016.)

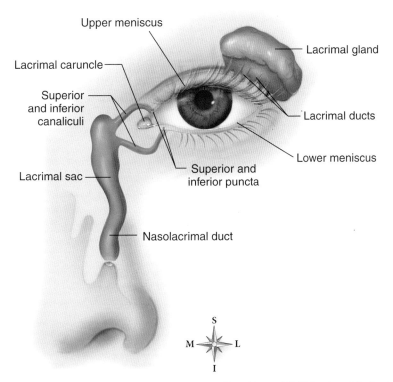

• **Figure 4-31** Depiction of the Nasolacrimal Apparatus. (From Patton KT, Thibodeau GA. *Anatomy and Physiology*. 8th ed. St Louis: Mosby; 2013.)

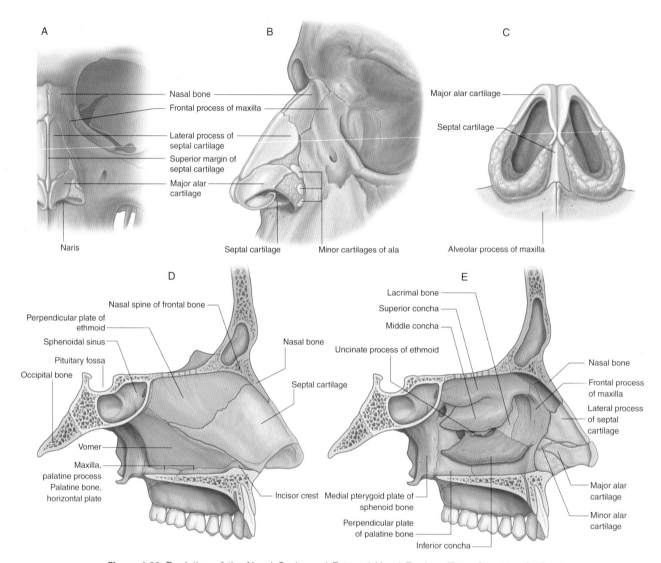

• **Figure 4-32** Depiction of the Nasal Cavity and External Nasal Region. (From Standring S. *Gray's Anatomy: The Anatomical Basis of Clinical Practice*. 41st ed. Philadelphia: Churchill Livingstone; 2016.)

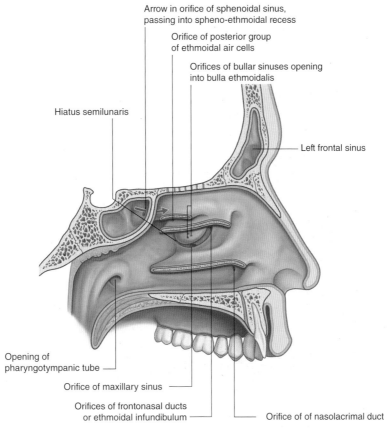

Arrow in orifice of sphenoidal sinus, passing into spheno-ethmoidal recess

Orifice of posterior group of ethmoidal air cells

Orifices of bullar sinuses opening into bulla ethmoidalis

Hiatus semilunaris

Left frontal sinus

Opening of pharyngotympanic tube

Orifice of maxillary sinus

Orifices of frontonasal ducts or ethmoidal infundibulum

Orifice of of nasolacrimal duct

• **Figure 4-33** Lateral Nasal Wall Openings of the Sinuses and Nasolacrimal Duct Ostia. (From Drake RL, Vogl AW, Mitchell AWM. *Gray's Anatomy for Students*. 3rd ed. Philadelphia: Churchill Livingstone; 2015.)

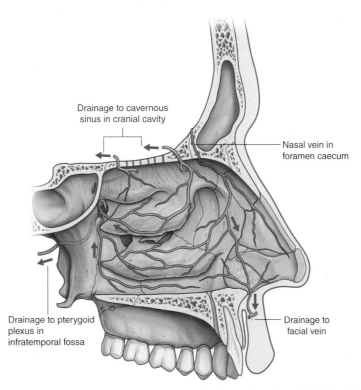

Drainage to cavernous sinus in cranial cavity

Nasal vein in foramen caecum

Drainage to pterygoid plexus in infratemporal fossa

Drainage to facial vein

• **Figure 4-34** Venous Drainage of the Nasal Cavity. (From Drake RL, Vogl AW, Mitchell AWM. *Gray's Anatomy for Students*. 3rd ed. Philadelphia: Churchill Livingstone; 2015.)

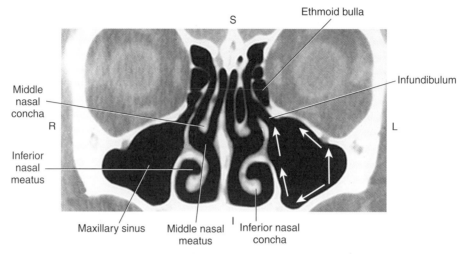

• **Figure 4-35** Coronal Computed Tomography of the Osteomeatal Complex and the Depiction of Mucociliary Flow *(white arrows)*. (From Patton KT, Thibodeau GA. *Anatomy and Physiology.* 8th ed. St Louis: Mosby; 2013.)

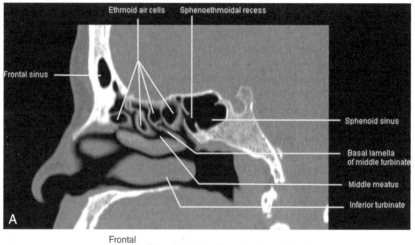

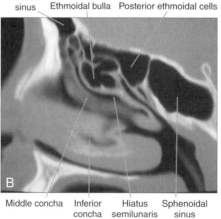

• **Figure 4-36** **A** and **B,** Sagittal section computed tomography of paranasal sinuses. (**A,** From Dym RJ, Masri D, Shfteh K. Imaging of the paranasal sinuses. *Oral Maxillofac Surg Clin North Am.* 2012;24[2]: 175-189; **B,** From Standring S. *Gray's Anatomy: The Anatomical Basis of Clinical Practice.* 41st ed. Philadelphia: Churchill Livingstone; 2016.)

canal, cavernous sinus, internal carotid artery, cranial nerves (III, IV, V1, V2, and VI), and the nasal cavity. The lymphatic drainage is to the retropharyngeal lymph nodes.

The health of the paranasal sinuses depends on immunity, mucociliary clearance, and aeration of the sinuses. The middle meatus forms the common drainage pathway for the anterior ethmoidal, frontal, and maxillary sinuses, and it can be readily examined with a fiberoptic endoscope. The posterior ethmoidal and sphenoidal sinuses drain into the superior meatus and sphenoethmoidal recess. Endoscopic examination will usually show infected mucus draining from these areas. Maxillary sinus infection can also spread from infected teeth. Although the sinus cavities are all intimately associated, infections originating in any of the sinuses can readily transform into pansinus disease.

Pharynx

The pharynx is a 5-inch-long muscular tube whose posterior wall borders the prevertebral fascia (Figure 4-37). It extends from the skull base to the inferior border of the cricoid cartilage at the sixth cervical vertebra (C6). It lies posterior to the larynx and oral and nasal cavities, and it is divided into three areas: nasopharynx, oropharynx, and laryngopharynx.

The nasopharynx is posterior to the nasal cavity and superior to the soft palate. The posterior nasal aperture transitions to the nasopharynx. The pharyngeal tonsil is housed by the mucosa above the pharyngeal recess. The pharyngotympanic tube opening connects the middle ear to the nasopharynx, anterior to the salpingopharyngeal fold.

Waldeyer's Ring

This parapharyngeal lymphatic tissue consists of the pharyngeal tonsils (adenoids), the lingual tonsils, and the palatine tonsils. The lateral tonsillar area drains into the main tonsil lymph node in the angle formed by the junction of the facial vein and the internal jugular vein. It is below the lower jaw angle, and drainage includes lymph nodes in the posterior suprahyoid region. Lymph drains to the superior pharyngeal lymphoid tissue from the pharyngeal tonsils. Tongue base lymphoid tissue drains into the deep cervical nodal chain between the posterior belly of the digastric and the omohyoid muscles. The "adenoid glands" are part of the upper vertical deep cervical chain. The posterior submandibular lymph nodes lie close to the spinal accessory nerve deep to the sternocleidomastoid.

The laryngopharynx is posterior to the larynx. It extends from the hyoid bone to the inferior border of cricoid cartilage, with the epiglottis and the aditus of the larynx found in the midline. The larynx, thyroid cartilage, and the inferior pharyngeal constrictor muscle border the lateral piriform recess. The overlapping constrictor muscles create four potential channels (gaps) in the pharyngeal muscles, through which varying structures traverse (Figure 4-38 and Box 4-3).

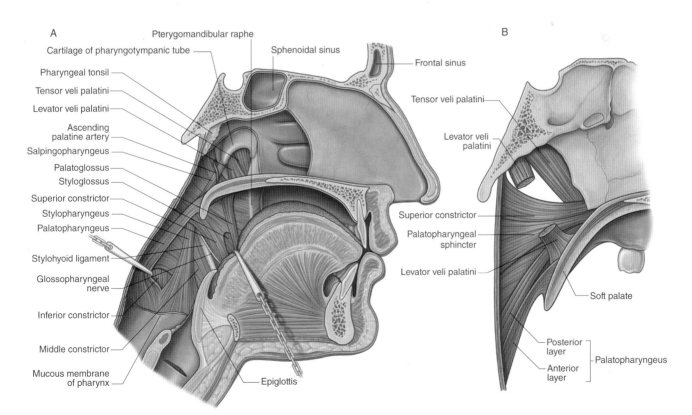

• **Figure 4-37** Pharynx Interior With the Lining Mucosa Removed. (From Standring S. *Gray's anatomy: the anatomical basis of clinical practice.* 41st ed. Philadelphia: Churchill Livingstone; 2016.)

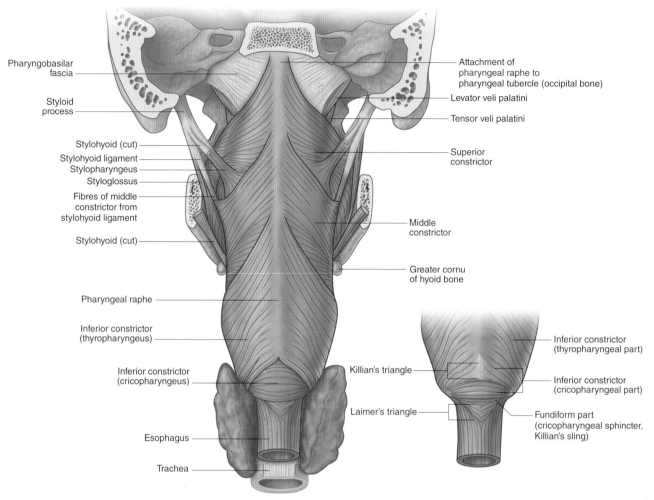

• **Figure 4-38** Posterior View of the Pharynx and the Overlapping Constrictor Muscles. The pharyngobasilar fascia suspends the nasopharynx. (From Standring S. *Gray's Anatomy: The Anatomical Basis of Clinical Practice.* 41st ed. Philadelphia: Churchill Livingstone; 2016.)

• BOX 4-3 **Pharyngeal Muscle Gap Regions and Contents**

Skull Base-Superior Constrictor M: Pharyngotympanic tube–Levator veli palatini m-Ascending pharyngeal a-Ascending palatine a

Superior and Middle Constrictor Muscles: Stylopharyngeus m-Glossopharyngeal m-Ascending palatine artery tonsillar br-Stylohyoid lig

Middle and Inferior Constrictor M: Internal laryngeal n-Superior laryngeal a and v

Inferior border of the Inferior Constrictor M: Recurrent laryngeal n-Inferior laryngeal a and v

a, Artery; *m*, muscle; *v*, vein.

Venous drainage is via the pharyngeal plexus in the buccopharyngeal fascia. The pharyngeal vein drains into the internal jugular vein and communicates with the pterygoid venous plexus in the infratemporal fossa lateral to the lateral pterygoid muscle.

Infections within the pharynx can involve an isolated area or spread to involve all three regions and their structures. Infections in this area pose a direct threat to the patency of the airway and should be treated urgently and aggressively (Figure 4-39).

Salivary Glands

Parotid

The parotid gland is entirely serous and pyramidal in shape, with a relatively thick capsule arising from the investing layer of DCF and the superficial layer of investing fascia (Figure 4-40, *A*). The majority (75%) of the gland overlies the masseter muscle, with the remainder occupying a retromandibular location. The facial nerve enters the gland by coursing between the posterior belly of the digastric muscle and the stylohyoid muscle. The carotid sheath contents lie posteromedial to these muscles. The posteromedial border is composed of the stylohyoid muscle and the posterior belly of the digastric muscle. The nerve splits the gland into

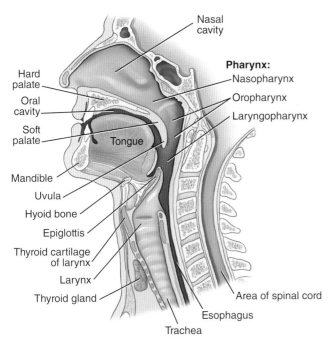

Nasal cavity

Hard palate

Oral cavity

Soft palate

Tongue

Mandible

Uvula

Hyoid bone

Epiglottis

Thyroid cartilage of larynx

Larynx

Thyroid gland

Esophagus

Trachea

Pharynx:

Nasopharynx

Oropharynx

Laryngopharynx

Area of spinal cord

• **Figure 4-39** Depiction of the Pharyngeal Regions of the Upper Aerodigestive Tract. (From Bontrager k, Lampignano J. *Textbook of Radiographic Positioning and Related Anatomy.* 8th ed. St Louis: Mosby; 2014.)

the superficial and deep lobe with a connecting isthmus. The buccal and zygomatic branches form an anastomosing loop superficial to the parotid duct (i.e., Stensen's duct). Bacterial parotitis may initially be contained by the parotid capsule, but eventually a fistula from the gland or duct may extend into the oral cavity or skin with or without sialocele formation.

The lymph node groupings for the parotid gland are superficial and deep. The superficial nodes lie external to the gland capsule, and the deep nodes are intraglandular. They receive drainage from the external ear, eyelids, forehead, and temporal scalp area. The efferent drainage goes to the deep cervical nodes below the mandibular angle. The deep nodes receive drainage from the middle ear, pharyngotympanic tube, hard and soft palate, nose, pterygopalatine fossa, external ear, and parotid parenchyma. Efferent drainage goes to the deep cervical nodes adjacent to the internal jugular vein, where it is crossed by the accessory nerve. Nodes in the deep retromandibular space drain to the deep fossa of the face, and to the deep vertical chain of cervical nodes crossing the omohyoid muscle.

Submandibular

The submandibular gland is in the submandibular triangle with an extension that wraps around the posterior mylohyoid muscle border to enter the oral cavity floor and lie between the hyoglossus muscle and the mandible (see Figure 4-40, *B*). It is surrounded by the investing layer of DCF. The facial artery courses between the gland and the

mandible, and the vein usually lies superficial to the gland. The submental artery usually branches from the facial artery anterior to the gland.

The submandibular lymph nodes are arranged in three main groupings: extracapsular nodes (superficial and lateral), subcapsular nodes, and intraglandular nodes. They receive lymph drainage from the submental nodes and higher drainage system; the mouth floor; the mandibular teeth, gingiva, and mucosa; mouth commissure; superficial parotid nodes; lateral upper and lower lips; the cheek; and the tongue tip. The deep posterior cervical lymph nodes are in close proximity to the bifurcation nodes around the common facial vein trunk, and submandibular nodes.

Floor of the Mouth (FOM) and Sublingual

The sublingual gland is located in the floor of the anterior oral cavity between the mucosa and the mylohyoid muscle, and the mandible sublingual fossa and the genioglossus muscle (see Figure 4-40, *C*). The floor is formed by the anterior mylohyoid muscle and posterior hyoglossus muscle. These muscles separate the FOM from the submandibular and submental neck regions. The posterior sublingual area is the anterior tonsillar pillar. The anterior boundary is the lingual mandible posterior and lateral to the symphysis. Infection in this area can rapidly pass by direct extension between the mylohyoid and hyoglossus muscles or lymphatic spread to the submental and submandibular gland projection, Wharton's duct, the excretory duct of the sublingual (SL) gland, lingual and hypoglossal nerves, and the SL blood vessels and lymphatics. Lymphatic drainage travels to the suprahyoid, submental, and submandibular nodes, and then to the superior deep cervical chain.

Neck

Larynx

The larynx is a complex organ that connects the oropharynx with the trachea. The superior laryngeal vein drains into the internal jugular vein. The inferior laryngeal vein drains into the left brachiocephalic vein via the inferior thyroid vein or the anterior tracheal venous plexus. The lymphatic vessels superior to the vocal folds drain into the superior deep cervical lymph nodes. The lymphatic vessels inferior to the vocal folds drain into the inferior deep cervical lymph nodes via the paratracheal or pretracheal lymph nodes.

Thyroid

The thyroid gland is positioned below the cricoid cartilage, anterior to the trachea, and surrounded by fibrous tissue that fuses with the visceral portion of the pretracheal layer of the DCF. It wraps around the trachea to border the carotid sheath and buccopharyngeal fascia. The external surface of the thyroid is covered by a rich anastomosing plexus of lymphatic vessels, as well as thyroid and parathyroid

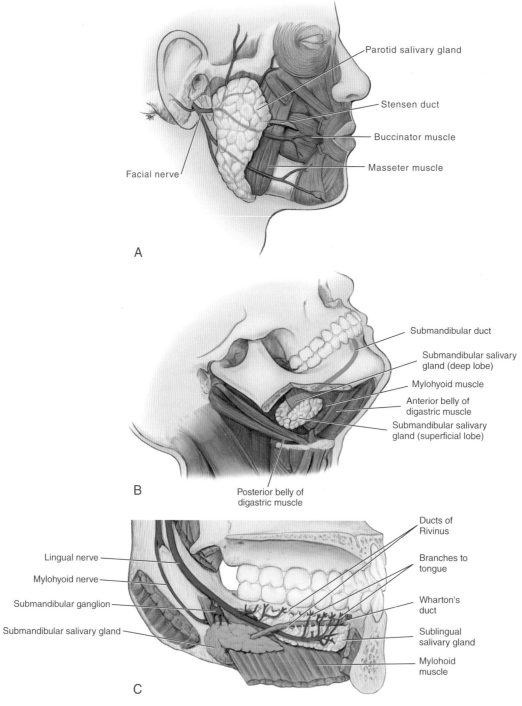

• **Figure 4-40** Depiction of the Major Salivary Glands. **A,** Parotid gland. **B,** Submandibular gland. **C,** Sublingual gland. (Modified from Fehrenbach MF, Herring SW. *Illustrated Anatomy of the Head and Neck.* 4th ed. St Louis: Saunders; 2012.)

nodes. The larger extraglandular collecting trunks drain the plexus and nodes into the paratracheal nodes.

Lymphatic System

Regional lymph nodes that are associated with particular organs or anatomic areas serve a primary filtering function, as compared with collecting lymph nodes that receive lymph fluid from multiple regional lymph node groups (Figure 4-41). In the head and neck, lymph draining to scattered regional nodes flows through the deep cervical collecting lymph nodes (Figure 4-42). The two main areas where lymphatic pathways intersect are the jugulofacial venous junction and the jugulosubclavian venous junction. There are no lymphatic structures in the cranial cavity.

Superficial nodes surround the neck from the inferior border of the mandible on one side and extend around the back of the neck to the corresponding location on the contralateral side. Deep nodes are positioned along the deep vessels of the head and neck. They constitute submental and submandibular nodes, nodes along the internal jugular vein, posterior cervical triangle nodes, and anterior cervical nodes.

Lymphatic vessels of the head drain to the superficial ring of nodes, and then to the superior deep cervical nodes. Facial nodes drain to the submandibular group before draining to the superior deep cervical nodes. Eight lymph node groups drain the head (Figure 4-43 and Table 4-3).

Lymph fluid from the occipital, retroauricular, preauricular, facial, and deep parotid nodes travels to the superior deep cervical nodes. The neck nodal groups, including the superficial cervical, retropharyngeal, submandibular, submental, deep facial, and jugulodigastric nodes, all drain to the superior deep cervical nodes. Tongue drainage is to the submandibular, suprahyoid, superior deep cervical, inferior deep cervical, and jugulo-omohyoid nodal groups (Figure 4-44). The anterior cervical nodes, both superficial and deep (prelaryngeal–pretracheal), drain to the superior deep cervical nodes. Lymph drainage from the tongue is via four major lymph channels. The apical draining the tongue tip is to the submental and submandibular nodes, and to the deep cervical chain supraomohyoid nodes. Marginal channels drain the lateral tongue to submandibular and then to deep cervical nodes. Central channels drain the central raphe area downward between the genioglossus muscles to affect the deep cervical chains. Basal channels drain the posterior tongue to enter the deep cervical nodes that mainly lay between the posterior digastric belly and the omohyoid muscle.

The laryngeal pharynx and upper esophagus drain to the inferior deep cervical nodes. The jugulo-omohyoid nodes

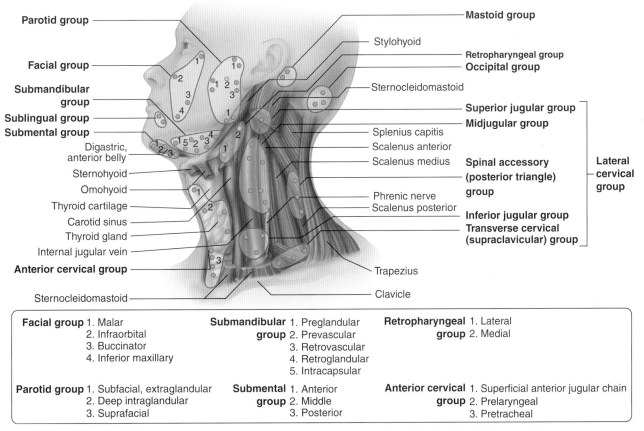

| Facial group | 1. Malar
2. Infraorbital
3. Buccinator
4. Inferior maxillary | Submandibular group | 1. Preglandular
2. Prevascular
3. Retrovascular
4. Retroglandular
5. Intracapsular | Retropharyngeal group | 1. Lateral
2. Medial |
| Parotid group | 1. Subfacial, extraglandular
2. Deep intraglandular
3. Suprafacial | Submental group | 1. Anterior
2. Middle
3. Posterior | Anterior cervical group | 1. Superficial anterior jugular chain
2. Prelaryngeal
3. Pretracheal |

• **Figure 4-41** Head and Neck Lymph Node Groups. (From Standring S. *Gray's Anatomy: The Anatomical Basis of Clinical Practice*. 41st ed. Philadelphia: Churchill Livingstone; 2016.)

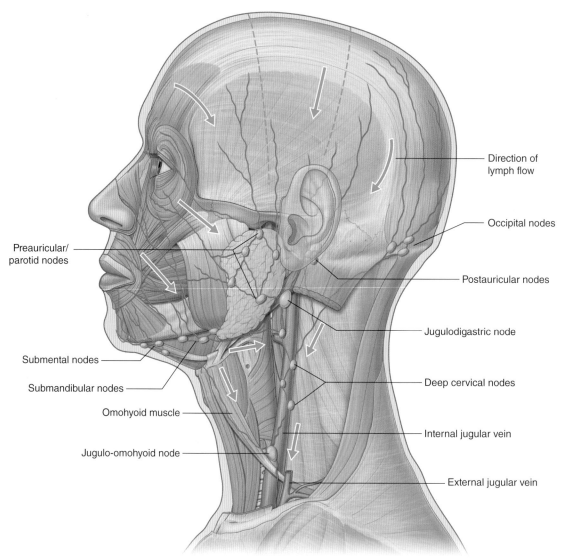

Preauricular/
parotid nodes

Submental nodes

Submandibular nodes

Omohyoid muscle

Jugulo-omohyoid node

Direction of
lymph flow

Occipital nodes

Postauricular nodes

Jugulodigastric node

Deep cervical nodes

Internal jugular vein

External jugular vein

• **Figure 4-42** Lymphatic Drainage of the Head and Neck. (Redrawn from Robinson JK. Basic cutaneous surgery concepts. In Robinson JK, Arndt KA, LeBoit PE, Wintroub BU, eds. *Atlas of Cutaneous Surgery*. Philadelphia: Saunders; 1996.)

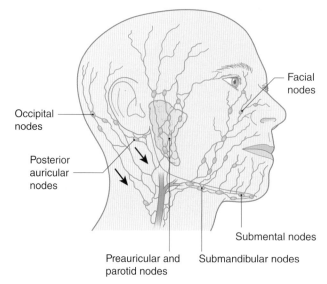

Occipital
nodes

Posterior
auricular
nodes

Facial
nodes

Preauricular and
parotid nodes

Submandibular nodes

Submental nodes

• **Figure 4-43** Face and Scalp Lymphatic Drainage. *Arrows* indicate drainage to the upper cervical nodes. (From Nouri K, Leal-Khouri S, Khouri R. *Techniques in Dermatologic Surgery*. St Louis: Mosby; 2003.)

TABLE 4-3   Lymphatic Drainage of Head and Neck

Structure	Position	Nodes
Face and scalp	Anterior Lateral	Facial → Submandibular → Deep cervical Parotid → Deep cervical
Scalp	Posterior	Occipital → Deep cervical
Eyelids	Medial Lateral	Submandibular → Deep cervical Parotid → Deep cervical
Chin		Submental → Submandibular → Deep cervical
External ear	Anterior Posterior	Parotid → Deep cervical Post-auricular → Deep cervical
Middle ear		Parotid → Deep cervical
Neck	Superficial Deep	Superficial cervical (ant, lat, and post) → Deep cervical Deep cervical
Floor of mouth	Anterior, lower incisors Lateral, teeth except incisors	Submental → Submandibular → Deep cervical or Submental → Deep cervical
Palatine tonsil Pharyngeal tonsil Nasopharynx Paranasal sinuses Soft palate Nasal cavity	Anterior Posterior	Jugulodigastric → Deep cervical Retropharyngeal → Deep cervical Submandibular → Deep cervical Retropharyngeal → Deep cervical
Larynx	Above cords Below cords	Superior deep cervical Laryngeal and tracheal → Inferior deep cervical
Oropharynx		Deep cervical
Cervical esophagus	C6-Superior posterior mediastinum	Tracheal plexus/deep cervical LN in this area if connections exist
Thyroid	Upper part Lower part	Laryngeal → Deep cervical Tracheal or superior mediastinal
Tongue	Tip bilateral	Submental → Submandibular → Deep cervical and jugulo-omohyoid
	Lateral borders	Submandibular → Deep cervical and jugulo-omohyoid

From Hutchings RT, Logan BM, Reynolds P. *McMinn's Color Atlas of Head and Neck Anatomy*. 3rd ed. St Louis: Mosby; 2003:103.

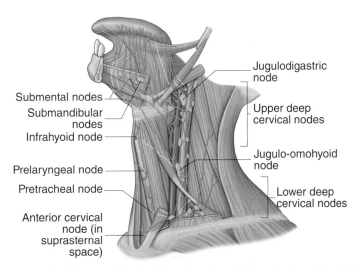

• **Figure 4-44** Lymphatic Drainage of Tongue. (From Standring S. *Gray's Anatomy: The Anatomical Basis of Clinical Practice*. 41st ed. Philadelphia: Churchill Livingstone; 2016.)

drain to the jugular trunk. The jugular trunk on the right side ends at the internal jugular and subclavian junction, or right lymphatic duct. The left side ends in the thoracic duct.

Mucosa-associated lymphoid tissue is distributed along the internal mucosal lining and constitutes the most extensive component of human lymphoreticular tissue. These specialized tissues protect the body from an enormous plethora of antigens. The tonsils, Peyer patches of the small intestine, and the vermiform appendix are examples of mucosa-associated lymphoid tissue.

Bibliography

Agur AMR, Dalley AF. *Grant's Atlas of Anatomy.* 13th ed. Philadelphia: Lippincott Williams and Wilkins; 2012.

Hupp JR, Ellis E, Tucker M. *Contemporary Oral and Maxillofacial Surgery.* 6th ed. St Louis: Elsevier; 2014.

Janfaza P, Nadol J Jr, Galla R, et al., eds. *Surgical Anatomy of the Head and Neck.* Philadelphia: Lippincott Williams and Wilkins; 2000.

Kumar V, Abbas AK In: Kumar V, ed, et al. *Robbins and Cotran Pathologic Basis of Disease.* 9th ed. St Louis: Elsevier Saunders; 2015.

Lindner H. *Clinical Anatomy.* New York: Lange; 1992.

Logan B, Reynolds PA, Rice S, Hutchings RT. *McMinn's Color Atlas of Head and Neck Anatomy.* 5th ed. St Louis: Mosby Elsevier; 2016.

Möeller TB, Reif E. *Pocket Atlas of Sectional Anatomy: Head and neck.* 3rd ed. Vol 1. New York: Thieme; 2007.

Moore KL, Agur AMR, Dalley AF. *Clinically Oriented Anatomy.* 7th ed. Philadelphia: Wolters Kluwer; 2013.

Netter FH. *Atlas of Human Anatomy.* 6th ed. St Louis: Saunders Elsevier; 2013.

Norton NS. *Netter's Head and Neck Anatomy for Dentistry.* 3rd ed. St Louis: Saunders Elsevier; 2017.

Rohen JW, Lutjen-Drecoll E, Yokochi C. *Color Atlas of Anatomy.* Philadelphia: Lippincott Williams & Wilkins; 2011.

Romanes GJ. *Cunningham's Manual of Practical Anatomy, Head Neck and Brain.* 16th ed. Vol. III. Oxford: Oxford Medical Publications; 2018.

Rosse C, Gaddum-Rosse P. *Hollinshead's Textbook Of Anatomy.* 5th ed. Philadelphia: Lippincott; 1997.

Ryan S. *Anatomy for Diagnostic Imaging.* 3rd ed. St Louis: Saunders Elsevier: 2010.

Sandring S. *Gray's Anatomy: The Anatomical Basis of Clinical Practice.* 40th ed. Philadelphia: Churchill-Livingstone Elsevier; 2008.

Schuenke M, Schulte E, Schumacher U. In: Baker EW, ed. *Head and Neck Anatomy for Dental Medicine.* Stuttgart: Thieme; 2010.

5

Introduction to the Laboratory Diagnosis of Infectious Diseases

THOMAS S. MURRAY, NEIL HAYCOCKS, AND SUSAN L. FINK

The accurate diagnosis of an infectious etiology of diseases of the head and neck relies in part on appropriate specimen collection, rapid transportation to the medical microbiology laboratory, and effective communication between the clinical care team and laboratory personnel (Figure 5-1).[1,2] A number of different modalities are used in microbial diagnostics, integrating specialized laboratory services, including clinical immunology for serologic testing, the pathology laboratory for direct visualization of histopathologic specimens and microorganisms in primary tissue, and the clinical microbiology laboratory for the detection, by nucleic acid or antigen testing, and cultivation of microorganisms. This chapter reviews the various tools available for determining the microbiology of infectious diseases affecting the head, neck, and orofacial regions.

In 2018, the Infectious Disease Society of America and the American Society for Microbiology jointly published updated recommendations for the laboratory diagnosis of infectious diseases organized by organ systems.[1,2] This publication is an excellent reference for clinicians and laboratorians to help with ordering the appropriate diagnostic tests when evaluating a patient with a possible head, neck, or orofacial infection.[1,2]

Anatomic pathology is the discipline that relies on direct visualization of human tissue, both grossly and microscopically, to render appropriate diagnoses. Many so-called special stains have been developed, some dating back to the 1800s, for the purpose of identifying and classifying microorganisms in biopsy or excisional specimens. Gram stain and various acid-fast stains still have broad usage for detecting bacteria and mycobacteria, respectively. Periodic acid–Schiff is a common stain capable of elucidating viable fungal elements (Figure 5-2) and certain bacteria (e.g., *Tropheryma whipplei*). Grocott methenamine silver is also commonly used and will highlight viable and nonviable fungal cells. Immunohistochemistry, which relies on the application of labeled antibodies to histologic specimens, has become more prevalent as a diagnostic tool for infectious agents. Commercially available immunohistochemistry stains that target bacteria (e.g., *Bartonella henselae*, *Mycobacterium tuberculosis*), viruses (e.g., Epstein-Barr virus [EBV], herpes simplex virus 1 and 2), and parasites (e.g., *Toxoplasma gondii*) are readily available (Figure 5-3). In some instances, these stains have essentially replaced older, silver-based stains, such as Warthin-Starry, for the visualization of specific microbes. In situ hybridization using nucleic acid probes has become more common as well, with the detection of EBV-encoded small RNA being a prototypical example (Figure 5-4).

Serologic testing identifies pathogen-specific antibodies produced during an immune response, as a diagnostic indicator of acute infection, prior infection, or vaccination. Serologic study is typically most useful in the diagnosis of infections involving organisms that are difficult to culture or detect by other means. Immunoglobulin (Ig) M is the first class of antibodies produced during an initial immune response and the presence of pathogen-specific IgM often indicates acute or recent infection. IgM antibodies are limited in their specificity and can be cross-reactive, producing false-positive results. IgG responses take longer to develop and may reflect prior infection or vaccination.

Clinical microbiology laboratories use a number of rapid tests to detect specific microbial antigens or nucleic acids in primary nontissue specimens. For example, *Cryptococcus* antigen testing can be performed on cerebral spinal fluid (CSF), and antigen testing for respiratory viruses can be performed on nasopharyngeal specimens. Molecular techniques are being used increasingly in clinical laboratories to detect pathogen-specific nucleic acids and have most notably been applied to virologic diagnosis, as discussed later. The introduction and rapid expansion of molecular techniques, especially nucleic acid detection methods such as polymerase chain reaction (PCR)/DNA amplification, to the identification of infectious agents requires clinicians to be familiar with the properties of these diagnostic tests.

In addition, the clinical microbiology laboratory is responsible for growing microorganisms from primary specimens

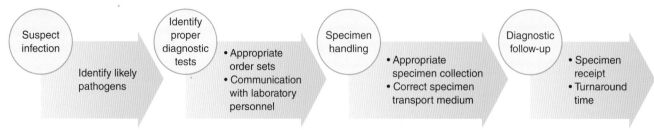

• **Figure 5-1** Initial approach to diagnostics for infectious diseases. Proper ordering, collection, and transport of primary specimens offer the best chance at recovering the etiologic agent.

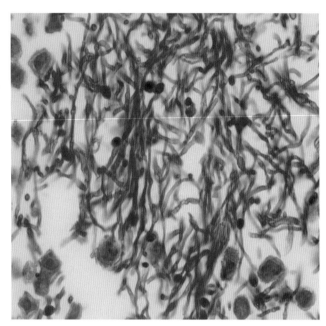

• **Figure 5-2** Periodic acid–Schiff stain for viable fungal hyphae. Positive special staining for viable fungal elements, which contrast sharply with the background of inflammatory exudate.

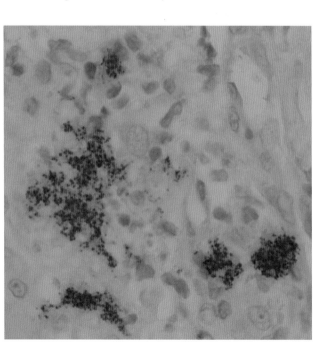

• **Figure 5-3** Immunohistochemistry bacterial staining. Positive immunohistochemical staining for *Bartonella henselae,* the etiologic agent of cat scratch disease. This preparation used a red chromophore directed against a *B. henselae* antigen.

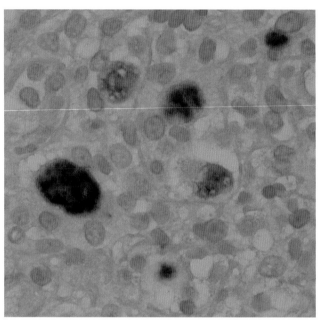

• **Figure 5-4** Epstein-Barr virus (EBV) diagnosed with in situ hybridization. In situ hybridization for EBV-encoded small RNA (EBER). This patient was positive for HIV and had persistent fever and lymphadenopathy, which was ultimately found to be EBV-positive Hodgkin lymphoma.

and identifying those most likely to be pathogenic.[3] In the virology laboratory, this requires the use of specific mammalian cell lines necessary for viral replication, whereas in the bacteriology and mycology laboratories, a variety of culture media with different nutritional components and different growth conditions (aerobic and anaerobic) are used to maximize the recovery of viable organisms. An advantage of cultivation over molecular techniques is that in most cases the susceptibility of a pathogen to a panel of antimicrobials can be determined by examining growth inhibition in the presence of a drug.

Specimen Collection and Test Ordering

Regardless of the specimen type, the first step toward the correct diagnosis involves ordering the proper diagnostic tests (see Figure 5-1). Initially, the likely organisms responsible for the presenting clinical syndrome are identified to determine the most sensitive and specific tests for those pathogens. An organism that is difficult to grow in the microbiology laboratory can be best diagnosed by alternative approaches, including molecular techniques or serologic studies, if available. The treating provider must be aware of which organisms will be identified from the specimen based on the type of laboratory order. For example, ordering a routine bacterial culture and susceptibility on a specimen typically does not result in an attempt to identify and grow mycobacteria, because these organisms have specialized growth requirements; an order for a separate test specific for mycobacteria is required. *Bordetella pertussis* is another example of a respiratory pathogen that requires unique growth conditions; therefore, it will not be recovered from routine bacterial cultures. In addition, if the patient has an underlying condition that puts him or her at increased risk for certain infectious agents, this information should also be conveyed to the clinical laboratory through either the order set or the label. For example, many laboratories have unique order sets for respiratory specimens from patients with cystic fibrosis that optimize the recovery of known cystic fibrosis pathogens such as *Burkholderia cepacia*. If this information is not conveyed to the laboratory, the specimen might not be plated to selective media for growth of these organisms.

Having a list of the potential pathogens is also important in determining the appropriate transport media as samples tested for viruses are transported under different conditions than samples sent for bacterial isolation (discussed later). Because many microorganisms are fastidious and may die rapidly when exposed to oxygen, rapid transport to the microbiology laboratory is of critical importance to give the microbiology laboratory the best opportunity to recover viable organisms for identification and antimicrobial susceptibility testing. If the clinical team is unsure about either the appropriate tests to order or the best method to collect and transport the specimen, direct consultation with staff members at the clinical laboratory can ensure that the patient samples are handled optimally. If unusual organisms are suspected, communication with laboratory personnel is critical before specimen collection to ensure optimal collection, transport, and growth conditions in the microbiology laboratory to maximize the chances of recovering viable organisms.

After the appropriate tests have been ordered, the next step is the proper collection of the sample (see Figure 5-1). The recovery of viable pathogens is optimized if sample collection occurs before initiating antimicrobial therapy. If collection of the material requires incision and drainage, sterilization of the skin with chlorhexidine is the preferred method.[1] In many cases, to get to the infected area, the clinician must either sample from or pass through a site that is not normally sterile, such as the oral cavity or nasal sinuses. Care must be taken to try to limit contamination with commensal flora. If the sample is not collected in a sterile manner, this important information should be conveyed to the clinical laboratory to assist in the interpretation of the growth of microorganisms from the sample.

As a general rule for patient samples when bacteria or fungi are the suspected cause of the pathologic process, pus or tissue is highly preferred to a swab of the infected area.

Although flocked swabs demonstrate improved recovery of organisms compared with conventional swabs, swabs tend to absorb small amounts of sample, and bacteria and fungi may cling to the swab when plated for growth. When a viral cause is suspected and molecular diagnostic approaches will be used, in many cases a swab of the appropriate patient material is sufficient to make the diagnosis. Another general rule is that the more volume of sample that is collected, the more the likelihood of recovering an organism from the sample increases. An important exception regarding direct sample collection is the unstable airway in epiglottitis where blood culture is the preferred diagnostic technique. Sampling directly from the epiglottis may result in tracheal occlusion and should be performed only after the airway has been secured.[1]

Once the sample has been collected into the appropriate transport media, the sample should be labeled appropriately (see Figure 5-1). In addition to the correct patient information, specimen information should include the location of the lesion, the specimen type (e.g., pus, tissue, prosthetic material), and how it was collected (e.g., needle aspiration, open incision, biopsy, swab). If there are multiple lesions or specimens collected differently, labeling which specimen came from each lesion is critical to ensure the reporting of accurate results. For example, superficial drainage from an open wound cultured at the beginning of a surgical procedure (potentially contaminated with skin flora) may yield organisms that are different from those in an intraoperative deep biopsy specimen from what should be a sterile site. The labels of these specimens should reflect these differences in collection, even from the same lesion.

Specimens sent to an anatomic pathology laboratory are often submitted in formalin, which fixes and preserves the tissue for processing and examination. Other options include submitting tissue fresh, in sterile saline, or in a defined cell growth medium, such as Roswell Park Memorial Institute medium (RPMI-1640). These latter options enable the anatomic laboratory staff member to reserve some viable tissue for ancillary studies, which may include flow cytometric analysis, fluorescent in situ hybridization analysis, or cytogenetic analysis. This can be particularly helpful if the specimen is a lymph node, because lymphoma is often in the differential diagnosis of a possible infection. In general, it is advisable to send some or all collected lymph node tissue in RPMI, with the clinical suspicion clearly explained on the requisition form. If the tissue is collected during off hours or in an office setting and is at risk of being processed the following day, the submitting clinician should contact the laboratory and arrange for appropriate handling of the specimen.

Virology

Laboratory diagnosis of viral infection relies on four principal modalities: culture, antigen detection, nucleic acid detection, and serology. Each method has particular advantages and limitations, and recent improvements in technology have led to increasing dominance of nucleic acid–based testing.

Because viruses are obligate intracellular pathogens, their detection with culture-based techniques requires inoculation of viable virions into susceptible host cells. Growth of specific viruses produces characteristic cytopathic changes or can be detected by staining the cell monolayer for specific viral antigens using fluorescently labeled antibodies. Although detection of viral pathogens by tissue culture methods has been the traditional means of diagnosis, viral culture requires technical proficiency, is labor intensive, generally has a longer turnaround time than newer methods do, and is frequently less sensitive than nucleic acid–based detection methods. An advantage of culture is that it can sometimes identify viruses that may not have been clinically suspected and can provide a somewhat unbiased approach to viral diagnosis. Shell vial culture is a modification of traditional culture techniques that allows detection after a shortened incubation period (1 to 3 days) and can be used for cytomegalovirus (CMV).

Many viruses can be rapidly identified directly from patient samples using antibody reagents specific for viral antigens. For example, in direct fluorescent antibody (DFA) tests, the patient's primary specimen is stained with specific fluorescently labeled antibodies and examined microscopically (Figure 5-5). DFA tests may be performed on mucosal and skin lesions for herpes simplex virus and varicella-zoster virus, as well as on ocular specimens for identification of herpes simplex virus and adenovirus. Respiratory DFA

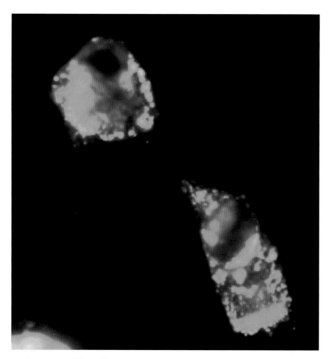

• **Figure 5-5** Direct fluorescent antibody (DFA) testing for respiratory viruses. In this example, the DFA test detects parainfluenza infection of respiratory epithelial cells from a nasal swab specimen. A fluorescence-labeled antibody that recognizes a parainfluenza antigen is detected using fluorescence microscopy.

panels have been used to detect multiple common viral respiratory pathogens, including influenza A and B, respiratory syncytial virus, adenovirus, parainfluenza viruses, and metapneumovirus. However, DFA procedures can be labor intensive and require a certain level of technical expertise for accurate interpretation, and, although more rapid than culture, they have largely been replaced by nucleic acid testing for respiratory specimens. With the SARS-CoV-2 pandemic, lateral flow colorimetric point-of-care rapid antigen testing for SARS-CoV-2 is now widely available. This test, while it can be performed at home, has varying sensitivity and specificity depending on the patient population and is less sensitive than the gold standard nucleic acid–based tests to diagnose SARS-CoV-2 infection.[4]

Nucleic acid–based testing is routinely available for sensitive and specific detection of viral DNA and RNA and has become the dominant method of testing for many viral pathogens. Detection of small quantities of viral nucleic acid is accomplished by target amplification methods, including PCR or signal amplification technologies such as hybrid capture. Nucleic acid–based methods do not rely on propagation of viable infectious virions, which allows greater latitude in specimen collection and transport and has expanded testing to viruses that have been difficult to grow in culture. These tests can generally be performed rapidly, often with results within several hours. Automation and the ability to combine several viral nucleic acid tests in a single multiplex assay has greatly accelerated throughput. A variety of commercial multiplex molecular panels allow for the detection of multiple respiratory viral pathogens from a single nasopharyngeal swab, each performing slightly differently.[5] For certain viruses such as adenovirus or HIV in the blood, real-time PCR permits not only detection but also accurate quantitation, and it is used to monitor viral loads and provide assessment of therapeutic response. Nucleic acid–based methods are also increasingly available to detect mutations associated with antiviral resistance.

Viral serology involves detecting pathogen-specific antibodies produced by infected patients; it can be useful for diagnosing recent infection and determining immunity. Serology is most often used for diagnosis when nucleic acid–based or other methods are not available or for infections in which viral titer decreases before clinical symptoms develop.

EBV infection induces not only virus-specific antibodies but also non-EBV heterophile antibodies. These broadly reactive antibodies agglutinate horse red blood cells, the basis of the monospot test. Other viruses for which serologic study is often part of the diagnostic evaluation include CMV, HIV, hepatitis viruses, measles, mumps, rubella, West Nile virus, and other arboviruses.

Bacteriology

As discussed previously, a wide variety of bacterial species are present at diverse anatomic sites as normal microbiota, and these may be recovered in clinical specimens. These organisms may be present along with pathogens, and some members of the normal microbiota are themselves capable of causing disease. Specimen collection that minimizes contamination of normal microbiota is optimal, but many sites are inherently nonsterile and appropriate interpretation of the clinical significance of bacteria recovered from specimens is essential.

The first test for the majority of laboratory specimens sent to the microbiology laboratory for bacterial culture and susceptibility is the Gram stain. This rapid test is used for primary specimens, and although the genus and species are not identified from the Gram stain, the type of staining (Gram positive is purple, Gram negative is pink) and the morphology of the organisms, cocci or rod-shaped, in pairs, clusters, or chains provide the first information about possible pathogens (Figure 5-6). The value of the Gram stain is in directing empiric antibiotic therapy specifically against either gram-positive or gram-negative organisms while awaiting final bacterial identification and susceptibility testing. In general, a Gram stain result is used only to expand antibiotic coverage, rather than narrow empiric therapy, pending the culture results.

In addition to the Gram stain, bacteria are primarily detected in clinical specimens by growth in culture. Media for culturing a given specimen type are chosen to optimize growth of the pathogens commonly encountered at a particular site and with consideration for the need to identify pathogenic bacteria within a mixed population of normal flora. In most cases, specimens are simultaneously inoculated on multiple types of media to maximize recovery and differentiation of organisms. Agar plates supplemented with blood allow growth of most medically significant bacteria and reveal patterns of hemolysis that aid in the identification of organisms. Chocolate agar contains blood that has been heated to release factors that aid in the growth of fastidious bacteria, most notably *Haemophilus* and *Neisseria* species. Selective media inhibit the growth of certain organisms, while allowing growth of others. An example is 5% sheep blood agar plates with colistin and nalidixic acid, which inhibits the growth of gram-negative bacilli while permitting gram-positive bacteria to grow. Differential media have properties that allow certain organisms to produce characteristic changes or growth patterns that aid in identification. Head, neck, and orofacial infections may be caused by strictly anaerobic bacteria such as *Fusobacterium* species that are killed by normal atmospheric concentrations of oxygen. If an anaerobic organism is suspected, the sample should be collected and cultured under anaerobic conditions.

Bacterial cultures generally require 18 to 24 hours of incubation for growth to be visible, with longer incubations required for some fastidious organisms and anaerobes. Anaerobic bacterial growth may not be checked for 48 hours, such that any reported results before this time should be interpreted with caution. Agar plates are carefully examined not only for the presence of growth, but to distinguish normal flora from potential pathogens (Figure 5-7). Accurate and precise knowledge of the anatomic site sampled is critical for laboratory staff to appropriately interpret bacterial culture results. The specimen type, as identified by the order and label, determines in part how the microbiology laboratory interprets the recovery of viable bacteria. For sites considered sterile, such as the CSF, the growth of any organism in any amount is reported, and antimicrobial susceptibility testing is performed. In many ENT infections, the site of infection connects either directly or indirectly to a nonsterile location with commensal flora (e.g., the oral cavity). For these specimens, there is an a priori expectation that bacteria will grow from the specimen, even in the absence of a known infectious process. In these cases, the microbiology

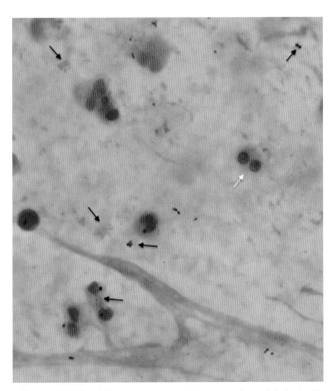

• **Figure 5-6** Mixed flora from a respiratory specimen labeled with Gram stain. The *black arrows* show both gram-positive *(dark, purple)* and gram-negative *(light, pink)* bacteria of varying morphologies. The *white arrow* indicates a neutrophil showing an ongoing inflammatory process in the host, consistent with infection.

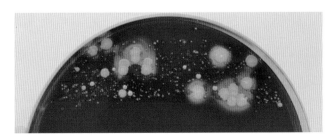

• **Figure 5-7** Growth of mixed flora from a primary specimen. Multiple colony morphologies are present after growth on a blood agar plate. The presence of β-hemolysis (complete lysis of red cells producing transparency) is used to distinguish pathogenic bacteria from commensal flora.

laboratory must attempt to determine whether the growth is mixed normal flora or a pathogen is growing among the normal bacteria (see Figure 5-7). An example of a bacterial characteristic laboratories use to identify pathogens is the presence of β-hemolysis around a colony. *Staphylococcus aureus, Streptococcus pyogenes,* and *Pseudomonas aeruginosa* are examples of pathogens that produce hemolysins that allow their identification from mixed growth (see Figure 5-7). Bacterial colonies are now commonly rapidly identified to the species level by mass spectrometry or using biochemical tests in rapid simple benchtop procedures or in automated systems that recognize the pattern of multiple biochemical reactions.

Antimicrobial therapy can be refined based on Gram stain results and the identification of pathogenic bacteria. For some bacteria, antimicrobial susceptibility is highly predictable and susceptibility testing is not performed. For others, variable resistance necessitates laboratory antimicrobial susceptibility testing, which is most often performed with agar diffusion tests and broth dilution tests. Agar diffusion tests involve growing a standardized inoculum of bacteria on agar plates in the presence of disks or strips impregnated with antibiotics. Inhibited growth surrounding the antibiotic correlates with susceptibility, and clinical guidelines are used to correlate in vitro susceptibility to clinical response. Broth dilution tests are performed in automated systems and similarly rely on growth of a standardized bacterial inoculum in liquid medium with varying concentrations of antibiotic. The antibiotic concentration required to inhibit growth is referred to as the *minimum inhibitory concentration*. As with agar diffusion tests, results of broth dilution tests must be interpreted using clinical guidelines to predict responsiveness to treatment. In a few instances, antibiotic resistance is due to a single gene, and molecular tests have been developed to rapidly identify resistance without the need for bacterial growth required for phenotypic tests. Molecular tests to detect methicillin-resistant *S. aureus* (MRSA) are the most common example. For many organisms, particularly gram-negative rods, antibiotic resistance can be conferred with numerous mechanisms and may be more challenging to detect.

For a few clinical syndromes, specific bacterial antigen testing has been developed for common pathogens. For example, rapid diagnosis of *S. pyogenes* pharyngitis can be easily established by simple antigen tests. However, these tests have imperfect sensitivity and negative rapid antigen tests should be confirmed by culture.[6] In addition, many laboratories now use a rapid molecular test for *S. pyogenes* with sufficient sensitivity to obviate culture for a negative result. Unlike most bacteria, the *Chlamydia* species are obligate intracellular pathogens, and they cannot replicate in standard bacterial culture. Like viral pathogens, DFA or nucleic acid–based tests are most commonly used for these organisms.

Mycobacteria have a unique cell wall rich in mycolic acids, which causes resistance to decolorization by acids during special staining procedures (i.e., Ziehl-Neelsen stain) and leads to their characterization as acid-fast bacilli. Many medically important mycobacteria are also slow growing, often requiring weeks of incubation rather than days, and require special techniques for growth in the microbiology laboratory, necessitating separate culture orders. Specimens for mycobacterial culture from sites containing normal flora are processed with a decontamination step before inoculation of media to prevent normal flora from overgrowing, and cultures are held for extended periods to allow detection of slow-growing organisms. Nucleic acid amplification techniques have enabled rapid detection of *M. tuberculosis* from primary specimens, most notably from sputum. In addition to testing for the presence of mycobacterial organisms, diagnosis of exposure to mycobacterial antigens, as occurs in patients with latent tuberculosis, can be performed using either a tuberculin skin test (TST) or an interferon-γ release assay (IGRA). IGRAs are particularly useful in the setting of Bacillus Calmette-Guérin vaccination for TB as they, in contrast to the TST, do not cross react with the vaccine immune response, reducing the chance of false-positive results.

Mycology

If fungal pathogens are suggested based on the clinical presentation, a separate order is required for mycology processing. Most yeasts, such as *Candida* species and some fungi, will grow on a standard blood agar plate; however, best practice is to include additional diagnostic testing to isolate fungi that grow as molds. This is particularly important for patients with immune system dysfunction, such as those receiving bone marrow transplants and patients with chronic diseases, such as diabetes. As many important fungal pathogens cause invasive disease in regions of the head and neck, tissue obtained by biopsy is often the specimen of choice, and swabs are discouraged because they might not accurately capture the deeper infectious process. Tissue specimens should be placed in a properly labeled, sealed, sterile aerobic container and transported to the microbiology laboratory at room temperature. Drying or freezing of the specimen should be avoided, because it will prevent recovery of viable organisms. If a delay in transport is expected or the tissue sample is small, as in a fine-needle biopsy specimen, sterile gauze moistened with sterile normal saline should be included in the container to prevent dehydration. Ideally, tissue should be sent to both the anatomic pathology laboratory for evidence of invasive fungal disease in fixed tissue and to the microbiology laboratory for recovery and identification of the organism. If limited tissue is available and the index of suspicion for infection is high, material should be sent to the microbiology laboratory for recovery and identification of the offending organism. Although the pathology laboratory can often identify fungal elements when staining tissue that suggest the cause of infection (Figure 5-2), confirmation and definitive diagnosis require growth and identification of the organism. When *Aspergillus* species is suggested in sinus disease, an aspirate from an antral puncture can be collected and transported with a vacuum aspirator.[1]

Common yeasts such as *Candida* species are readily visible with a standard bacterial Gram stain. An exception is *Cryptococcus neoformans,* which stains poorly with Gram stain and is better seen with traditional stains used for fungi. *C. neoformans* is also urease positive when grown and has a thick capsule when visualized with India ink stain. Identification of fungal elements in primary specimens requires additional stains, two of the most common being the Calcofluor-KOH that binds the chitin of fungal cell walls and the previously described periodic acid–Schiff stain that colors the organisms pink because of the presence of hexose.

Ideally, specimens for fungal culture are not ground with pestle and mortar, because this may destroy hyphal elements making fungi nonviable. If a single, small specimen is sent for both bacterial and fungal culture, it may be unavoidable to enhance recovery of bacterial pathogens. Ideally, primary tissue sent for mycology culture should be cut into tiny pieces with scissors or a scalpel to preserve hyphae and viability. Specimens are inoculated to several different media to optimize the recovery of pathogenic fungi. Examples include Sabouraud dextrose with and without chloramphenicol and cycloheximide. The latter antimicrobials are added to prevent growth of bacteria and environmental fungi less likely to be pathogenic. Specimens are also added to a rich brain-heart infusion broth that promotes growth of fastidious fungi. Plates and broth inoculated for fungal growth are incubated at 30°C. Dimorphic fungi such as *Histoplasma capsulatum* grow as a mold at lower temperatures, room temperature to 30°C, and as yeast at higher temperatures similar to body temperature (37°C). When a dimorphic fungus is suspected, increasing the incubation temperature will convert growth from a mold to a yeast form. Because fungal growth rates are generally much slower than bacterial rates, the plates are kept in the laboratory much longer than for bacterial growth, usually up to 28 days before a final determination of no growth.[7]

When growth occurs, the rate of growth and phenotype of the colony provide initial clues to identification. The colony is examined for its color and texture. For example, the colonies of many zygomycetes have a white cotton appearance on the plate. When the colony matures, the morphology of the mold and its fruiting bodies are used for the final identification. To preserve the fungal structures, Scotch tape is lightly pressed on the colony and removed to a drop of lactophenol cotton blue for examination under the light microscope (Figure 5-8). Characteristics of filamentous fungi that aid in identification include the presence or absence of septa, the thickness and angle of hyphal branching, and the morphology of conidia and spores. Two classes of medically important fungi that must be contrasted are the *Aspergillus* species and the zygomycetes (Figure 5-8). *Aspergillus* species typically produce septate hyphae with branching at 45-degree angles with distinctive macroconidia. In contrast, zygomycetes, such as *Mucor* and *Rhizopus* species, are generally aseptate with 90-degree branching of hyphal structures. The vast majority of pathogenic fungi

can be identified based on the morphology of both the colony and the fungal elements. Yeast can be identified by matrix-assisted laser desorption ionization time of flight (MALDI-TOF) mass spectrometry or commercial identification systems based on biochemical properties. Some commercial systems fail to correctly identify *Candida auris,* an increasingly important pathogenic *Candida* species that is often resistant to multiple antifungal agents.[8] If *C. auris* is suspected, the clinical microbiology laboratory should be alerted. Molecular methods can be applied in the mycology laboratory with DNA sequencing of rRNA ribosomal genes of the patient isolate compared with a known database of fungal sequences to identify the pathogen.[7] This technique has been successful in identifying the majority of important pathogenic molds. On occasion, a mold grown from a primary specimen cannot be identified based on morphology because of the lack of distinctive morphology. Some of these unusual organisms can be identified using these molecular techniques, assuming they are represented in the reference database. Given the ubiquitous presence of a diverse population of fungal spores in the environment, it can be difficult to assess whether more unusual fungi are true pathogens. This requires clinical correlation and communication with the mycology laboratory.

As mycology laboratories have improved in identifying both the genus and species of fungi, unusual, environmental fungi are reported in the literature as causing human disease. These reports emphasize that communication between the clinical laboratory and patient care team becomes even more important in determining whether an identified organism is a true pathogen. If the clinician is unfamiliar with the identified mold or yeast or is unsure of the pathogenic potential in the clinical setting, the mycology laboratory can be a resource to provide additional information about the taxonomy of the fungus.

Although the vast majority of invasive fungal diseases are diagnosed based on culture, other tools are also used in the diagnosis of invasive molds and yeasts. Serology from both the serum and CSF aids in the diagnosis of *C. neoformans* and several of the dimorphic fungi such as *H. capsulatum* and *Coccidioides immitis.* More recently, antigen tests for the presence of fungal cell wall components shed into the serum have been used for the detection of invasive fungal disease in immunosuppressed patients. Galactomannan is a polysaccharide shed by *Aspergillus* species during invasive growth and can be a marker for both the presence of *Aspergillus* species and patient response to antifungal therapy, particularly after bone marrow transplant. The sensitivity and specificity of this test varies depending on the population studied, and false-positive (with antibiotic use) and false-negative results are well documented. Another antigen detected in serum, β-D-glucan, is shed by fungi, including but not limited to *Candida* species, *Aspergillus* species, *H. capsulatum,* and *C. immitis* and is used as a diagnostic aid for invasive fungal disease. Importantly, zygomycetes are not detected with either of the above antigen tests.

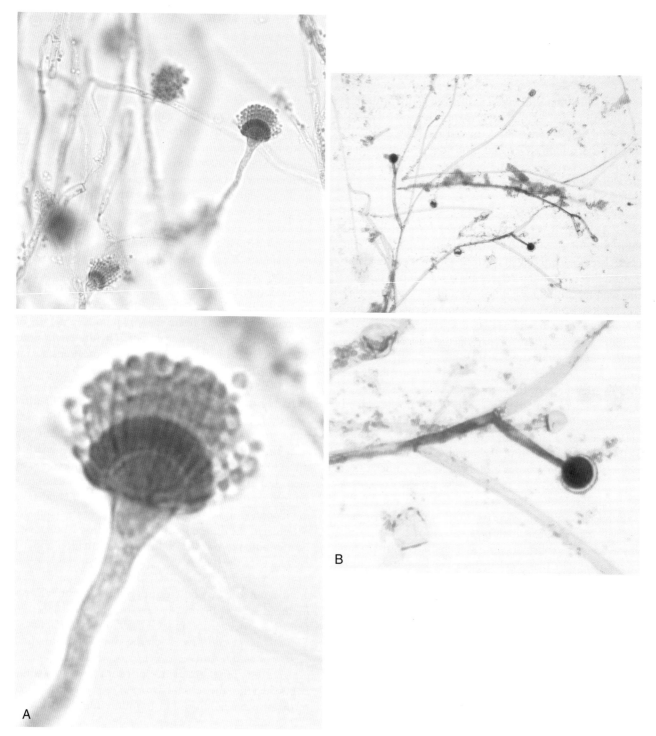

• **Figure 5-8** Morphology and the identification of pathogenic fungi. Fungi stained with lactophenol cotton blue after a Scotch tape preparation from colonies growing on agar plates. **A,** *Aspergillus fumigatus.* Note the circular conidia at the top of the stalk (conidiophore). **B,** The zygomycetes, *Mucor* species. Note the lack of septa and 90-degree branching. Conidia are also absent, which is consistent with a zygomycetes. (Images courtesy Mark Lewis, Yale New Haven Hospital.)

Advances in Diagnostics

Recent advances in technology have led to significant changes in the laboratory diagnosis of microbial infections, and continued advances in the coming years are likely to further change and improve diagnostic testing.[9] Nucleic acid–based testing of primary specimens has fundamentally changed how the clinical microbiology rapidly identifies viral pathogens and some bacterial pathogens. These tests are becoming widespread, easier for smaller laboratories to implement, and more widely applied to bacterial, fungal, and parasitic infections that are difficult to culture. Furthermore, nucleic acid–based tests require only knowledge of conserved sequences characteristic of given pathogens and not laborious development of specialized reagents, such as antibodies. For this reason, they are readily applicable to emerging infections as exemplified by the COVID-19 pandemic. Because of the presence of normal flora, nucleic acid–based testing of primary specimens relies on identification of sequences specific for a given pathogen. Although multiplex assays enable testing for multiple organisms, unlike culture, nucleic acid identification is limited to the specific sequence sought.

Proteomic tools, such as mass spectrometry, have revolutionized clinical microbiology. MALDI-TOF mass spectrometry is increasingly used by clinical microbiology laboratories for the identification of bacteria and yeast isolated in culture.[10] This technique involves generating a proteomic spectrum from abundant peptides and proteins in the sample, particularly ribosomal proteins. Software is used to compare this spectrum to those in a database to identify the organism. Initial databases were focused on medically important bacteria, but with expansion and improvement of databases, identification has been extended to mycology. This technology allows for fast and inexpensive organism identification. In many large hospital laboratories and academic centers, MALDI-TOF has replaced conventional phenotypic methods for pathogen identification.

The latest innovation in the clinical microbiology laboratory is the introduction of next-generation whole-genome DNA sequencing of pathogens.[9] This technology is in its early days of clinical use, but examples of its potential include determining viral variants circulating in a community, whether bacterial isolates recovered in hospital-onset infections are genetically related, suggesting a common source outbreak, and what antibiotic resistance genes are present in a primary specimen. Another area of intense future interest is the development of phenotypic antibiotic susceptibility testing that reduces the turnaround time, quickly identifying resistant bacteria so the appropriate antibiotics can be prescribed.[9]

Acknowledgments

The authors thank Mark Lewis from the Yale New Haven Clinical Microbiology Laboratory for critical evaluation of the chapter and for supplying mycology images.

References

1. Miller JM, Binnicker MJ, Campbell S, et al. A guide to utilization of the microbiology laboratory for diagnosis of infectious diseases: 2018 update by the Infectious Diseases Society of America and the American Society for Microbiology. *Clin Infect Dis.* 2018;67(6):e1-e94. Available at: https://doi.org/10.1093/cid/ciy381.

2. Miller JM, Binnicker MJ, Campbell S, et al. A guide to utilization of the microbiology laboratory for diagnosis of infectious diseases: 2018 update by the Infectious Diseases Society of America and the American Society for Microbiology. *Clin Infect Dis.* 2018;67(6):813-816. Available at: https://doi.org/10.1093/cid/ciy584.

3. Lagier JC, Edouard S, Pagnier I, et al. Current and past strategies for bacterial culture in clinical microbiology. *Clin Microbiol Rev.* 2015;28(1):208-236. Available at: https://doi.org/10.1128/CMR.00110-14.

4. Truong TT, Dien Bard J, Butler-Wu SM. Rapid antigen assays for SARS-CoV-2: promise and peril. *Clin Lab Med.* 2022;42(2):203-222. Available at: https://doi.org/10.1016/j.cll.2022.03.001.

5. Popowitch EB, Kaplan S, Wu Z, et al. Comparative performance of the Luminex NxTAG Respiratory Pathogen Panel, GenMark eSensor Respiratory Viral Panel, and BioFire FilmArray Respiratory Panel. *Microbiol Spectr.* 2022;10(4):e0124822. Available at: https://doi.org/10.1128/spectrum.01248-22.

6. Shulman ST, Bisno AL, Clegg HW, et al. Clinical practice guideline for the diagnosis and management of group A streptococcal pharyngitis: 2012 update by the Infectious Diseases Society of America. *Clin Infect Dis.* 2012;55(10):e86-e102. Available at: https://doi.org/10.1093/cid/cis629.

7. Kozel TR, Wickes B. Fungal diagnostics. *Cold Spring Harb Perspect Med.* 2014;4(4):a019299. Available at: https://doi.org/10.1101/cshperspect.a019299.

8. Centers for Disease Control and Prevention. *Identification. Candida auris: A Drug-Resistant Yeast that Spreads in Healthcare Facilities.* Available at: https://www.cdc.gov/fungal/candida-auris/identification.html.

9. Doern CD, Miller MB, Alby K, et al. Proceedings of the Clinical Microbiology Open 2018 and 2019: a discussion about emerging trends, challenges, and the future of clinical microbiology. *J Clin Microbiol.* 2022;60(7):e0009222. Available at: https://doi.org/10.1128/jcm.00092-22.

10. Tsuchida S, Umemura H, Nakayama T. Current status of matrix-assisted laser desorption/ionization-time-of-flight mass spectrometry (MALDI-TOF MS) in clinical diagnostic microbiology. *Molecules.* 2020;25(20):4775.

6

Imaging for Maxillofacial Infections

DANIEL P. CARUSO AND ZACHARY S. PEACOCK

Imaging has become an essential component of the practice of maxillofacial surgery. Since the advent of roentgenography at the end of the seventeenth century, plain films and later tomograms were used to visualize the hard and soft tissues in the maxillofacial region.[1] In the late 1970s, computed tomography (CT) and magnetic resonance imaging (MRI) became available, allowing the surgeon to use cross-sectional images. In recent years improvements in imaging techniques, speed, resolution, and cost have resulted in a wide range of applications, decreased radiation exposure, real-time imaging, and assessment of specific physiologic processes.

Imaging is currently used for diagnosis, treatment planning, intraoperative guidance, and posttreatment evaluation of a variety of maxillofacial infections.[1,2] Various imaging modalities including CT, MRI, ultrasound (US), and nuclear medicine techniques have a role in the management of infectious processes of the head and neck.[3] The purpose of this chapter is to describe the various methods of imaging and to provide the practitioner with a framework for choosing the appropriate study in specific clinical scenarios.

Imaging Modalities

To determine the appropriate imaging study for a clinical situation, a basic understanding of the individual techniques is necessary. The ordering clinician should understand the utility, benefits, and relative risks for each imaging procedure.

Plain Film and Tomography

Plain films are obtained by using x-rays, a type of electromagnetic radiation that can pass through biologic tissues. An x-ray tube (source) emits x-ray photons, which pass through an object of interest and are absorbed by radiographic film or a digital detector. The resultant image is due to the differential absorption of x-ray photons by different tissue types. High-density tissues (bone) absorb most of the emitted photons and thus appear white on film. Low-density tissues (lungs) are poorly absorbing, allowing most photons to pass through, and appear black on film. Plain films used for the assessment of maxillofacial infections include dental radiographs (bitewing, periapical, occlusal), cephalograms (anterior-posterior [AP], lateral), and cephalometric studies with variant views (Waters, Townes, Caldwell, and submentovertex).

The tomogram is a related type of image that also uses x-ray photons. The technique involves synchronous movement in opposite directions of an x-ray tube and film detector placed on either side of a patient's head. As the apparatus rotates, serial radiographs are taken at various angles to create a two-dimensional (2D) image. The most common tomogram used in maxillofacial surgery is the orthopantogram (OPG), or panoramic radiograph.

Plain films and OPGs are fast, readily available, and require minimal equipment. These images are helpful for localizing the source of odontogenic infections and allow for evaluation of the teeth, jaws, and maxillary sinuses. Lateral and AP cephalograms can also be obtained expeditiously and provide objective evidence regarding the severity of airway compromise in patients demonstrating stridor and suspected deep space infections (Figure 6-1).[3]

Computed Tomography

CT has become the most-used imaging modality for maxillofacial infections.[1-3] The CT scan was created through the combined efforts of Hounsfield and Cormack, which earned them the Nobel Prize in Physiology/Medicine in 1979. CT images are a computer-generated digitization of multiple x-rays obtained as the x-ray source and detector rotate around a patient.[1] The detector measures the varying attenuations of the x-rays as they pass through the patient's body, and the resultant data are processed by a series of complex formulas to calculate the amount of absorption of individual 3D cubes termed *voxels*. The relative radiodensity of each voxel is given a numerical value known as a Hounsfield unit (HU), which is a standardized unit based on the relative uptake of x-ray energy in comparison to water. As a reference point, some common HUs are air (−1000), fat (−80 to −100), water (0), blood (60 to 110), and bone (1000). The algorithm-driven tomographic reconstruction process generates cross-sectional axial images that can be reformatted into other sequences, including coronal, sagittal, and 3D images. The *window width*

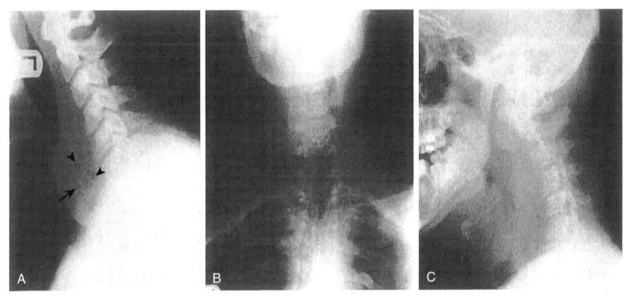

• **Figure 6-1** Lateral neck view **(A)** with windowing to highlight soft tissue pathologic condition from a patient who ingested a plastic foreign body *(large arrow)* 5 days before clinical presentation. There is significant thickening of the prevertebral soft tissue with retrotracheal and retrolaryngeal air *(arrowheads)* causing significant narrowing and anterior displacement of the airway. Anteroposterior **(A)** and lateral neck **(B)** and **(C)** lateral cervical films of a patient with an abscess involving the submandibular, parapharyngeal, and retropharyngeal deep neck spaces. Note the displacement of the airway column to the left in the anteroposterior view as well as significant narrowing with increased prevertebral and retroglossal soft tissue in the lateral view. (From DelBalso AM, Hall RE. Diagnostic imaging of maxillofacial and fascial space infections. In: *Oral and Maxillofacial Infections*. 4th ed. Philadelphia: Saunders; 2002.)

describes the range of HUs being displayed at any one time. Manipulation of the window width, or "windowing," allows the clinician to create greater contrast between structures within the chosen range of HUs (e.g., bone, soft tissue, or lung windows).

Intravenous (IV) iodinated contrast agents can be used to better visualize vascular structures, enhance areas of inflammation, localize sources of active bleeding, and identify abscess formation (Figure 6-2). The main concern when using intravenous contrast is the risk for contrast-induced nephropathy, which is defined as a 25% increase in serum creatinine 2 to 7 days after contrast exposure.[4] There is an increased risk for nephropathy in patients with preexisting renal impairment (creatinine >1.3 and 1.0 in men and women, respectively), hypertension, hemodynamic instability, age older than 60 years, or congestive heart failure and for those receiving a high contrast load.[5] Predictor models, such as the Roxana Mehran score, have been developed to calculate an individual patient's potential risk and thus the need for preventive measures. If contrast is deemed necessary based on the clinical scenario, the following methods can be used to decrease the risk of nephropathy: minimize contrast load, use low- or iso-osmolar contrast agents, discontinue nephrotoxic drugs, and prehydrate for volume expansion using intravenous fluids.[6,7] Treatment for contrast-induced nephropathy is mostly supportive, focusing on elimination of contrast, avoiding further kidney injury, adjusting medication doses, and ensuring appropriate fluid and electrolyte balance.[8] There are variable levels of evidence for other therapeutics such as

vitamin C, sodium bicarbonate, *N*-acetylcysteine, and prophylactic hemodialysis, and therefore they are not commonly used.[8-10] Antihistamines and corticosteroids can be used in patients who have had previous minor allergic reactions to IV contrast (i.e., rash or pruritus).[11]

Early CT scans could take 30 minutes or longer to obtain and resulted in large radiation exposures.[1-3] With increased detector sensitivity, optimization of beam characteristics (i.e., helical or spiral), and enhanced computer processing power, the speed of acquisition and radiation dose has decreased significantly.[3] This is especially important for children and for patients who require multiple scans, are medically unstable, or cannot tolerate prolonged periods in a scanner.

Cone-Beam Computed Tomography

Cone-beam CT (CBCT), synonymous with digital volume tomography, is an imaging modality with many features similar to traditional fan-beam CT but with some key differences, mainly involving the imaging reconstruction process. It is popular among dentists and maxillofacial surgeons because of the ability to obtain 3D imaging expeditiously in an office setting and is becoming the standard of care.[3,12] The technique relies on a cone-shaped, divergent, x-ray beam and multidimensional detectors.[2,3] Similar to traditional CT, software computes digital volumes made up of 3D voxels that can be manipulated. CBCT scanners are relatively inexpensive, have a small footprint, and can

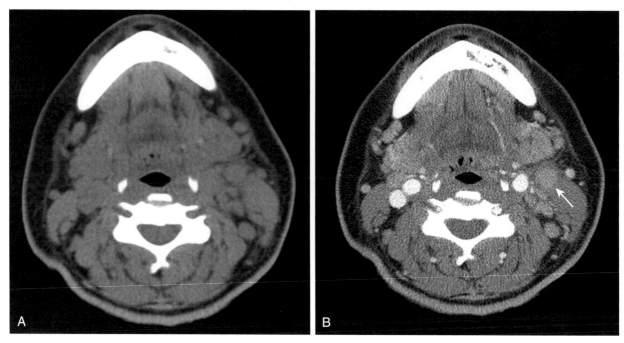

• **Figure 6-2** Axial computed tomographic images at the same level **(A)** before and **(B)** after intravenously administered contrast that is used to enhance structures with high vascularity. In **(B)**, note the prominence of venous and arterial structures, salivary glands, and lymph nodes. The *white arrow* shows an enhancing left neck mass consistent with lymphadenitis.

obtain images faster and with less radiation than a medical-grade CT.[13] CBCT is most useful for visualizing high-contrast tissues such as teeth and bone. Soft tissue changes associated with infectious processes are not well delineated because of the wide collimation of the x-ray beam causing increased scatter radiation and subsequent loss of contrast required for detailed soft tissue analysis.[12,14]

Radiation Safety

With the increased use of imaging modalities based on ionizing radiation there is substantial interest regarding the effects of elevated radiation exposures on both the patient and operator. The use of CT imaging has more than doubled since 1996.[15] Over 75% of CT images are obtained in the acute care setting, which includes maxillofacial scans for infections.[15,16] Medical imaging now accounts for approximately half of the radiation exposure experienced by the population of the United States.[17] Ionizing radiation causes free radical production leading to destruction of enzymes and damage to DNA structure. This damage has been linked to harmful effects, including radiation-induced malignancy, cataract formation, shortened lifespan, and damage to gametes with hereditary consequences.[15,17-19] The amount of cell turnover and level of differentiation within tissue types determines the susceptibility to radiation damage. In the maxillofacial region, areas of high susceptibility include lymphatic tissue, skin, the lens/cornea of the eye, thyroid, salivary glands, and oral mucosa.[17,20] Less susceptible tissues include muscle, bone, spinal cord, and the brain.[17,20]

Determining the real-time risk of radiation exposure in individual patients is challenging because there are a variety of contributing factors (i.e., environmental, genetic) and the outcomes can be delayed for decades after the exposure.[17] Many different models have been used in the attempt to quantify the risk of radiation exposure from medical imaging, most of which use extrapolated data from survivors of nuclear warfare. The theory most widely accepted assumes a linear relationship between exposure and probability of malignancy without a threshold level of exposure.[18] Several groups, including the American Society of Radiologic Technologists, have developed risk calculators that clinicians and patients can use to calculate the risk of an individual.[19] Caution must be used because the effective radiation dose may differ significantly based on several factors, including scanner variability and the weight of the patient. Individual studies show that the risk of developing a malignancy is low but increases in children and those subjected to multiple high-radiation dose studies.[21] It is important that clinicians weigh the risks and benefits of a particular study and use as little ionizing radiation as possible. The American College of Radiology provides "appropriateness" guidelines for selecting imaging studies in a variety of clinical scenarios; however, no guidelines exist for the majority of maxillofacial infections.

Magnetic Resonance Imaging

The first MR image was described by Lauterbur in 1973 and was further developed by Mansfield, ultimately earning them both the Nobel Prize in 2003.[22,23] MRI has been used in clinical practice since the 1980s and has a major advantage of not relying on ionizing radiation, but instead using strong magnetic fields and radio waves.[2,22] The MRI scanner creates a constant magnetic field that causes protons within the patient to align with the field. Radiofrequency (RF) pulses are then broadcast to the patient causing a transient change in the magnetic field as a result of absorption of the RF pulse by the protons. When the RF pulse is stopped, the protons again realign with the constant magnetic field. The transitional change in the proton state produces energy that is detected by the MR receiver coil, which is then translated into an image. The MRI signal intensity depends on the concentration of protons and their freedom of movement. This means that tissues with high concentrations of loosely bound protons (fat) have a much higher signal than tissue with tightly bound hydrogen atoms (bone). Relaxation of protons to a lower energy state occurs through two different mechanisms: (1) T1 relaxation is the transfer of energy from the protons (spin) to the other surrounding atoms (lattice); (2) T2 relaxation is the interference of signal between adjacent protons. T1 and T2 relaxation times occur in a predictable fashion in different tissue types.

Imaging sequences are generated by varying the time between the RF pulse and the point where the signal is read. T1-weighted images are generated by short repetition and echo times to emphasize differences between T1 values in tissue. In these images, tissue with short T1 decay constants will appear bright (fat) and those with long T1 constants will appear dark (fluid/CSF). T2 images are produced with long repetition and echo times. In these images, tissue with long T2 constants will appear bright (CSF, fluid) and those with short T2 constants will be dark (fat). T2-weighted images highlight inflammatory or pathologic changes. There are other more complex sequences such as fat suppression and diffusion-weighted imaging that also can be acquired. Additionally, intravenous contrast agents (e.g., gadolinium) can shorten the T1 relaxation times of the tissues where it is absorbed (e.g., tumors, sites of hyperemia).

The advantages of MRI are increased soft tissue resolution and contrast. T1 and T2 relaxation times between soft tissues vary more than x-ray attenuation coefficients in CT. Images can be obtained in multiple planes without repositioning the patient, but image acquisition time is much longer than with CT. Having an implanted ferromagnetic metal (e.g., pacemakers, vascular clips, foreign bodies) is an absolute contraindication to MRI. Gadolinium is often considered safer than iodinated contrast, but can result in nephrogenic systemic fibrosis in patients with existing severe renal disease.[24,25]

Ultrasound

As with MRI, ultrasonography gained popularity because it does not rely on ionizing radiation. US waves are pressure waves of a greater frequency than can be heard by the human ear (>20 KHz).[23] The US transducer produces electrical current that is passed through piezoelectric crystals causing them to rhythmically change shape and thus create pressure waves. As the transducer is held against a patient's skin some of the sound waves reflect back toward the transducer, causing an additional change in the size of the piezoelectric crystals. This generates an electric signal that can be amplified and displayed as an image on a monitor. Contrast is derived from the varied acoustic impedance patterns in different tissue types. High-density tissues reflect more sound waves than low-density tissues.

US is used extensively in obstetrics and for imaging of the liver, heart, and abdomen. Images can be obtained in real time at the bedside, making US an ideal modality for assessing acute thoracoabdominal injuries in unstable trauma patients. A technique known as the focused assessment with sonography for trauma (FAST) has been used in the United States since the 1980s and is the preferred imaging modality in the Advanced Trauma Life Support (ATLS) protocol developed by the American College of Surgeons.[26] The FAST examination uses US to examine the abdominal cavity and mediastinum for free fluid and also to evaluate the thoracic cavity for pneumothorax and hemothorax.[27]

Several groups have assessed the use of US to evaluate and treat the upper airway and deep anatomic structures of the neck.[28-38] In clinical practice, US is mainly used for visualization of superficial infections and surgical guidance for abscesses drainage.[2,34] Utilization in the maxillofacial region is not universal because of lack of familiarity with the technique, wide availability of CT scanners, limited comparative studies with other techniques, and inability to assess structures deep to tissues with high acoustic impedance (i.e., bone).[2] US provides excellent soft tissue contrast, which is helpful for distinguishing fluid-filled cavities such as abscesses. Bedside US has the potential to be an important imaging modality to diagnose and treat many of the infectious and inflammatory conditions of the head and neck without added radiation.

Nuclear Techniques

CT, MRI, and US yield macroscopic images for anatomic and pathologic diagnoses but do not provide molecular or biochemical information. Nuclear imaging is a combination of multiple imaging techniques that uses radionuclides, which are unstable molecules that emit gamma radiation.[39] Molecular and biochemical abnormalities often occur before morphologic change, which allows for earlier detection of disease processes. Nuclear imaging is used to detect malignancies throughout the body, pathologic processes of the thyroid or brain, and several maxillofacial inflammatory conditions.[39] After uptake of the radionuclide by tissue, photons emitted from decay are captured by a γ-scintillation (Anger) camera. The captured energy is first converted to light and subsequently to a voltage signal, which gets amplified and displayed. Imaging can be obtained in a planar fashion or with tomographic views using cameras rotated around the patient (i.e., single-photon emission computed tomography [SPECT]).

Two of the most commonly used radiotracers are iodine-131 (^{131}I) and technetium 99m (^{99m}Tc). ^{99m}Tc is a metastable intermediate formed by the transition of molybdenum-99 to technetium-99. It is used in approximately 85% of nuclear medicine scans today because of its short half-life (6 hours), ease of production, and excellent tissue penetration of emitted photons that can be collimated for visualization.[40] ^{99m}Tc can be injected intravenously and also can be combined with a variety of carrier molecules specifically tailored to image almost every organ in the body.[39,41]

Nuclear imaging using ^{99m}Tc has several applications in the head and neck. A pertechnetate radiotracer variant can be used to image the thyroid, salivary glands, and gastric mucosa by substituting for iodine in the Na/I symporter.[2,23,42] ^{99m}Tc bound to phosphate compounds (e.g., methylene diphosphonate [MDP]) can be administered intravenously and are absorbed in areas of high metabolic activity allowing for visualization of skeletal growth centers, neoplasms, and inflammatory processes (e.g., osteomyelitis) in the maxillofacial region (Figure 6-3).[23,43-45]

Head and neck images using MDP are obtained in the following phases: Phase 1 ("radionuclide angiogram")—obtained shortly after injection of the radiotracer (within 60 to 90 seconds) and consists of flow and blood pool images. Phase 2 (scintigraphy phase)—obtained 2 to 3 hours after injection when the tracer has been absorbed by the skeleton. Phase 3—obtained 5 hours after injection and may show abnormal persistent metabolic activity; in osteomyelitis, uptake persists during phase 3 allowing for

differentiation from surrounding healthy bone where tracer activity has decreased. Phase 4—obtained 24 hours after injection; osteomyelitis will show persistent activity.

^{99m}Tc scintigraphy has the potential for early detection of inflammatory conditions of the maxillofacial skeleton, but high ionizing radiation and lack of diagnostic specificity limit its use.[46] An increase in phase 1 signal is seen in soft tissue trauma, infections, and vascular abnormalities because of increased blood flow. Increased uptake in later phases is seen after fractures, neoplasms, tooth extractions, and other diseases with altered bone turnover (e.g., hyperthyroidism, Paget's disease, and fibrous dysplasia).[46,47] Additional radiotracers that have been used to enhance the specificity for inflammatory conditions include gallium, tagged white cells (indium or hexamethylpropylenamin oxime), and ^{99m}Tc-tagged nanocolloids.[47] These types of scans are rarely used in clinical practice, but are potentially useful for detecting infected hardware in patients with a contraindication for MRI.

Positron emission tomography (PET) is a related nuclear imaging modality that relies on positron-emitting radionuclides (nitrogen-13 [^{13}N], oxygen-15 [^{15}O], fludeoxyglucose-18 [^{18}F]) combined with carrier molecules (e.g., glucose). When the emitted positron interacts with a free electron, the positron and electron are annihilated, producing two photons emitted at 180 degrees from each other, which are then detected by the PET scanner. PET is more sensitive than other nuclear images (100× more sensitive than SPECT) and can be combined with CT scans for localization of metastatic tumors and lymph node infiltration.[23]

Imaging for Common Inflammatory Disease Processes

The purpose of this section is to guide the clinician in prescribing the correct imaging modality based on the disease process in question. Multiple factors must be considered when choosing appropriate imaging. Although it is not possible to include all clinical scenarios, several principles will be reviewed to aid clinical decision-making. The surgeon should obtain imaging only when the information obtained from the study will directly affect clinical care. For example, a vestibular abscess apical to a carious maxillary canine would require plain films to determine the tooth of origin, but a CT scan would not change the decision to perform incision and drainage followed by tooth extraction or root canal treatment. Alternatively, if periorbital inflammation or vision changes were present, a CT scan with contrast may determine if emergent incision and drainage of an orbital infection is necessary. The ease, availability, and rapidity of CT scans have led to a massive increase in use, but may also be a result of practicing "defensive medicine." It is important to weigh the risks of radiation relative to the benefits in each case.

Imaging can be used for complex maxillofacial infections to monitor disease progression and resolution. Ideally, the same imaging modality used for diagnosis also would be

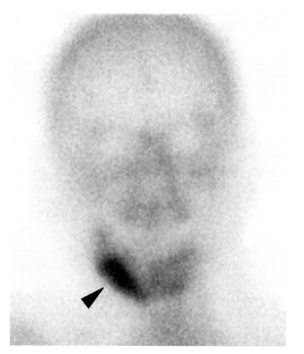

• **Figure 6-3** Anteroposterior image of a ^{99m}Tc radionuclide bone scan (bone phase) showing an area of increased uptake in the right mandibular body–symphyseal region *(arrowhead)* in a patient who later received a diagnosis of osteomyelitis. (From Koorbusch GF, Deatherage JR. How can we diagnose and treat osteomyelitis of the jaws as early as possible? *Oral Maxillofac Surg Clin North Am.* 2011;23:557-567.)

used in follow-up direct comparison. In patients requiring serial imaging, the clinician should use a modality that is cost effective, readily available, easy to interpret, and uses the least ionizing radiation as possible. For inflammatory processes in many other areas of the body, US is used, but as discussed above, its application is limited for head and neck infections. If plain films are deemed useful in the diagnostic process, they should be obtained as a baseline to allow comparisons using this lower radiation modality.

Local Odontogenic Infections

As many as 90 to 95% of oral cavity infections are odontogenic in origin.[48] These infections can range from caries, periodontal disease, and periapical periodontitis to more advanced disease states including deep space infections, sinus infections, and osteomyelitis. Oral infections are often polymicrobial in nature and the source can often be identified with clinical and radiological exam. Intraoral dental radiographs (i.e. bitewings and periapicals) are the most useful images to obtain for detecting dental caries and periodontal disease (Figure 6-4). These images are easily obtained, inexpensive, and can identify the involved tooth and amount of demineralization. However, patients must be cooperative and the ability to obtain these images can be hindered by limited mouth opening and physical impediments such as frenal attachments, tori, and floor of mouth swelling. Furthermore, intraoral dental imaging is typically

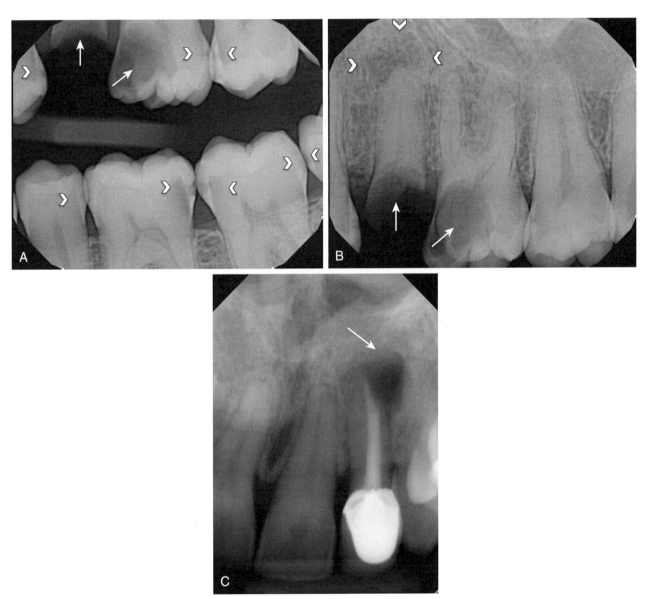

• **Figure 6-4** **A,** Intraoral bitewing radiograph showing extensive interproximal *(white arrowheads)* and severe decay *(white arrows)*. **B,** Maxillary periapical radiograph of the same patient again shows extensive decay *(white arrows)* and associated periapical rarefying osteitis *(white arrowhead)*. **C,** Periapical radiograph of an endodontically treated lateral incisor, demonstrating a well-defined radiolucent lesion determined to be a periapical cyst *(white arrow)*.

not available in emergency departments. When intraoral imaging cannot be completed, extraoral plain films such as a four-view mandibular series or a panoramic radiograph can be obtained as they are generally easier to perform and better tolerated by patients. Panoramic radiographs can be used as a screening tool for the dentition, mandible (including the temporomandibular joints), maxilla, and maxillary sinuses. The main disadvantage is that the resolution is not as high as intraoral radiographs, and therefore may not detect small carious or osseous lesions.[23]

Osteomyelitis

Osteomyelitis is an infection of medullary bone that can involve cortical plates. In the maxillofacial skeleton, it usually occurs through contiguous spread from an odontogenic infection. Other inciting factors include fractures, tooth extractions, vascular insufficiency episodes, or adjacent soft tissue infections. Bacteria can spread into the marrow space locally via the periodontal ligament or more globally via hematogenous dissemination.[2] In the maxillofacial region, osteomyelitis most commonly affects the mandible. The maxilla is almost never involved because of its significant vascular supply and thin cortical bone.[46,49] Osteomyelitis is described as either suppurative (pus-forming) or non-suppurative and is further defined as acute (<1 month duration) or chronic (>1 month).[49] Other diseases of the maxillofacial skeleton with an element of classic osteomyelitis include osteoradionecrosis, medication-related osteonecrosis of the jaw, Garré osteomyelitis, and chronic sclerosing osteomyelitis.[23,46,47,49]

The choice of imaging modality can be challenging for diagnosis and treatment of osteomyelitis. It is recognized that early diagnosis (shorter duration of pretreatment symptoms) is associated with higher cure rates.[46,50] The imaging protocol preferred by the authors is listed in Figure 6-5. Because osteomyelitis of the maxillofacial skeleton is often odontogenic in origin, intraoral or extraoral plain films should be obtained to identify potential infectious sources (e.g., caries, periodontitis, fracture, etc.).[2] Some of the characteristic signs of the spread of an odontogenic infection into the surrounding marrow cavity include loss of the trabecular bony lattice; widening of the periodontal ligament space; loss of the lamina dura; and loss of contrast between bone and normal anatomic structures, including the mandibular canal, maxillary sinuses, and nasal cavities.[50] These findings are often subtle, and comparison to the contralateral side can be helpful to delineate any true differences. In later stages of osteomyelitis, plain films may demonstrate a mixed radiolucent/radio-opaque pattern, bony sequestration, and periosteal reaction (Figure 6-6).[50] Plain films are insensitive for detection of early osteomyelitis because approximately 50% of bony demineralization is needed before becoming radiographically apparent. This process may take as long as 3 weeks after symptom onset.[46] Because of this, advanced imaging techniques are favored when osteomyelitis is suspected.

CT and MRI are the most commonly used advanced imaging modalities for osteomyelitis. CT scans obtained for diagnosis may also be used for presurgical planning. CT is more sensitive than plain radiographs in the detection of bony demineralization and is able to demonstrate cortical perforations, abscesses, sinus tract formation, soft tissue edema, and associated lymphadenopathy (Figure 6-7). Findings suggestive of chronic osteomyelitis include medullary sclerosis, periosteal bone formation, and sequestrum formation (Figure 6-8).

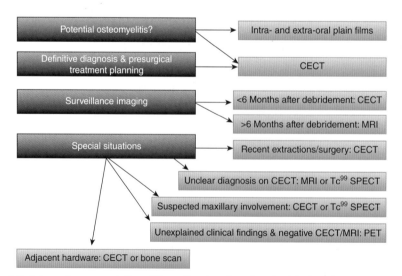

• **Figure 6-5** Schematic representation of the authors' preferred method for imaging maxillofacial osteomyelitis. The decision to obtain plain films, contrast-enhanced computed tomography *(CECT)*, magnetic resonance imaging *(MRI)*, or positron emission tomography *(PET)*, is often multifactorial and requires careful consideration. The clinical scenarios and subsequent imaging recommendations are provided to aid the clinician in obtaining adequate imaging for both common and challenging situations encountered in the workup of osteomyelitis. *SPECT,* Single-photon emission computed tomography.

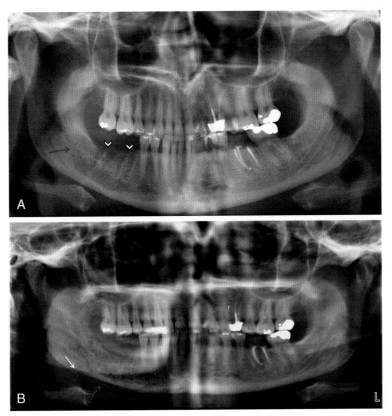

• **Figure 6-6** Subacute suppurative osteomyelitis. Patient with persistent pain and swelling after extraction of right mandibular molars. **A,** Orthopantogram demonstrating extraction sites with ill-defined borders *(white arrowheads),* loss of definition of the mandibular canal *(red arrow),* and mixed radiolucent–radiopaque appearance of the surrounding bone in comparison with the contralateral hemimandible. **B,** A follow-up orthopantogram 3 weeks later after intraoral debridement and antibiotic therapy shows a postsurgical decrease in alveolar bone height, increase extension of mixed radiolucent–radiopaque appearance to the inferior border with extension in the anteroposterior dimension, further loss of definition of the mandibular canal and inferior cortical margin *(white arrow),* and periosteal new bone formation *(red arrow).*

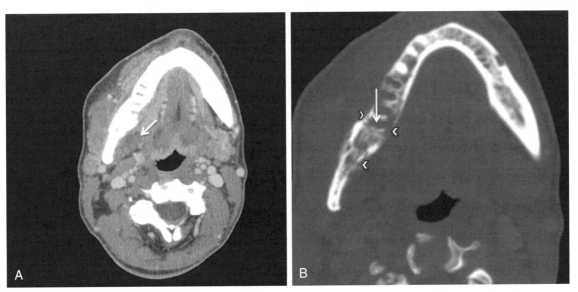

• **Figure 6-7** Contrast-enhanced computed tomographic scan obtained in a patient with acute on chronic suppurative osteomyelitis. **A,** Axial contrast-enhanced image with soft tissue windowing demonstrating a masticator space phlegmon *(arrow)* and masseter and medial pterygoid myositis. **B,** Axial image in bone window demonstrating mottled-appearing bone surrounding the extraction site *(arrow)* and thinning and perforation *(arrowheads)* of the bone cortex.

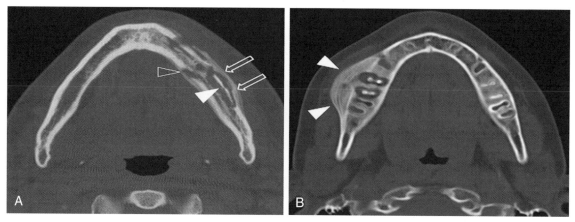

• **Figure 6-8 A,** Noncontrast maxillofacial computed tomographic (CT) axial view bone window of a patient with chronic suppurative osteomyelitis demonstrating bony sequestrum *(solid white arrowhead),* involucrum *(arrows),* and erosion of the lingual cortex *(open arrowhead).* **B,** Noncontrast maxillofacial CT axial view bone window of a child with osteomyelitis caused by actinomycosis and demonstrating buccal periosteal new bone formation in a lamellar pattern *(arrowheads).* (From Koorbusch GF, Deatherage JR. How can we diagnose and treat osteomyelitis of the jaws as early as possible? *Oral Maxillofac Surg Clin North Am.* 2011;23:557-567.)

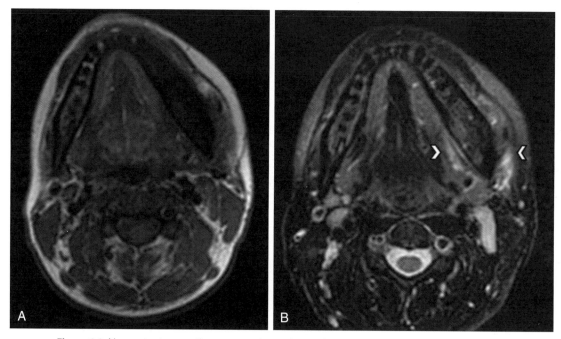

• **Figure 6-9** Noncontrast magnetic resonance image in a patient with chronic left mandibular osteomyelitis. **A,** T1-weighted axial image showing enlarged left hemimandible with decreased bone marrow signal. **B,** On this axial T2, fat-suppressed image, there is hyperintense signal in the soft tissue surrounding the mandible *(arrowheads),* indicating an edematous inflammatory reaction.

MRI is even more sensitive than CT for osteomyelitis and often demonstrates larger areas of disease, because the inflammatory reaction occurring within the marrow alters the MR signal.[46] However, MRI is less specific than CT and operative planning based on this larger area altered signal could lead to overtreatment. Bone affected by acute osteomyelitis has a decreased marrow signal on T1 sequences because the normally fatty marrow (bright on T1) is altered by inflammation (Figure 6-9).[46] Additional MR sequences including contrast enhanced T1 and short tau inversion recovery (STIR) allow detection of vascularity and water content, respectively (Figure 6-10). Changes in marrow signal on MRI can take as long as 6 months to resolve after treatment, so MRI is not an ideal modality to determine short-term response to treatment. MRI can be useful for long-term surveillance owing to its increased sensitivity in detection of disease recurrence when compared to CT.[46]

Nuclear imaging, including triphasic ^{99m}Tc scans, can show evidence of osteomyelitis as soon as 3 days after symptom onset (Figure 6-11). As with MRI, these scans lack

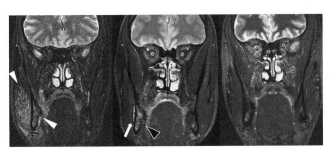

• **Figure 6-10** Serial contrast-enhanced magnetic resonance images and short tau inversion recovery sequence coronal images in a patient with right mandibular osteomyelitis at initial presentation, 2 months later, and 1 year follow-up (from *right* to *left,* respectively). Initial images demonstrate edema within the masseter and medullary bone of the right mandible *(arrowheads).* Two-month follow-up images show significant improvement of the soft tissue edema, but with persistent hyperintense signal in the subperiosteal region *(arrow)* and medullary bone *(arrowhead).* At 1-year follow-up, there is complete resolution of the radiographic abnormalities. (From Koorbusch GF, Deatherage JR. How can we diagnose and treat osteomyelitis of the jaws as early as possible? *Oral Maxillofac Surg Clin North Am.* 2011;23:557-567.)

specificity and spatial localization required for operative planning.[47,51] Skeletal scintigraphy provides a sensitive means for monitoring disease progression/treatment response and is useful for patients with contraindications to MRI/CT scans or who have hardware that would distort image quality.[46]

Currently there is no single evidence-based imaging approach for maxillofacial osteomyelitis. The modality preferred by the authors is panoramic imaging and contrast-enhanced CT. CT has a high sensitivity and specificity while also acting as an excellent tool for planning resection margins when indicated.

Deep Space Neck Infections

Rapid diagnosis, tailored antibiotics, and surgical intervention for localized infections have made deep space neck infections (DSNIs) less common in the modern era.[52] However, when DSNIs do occur, the risk of life-threatening

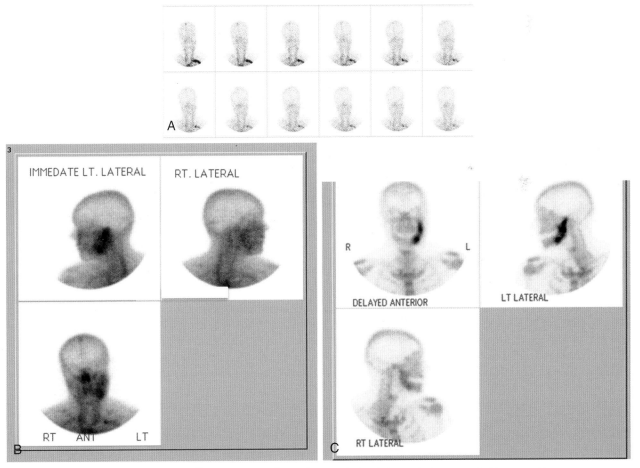

• **Figure 6-11** Triphasic ⁹⁹ᵐTc methylene diphosphonate single-photon emission computed tomographic scan. The patient had a biopsy-proven osteomyelitis that was treated conservatively with debridement and long-term intravenous antibiotics during pregnancy. The patient's symptoms stabilized, and antibiotics were stopped after magnetic resonance imaging showed no increased marrow signal indicating quiescent disease. She then had a recurrence of symptoms that prompted the team to obtain a bone scan. **A,** A nuclear angiography series obtained at 3-second intervals from left to right shows a minimally increased flow to the left mandible and surrounding soft tissues. **B,** In the immediate bone scan images and delayed images, there is increased radiotracer activity identified within the left mandible extending from the angle of the mandible to the condyle with no additional foci, consistent with active osteomyelitis.

complications can be as high as 10 to 20%.[53-56] DSNIs are a source of significant morbidity as well as financial burden.[52-56] The neck has an innate ability to obstruct the spread of infection because it is composed of anatomic compartments separated by cervical fascia (see Chapter 4).[56,57] When these tissue planes are violated, infection can spread to adjacent compartments leading to rapid clinical decline, airway compromise, mediastinitis, and involvement of nearby neurologic/vascular structures.[56]

There are multiple causes of DSNIs and the demographic characteristics vary with patient age, socioeconomic status, and immune competence.[56,58] DSNIs most commonly result from contiguous or lymphatic spread emanating from the dentition, salivary glands, sinuses, or middle ear.[2,56] Despite advances in imaging, up to 67% of cases have an unidentified source.[56,59] DSNIs often begin as an isolated cellulitis from a local infection or from lymph node perforation spreading into adjacent tissues. In many cases the host reacts to the infection by forming an abscess to "wall off" and limit the spread of infection. If untreated, the infection will spread, initially within the confines of the fascial space of origin and ultimately to adjacent or communicating compartments. The most concerning spaces of involvement are those that are vertically oriented (parapharyngeal, retropharyngeal, carotid, danger, preverterbral) and are in close proximity to or contain critical structures, including the aerodigestive tract, cranial nerves, and large-caliber vasculature.[56,58]

Patients with DSNIs have varied clinical presentations, with findings ranging from those common to superficial infections (i.e., pain, lethargy, fever, elevated inflammatory markers) to more worrisome signs/symptoms, including trismus, limited neck mobility, dysphagia, voice changes, and mental status changes. Because of the many potential infectious sources and wide-ranging clinical presentations, a detailed physical examination should be completed to localize the area of concern and help direct further care. The potential for rapid decompensation in these patients should be relayed to the entire treatment team. The clinician must maintain a high index of suspicion and a detailed understanding of anatomic spaces, including the pathways of spread for appropriate diagnosis and treatment.

The purpose of imaging for DSNIs includes differentiating cellulitis from abscess, determining the extent of disease, identifying complicating factors, surgical treatment planning, and monitoring disease progression. A variety of modalities are used, including plain films, US, CT, and MRI.

Plain films, which provide limited soft tissue resolution, remain helpful in diagnosis and management of deep space infections. It is now common to obtain advanced imaging (i.e., CT scans) before plain films with concerns for DNSIs. Plain films do allow for a quick assessment of the severity of airway obstruction and in some cases identification of the infectious source (e.g., the dentition or maxillary sinuses). AP and lateral neck films allow for examination of bony structures, localization of foreign bodies, and the soft tissues surrounding the airway, particularly in children (Figure 6-4).

Findings associated with deep space infections include narrowing or displacement of the airway, thickening of the retropharyngeal soft tissues, and soft tissue emphysema. The lateral neck film is most useful in evaluating airway patency and the prevertebral soft tissue. The maximal thickness of the prevertebral soft tissue on a lateral neck film in neutral position should not exceed 10 mm at C1, 7 mm at C3, and 20 mm at C7 in adults; in adolescents the measurements include 6 mm at C2 and 15 mm at C6. On AP films, the clinician can evaluate airway symmetry and detect narrowing especially in the subglottic region.

Advanced imaging can characterize the source, severity, and extent of the deep space infection. Advanced imaging should be obtained in patients with a high pretest probability of disease, including those with negative findings on plain films. For example, plain films have a sensitivity of 83% in detection of retropharyngeal abscess compared to nearly 100% with contrast-enhanced CT scans.[60]

US has become increasingly implemented in facilities where available and is becoming the gold standard for diagnosing superficial neck abscesses (Figure 6-12).[32-34,56] When possible and adequate for diagnosis, US is a preferred imaging modality in children to avoid radiation and can usually be obtained without sedation. Additionally, pediatric patients typically have smaller necks allowing for better visualization of deep structures. The limitations of US for DSNIs are discussed previously.[33] With increasing familiarity and development of alternative views (e.g., intraoral, sublingual), use of US for diagnosis will likely increase. US-guided drainage and catheter placement can be used in select patients with unilocular DSNIs as an alternative to incision and drainage.[30,34,61] Patients treated in this manner were found to have success rates ranging between 73 and 100%.[30,34,61] The potential benefits of US-guided treatment include avoidance of general anesthesia, decreased risk of damage to major neurovascular structures, decreased length of hospital stay, and decreased cost.[34]

CT is the most widely used modality for evaluation of deep space infections.[62,63] CT can provide detailed information regarding localization of an infectious source, extent of spread to adjacent tissues, involvement of nearby structures, and any mass effect affecting airway caliber or position.[34] Differentiating cellulitis from abscess is important, because cellulitis may respond to antibiotic treatment alone, whereas abscesses require surgical drainage in addition to antibiosis.[64,65] The use of intravenous contrast enhances the rim surrounding an abscess cavity, aiding in diagnosis, and can determine compromise of surrounding vasculature (see Figure 6-2).[56] The recommended protocol is a fine-cut CT scan (1-mm slice thickness) with intravenous iodinated contrast and includes coronal and sagittal reformats. Contrast-enhanced CT has a reported sensitivity of 80 to 90% and specificity of 75% in the detection of drainable abscess collections.[56,65-67] Specificity of CT in abscess detection is increased for adults, cavities larger than 3.5 cm, and when gas formation is detected.[56,66,68] When contrast is not used, sensitivity for detecting inflammatory conditions is reduced.

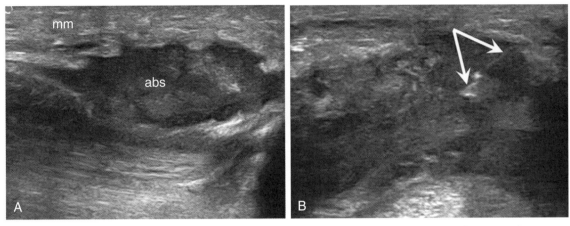

• **Figure 6-12** Ultrasound images obtained in a patient with an odontogenic abscess. **A,** Pretreatment image shows a hypoechoic abscess cavity *(abs)* and masseter muscle *(mm)*. **B,** Aspiration image of the same abscess shows hyperechoic needle (along *arrows*) within the abscess cavity. (From Maroldi R, Farina D, Ravanelli M, et al. Emergency imaging assessment of deep neck space infections. *Semin Ultrasound CT MR.* 2012;33:432-442.)

In cases with equivocal findings, an MRI may be warranted to further delineate the diagnosis.

Typical CT findings in DSNIs include cellulitis, fasciitis, myositis, abscess formation, airway deformation, and lymphadenopathy.[69] Cellulitis is characterized by fat stranding, edema, and loss of normal tissue architecture (Figure 6-13). If the infection progresses, a phlegmon may form, which is visualized as an area of soft tissue or fluid density effacing/displacing tissue planes with variable contrast enhancement. Abscesses are a result of the body isolating an infection and are characterized by a central area of low attenuation surrounded by an exteriorly enhanced rim (Figure 6-13). Advanced disease may demonstrate airway deviation/deformation/narrowing, mediastinal involvement, internal jugular vein thrombosis, and/or carotid artery erosions (Figure 6-14). Intraoperative CT imaging can localize difficult-to-assess abscess cavities and ensure appropriate drainage or cannulation (i.e., paravertebral or prevertebral abscesses). Real-time imaging also can be useful for drainage of residual infections or for multilocular disease.

The use of MRI in DSNIs may allow for more precise diagnosis; however, its use has been limited because of decreased scanner availability in emergency settings and long acquisition times requiring patient cooperation.[56] MRI may be indicated in stable patients who cannot receive CT contrast agents or those with possible intracranial/intraspinal involvement (Figure 6-15).

Infections of the Salivary Glands

Salivary gland pathologic conditions can be divided into neoplastic and nonneoplastic. Nonneoplastic disease most commonly affects the major salivary glands (parotid, submandibular, sublingual) and include infectious/inflammatory conditions and sialolithiasis. Depending on the clinical scenario, various imaging modalities, including sialography, US,

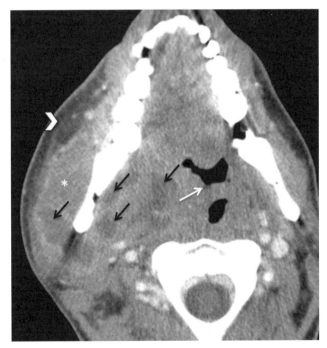

• **Figure 6-13** Contrast-enhanced maxillofacial computed tomographic scan of a 38-year-old patient with deep space neck infection arising from a right mandibular third molar. Axial soft tissue image shows a multiloculated abscess *(black arrows)* involving the masseteric, pterygoid, and retropharyngeal spaces with myositis of the masseter *(asterisk)*, airway deviation away to the left *(white arrow)*, and fat stranding *(white arrowhead)* indicating cellulitis.

CT, MRI, and PET, can be used to assess swelling around the major salivary glands.[70]

The most common causes of acute sialadenitis are bacterial infection, sialolithiasis, and viral infection. Imaging may not be needed if a stone is readily palpable or if a viral cause is suspected. However, imaging should be obtained in cases of recurrent disease, suspected sialolithiasis without

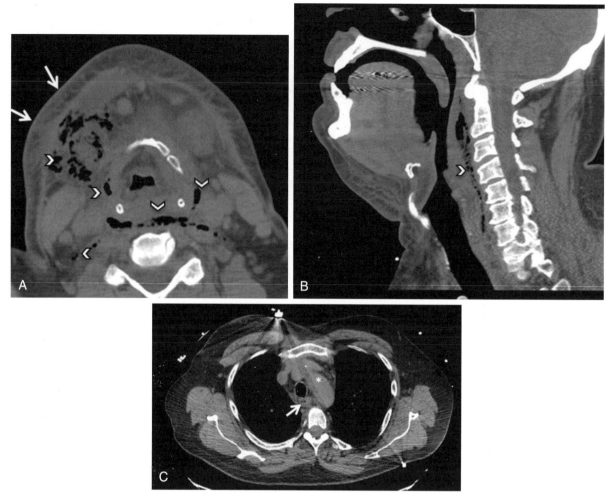

• **Figure 6-14** Noncontrast computed tomographic scan of a patient with an acute deep space neck infection of odontogenic origin caused by gas-forming organisms. **A,** Axial images show skin thickening and cellulitis *(arrow)* and soft tissue emphysema *(white arrowheads)* in the submandibular carotid, parapharyngeal, and retropharyngeal spaces. **B,** Sagittal image shows thickened prevertebral soft tissue and emphysema *(white arrowhead)* tracking along the prevertebral space. **C,** Axial image through the mediastinum shows emphysema within the posterior mediastinum *(white arrowhead)* adjacent to the aortic arch *(asterisk)*.

palpable stones, and when there is concern for abscess formation requiring drainage.

Chronic salivary gland inflammation occurs with chronic untreated sialolithiasis, intraglandular strictures, autoimmune disorders, granulomatous disease from fungal or acid-fast bacterial infections, syphilis, sarcoidosis, and granulomatosis with polyangiitis.[70] These conditions are best imaged with contrast-enhanced CT or MRI.

Obstructing salivary disease can be a result of sialolithiasis or intraglandular strictures.[70] Nearly 1% of the population has salivary stones, but very few cause symptomatic disease.[71] Plain films were the first imaging technique used to assess for the presence of salivary stones (Figure 6-16). They are now rarely used because overlying osseous structures may obstruct visualization of stones and presence of an accompanying abscess or neoplasm cannot be detected.[72,73] Noncontrast CT scans are typically used if a salivary stone is thought to be the cause of the obstruction because contrast can obscure

detection or mimic smaller stones (Figure 6-17). Stones are readily visualized because high attenuating masses within the salivary ducts and the gland parenchyma may be enlarged. In cases of true salivary gland infection, CT is best for visualizing abscess formation owing to the glandular high fat content (particularly the parotid gland) (Figure 6-18).[70]

In many institutions, high-resolution US has become the first-line modality to assess superficial parotid and submandibular gland obstruction. The sensitivity for detecting salivary stones (>2 mm), abscesses, and masses is approximately 90%.[70,74,75] If deep parotid pathologic condition or airway obstruction is suspected, a CT scan should be obtained (Figure 6-19). Contrast should be added if an abscess or neoplasm is suspected. Previously, digital subtraction sialography was implemented to evaluate salivary ducts in suspected cases of stricture, but newer techniques, including MR sialography, are less invasive and provide adequate sensitivity and specificity[76] (see Chapter 15).

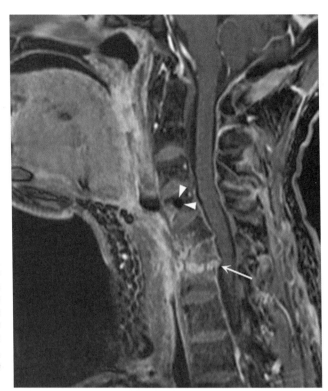

• **Figure 6-15** Magnetic resonance image with contrast obtained for a patient with a possible complicated deep space neck infection after a pharyngolaryngectomy. A sagittal reconstruction of an isotropic volumetric interpolated breath hold examination sequence. There is collapse of the C5-C6 vertebral bodies, enhancing discitis, and air within the C4 body *(arrowheads)*. In addition, there is dural thickening and enhancement *(arrow)* suggestive of a prevertebral abscess. (From Maroldi R, Farina D, Ravanelli M, et al. Emergency imaging assessment of deep neck space infections. *Semin Ultrasound CT MR.* 2012;33:432-442.)

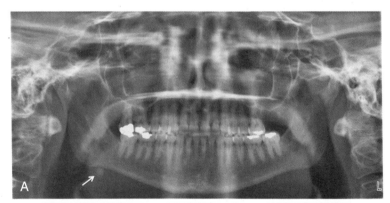

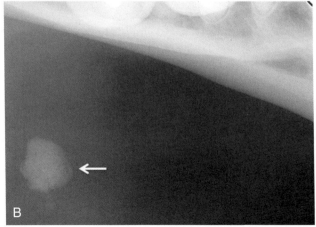

• **Figure 6-16** Right submandibular sialolith in a patient with a history of intermittent right facial swelling. **A,** An orthopantogram shows a well-defined radiolucent sialolith below the inferior border of the mandible *(arrow)*. **B,** Three-dimensional localization was obtained with a follow-up occlusal film showing the sialolith *(arrow)* on the lingual side of the mandible adjacent to the second molar.

Pathologic Conditions of the Paranasal Sinuses

The paranasal sinuses consist of four paired air-filled cavities that are named after the bones in which they originate (maxillary, sphenoidal, ethmoidal, and frontal). Each sinus is lined with respiratory epithelium and communicates with the nasal cavity via narrow ostia (natural openings within the bone). Paranasal sinus disease, including sinusitis and other pathologic conditions (e.g., mucoceles), are a frequent

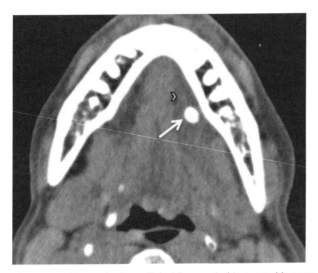

• **Figure 6-17** Noncontrast maxillofacial computed tomographic scan for a patient with left submandibular sialolithiasis and mild sialoadenitis. On axial view, there is a 4 × 8-mm sialolith at the anterior aspect of the right submandibular gland *(arrow)* with mild associated fat stranding *(arrowhead)*.

cause of maxillofacial pain. Inflammatory conditions may cause edema and subsequent blockage of these complexes leading to stasis, bacterial growth, and ultimately infection. Infection can also occur by direct spread from adjacent structures, such as the roots of the posterior maxillary dentition (odontogenic sinusitis).

The most common inflammatory condition affecting the sinuses is acute rhinosinusitis, affecting over 30 million adults in the United States each year.[77] The cause of acute rhinosinusitis is overwhelmingly viral (>98%).[78] Bacterial and fungal infections are more likely to occur in patients with predisposing risk factors such as allergies, immune dysfunction, impaired ciliary function (ciliary dyskinesia), thickened secretions (cystic fibrosis), odontogenic infections, and anatomically narrow ostia.[79,80]

Rhinosinusitis is a clinical diagnosis, and imaging is not usually needed. Cases that may warrant further diagnostic evaluation are those that are complicated, recurrent, chronic, or in immunocompromised patients.[81] Other factors warranting imaging include vision changes, periorbital swelling, neurologic deficits/mental status changes, and treatment-resistant disease.[77-79,82] Sinus pathologic conditions may be asymptomatic and may be found incidentally on imaging for other indications.

Plain radiography is considered to have limited use in the management of sinusitis. The Water's or Caldwell's view has overlap of midface structures and therefore has a poor sensitivity (76%) and specificity (79%) for detecting mucosal disease.[2,83] These images can show sinus opacification, mucosal thickening, periosteal reaction, air-fluid levels, foreign bodies, and bony destruction (Figure 6-20). Although seen

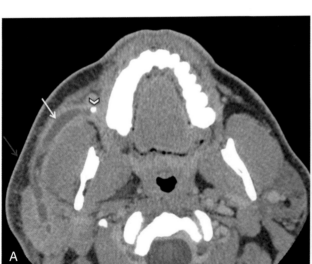
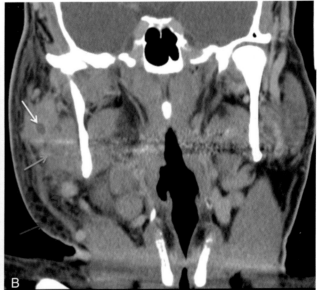

• **Figure 6-18** Contrast-enhanced computed tomographic image obtained for a patient with acute right-sided facial swelling. **A,** Axial image with soft tissue window showing a 4 × 4-mm stone within the parotid duct *(arrowhead)*, with significant ductal dilatation *(white arrow)* with associated soft tissue edema and fat stranding *(red arrow)*. **B,** Coronal image soft tissue window, showing enlarged lymph node *(red arrowhead)*, ductal dilatation *(white arrow)*, fat stranding *(red arrow)*, and significant enlargement of the parotid gland *(blue arrow)*.

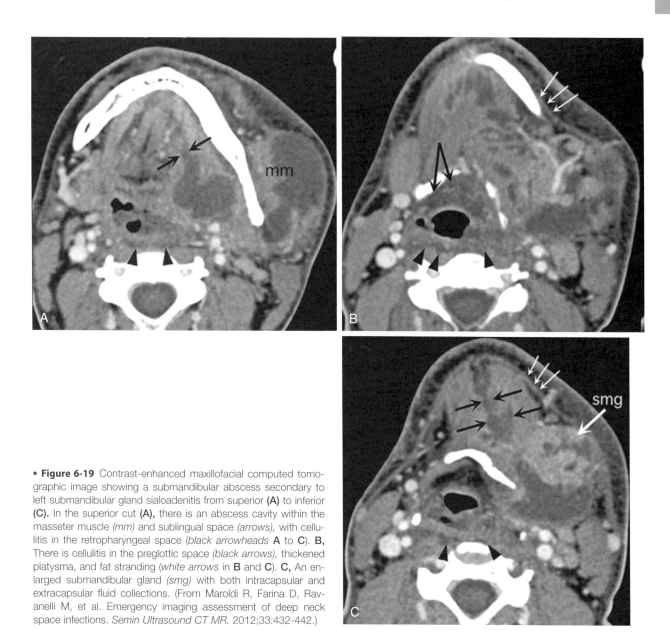

• **Figure 6-19** Contrast-enhanced maxillofacial computed tomographic image showing a submandibular abscess secondary to left submandibular gland sialoadenitis from superior **(A)** to inferior **(C)**. In the superior cut **(A)**, there is an abscess cavity within the masseter muscle *(mm)* and sublingual space *(arrows),* with cellulitis in the retropharyngeal space *(black arrowheads* **A** to **C**). **B,** There is cellulitis in the preglottic space *(black arrows),* thickened platysma, and fat stranding *(white arrows* in **B** and **C**). **C,** An enlarged submandibular gland *(smg)* with both intracapsular and extracapsular fluid collections. (From Maroldi R, Farina D, Ravanelli M, et al. Emergency imaging assessment of deep neck space infections. *Semin Ultrasound CT MR.* 2012;33:432-442.)

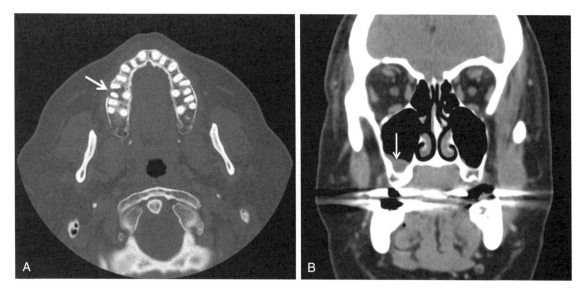

• **Figure 6-20** Noncontrast computed tomographic scan obtained for a patient with recurrent right maxillary pain. **A,** In the axial image, there is a periapical abscess *(arrow)* with loss of the buccal cortex. **B,** In the coronal view, there is an air-fluid level within the right maxillary sinus *(arrow)* indicating sinus disease.

in a majority of sinusitis cases, mucosal thickening is non-specific, while air-fluid levels and opacification are seen less frequently, but are more specific. Plain films are best used as a quick screening tool in questionable diagnoses before antibiotic trials. An OPG may be useful in cases of suspected odontogenic sinusitis, because it allows for evaluation of both the dentition and a screen of the maxillary sinuses.[32] Ultimately, plain films are unable to provide the detailed anatomy necessary for decision-making or planning for surgical intervention and false positive results arise from benign entities, including mucoceles and nasal polyps.[32]

CT scans provide much more anatomic detail of the paranasal sinuses and are more sensitive for detecting pathologic conditions. CT imaging should not be obtained routinely, but rather when indicated, as detailed earlier. CT is needed to determine blockage of ostia and delineating anatomy before operative intervention.[82] Contrast should be added to evaluate for infectious complications.

MRI is also used for imaging of the sinuses and is indicated to rule out neoplastic soft tissue conditions. It provides a detailed examination of the orbits and intracranial structures in complicated sinus disease.[32] MRI provides better soft tissue differentiation, but with less differentiation of bony anatomy, has an increased cost, takes longer to complete, and is not as readily available as CT (see Chapter 14).

References

1. Ouyang T, Branstetter BF. Advances in head and neck imaging. *Oral Maxillofac Surg Clin North Am*. 2010;22(1):107-115. Available at: https://doi.org/10.1016/j.coms.2009.10.002.

2. Topazian RG, Goldberg MH, Hupp JR, eds. *Oral and Maxillofacial Infections*. 4th ed. Philadelphia: Saunders; 2002.

3. Boeddinghaus R, Whyte A. Current concepts in maxillofacial imaging. *Eur J Radiol*. 2008;66(3):396-418. Available at: https://doi.org/10.1016/j.ejrad.2007.11.019.

4. Bellomo R, Ronco C, Kellum JA, Mehta RL, Palevsky P, Acute Dialysis Quality Initiative workgroup. Acute renal failure: definition, outcome measures, animal models, fluid therapy and information technology needs—the Second International Consensus Conference of the Acute Dialysis Quality Initiative (ADQI) Group. *Crit Care*. 2004;8(4):R204-R212. Available at: https://doi.org/10.1186/cc2872.

5. Gurm HS, Seth M, Kooiman J, Share D. A novel tool for reliable and accurate prediction of renal complications in patients undergoing percutaneous coronary intervention. *J Am Coll Cardiol*. 2013;61(22):2242-2248. Available at: https://doi.org/10.1016/j.jacc.2013.03.026.

6. Pannu N, Wiebe N, Tonelli M, Alberta Kidney Disease Network. Prophylaxis strategies for contrast-induced nephropathy. *JAMA*. 2006;295(23):2765-2779. Available at: https://doi.org/10.1001/jama.295.23.2765.

7. Asif A, Epstein M. Prevention of radiocontrast-induced nephropathy. *Am J Kidney Dis*. 2004;44(1):12-24. Available at: https://doi.org/10.1053/j.ajkd.2004.04.001.

8. Rudnick MR. Contrast-associated and contrast-induced acute kidney injury: clinical features, diagnosis, and management. In: Palevsky PM, Forman JP, eds. *UpToDate*. Wolters Kluwer; 2023:7241.

9. Weisbord SD, Gallagher M, Jneid H, et al. Outcomes after angiography with sodium bicarbonate and acetylcysteine. *N Engl J Med*. 2018;378(7):603-614. Available at: https://doi.org/10.1056/NEJMoa1710933.

10. Cruz DN, Goh CY, Marenzi G, Corradi V, Ronco C, Perazella MA. Renal replacement therapies for prevention of radiocontrast-induced nephropathy: a systematic review. *Am J Med*. 2012;125(1):66-78.e3. Available at: https://doi.org/10.1016/j.amjmed.2011.06.029.

11. Khwaja A. KDIGO clinical practice guidelines for acute kidney injury. *Nephron Clin Pract*. 2012;120(4):c179-c184. Available at: https://doi.org/10.1159/000339789.

12. Dammann F, Bootz F, Cohnen M, Hassfeld S, Tatagiba M, Kösling S. Diagnostic imaging modalities in head and neck disease. *Dtsch Arztebl Int*. 2014;111(23-24):417-423. Available at: https://doi.org/10.3238/arztebl.2014.0417.

13. De Vos W, Casselman J, Swennen GRJ. Cone-beam computerized tomography (CBCT) imaging of the oral and maxillofacial region: a systematic review of the literature. *Int J Oral Maxillofac Surg*. 2009;38(6):609-625. Available at: https://doi.org/10.1016/j.ijom.2009.02.028.

14. Horner K, O'Malley L, Taylor K, Glenny AM. Guidelines for clinical use of CBCT: a review. *Dentomaxillofac Radiol*. 2015;44(1):20140225. Available at: https://doi.org/10.1259/dmfr.20140225.

15. Lee J, Kirschner J, Pawa S, Wiener DE, Newman DH, Shah K. Computed tomography use in the adult emergency department of an academic urban hospital from 2001 to 2007. *Ann Emerg Med*. 2010;56(6):591-596. Available at: https://doi.org/10.1016/j.annemergmed.2010.05.027.

16. Smith-Bindman R, Miglioretti DL, Johnson E, et al. Use of diagnostic imaging studies and associated radiation exposure for patients enrolled in large integrated health care systems, 1996-2010. *JAMA*. 2012;307(22):2400-2409. Available at: https://doi.org/10.1001/jama.2012.5960.

17. Brenner DJ, Hall EJ. Computed tomography: an increasing source of radiation exposure. *N Engl J Med*. 2007;357(22):2277-2284. Available at: https://doi.org/10.1056/NEJMra072149.

18. Pierce DA, Preston DL. Radiation-related cancer risks at low doses among atomic bomb survivors. *Radiat Res*. 2000;154(2):178-186. Available at: https://doi.org/10.1667/0033-7587(2000)154[0178:rrcral]2.0.co;2.

19. Smith-Bindman R, Lipson J, Marcus R, et al. Radiation dose associated with common computed tomography examinations and the associated lifetime attributable risk of cancer. *Arch Intern Med*. 2009;169(22):2078-2086. Available at: https://doi.org/10.1001/archinternmed.2009.427.

20. Rubin P, Casarett GW. Clinical radiation pathology as applied to curative radiotherapy. *Cancer*. 1968;22(4):767-778. Available at: https://doi.org/10.1002/1097-0142(196810)22:4<767::aid-cncr2820220412>3.0.co;2-7.

21. Brenner D, Elliston C, Hall E, Berdon W. Estimated risks of radiation-induced fatal cancer from pediatric CT. *AJR Am J Roentgenol*. 2001;176(2):289-296. Available at: https://doi.org/10.2214/ajr.176.2.1760289.

22. Westbrook C, Talbot J. *MRI in Practice*. 5th ed. Hoboken NJ: Wiley Blackwell; 2018.

23. Mallya SM, Lam EWN, White SC, Pharoah MJ. *White and Pharoah's Oral Radiology: Principles and Interpretation*. 8th ed. St Louis: Elsevier; 2019.

24. Weinreb JC. Which study when? Is gadolinium-enhanced MR imaging safer than iodine-enhanced CT? *Radiology*. 2008;249(1):3-8. Available at: https://doi.org/10.1148/radiol.2493200803.

25. Weinreb JC, Abu-Alfa AK. Gadolinium-based contrast agents and nephrogenic systemic fibrosis: why did it happen and what have we learned? *J Magn Reson Imaging*. 2009;30(6):1236-1239. Available at: https://doi.org/10.1002/jmri.21979.

26. Scalea TM, Rodriguez A, Chiu WC, et al. Focused assessment with sonography for trauma (FAST): results from an international consensus conference. *J Trauma*. 1999;46(3):466-472. Available at: https://doi.org/10.1097/00005373-199903000-00022.

27. Roberts JR, Custalow CB, Thomsen TW, eds. *Roberts and Hedges' Clinical Procedures in Emergency Medicine and Acute Care*. 7th ed. St Louis: Elsevier; 2019.

28. Ariji E, Ariji Y, Yoshiura K, Kimura S, Horinouchi Y, Kanda S. Ultrasonographic evaluation of inflammatory changes in the masseter muscle. *Oral Surg Oral Med Oral Pathol*. 1994;78(6): 797-801. Available at: https://doi.org/10.1016/0030-4220(94) 90098-1.

29. Thiruchelvam JK, Songra AK, Ng SY. Intraoperative ultrasound imaging to aid abscess drainage: a technical note. *Int J Oral Maxillofac Surg*. 2002;31(4):442-443. Available at: https://doi.org/10.1054/ijom.2001.0188.

30. Yusa H, Yoshida H, Ueno E, Onizawa K, Yanagawa T. Ultrasound-guided surgical drainage of face and neck abscesses. *Int J Oral Maxillofac Surg*. 2002;31(3):327-329. Available at: https://doi.org/10.1054/ijom.2002.0233.

31. Abbasi M, Bayat M, Beshkar M, Momen-Heravi F. Ultrasound-guided simultaneous irrigation and drainage of facial abscess. *J Craniofac Surg*. 2012;23(2):558-559. Available at: https://doi.org/10.1097/SCS.0b013e31824cd63a.

32. Jehle D, Davis E, Evans T, et al. Emergency department sonography by emergency physicians. *Am J Emerg Med*. 1989;7(6): 605-611. Available at: https://doi.org/10.1016/0735-6757(89) 90283-0.

33. Parmar SB, Mehta HK, Shah NK, Parikh SN, Solanki KG. Ultrasound: a novel tool for airway imaging. *J Emerg Trauma Shock*. 2014;7(3):155-159. Available at: https://doi.org/10.4103/0974-2700.136849.

34. Biron VL, Kurien G, Dziegielewski P, Barber B, Seikaly H. Surgical vs ultrasound-guided drainage of deep neck space abscesses: a randomized controlled trial: surgical vs ultrasound drainage. *J Otolaryngol Head Neck Surg*. 2013;42:18. Available at: https://doi.org/10.1186/1916-0216-42-18.

35. Prasad A, Yu E, Wong DT, Karkhanis R, Gullane P, Chan VWS. Comparison of sonography and computed tomography as imaging tools for assessment of airway structures. *J Ultrasound Med*. 2011;30(7):965-972. Available at: https://doi.org/10.7863/jum.2011. 30.7.965.

36. Singh M, Chin KJ, Chan VWS, Wong DT, Prasad GA, Yu E. Use of sonography for airway assessment: an observational study. *J Ultrasound Med*. 2010;29(1):79-85. Available at: https://doi.org/10.7863/jum.2010.29.1.79.

37. Nicholls SE, Sweeney TW, Ferre RM, Strout TD. Bedside sonography by emergency physicians for the rapid identification of landmarks relevant to cricothyrotomy. *Am J Emerg Med*. 2008;26(8): 852-856. Available at: https://doi.org/10.1016/j.ajem.2007.11.022.

38. Ko DR, Chung YE, Park I, et al. Use of bedside sonography for diagnosing acute epiglottitis in the emergency department: a preliminary study. *J Ultrasound Med*. 2012;31(1):19-22. Available at: https://doi.org/10.7863/jum.2012.31.1.19.

39. Mettler FA, Guiberteau MJ. *Essentials of Nuclear Medicine and Molecular Imaging*. 7th ed. St. Louis: Elsevier; 2019.

40. Eckelman WC. Unparalleled contribution of technetium-99m to medicine over 5 decades. *JACC Cardiovasc Imaging*. 2009; 2(3):364-368. Available at: https://doi.org/10.1016/j.jcmg. 2008.12.013.

41. Eckelman WC, Reba RC, Kelloff GJ. Targeted imaging: an important biomarker for understanding disease progression in the era of personalized medicine. *Drug Discov Today*. 2008;13 (17-18):748-759. Available at: https://doi.org/10.1016/j.drudis. 2008.05.009.

42. Ryo UY, Vaidya PV, Schneider AB, Bekerman C, Pinsky SM. Thyroid imaging agents: a comparison of I-123 and Tc-99m pertechnetate. *Radiology*. 1983;148(3):819-822. Available at: https://doi.org/10.1148/radiology.148.3.6308711.

43. Treves ST, ed. *Pediatric Nuclear Medicine and Molecular Imaging*. 4th ed. New York: Springer; 2014.

44. Peacock ZS, Lawler ME, Fahey FH, Kaban LB. The role of skeletal scintigraphy in the diagnosis and management of mandibular growth abnormalities and asymmetry. In: Treves ST, ed. *Pediatric Nuclear Medicine and Molecular Imaging*. New York: Springer; 2014:407-427. Available at: https://doi.org/10.1007/978-1-4614-9551-2_18.

45. Chiang S. Nuclear medicine imaging studies in the diagnosis of head and neck disease. *Oral Maxillofac Surg Clin North Am*. 2014;26(2):239-245. Available at: https://doi.org/10.1016/j. coms.2014.02.001.

46. Koorbusch GF, Deatherage JR, Curé JK. How can we diagnose and treat osteomyelitis of the jaws as early as possible? *Oral Maxillofac Surg Clin North Am*. 2011;23(4):557-567, vii. Available at: https://doi.org/10.1016/j.coms.2011.07.011.

47. Gotthardt M, Bleeker-Rovers CP, Boerman OC, Oyen WJG. Imaging of inflammation by PET, conventional scintigraphy, and other imaging techniques. *J Nucl Med*. 2010;51(12): 1937-1949. Available at: https://doi.org/10.2967/jnumed.110. 076232.

48. Fragiskos FD. *Oral Surgery*. New York: Springer; 2007.

49. Baltensperger MM, ed. *Osteomyelitis of The Jaws: 47 Tables*. New York: Springer; 2009.

50. Schuknecht B, Valavanis A. Osteomyelitis of the mandible. *Neuroimaging Clin N Am*. 2003;13(3):605-618. Available at: https://doi.org/10.1016/s1052-5149(03)00044-3.

51. Reinert S, Widlitzek H, Venderink DJ. The value of magnetic resonance imaging in the diagnosis of mandibular osteomyelitis. *Br J Oral Maxillofac Surg*. 1999;37(6):459-463. Available at: https://doi.org/10.1054/bjom.1999.0200.

52. Hall JB, Schmidt GA. *Principles of Critical Care*. 4th ed. New York: McGraw-Hill Education; 2015.

53. Boscolo-Rizzo P, Stellin M, Muzzi E, et al. Deep neck infections: a study of 365 cases highlighting recommendations for management and treatment. *Eur Arch Otorhinolaryngol*. 2012;269 (4):1241-1249. Available at: https://doi.org/10.1007/s00405-011-1761-1.

54. Bakir S, Tanriverdi MH, Gün R, et al. Deep neck space infections: a retrospective review of 173 cases. *Am J Otolaryngol*. 2012;33(1):56-63. Available at: https://doi.org/10.1016/j.amjoto. 2011.01.003.

55. Kinzer S, Pfeiffer J, Becker S, Ridder GJ. Severe deep neck space infections and mediastinitis of odontogenic origin: clinical relevance and implications for diagnosis and treatment. *Acta Otolaryngol*. 2009;129(1):62-70. Available at: https://doi.org/10.1080/00016480802008181.

56. Maroldi R, Farina D, Ravanelli M, Lombardi D, Nicolai P. Emergency imaging assessment of deep neck space infections. *Semin Ultrasound CT MR*. 2012;33(5):432-442. Available at: https://doi.org/10.1053/j.sult.2012.06.008.

57. Vieira F, Allen SM, Stocks RMS, Thompson JW. Deep neck infection. *Otolaryngol Clin North Am.* 2008;41(3):459-483, vii. Available at: https://doi.org/10.1016/j.otc.2008.01.002.

58. Hasegawa J, Hidaka H, Tateda M, et al. An analysis of clinical risk factors of deep neck infection. *Auris Nasus Larynx.* 2011;38(1):101-107. Available at: https://doi.org/10.1016/j.anl.2010.06.001.

59. Parhiscar A, Har-El G. Deep neck abscess: a retrospective review of 210 cases. *Ann Otol Rhinol Laryngol.* 2001;110(11):1051-1054. Available at: https://doi.org/10.1177/000348940111001111.

60. Nagy M, Backstrom J. Comparison of the sensitivity of lateral neck radiographs and computed tomography scanning in pediatric deep-neck infections. *Laryngoscope.* 1999;109(5):775-779. Available at: https://doi.org/10.1097/00005537-199905000-00017.

61. Chang KP, Chen YL, Hao SP, Chen SM. Ultrasound-guided closed drainage for abscesses of the head and neck. *Otolaryngol Head Neck Surg.* 2005;132(1):119-124. Available at: https://doi.org/10.1016/j.otohns.2004.08.004.

62. Holliday RA, Prendergast NC. Imaging inflammatory processes of the oral cavity and suprahyoid neck. *Oral Maxillofac Surg Clin North Am.* 1992;4(1):215-240. Available at: https://doi.org/10.1016/S1042-3699(20)30578-1.

63. Nyberg DA, Jeffrey RB, Brant-Zawadzki M, Federle M, Dillon W. Computed tomography of cervical infections. *J Comput Assist Tomogr.* 1985;9(2):288-296. Available at: https://doi.org/10.1097/00004728-198503000-00011.

64. Elden LM, Grundfast KM, Vezina G. Accuracy and usefulness of radiographic assessment of cervical neck infections in children. *J Otolaryngol.* 2001;30(2):82-89. Available at: https://doi.org/10.2310/7070.2001.20808.

65. Vural C, Gungor A, Comerci S. Accuracy of computerized tomography in deep neck infections in the pediatric population. *Am J Otolaryngol.* 2003;24(3):143-148. Available at: https://doi.org/10.1016/s0196-0709(03)00008-5.

66. Lazor JB, Cunningham MJ, Eavey RD, Weber AL. Comparison of computed tomography and surgical findings in deep neck infections. *Otolaryngol Head Neck Surg.* 1994;111(6):746-750. Available at: https://doi.org/10.1177/019459989411100608.

67. Smith JL, Hsu JM, Chang J. Predicting deep neck space abscess using computed tomography. *Am J Otolaryngol.* 2006;27(4):244-247. Available at: https://doi.org/10.1016/j.amjoto.2005.11.008.

68. Freling N, Roele E, Schaefer-Prokop C, Fokkens W. Prediction of deep neck abscesses by contrast-enhanced computerized tomography in 76 clinically suspect consecutive patients. *Laryngoscope.* 2009;119(9):1745-1752. Available at: https://doi.org/10.1002/lary.20606.

69. Lyle NJ, Rutherford EE, Batty VB. A pain in the neck: imaging in neck sepsis. *Clin Radiol.* 2011;66(9):876-885. Available at: https://doi.org/10.1016/j.crad.2011.03.016.

70. Burke CJ, Thomas RH, Howlett D. Imaging the major salivary glands. *Br J Oral Maxillofac Surg.* 2011;49(4):261-269. Available at: https://doi.org/10.1016/j.bjoms.2010.03.002.

71. Williams MF. Sialolithiasis. *Otolaryngol Clin North Am.* 1999; 32(5):819-834. Available at: https://doi.org/10.1016/s0030-6665(05)70175-4.

72. Sobrino-Guijarro B, Cascarini L, Lingam RK. Advances in imaging of obstructed salivary glands can improve diagnostic outcomes. *Oral Maxillofac Surg.* 2013;17(1):11-19. Available at: https://doi.org/10.1007/s10006-012-0327-8.

73. Hoffmann B. Sonographic bedside detection of sialolithiasis with submandibular gland obstruction. *Am J Emerg Med.* 2011; 29(5):574.e5-574.e7. Available at: https://doi.org/10.1016/j.ajem.2010.05.020.

74. Murray ME, Buckenham TM, Joseph AE. The role of ultrasound in screening patients referred for sialography: a possible protocol. *Clin Otolaryngol Allied Sci.* 1996;21(1):21-23. Available at: https://doi.org/10.1111/j.1365-2273.1996.tb01019.x.

75. Yousem DM, Kraut MA, Chalian AA. Major salivary gland imaging. *Radiology.* 2000;216(1):19-29. Available at: https://doi.org/10.1148/radiology.216.1.r00jl4519.

76. Kalinowski M, Heverhagen JT, Rehberg E, Klose KJ, Wagner HJ. Comparative study of MR sialography and digital subtraction sialography for benign salivary gland disorders. *AJNR Am J Neuroradiol.* 2002;23(9):1485-1492.

77. Rosenfeld RM, Andes D, Bhattacharyya N, et al. Clinical practice guideline: adult sinusitis. *Otolaryngol Head Neck Surg.* 2007;137(suppl 3):S1-31. Available at: https://doi.org/10.1016/j.otohns.2007.06.726.

78. Gwaltney JM. Acute community-acquired sinusitis. *Clin Infect Dis.* 1996;23(6):1209-1223; quiz 1224-1225. Available at: https://doi.org/10.1093/clinids/23.6.1209.

79. Scheid DC, Hamm RM. Acute bacterial rhinosinusitis in adults: part I. Evaluation. *Am Fam Physician.* 2004;70(9):1685-1692.

80. Fokkens W, Lund V, Mullol J, European Position Paper on Rhinosinusitis and Nasal Polyps Group. EP3OS 2007: European position paper on rhinosinusitis and nasal polyps 2007: a summary for otorhinolaryngologists. *Rhinology.* 2007;45(2):97-101.

81. Kroll H, Hom J, Ahuja N, Smith CD, Wintermark M. R-SCAN: imaging for uncomplicated acute rhinosinusitis. *J Am Coll Radiol.* 2017;14(1):82-83.e1. Available at: https://doi.org/10.1016/j.jacr.2016.08.018.

82. Osguthorpe JD, Hadley JA. Rhinosinusitis. current concepts in evaluation and management. *Med Clin North Am.* 1999;83(1): 27-41, vii-viii. Available at: https://doi.org/10.1016/s0025-7125(05)70085-7.

83. Mafee MF, Tran BH, Chapa AR. Imaging of rhinosinusitis and its complications: plain film, CT, and MRI. *Clin Rev Allergy Immunol.* 2006;30(3):165-186. Available at: https://doi.org/10.1385/CRIAI:30:3:165.

7

Principles of Surgical and Medical Management of Infections of the Head and Neck Region

RABIE M. SHANTI, ODAI ABUSHANAB, VINCENT B. ZICCARDI, AND THOMAS R. FLYNN

In our modern antibiotic era, the incidence of infections of the head and neck region has been greatly reduced. Nonetheless, infections of the head and neck region are still routinely encountered and pose a significant burden to the health care system.[1,2] The majority of infections of the head and neck region are of odontogenic origin and will present with the classic signs and symptoms of an infectious disease process (e.g., pain, swelling, heating, surface erythema, and limitation of function). The patient in Figure 7-1 demonstrates trismus as a result of limitation of function of the muscles of mastication. Typically, these patients are managed in an outpatient setting with incision and drainage and removal of source, including tooth extraction or pulpectomy followed by a predictable clinical course. Even with the significant recent advancements in airway management, rapid diagnostic imaging, and antimicrobial agents that have occurred over the past several decades, infections of the head and neck region still carry a significant risk of morbidity and potentially mortality because of their close proximity to vital anatomic structures, airway obstruction, and increasing microbial antibiotic resistance.

Life-threatening head and neck infections are encountered in patients with compromised host defense mechanisms such as diabetes mellitus and primary immunodeficiency disorders. In the past, death from head and neck infection resulted most frequently from acute upper airway obstruction.[3,4] Airway security alone is not sufficient, because most deep fascial space infections of the head and neck, especially odontogenic ones, are caused by inherently abscess-forming bacteria creating obstruction from mass effect. Surgical drainage of deep fascial spaces involved by abscess or cellulitis prevents further spread of the infection into deeper anatomic spaces and hastens resolution.[5,6]

Other life-threatening complications of head and neck infection include invasive streptococcal infections, streptococcal or staphylococcal toxic shock, necrotizing fasciitis, descending necrotizing mediastinitis (perhaps the same process as necrotizing fasciitis, occurring in a deeper anatomic plane),[7] internal jugular vein thrombosis,[8] cavernous sinus thrombosis,[9] carotid artery pseudoaneurysm/rupture,[10] and systemic inflammatory response syndrome (SIRS). The diagnostic criteria for SIRS are listed in Box 7-1.

In this chapter we aim to provide a comprehensive stepwise approach to the medical and surgical care of patients with soft tissue fascial plane infections of the head and neck region beginning from initial patient assessment and then progressing to principles of medical and surgical management and follow-up care. Box 7-2 lists the eight steps in the management of severe head and neck infections. Although conscientiously following these steps cannot guarantee a favorable outcome, they can reassure the clinician that the standard of care has been met.

Principles of Surgical and Medical Management of Head and Neck Infections

Step 1: Determine the Severity of Infection

Determining the severity of an infection requires assessment of three main factors: (1) airway patency, (2) anatomic location, and (3) rate of progression.

Airway Patency

The initial assessment of head and neck infection is immediately directed to airway status. This concept dates back to the 1940s, when Dr. Ashbel Williams of Boston City Hospital presented a series of 37 patients with Ludwig's angina. In his patient cohort, 54% of patients succumbed to their infection. The most common cause of death was airway compromise.[3] Only 3 years later, Drs. Williams and Walter Guralnick published a series of 20 cases of Ludwig's angina in which the incidence of mortality was reduced to 10%.[4] The authors had changed their airway management protocol from expectant observation for the development of

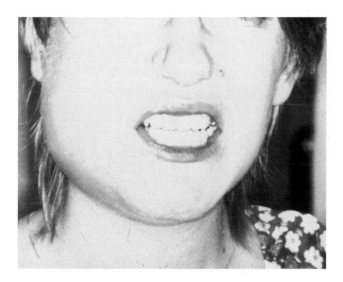

• **Figure 7-1** Trismus (inability to open the mouth widely) resulting from right submasseteric abscess, causing inflammation in the masseter muscle. Note the swelling over the ascending ramus of the mandible, anterior to and obscuring the right ear. (From Flynn TR, Topazian RG. Infections of the oral cavity. In: Waite D, ed. *Textbook of practical oral and maxillofacial surgery.* Philadelphia: Lea & Febiger; 1987:300. Used with permission.)

BOX 7-1	Diagnostic Criteria for Systemic Inflammatory Response Syndrome (SIRS)

If Two or More of the Following Exist:

- 36°C < temperature > 38°C
- Pulse >90
- Respiratory rate >20
- Mean arterial pressure < 32
- 4 < white blood cell count >12
- Bands >10%

Look for Organ Damage in:

- Kidneys
- Liver
- Lungs
- Brain
- Extremities

BOX 7-2	Principles of Management of Odontogenic Infections

1. Determine severity
2. Evaluate host defenses
3. Determine the setting of care
4. Treat surgically
5. Support medically
6. Choose and prescribe appropriate antibiotic(s)
7. Administer antibiotic appropriately
8. Reevaluate frequently

Modified from Flynn TR. Principles and surgical management of head and neck infections. In: Bagheri SC, Bell RB, Khan HA, eds. *Current Therapy in Oral & Maxillofacial Surgery.* St. Louis: Elsevier; 2011:1084. Used with permission.

airway compromise to prompt initial airway stabilization with endotracheal intubation or tracheotomy followed immediately by aggressive open surgical drainage of all infected anatomic spaces. Of note, this dramatic reduction in the mortality of Ludwig's angina was achieved before penicillin was available to civilians by an approach focused on airway protection and early, aggressive surgical management and debridement.

This historic case series highlights the value of prioritizing airway stabilization as the first step in assessing head and neck infections. Signs of impending upper airway obstruction include inability to tolerate oral secretions, use of the accessory muscles of inspiration, orthopnea, dyspnea, stridor, and the tripod position illustrated in Figure 7-2. If a patient develops signs of impending upper airway obstruction, this should alert the practitioner to the urgency of securing the patient's airway. For example, if such a patient is being evaluated in an outpatient setting, it is imperative to activate the emergency medical system and transfer the patient to the nearest appropriate facility equipped to manage a difficult airway. Additionally, if the patient is being evaluated in an emergency department/acute care setting, the practitioner can proceed with immediate transfer to the operating room for securing the patient's airway if logistically feasible. If not, the practitioner should consider securing the patient's airway in the emergency department/acute care setting. In the setting of impending airway obstruction, one must always be prepared to establish and secure a surgical airway by cricothyrotomy or tracheotomy. Today, with advanced airway techniques securing the difficult airway can usually be performed in a noninvasive and predictable manner. For instance, Wolf et al. reported a series of 29 patients with Ludwig's angina and deep neck infections, with 19

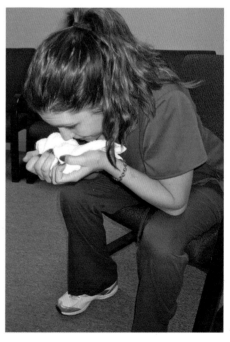

• **Figure 7-2** The tripod position, leaning forward with the elbows on the knees, drooling into a towel.

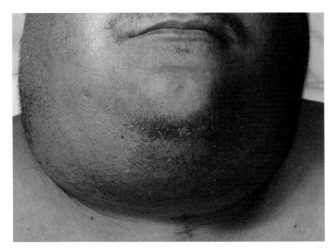

• **Figure 7-3** Marks over the deviated cricothyroid membrane and trachea in a patient with right lateral pharyngeal space abscess.

TABLE 7-1	Synonyms For the Deep Fascial Spaces of the Head and Neck
Name Used in This Text	**Synonym**
Space of the body of the mandible	Mandibular space
Submandibular space	Submaxillary space Submylohyoid space
Masticator space	Masticatory space Masseteric space
Temporal spaces (superficial and deep)	Temporal pouches
Infratemporal space	Postzygomatic space
Buccal space	Buccinator space
Infraorbital space	Canine space
Lateral pharyngeal space	Parapharyngeal space Pharyngomaxillary space
Retropharyngeal space	Retroesophageal space
Pretracheal space	Perivisceral space Paravisceral space Paratracheal space
Carotid sheath	Visceral vascular space

Adapted from Flynn TR. Anatomy and surgery of deep fascial space infections. In: Kelly JJ, ed. *Oral and Maxillofacial Surgery Knowledge Update 1994*. Rosemont, IL: American Association of Oral and Maxillofacial Surgeons; 1994:82. Used with permission.

(65.5%) patients exhibiting evidence of airway compromise.[11] Of the patients with airway compromise, 8 (42%) required an advanced airway technique to secure their airway and no patients in this report required a surgical airway. Nonetheless, the surgeon must always be prepared to establish a surgical airway in case the anesthesia team is unable to secure the airway with noninvasive airway techniques. In cases of potential airway obstruction, the surgeon can identify and mark the landmarks for a cricothyrotomy (thyroid cartilage, cricoid cartilage, and cricothyroid membrane), followed by marking an incision along the cricothyroid membrane, as shown in Figure 7-3. The surgical airway armamentarium should be readily available in the operating room during conventional airway instrumentation. In the cannot intubate, cannot ventilate situation, any delay in the establishment of a surgical airway could prove fatal. Vigilance and preparation is required. In summary, in all patient encounters the airway must always be assessed and appropriately managed first. Once this has been accomplished, a thorough history and physical examination may ensue.

Anatomic Location

Surgeons of varying disciplines may have different names for the deep fascial spaces of the head and neck. Table 7-1 lists various synonyms for these spaces, and for purposes of clarity, the borders, and contents of the deep fascial spaces of the head and neck, along with their anatomic relations and surgical approaches for incision and drainage, are listed in Tables 7-2 and 7-3. Anatomic diagrams of the masticator, submandibular and sublingual, lateral pharyngeal, and retropharyngeal spaces are also included in Figures 7-4 to 7-7.

Infections of each of the deep fascial spaces of the head and neck manifest with characteristic subjective complaints and objective signs,[6] which can aid in identifying the spaces involved. Accurate determination of the anatomic location of the infection allows the surgeon to stratify the severity of the infection into low, moderate, and high categories, based on the likelihood of swelling in the involved anatomic space(s) causing airway deviation, effacement, or obstruction;

hindering access to the airway for intubation; or directly impinging upon vital structures such as the brain or heart.[6] The severity rankings of the various deep fascial spaces of the head and neck are listed in Table 7-4. For instance, vestibular space infections have low severity because they are separated from the airway by the bony structures of the maxilla and mandible. In cases with a cooperative patient, vestibular space abscess can be easily managed in an outpatient setting (Figure 7-8, A and B).

When the masticator, submandibular, or sublingual spaces (Figure 7-8, C and D) are infected individually, the severity is moderate because of trismus or elevation of the tongue and floor of the mouth. Infections in the pterygomandibular space (part of the masticator space) may displace or even efface the airway space, and the associated trismus hinders airway access. Pterygomandibular space involvement was found in 60% of cases of severe odontogenic infection[6] and occurs more commonly than previously appreciated, probably because the associated trismus hinders visualization of the oropharynx, as shown in Figure 7-8, D.

Infection of both right and left submandibular and sublingual spaces along with the submental space between them in the midline constitutes Ludwig's angina, a high-severity infection because of the great risk of airway obstruction as a result of displacement of the tongue and the propensity to rapidly spread into the deeper spaces of the neck. Such a case is illustrated in Figure 7-9, A and B.

TABLE 7-2 Borders of the Deep Fascial Spaces of the Head and Neck

Space	Anterior	Posterior	Superior	Inferior	Superficial or Medial§	Deep or Lateral*
			BORDERS			
Buccal	Corner of mouth	Masseter m. Pterygoman dibular sp.	Maxilla Infraorbital space	Mandible	Subcutaneous tissue and skin	Buccinator m.
Infraorbital	Nasal cartilages	Buccal space	Quadratus labii superioris m.	Oral mucosa	Quadratus labii superioris m.	Levator anguli oris m. Maxilla
Submandibular	Ant. belly digastric m.	Post. belly digastric m. Stylohyoid m. Stylopharyngeus m.	Inf. and medial surfaces of mandible	Digastric tendon	Platysma m., Investing fascia	Mylohyoid, Hyoglossus, Sup. constrictor muscles
Submental	Inf. border of mandible	Hyoid bone	Mylohyoid m.	Investing fascia	Investing fascia	Ant. bellies digastric mm.*
Sublingual	Lingual surface of mandible	Submandibular space	Oral mucosa	Mylohyoid m.	Muscles of tongue†	Lingual surface of mandible*
Pterygomandibular	Buccal space	Parotid gland	Lateral pterygoid m.	Inf. border of mandible	Med. pterygoid muscle†	Ascending ramus of mandible*
Submasseteric	Buccal space	Parotid gland	Zygomatic arch	Inf. border of mandible	Ascending ramus of mandible†	Masseter m.*
Lateral pharyngeal	Sup. and mid. Pharyngeal constrictor mm.	Carotid sheath and scalene fascia	Skull base	Hyoid bone	Pharyngeal constrictors and Retropharyngeal space†	Medial pterygoid m.*
Retropharyngeal	Sup. and mid. Pharyngeal constrictor mm.	Alar fascia	Skull base	Fusion of alar and vertebral fasciae at C6-T4		Carotid Sheath and lateral pharyngeal space*
Pretracheal	Sternothyroid-thyrohyoid fascia	Retropharyngeal space	Thyroid cartilage	Superior mediastinum	Sternothyroid-thyrohyoid fascia	Visceral fascia over trachea and thyroid gland

*Medial border; *m.*, muscle; *Ant.*, anterior; *Inf.*, inferior; *Med.*, medial.
†Lateral border; *Sp.*, Space; *Post.*, posterior; *Sup.*, superior; *Lat.*, lateral.
§Superficial or Medial Borders

Reproduced with permission from Flynn TR, Topazian RG. Infections of the oral cavity. In: Waite D, ed. *Textbook of Practical Oral and Maxillofacial Surgery*. Philadelphia: Lea & Febiger; 1987:296. Used with permission.

TABLE 7-3 **Relations of Deep Spaces in Head and Neck Infections**

Space	Likely Causes	Contents	Neighboring Spaces	Approach For Incision and Drainage
Buccal	Upper bicuspids Upper molars Lower bicuspids	Parotid duct Ant. facial a. and v. Transverse facial a. and v. Buccal fat pad	Infraorbital Pterygomandibular Infratemporal	Intraoral (small) Extraoral (large)
Infraorbital	Upper cuspid	Angular a. and v. Infraorbital n.	Buccal	Intraoral
Submandibular	Lower molars	Submandibular gland Facial a. and v. Lymph nodes	Sublingual Submental Lateral pharyngeal Buccal	Extraoral
Submental	Lower anterior fracture of symphysis	Ant. jugular v. Lymph nodes	Submandibular (on either side)	Extraoral
Sublingual	Lower bicuspids Lower molars Direct trauma	Sublingual glands Wharton's ducts Lingual n. Sublingual a. and v.	Submandibular Lateral pharyngeal Visceral (trachea and esophagus)	Intraoral Intraoral-extraoral
Pterygomandibular	Lower third molars Fracture of angle of mandible	Mandibular div. of trigeminal n. Inf. alveolar a. and v.	Buccal Lateral pharyngeal Submasseteric Deep temporal Parotid Peritonsillar	Intraoral Intraoral-extraoral
Submasseteric	Lower third molars Fracture of angle of mandible	Masseteric a. and v.	Buccal Pterygomandibular Superficial temporal Parotid	Intraoral Intraoral-extraoral
Infratemporal and deep temporal	Upper molars	Pterygoid plexus Int. max. a. and v. Mand. div. of trigeminal n. Skull base foramina	Buccal Superf. temporal Inf. petrosal sinus	Intraoral Extraoral Intraoral-extraoral
Superficial Temporal	Upper molars Lower molars	Temporal fat pad Temporal branch of facial n.	Buccal Deep temporal	Intraoral Extraoral Intraoral-extraoral
Lateral	Lower third molars	Carotid a.	Pterygomandibular	Intraoral
Pharyngeal	Tonsils Infection in neighboring spaces	Internal jugular v. Vagus n. Cervical sympathetic chain	Submandibular Sublingual Peritonsillar Retropharyngeal	Intraoral-extraoral

Reproduced with permission from Flynn TR, Topazian RG. Infections of the oral cavity. In: Waite D, ed. *Textbook of Practical Oral and Maxillofacial Surgery*. Philadelphia: Lea & Febiger; 1987:297. Used with permission.

The deep neck spaces, such as the retropharyngeal, lateral pharyngeal, and prevertebral spaces also carry high severity, because swelling in these spaces can readily displace, efface, or obstruct the airway. Further, infection in the deep neck spaces can rapidly spread inferiorly to threaten the mediastinum and its contents or superiorly to threaten the brain, especially by involvement of the internal jugular vein or other connections to the intracranial venous sinuses.

The most common subjective complaint in patients with head and neck infection is dysphagia (difficulty swallowing),

present in 78% of patients.[6] Trismus occurred in 73% of patients in the same cohort. Similarly, Plaza Mayor et al. reported that odynophagia (pain on swallowing) and dysphagia were the most common presenting symptoms, occurring in 84% and 71% of patients, respectively.[12] Trismus is also likely, which is indicative of involvement of masticator space, whose components are the submasseteric, superficial temporal, deep temporal, and pterygomandibular spaces, as diagrammed in Figure 7-4, and seen clinically in Figure 7-10. Trismus is an inherently protective reflex

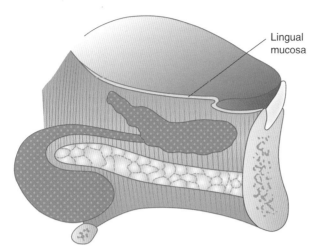

• **Figure 7-4** Parasagittal diagram of the relationship between the submandibular and sublingual spaces, which communicate at the posterior edge of the mylohyoid muscle. (From, Hollinshead WH: Anatomy for surgeons, vol. 1, ed. 2, Hagerstown, MD, 1968, Harper & Row. Used with permission.)

that may limit movement and limit spread of infection. Facial or neck swelling is also frequently observed in patients with head and neck infections.

The clinical presentation of the patient is dependent on the involved anatomic space(s).[13] Figures 7-8 to 7-15 illustrate the typical clinical appearance of infection in the various deep fascial spaces of the head and neck. Unfortunately, when assessing patients with severe infections of the head and neck, clinical examination is often limited by swelling, trismus, and pain. Reactive adenopathy may mimic abscess or cellulitis. Deeper spaces, such as the lateral pharyngeal, retropharyngeal, and pterygomandibular spaces, can be difficult to fully

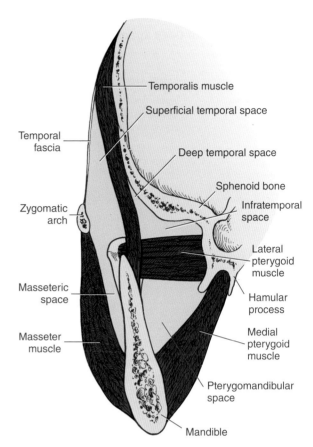

• **Figure 7-5** Coronal diagram of the masticator space, with a section through the ascending ramus of the mandible, zygomatic arch, and temporal bone. All four compartments of the masticator space are illustrated. (From Flynn TR. Complex odontogenic infections. In: Ellis E, Hupp JR, Tucker MR, eds. *Contemporary Oral and Maxillofacial Surgery*. 6th ed. St. Louis: Mosby; 2013:326. Used with permission.)

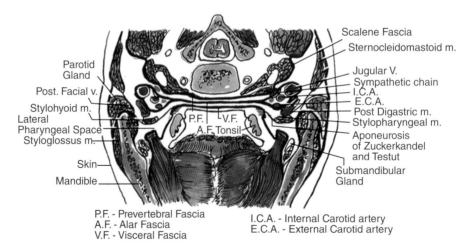

• **Figure 7-6** Diagrammatic oblique section through the ascending ramus and condylar neck of the mandible, illustrating the contents and relations of the lateral pharyngeal space and carotid sheath. (From Flynn TR. Anatomy and surgery of deep fascial space infections. In: Kelly JJ, ed. *Oral and Maxillofacial Surgery Knowledge Update 1994*. Rosemont, IL: American Association of Oral and Maxillofacial Surgeons; 1994:86. Used with permission.)

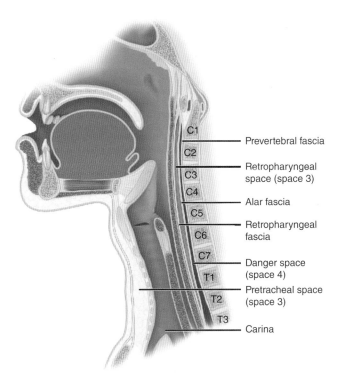

• **Figure 7-7** Sagittal section through the head and neck, illustrating the relationships of the pretracheal and retropharyngeal spaces and the danger space (space 4). (From Flynn TR. Principles and surgical management of head and neck infections. In: Bagheri SC, Bell RB, Khan HA, eds. *Current Therapy in Oral & Maxillofacial Surgery.* St. Louis: Elsevier; 2011:1086. Used with permission.)

TABLE 7-4	Severity of Fascial Space Infections	
Severity	**Anatomic Space**	
Low (low risk to airway or vital structures)	Vestibular Subperiosteal Space of the body of the mandible Infraorbital Buccal	
Moderate (moderate risk to airway or vital structures)	Submandibular Submental Sublingual Pterygomandibular Submasseteric Superficial temporal Deep temporal (or infratemporal)	
High (high risk to airway or vital structures)	Lateral pharyngeal Retropharyngeal Pretracheal Danger space (space 4) Mediastinum Intracranial infection	

Modified with permission from Flynn TR. Principles and surgical management of head and neck infections. In: Bagheri SC, Bell RB, Khan HA, eds. *Current Therapy in Oral & Maxillofacial Surgery.* St. Louis: Elsevier; 2011:1084. Used with permission.

examine because of their deep location within the neck with multiple superimposing anatomic structures. Similarly, trismus as a result of guarding from pain or from mechanical obstruction limits visualization of the oropharynx.

Differentiating postoperative edema from infection can be difficult. For example, a patient that is 3 days after third molar removal typically experiences pain, tenderness, swelling, dysphagia, odynophagia, and trismus, yet still may not have an infection. The trend of these parameters over time can help the clinician differentiate infection from postoperative inflammation; a worsening course after about 3 days may indicate infection, while postoperative inflammation generally is decreasing by roughly 3 days after surgery.

Additionally, the presentation of a malignancy as an abscess is a rare phenomenon that can be quite deceptive. Tumors can become secondarily infected or undergo central necrosis, manifesting as a swelling with suppuration. Misdiagnosis of a malignancy can result in treatment delay, which may therefore result in increased tumor size or allow regional or distant metastasis. Furthermore, surgical management of a malignant tumor as an infection, with incision and drainage may result in seeding of tumor cells and alteration of the normal lymphovascular networks, aiding dissemination of the tumor.[14]

Radiographic Evaluation

Plain film radiographs (e.g., orthopantogram, dental periapical x-rays) are limited to identification of the causative teeth in odontogenic infection. Computed tomography (CT) is generally used to identify otorhinologic infection and infection of the deeper structures, such as the deep fascial spaces and cranial cavity.

To accurately identify the anatomic location of the infection, we must rely on both a thorough clinical examination and advanced radiographic studies. Today, for severe infections of the head and neck, contrast-enhanced computed tomography (CECT) is the most widely used imaging modality. CECT is widely available. Magnetic resonance imaging (MRI) has longer acquisition time, and it therefore requires patients to lie in the supine position for an extended period, which may precipitate airway obstruction in the patient with an infection of moderate or high severity.

Ultrasound (US) offers the advantages of portability and avoiding radiation; however, US for deep neck structures is technique sensitive, requiring a level of expertise that is not as widely available as CECT. Most clinicians are not trained in the use or interpretation of US techniques. Furthermore, CECT allows assessment of the airway deviation, compression, and patency. Figure 7-16, A, depicts a patient with deviation and effacement of the airway to the right, whereas Figure 7-16, B, depicts tracheal deviation and loss of airway patency. This added radiographic information allows more accurate evaluation of the airway, which is most critical in assessing the severity of infection and the overall condition of the patient. Additionally, CECT allows one to differentiate cellulitis from abscess with rim enhancement of fluid collections indicating abscess formation. CECT

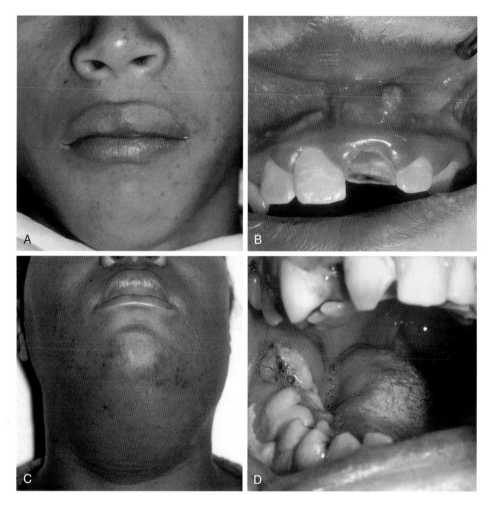

• **Figure 7-8** **A,** Frontal view of a patient with a vestibular space abscess, causing swelling of the upper lip and elevation of the left ala of the nose. **B,** Intraoral view of the same patient, with a fractured maxillary left central incisor, swelling in the maxillary alveolar mucosa and vestibule, and a draining parulis in the mucobuccal fold. **C,** Submentovertex view of a patient with a cellulitis of the left submandibular and submental spaces. **D,** Intraoral view of a right pterygomandibular space infection due to a fractured and carious lower right molar. Note the deviation of the uvula to the opposite side and the swelling of the right anterior tonsillar pillar. Trismus has been overcome under general anesthesia, enabling this view. (A and B, From Flynn TR. Anatomy of oral and maxillofacial infections. In: Topazian RG, Goldberg MH, Hupp JR, eds. *Oral and Maxillofacial Infections.* 4th ed. Philadelphia: WB Saunders; 2002:196. Used with permission. C, From Flynn TR. Surgical management of orofacial infections. *Atlas Oral Maxillofac Surg Clin North Am.* 2000;8:79. D, From Flynn TR, Topazian RG. Infections of the oral cavity. In: Waite D, ed. *Textbook of Practical Oral and Maxillofacial Surgery.* Philadelphia: Lea & Febiger; 1987:300. Used with permission.)

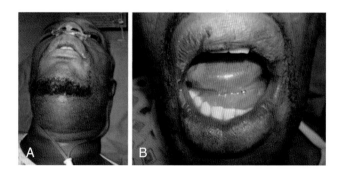

• **Figure 7-9** **A,** Ludwig's angina, with swelling of both submandibular and sublingual spaces, plus the submental space in the midline. **B,** The same patient, with sublingual swelling, elevation of the tongue and displacing it posteriorly into the oropharynx.

does have the disadvantage of using radiation, whereas MRI and US do not.

When contrast medium is used, it is necessary to assess renal function by measurement of serum creatinine. This could be a source of delay; however, unless the patient has an unstable airway that must be secured immediately in the operating room, obtaining a CT study, even without contrast, enables more accurate surgical planning than proceeding with surgery based on clinical examination alone. Miller et al. reported in 1999 on the accuracy of CECT combined with clinical examination in identifying a drainable collection of pus.[15] In this study, CECT alone had an accuracy of 77%, sensitivity of 95%, and specificity of 53%, whereas while clinical examination alone had an

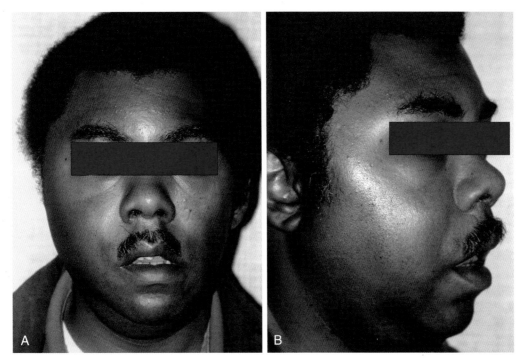

• **Figure 7-10** Frontal view of a patient with infection of the entire right masticator space, including the superficial and deep temporal spaces and the submasseteric and pterygomandibular spaces. Note the right temporal and masseteric swelling, and the inability to open the mouth widely. In this view, the masseteric swelling obscures the right ear. This infection was of 60 days' duration, indicating low virulence and good host resistance. **B,** Oblique view of the same patient. Note that the masseteric swelling stops anterior to the ear lobe, where the infection is contained by the parotideomasseteric fascia. Note also the flattening of the swelling over the zygomatic arch, where the temporalis fascia is tightly bound down to the underlying bone. (A, From Flynn TR. The swollen face. *Emerg Med Clin North Am.* 2000;15:481-519. Used with permission. B, From Flynn TR. Complex odontogenic infections. In: Ellis E, Hupp JR, Tucker MR, eds. *Contemporary Oral and Maxillofacial Surgery.* 6th ed. St. Louis: Mosby; 2013:329. Used with permission.)

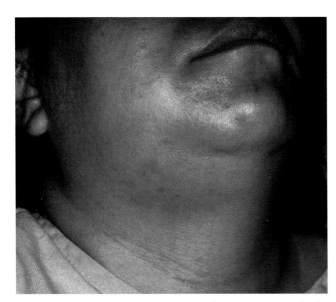

• **Figure 7-11** Oblique view of a patient with a right submandibular space abscess. Note the reddened swelling defined by the inferior border of the mandible, the anterior and posterior bellies of the digastric muscle, and the hyoid bone. (From Flynn TR. The swollen face. *Emerg Med Clin North Am.* 2000;15:481-519. Used with permission.)

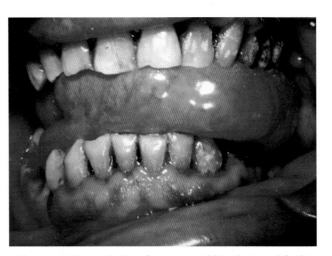

• **Figure 7-12** Intraoral view of a severe sublingual space infection, with the tongue forced superiorly, with the dorsal surface against the palate, exposing the ventral surface of the tongue and floor of the mouth. (From Flynn TR, Topazian RG. Infections of the oral cavity. In: Waite D, ed. *Textbook of Practical Oral and Maxillofacial Surgery.* Philadelphia: Lea & Febiger; 1987:300. Used with permission.)

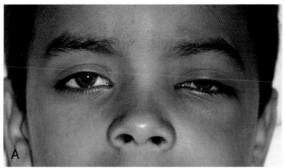

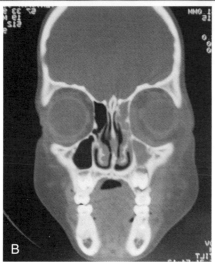

• **Figure 7-13 A,** Left subperiosteal orbital abscess as a result of maxillary and ethmoid sinusitis, associated with carious primary molars. Note the left periorbital erythema, partial ptosis, and lateral deviation of the left globe of the eye. **B,** Coronal CT of the same patient. Note the opacification of the left maxillary and ethmoid sinuses, thickening of the periosteum of the medial orbital wall, and lateral deviation of the globe. (From Simos C, Flynn TR, Piecuch JF, Topazian RG. Infections of the oral cavity. In: Feigin RD, Cherry JD, eds. *Textbook of pediatric infectious diseases*. 6th ed. Philadelphia: Saunders; 2007. Used with permission.)

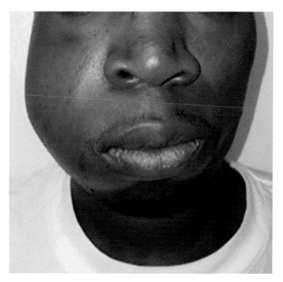

• **Figure 7-14** Right buccal space infection. Note the limitation of swelling at the zygoma, the inferior border of the mandible, and the corner of the mouth.

accuracy of 63%, sensitivity of 55%, and a specificity of 73%. However, the combination of CECT and clinical examination had an accuracy of 89%, sensitivity of 95%, and specificity of 80%. This study and others have provided clear evidence that in combination, CECT and clinical examination have the best accuracy, sensitivity, and specificity in identifying drainable collections of pus.[15,16] Clinicians treating deep space fascial infections should be well versed in anatomy and be able to diagnose fascial spaces involved based on clinical examination.

In severe infection of the deep neck spaces, such as in retropharyngeal space abscess or Ludwig's angina, the patient may not be able to lie supine without experiencing airway obstruction, even for the duration of a CT scan. A patient

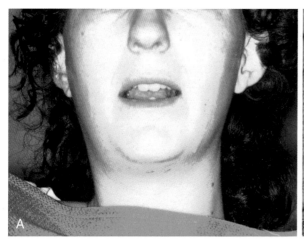

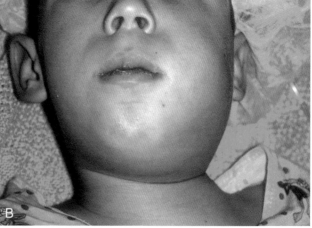

• **Figure 7-15 A**, Left lateral pharyngeal space infection. Note the swelling at the anterior border of the sternocleidomastoid muscle above the hyoid bone, and the mild trismus **B**, A boy with a left buccal, submandibular, and lateral pharyngeal space infection. Note the deviation of the trachea to the right, as the child positions his head to the right, to position the upper airway over the deviated trachea. (From Flynn TR. Anatomy of oral and maxillofacial infections. In: Topazian RG, Goldberg MH, Hupp JR, eds. *Oral and Maxillofacial Infections*. 4th ed. Philadelphia: Saunders; 2002:206. Used with permission.)

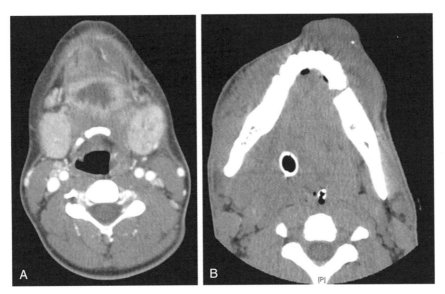

• **Figure 7-16 A,** Axial CT image at the level of the hyoid bone. Note the deviation of the airway to the right, with effacement of the left pyriform recess. **B,** Axial CT image at the level of the mandible. Note the complete obstruction of the oropharyngeal airway, which is tightly enclosed around the endotracheal and nasogastric tubes.

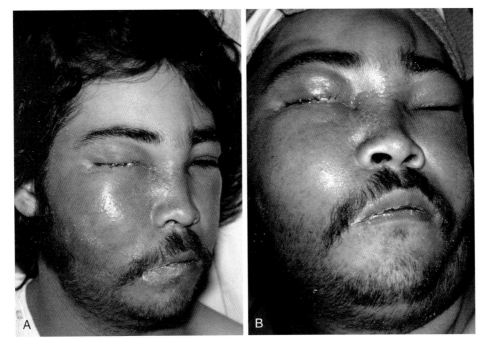

• **Figure 7-17 A,** Oblique view of a patient with a right buccal, infraorbital, and periorbital infection. **B,** The same patient 4 hours later. Note the extension of the swelling to the forehead, the superficial temporal space, and the left periorbital space. Incipient cavernous sinus thrombosis was diagnosed, resulting from congestion of the retinal veins in the left eye. (From Flynn TR, Topazian RG. Infections of the oral cavity. In: Waite D, ed. *Textbook of Practical Oral And Maxillofacial Surgery.* Philadelphia: Lea & Febiger; 1987:301. Used with permission.)

who is too unstable to lie supine even for a brief study, such as a CT scan of the neck, should have the airway immediately secured, with definitive radiographic studies performed later.

Rate of Progression

Finally, when assessing severity, one must consider the infection's rate of progression. This portion of the assessment of severity of infection could be elucidated by obtaining the history of symptoms from the patient. For example, a patient with a massive swelling that started only in the past few hours has a more virulent infection than one with a similar swelling of longer duration. Figure 7-17 shows a patient demonstrating significant progression in 4 hours. The patient in Figure 7-10 had a 60-day history of facial

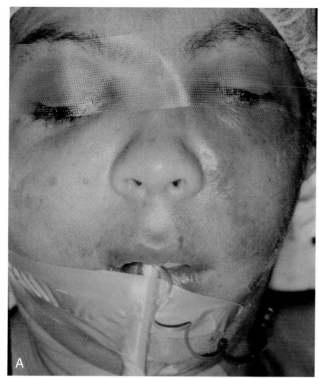

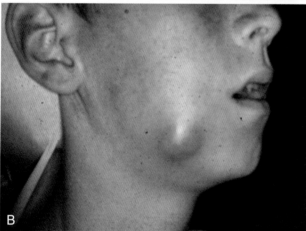

• **Figure 7-18** **A**, Cellulitis of the left infraorbital and periorbital spaces. This swelling is reddened, firm, and exquisitely tender. **B**, Fluctuant abscess of the right buccal space, about to drain subcutaneously near the inferior border of the mandible.

swelling. Figure 7-18 shows two other patients. The one with the localizing abscess about to drain through the skin has a less severe infection than the one with a brawny, indurated cellulitis. This is because cellulitis occurs during the accelerating portion of the clinical course, and abscess formation is a result of mounting host resistance and walling off of the infection by incipient encapsulation.

In summary, a rapid but accurate clinical assessment of the patient's airway stability, and evaluation of the recent history, symptoms, and clinical signs will allow the clinician to determine the severity of the infection and will guide decision-making about the setting and timing of care.

Step 2: Evaluate Host Defenses

Ascertaining the patient's medical history will allow the clinician to assess the patient's host defenses. Although a full history and physical examination may at times be limited in the critically ill patient or one with a compromised airway, the surgeon must always elucidate the presence of metabolic disorders (e.g., diabetes mellitus), immunodeficiency disorders (e.g., long-term steroid use, human immunodeficiency virus [HIV] infection, primary immunodeficiency disease), and/or the presence of renal dysfunction. Not only will awareness of metabolic and immunologic disorders enable appropriate medical management, but also these disorders can predispose to infection with atypical pathogens, such as *Klebsiella pneumoniae* in diabetes, intracellular pathogens in HIV infection, methicillin-resistant *Staphylococcus aureus* (MRSA) in drug abuse, and fungi in iatrogenic or oncologic immunodeficiency. Box 7-3 lists the most common immunocompromising diseases.

Infections of the head and neck region may appear at all ages; however, the average age of a patient with a severe odontogenic infection has been reported to be 34.9 to 36.2 years of age with a standard deviation of 13.7 to 15.8 years.[6,17] We must also consider that the proportion of the population aged 65 and over is also increasing in developed countries. Because the rate of edentulousness is decreasing, odontogenic infections remain the most common head and neck infection in elderly patients. Of note, due to a higher incidence of xerostomia from variety of causes, including polypharmacy, salivary gland infections are becoming more common in elderly patients. Chi et al. reported that 21.6% of 148 patients with deep neck infection were older than 65 years of age. The elderly population has more comorbid conditions and compromised host defenses than younger patients, which may explain the higher ratio of multiple space involvement, longer hospital stay, and a higher complication rate (e.g., upper gastrointestinal bleeding, jugular vein thrombosis, airway obstruction, and septic shock) seen in the elderly.[18]

•**BOX 7-3** **Immune System Compromise**

Conditions Associated With Immune System Compromise

Diabetes
Steroid therapy
Organ transplants
Malignancy
Chemotherapy
Chronic renal disease
Malnutrition
Alcoholism
End-stage AIDS

From Flynn TR. Principles and surgical management of head and neck infections. In: Bagheri SC, Bell RB, Khan HA, eds. *Current Therapy in Oral & Maxillofacial Surgery*. St. Louis: Elsevier; 2011;1087. Used with permission.

Systemic disease has been shown to significantly worsen clinical course. For instance, Chang et al. reported that multiple fascial space involvement occurred in 60% of their patients with diabetes and only in 27.3% of patients without diabetes.[19] Further, patients with diabetes had a much longer hospitalization, 28.9 days versus 15.4 days for those without diabetes. Likewise, Carey and Dodson reported a more intense hospital course for HIV-positive patients, prolonged period of fever over 38°C, and greater use of the intensive care unit.[20] Of note, Miller and Dodson did not find greater length of hospital stay or greater incidence of severe odontogenic infection in HIV-positive patients than in the general population.[21] In summary, a thorough yet concise review of the medical history will allow the clinician to not only appropriately manage patients' comorbidities but also to counsel them as to their expected hospital course.

Step 3: Determine the Setting of Care

The clinician's decision on the setting of care for each given case is based on the previous two steps and logically flows from them. This decision determines the safety and intensity of care and monitoring, the ability to adapt treatment to changing host response to the infection, and ultimately the cost of care. Box 7-4 lists the criteria for hospital admission for head and neck infections.

In general, low-severity infections in healthy patients can be managed with outpatient surgery, local anesthesia or conscious sedation, oral antibiotics and analgesics, and periodic follow-up. Moderate to severe infections, however, are usually managed in hospital, which allows for securing the airway, incision and drainage of deeper anatomic spaces, intravenous fluids and medications, advanced imaging, closer monitoring, and consultation with other specialists as indicated, including infectious diseases experts. Hospital admission for even low-severity infections may be indicated when general anesthesia is necessary or inpatient management of systemic conditions is required, such as control of diabetes or reversal of anticoagulation.

As examples of this decision-making process, a patient with a low-severity abscess of a perioral space, such as the infraorbital or vestibular space, but with poor diabetes control (e.g., plasma glucose >400 mg/dL) may warrant inpatient admission and administration of intravenous fluids, parenteral

antibiotics, and intravenous insulin therapy. Even though this patient's infection alone might be managed surgically in an outpatient setting, achieving glycemic control is necessary for an effective host response. On the other hand, a healthy young patient with a lateral pharyngeal space abscess will require hospitalization for surgical management of the infection under general anesthesia in an operating room setting, and will likely need prolonged tracheal intubation and ventilator support. An uncooperative child may require general anesthesia for management of an otherwise minor infection. In general, it is preferable to err on the side of hospital admission because of safety considerations.

Step 4: Support Medically

The mainstay of head and neck infections is surgical therapy; however, medical therapy cannot be overlooked. After diagnosis and evaluation of the systemic reserve and host defenses, medical therapy is aimed at supporting the host's systemic response to the infection and at correcting any systemic deficiencies that may interfere that response. The role of medical therapy in head and neck infections is primarily supportive of the surgical management and consists of appropriate antibiotic therapy, identification and management of existing comorbidities, and support of hydration and nutrition.

Step 5: Treat Surgically

The principles of the surgical management of head and neck infections are: (1) achieve source control, (2) incision and drainage of involved anatomic sites, and (3) continuous clinical reassessment (including radiographic reassessment when necessary). Figure 7-19 is an algorithm of the surgical management of deep fascial space infections of the head and neck that integrates these principles in a graphic format.

Source control is the removal of the cause of the infection. In odontogenic infection, the causative tooth or teeth are usually removed, although other therapies may occasionally be appropriate, such as pulpectomy or periodontal curettage. The mandibular third molar is most commonly involved, followed by other mandibular posterior teeth.[6] Although dental caries and pericoronitis (inflammation of the soft tissues surrounding an impacted tooth) are common predisposing conditions, one must not overlook periodontal disease as an etiologic factor.[6] Implanted alloplastic materials, such as bone plates and screws, dental implants, alloplastic cosmetic augmentation materials, or temporomandibular joint prostheses can serve as a nidus of infection and generally require removal of the involved foreign bodies. Similarly, in cases of osteomyelitis, debridement, and removal of necrotic bone is required for clinical resolution.

Source control in ear, sinus, and salivary infections generally includes the reestablishment of natural drainage pathways. For example, endoscopic surgery is used to reopen the ostium draining the maxillary sinus in addition to removing obstructing polyps and congested mucosa. Sialolithectomy

---

• BOX 7-4   Criteria for Hospital Admission

- Temperature >101°F
- Dehydration
- Threat to the airway or vital structures
- Infection in moderate or high-severity anatomic spaces
- Need for general anesthesia
- Need for inpatient control of systemic disease

From Flynn TR. Principles and surgical management of head and neck infections. In: Bagheri SC, Bell RB, Khan HA, eds. *Current Therapy in Oral & Maxillofacial Surgery*. St. Louis: Elsevier; 2011:1087. Used with permission.

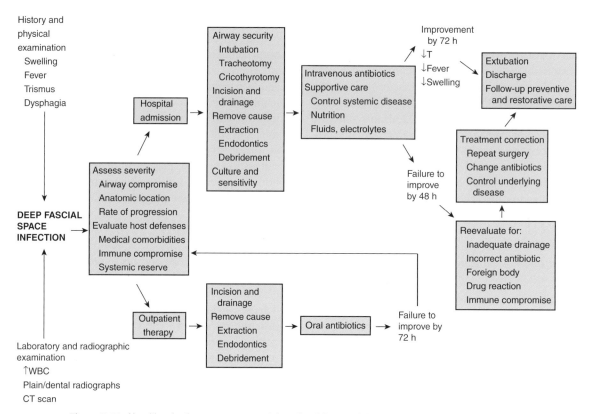

• **Figure 7-19** Algorithm for the management of deep fascial space infections of the head and neck. (From Flynn TR. Deep fascial space infections. In: Laskin DM, Abubaker AO, eds. *Decision Making in Oral and Maxillofacial Surgery*. Chicago: Quintessence; 2007:11. Used with permission.)

reestablishes salivary flow when the source gland has not irreversibly atrophied.

Even with all our advancements to date in diagnostic imaging, antimicrobial therapy, and medical supportive care, surgical incision and drainage remains the cornerstone of management of head and neck infections. The most likely explanation for this fact is that the flora of deep fascial space infections is largely composed of inherently abscess-forming pathogens. The incision and drainage procedure provides benefit to patients by draining painful abscesses, allowing placement of drains for continued irrigation, and increasing blood flow to surgical sites by inflammatory mechanisms enhancing systemic delivery of antibiotics to infection source.

Progression of Head and Neck Infections

Surgical therapy for head and neck infections is based on a thorough knowledge of the anatomy of the deep fascial spaces of the head and neck, as well as an appreciation of the predictable pathways of invasive infections as they progress into deeper anatomic spaces. For example, infections in the submandibular space often extend anteriorly around the anterior belly of the digastric muscle to enter the submental space. From there, the infection can extend around the contralateral anterior belly of the digastric muscle to involve the opposite submandibular space. When a submandibular space infection extends posteriorly, it can extend around the posterior belly of the digastric muscle to enter the lateral

pharyngeal space or superiorly around the posterior border of the mylohyoid muscle to involve the sublingual space. When both submandibular, both sublingual, and the submental spaces are infected with a brawny, indurated cellulitis, Ludwig's angina can be diagnosed.

Another predictable extension pathway for head and neck infections involves the confluence of spaces. This location is in the inferior portion of the anterior palatoglossal arch, just posterior to the floor of the mouth and just lateral to the tongue base. Here the sublingual and submandibular spaces meet at their posterior borders. Also, the anterior-inferior border of the pterygomandibular space forms the lateral boundary of the confluence of spaces. The posterior border of this confluence is the glossopharyngeal gap, where the styloglossus and stylohyoid muscles pass between the superior and middle pharyngeal constrictor muscles, as they extend from the styloid process in the lateral pharyngeal space to the tongue and hyoid bone.

At this anatomic interchange, infections can readily pass from any of the spaces that border it into any of the other spaces. Thus, a pterygomandibular space abscess can often spread into the submandibular or lateral pharyngeal spaces via the confluence of spaces, or a submandibular or sublingual abscess can similarly spread into the lateral pharyngeal space. Clinically, there will be confluence of the adjacent spaces and infections will not be able to skip fascial spaces.

There is no anatomic barrier between the lateral pharyngeal spaces on either side and the retropharyngeal space;

thus, lateral pharyngeal space infections can rapidly surround the oropharynx and hypopharynx via the retropharyngeal space. The retropharyngeal space ends inferiorly at the fusion of the retropharyngeal fascia with the alar fascia, at a variable level between the sixth cervical (C-6) and fourth thoracic (T-4) vertebrae. Once infection is in this location, inflammation and the negative inspiratory force aid in the rupture of the alar fascia, which separates the retropharyngeal space from the danger space, also known as space 4. The danger space extends from the base of the skull to the diaphragm and includes the posterior mediastinum. This is the pathway by which most descending neck infections enter the mediastinum.

Technique of Incision and Drainage

Surgical incision and drainage of the deep fascial spaces of the head and neck is fairly straightforward, once the anatomy of those spaces has been mastered. Figure 7-20 illustrates the external incisions that are used for drainage of the deep fascial spaces. Except, perhaps, in cases of necrotizing fasciitis or descending necrotizing mediastinitis, in which repeated surgical exploration, debridement, and drainage can be anticipated, long incisions and open dissection are usually not necessary. The dissection of the involved spaces can be done bluntly, with a closed hemostat inserted into the respective anatomic spaces. The hemostat is then opened and withdrawn through the incision, creating a pathway for the gravity-dependent egress of pus and infected tissue fluid. It is important to remove the hemostat in opened

position and not close internally potentially grabbing vital structures on withdrawal. This process is repeated multiple times to explore the entire extent of the target anatomic space and to open all loculations of abscess. The pathway created also allows for insertion of culture swabs for sampling of the infecting pathogens, followed by copious irrigation of the deep fascial space, to remove and dilute pathogens and necrotic tissue. At this point a drain can simply be inserted into the wound and sutured to the skin margin with a nonresorbable suture or suturing of safety pin to skin, allowing drains to be advanced and secured in their new position. Alternatively, the drain may pass from one incision to another and its two ends are sutured together, as shown in Figure 7-21, thus creating a through-and-through drain, which allows for easier egress of infected material and irrigation fluid.

Drainage of the lateral pharyngeal space can be accomplished by an incision placed at "D" in Figure 7-20. A patient with a submandibular and lateral pharyngeal space abscess, and the surgical approach to drainage of these spaces, is illustrated in Figure 7-22. The incision passes through skin, subcutaneous tissue, and the superficial fascia. The anterior, or investing, layer of the deep cervical fascia is followed superiorly and posteriorly until the anterior border of the sternocleidomastoid muscle and the angle of the mandible with the overlying masseter muscle and parotideomasseteric fascia are identified. Blunt dissection then can be carried through the fascia just anterior to the sternocleidomastoid muscle, and the palpating finger can enter and bluntly dissect the lateral pharyngeal space. The landmarks to be palpated are the angle of the mandible anterolaterally, the carotid sheath posterolaterally, the transverse processes of the cervical vertebrae posteromedially, and the endotracheal tube, if present, anteromedially. Caution must be taken not to perforate the posterior oropharyngeal wall by aggressive finger dissection toward the oropharynx, however. If desired, the superior portion of the retropharyngeal space can be dissected merely by continuing the finger dissection across the

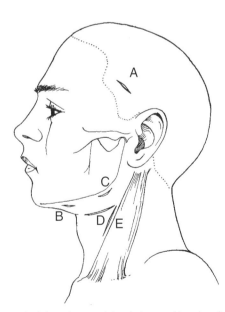

• **Figure 7-20** Incision placement for drainage of head and neck infections. **A,** Superficial or deep temporal spaces. **B,** Submental or submandibular spaces. **C,** Submandibular, submasseteric, or pterygomandibular spaces. **D,** Lateral pharyngeal space or superior portion of the retropharyngeal space. **E,** Retropharyngeal space. When both incisions at **B** and **C** are used, through-and-through drainage of the submandibular space can be achieved, as illustrated in Figure 7-21. (From Flynn TR. Surgical management of orofacial infections. *Atlas Oral Maxillofac Surg Clin North Am.* 2000;8:85.)

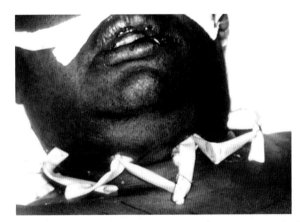

• **Figure 7-21** Through-and-through drainage of both submandibular spaces and the submental space, provided by bilateral incisions placed at **B** and **C** shown in Figure 7-20.

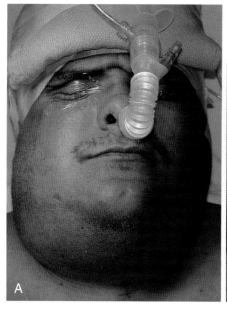
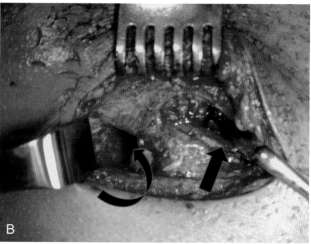

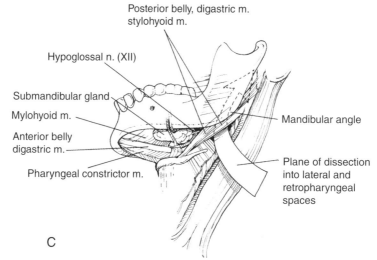

Posterior belly, digastric m.
stylohyoid m.

Hypoglossal n. (XII)

Submandibular gland

Mylohyoid m.

Anterior belly
digastric m.

Pharyngeal constrictor m.

Mandibular angle

Plane of dissection
into lateral and
retropharyngeal
spaces

C

• **Figure 7-22 A,** Frontal view of a patient with a right submandibular and lateral pharyngeal space infection. **B,** Intraoperative view of the same patient, with drainage of the right submandibular and lateral pharyngeal spaces through an incision placed at D shown in Figure 7-20. The anterior (investing) layer of the deep cervical fascia is divided between the submandibular gland and the inferior border of the mandible to drain the submandibular space *(straight arrow)*. The same fascial layer is divided just anterior to the sternocleidomastoid muscle to drain the lateral pharyngeal space *(curved arrow)*. **C,** Diagram of the dissection for drainage of the lateral pharyngeal space and superior portion of the retropharyngeal space. The significant landmarks include the anterior border of the sternocleidomastoid muscle, the posterior belly of the digastric muscle, the submandibular gland, the angle of the mandible, the carotid sheath, and the transverse processes and bodies of the cervical vertebrae. (A, From, Flynn TR. Complex Odontogenic Infections. In: Ellis E, Hupp JR, Tucker MR, editors. *Contemporary Oral and Maxillofacial Surgery.* 6 edition. St. Louis: Mosby; 2013, p. 322. Used with permission. B, From James R. Hupp, Edward Ellis, Myron R. Tucker. *Contemporary Oral and Maxillofacial Surgery*, 5th edition, 2008, Elsevier India. C, From, Flynn TR. Surgical management of orofacial infections. *Atlas of the oral and maxillofacial surgery clinics of North America* 2000;8(Mar):94.)

vertebral bodies posteriorly until the contralateral transverse vertebral bodies are reached.

Drainage of the inferior portion of the retropharyngeal space can be accomplished by an incision placed at "E" in Figure 7-20. The dissection is similar to that for the lateral pharyngeal space described previously, except that as the anterior border of the sternocleidomastoid muscle is exposed, it is retracted posteriorly to expose the carotid sheath, as diagrammed in Figure 7-23. The loose connective tissue lying between the esophagus and the carotid sheath is then bluntly dissected posteriorly and medially to expose the visceral fascia, which surrounds the esophagus, trachea, and

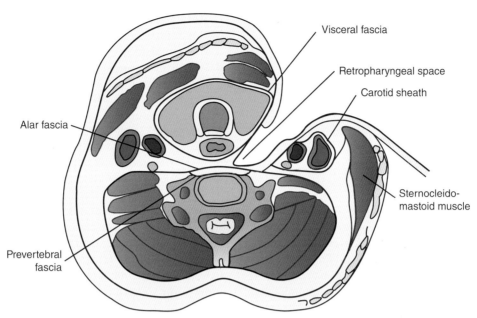

• **Figure 7-23** Diagram of the dissection for drainage of the retropharyngeal space. The significant landmarks include the anterior layer of the deep cervical fascia, the anterior border of the sternocleidomastoid muscle, the carotid sheath, the visceral fascia surrounding the trachea, esophagus and thyroid gland, and the transverse processes and bodies of the cervical vertebrae. (From Flynn TR. Anatomy and surgery of deep fascial space infections. In: Kelly JJ, ed. *Oral and Maxillofacial Surgery Knowledge Update 1994.* Rosemont, IL: American Association of Oral and Maxillofacial Surgeons; 1994:93. Used with permission.)

thyroid gland. The surgeon can then bluntly follow the visceral fascia into the retropharyngeal space. Multiple soft drains can then be placed into the retropharyngeal space. Soft drains are used to avoid erosion of any of the large vessels in the region.

Timing of Incision and Drainage

Most of the general surgery and otolaryngology literature follows the principle of watchful waiting for the development of a frank abscess before surgical drainage is attempted. This expectant approach may be based on an expectation that antibiotic therapy plus the host defenses may eradicate the infection without requiring surgery. On the other hand, the oral and maxillofacial surgery literature questions that approach, and some studies have been performed providing evidence that, at least with odontogenic infections, early incision and drainage of all deep fascial spaces affected by cellulitis or abscess may hasten resolution, appears to abort the spread of the infection into deeper anatomic spaces that involve a greater threat to the airway and other vital structures and is not associated with increased complications. In addition, release of pressure resulting from incision of cellulitic process provides pain relief to the patient. The collective experience of oral and maxillofacial surgeons in the management of severe odontogenic infections supports this approach as well.

Flynn et al. published a case series of 37 severe odontogenic infections treated with a protocol of incision and drainage as soon as possible after hospital admission, with time between admission and surgery of 5.1 + 7.3 hours,

with a range of 0.2 to 23.3 hours. All deep fascial spaces affected by cellulitis or abscess were surgically explored, and at least one drain was placed in each space. All subjects received intravenous penicillin G, except 3 penicillin-allergic patients, who received clindamycin. There were no deaths in the study. Pus was found at surgery (indicating abscess) in 76% of patients; and no pus (indicating cellulitis only) was found in 24%. Multivariate models were then constructed on these outcome variables: length of hospital stay, presence or absence of pus at surgical drainage, and complications. Length of hospital stay was predicted by the number of deep fascial spaces affected and by the occurrence of complications, namely by the need for reoperation and penicillin therapeutic failure (failure to improve after radiographically verified adequate drainage or repeat surgery, plus at least 48 hours of intravenous penicillin). The presence or absence of pus did not predict length of hospital stay, or any other outcome variable. On multivariate analysis, the only predictor of the presence or absence of pus was later identification of peptostreptococci in culture, which was associated with cellulitis, not abscess. No other clinical variable was predictive of abscess formation, including duration of symptoms, white blood cell count, temperature, or severity of infection. (It should be noted that radiographic findings were not included in this analysis.) These data allow us to conclude that early incision and drainage, in the cellulitis stage of infection, was not associated with an increased length of hospital stay or complications, such as the need for reoperation. Clinically, this appears to indicate that early incision and drainage does indeed serve to abort the spread of infection into deeper, more threatening anatomic spaces.[5,6]

Steps 6 and 7: Choose and Administer Appropriate Antibiotic Therapy

The appropriate choice and mode of administration of antibiotic therapy for head and neck infections is discussed fully in Chapter 8 of this text.

Step 8: Reevaluate Frequently

In severe head and neck infections, close clinical follow-up after the initial therapy is warranted because (1) infections can progress into deeper anatomic spaces even after thorough drainage of all spaces affected by cellulitis or abscess; (2) failure of host response to the infection may occur, especially in the setting of comorbidities that compromise the immune system or diminish systemic reserve; (3) the incidence of antibiotic-resistant bacteria in head and neck infections is increasing.

The need for frequent reevaluation in severe head and neck infections can be best illustrated by the experience of cardiothoracic surgeons in treating mediastinitis, clearly an even more severe infection than most head and neck infections, yet a possible complication of head and neck infections. Further, most mediastinitis cases are caused by the same flora as head and neck infections, with the exception that poststernotomy infections are generally due to a nosocomial flora predominated by MRSA.

In 1997, Corsten et al. reported that they were able to reduce the previously reported 47% mortality of mediastinitis to 19% with a policy of open thoracotomy and direct dependent mediastinal drainage. In 2000, Freeman et al. reported on 10 cases of mediastinitis with no mortality. Their policy was immediate open thoracotomy and dependent drainage supplemented by close follow-up with repeated CT scans every 2 to 3 days to examine for new or undrained loculations of pus. Reoperation for new drainage, redebridement, and washout of the surgical wounds was undertaken when extension of infection or clinical deterioration was detected. The subjects experienced an average of six surgeries and six CTs per case, with an average of four cervical incision and drainage procedures and two thoracic drainage procedures per case. The infection progressed through the diaphragm, requiring laparotomy in 30% of cases. Tracheotomy was performed in 40% of cases. The mean length of hospital stay was 46 days, with a range of 14 to 113 days.[22-23]

This dramatic improvement in the mortality of mediastinitis illustrates the therapeutic power of aggressive source control in severe infections, enabled by repeated postoperative CT imaging and close clinical monitoring, when combined with a commitment to the repeated surgical pursuit of infected tissue and necrotic material. Further, such repeated surgery allows the opportunity to sample the infection for new and resistant pathogens in a timely manner.

Although experimental data proving the effectiveness of this approach in head and neck infections are lacking, the results achieved in mediastinitis should encourage head and neck surgeons to adopt a policy of aggressive follow-up with repeated clinical examination, CT imaging, and reoperation when necessary, especially in patients that are not improving or are even deteriorating clinically. CT scans are clearly indicated when patients are not clinically improving, usually demonstrating new loculations or areas not addressed by initial incision and drainage procedures.

The criteria for hospital discharge are listed in Box 7-5. They include measures indicating a subsiding infection, stable airway, and recovery of autonomous function. Box 7-6 specifies the criteria for extubation. The ventilatory parameters measure functionality in the lower airway; yet in head and neck infection, obstruction of the upper airway is the prime concern. The gold standard in determining the stability of the upper airway is the air leak test. The air leak test is illustrated in Figure 7-24. The steps in performing the air leak test are listed in Box 7-7. By experience, we have found that identification of air space surrounding the endotracheal tube on CT is a late indicator of a stable upper airway.

Occasionally, the clinical course will deteriorate after initial therapy. Table 7-5 lists the most common potential causes of worsening fever, swelling, airway patency, white blood cell count, or C-reactive protein. When any of these parameters

---

• BOX 7-5   Criteria for Hospital Discharge

Extubation
T < 100° F for 24 h
Oral intake > 10 mL/kg/shift for two shifts
All drains out
Swelling decreasing
Minimal or no drainage
Adequate control of systemic disease
Ambulation

From Flynn TR. Principles and surgical management of head and neck infections. In: Bagheri SC, Bell RB, Khan HA (eds). *Current therapy in oral & maxillofacial surgery.* St. Louis: Elsevier; 2011:1088. Used with permission.

• BOX 7-6   Criteria for Extubation

- Recovery from general anesthesia and paralyzing agents
- Stable and acceptable vital signs
- Acceptable ventilatory parameters
  - Normal respiratory rate
  - Vital capacity >15 mL/kg
  - Inspiratory force >25 cm H_2O
  - Minute ventilation = 6-10 L/min
- Normal blood gases or oxygen saturation
- Normal end-tidal carbon dioxide
- Ability to swallow (tracheotomy patients)
- Positive air leak test

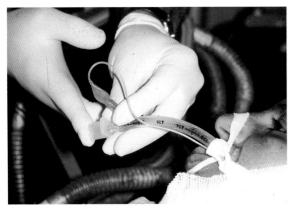

• **Figure 7-24** Air leak test. The technique is described in Box 7-7. (From Flynn TR. Principles and surgical management of head and neck infections. In: Bagheri SC, Bell RB, Khan HA, eds. *Current Therapy in Oral & Maxillofacial Surgery*. St. Louis: Elsevier; 2011:1088. Used with permission.)

• BOX 7-7 Air Leak Test Procedure

1. Reverse sedation.
2. Suction the mouth, oropharynx, and hypopharynx.
3. Suction the endotracheal/tracheotomy tube and trachea.
4. Consider topical lidocaine via the endotracheal tube for topical anesthesia.
5. Administer 100% oxygen for 3-5 min.
6. Deflate the cuff of the endotracheal/tracheotomy tube; allow coughing to subside.
7. Occlude the endotracheal/tracheotomy tube; observe for airway distress, oxygen desaturation, and the ability to breathe around the occluded tube.
8. If the patient can successfully maintain respiration around the occluded endotracheal/tracheotomy tube, reinflate its cuff and reconnect 100% oxygen for 3-5 min.
9. Suction the mouth, oropharynx, and hypopharynx and endotracheal/tracheotomy tube again.
10. Administer 100% oxygen for 3 min.
11. Insert a stylet or tube changer device down the entire length of the endotracheal/tracheotomy tube.
12. Deflate the cuff of the endotracheal/tracheotomy tube and allow coughing to subside. Oxygenate as necessary.
13. Withdraw the endotracheal/tracheotomy tube, leaving the stylet or tube changer in place. A nasoendotracheal tube can be withdrawn partially, with the tip of the tube remaining in the nasopharynx.
14. Observe for airway distress, oxygen desaturation, or airway obstruction for 20 min.
15. If the airway remains stable, the stylet or tube changer, plus the endotracheal tube if present, can be withdrawn fully. Observe for airway distress, oxygen desaturation, or airway obstruction for several hours.
16. If the airway does not remain stable, advance the endotracheal/tracheotomy tube over the stylet into the trachea and reinflate the cuff. Oxygenate as necessary. Consider reinstituting sedation.

TABLE 7-5 Causes of Treatment Failure

Cause	Example
Inadequate surgery	Undrained loculation of pus
Undiagnosed osteomyelitis	Recurrent soft tissue infection in perimandibular spaces
Depressed host defenses	Poorly controlled diabetes
Foreign body	Bone plate, dental implant
Tumor	Squamous cell carcinoma
Obstruction of anatomic drainage	Sialolithiasis, sinusitis
Antibiotic problems	
• Selection	Incorrect choice of empiric antibiotic
• Compliance	Patient cannot afford prescription
• Absorption	Dairy products interfere with fluoroquinolones
• Dosage	Incorrect dosage prescribed
• Allergy	Penicillin allergy
• Toxicity	Q-T interval prolongation with fluoroquinolones
Superinfection	Candidiasis following antibiotic prescription
Reinfection	Relapse of actinomycosis

Modified with permission from Flynn TR. Principles of management and prevention of odontogenic infections. In: Ellis E, Hupp JR, Tucker MR, eds. *Contemporary Oral and Maxillofacial Surgery*. 6th ed. St. Louis: Mosby; 2013:311. Used with permission.

are failing to improve, thorough clinical reassessment, possibly including CT imaging, may indicate the cause. Repeat radiographic imaging may identify a foreign body, an undrained loculation of pus, or extension of infection into a new location. When local soft tissue infection returns or worsens in spite of adequate initial therapy, a previously undiagnosed osteomyelitis, typically of the mandible, may represent an inadequately controlled source of infection.

When an anatomic cause of clinical deterioration cannot be identified, attention may then be directed to a microbiologic or systemic problem. This is when consultation with other specialists may be helpful. For example, the initial antibiotic selection may have been appropriate based on the usual sensitivity patterns of the pathogens identified in culture. However, an increasing proportion of many head and neck pathogens now are becoming resistant to the usual antibiotic choices. A given strain may also become resistant during the course of therapy; or new pathogens can be introduced during the course of therapy, such as nosocomial sinusitis after prolonged nasoendotracheal intubation. Nosocomial sinusitis is frequently caused by highly antibiotic-resistant bacteria, such as *Pseudomonas, Acinetobacter, Escherichia coli, S. aureus,* and *Candida* species.

Systemic causes of treatment failure include the immunosuppressive and metabolic diseases listed in Box 7-3.

For example, poorly controlled diabetes interferes with the chemotaxis of white blood cells toward invading bacteria, which decreases host response. Unusual pathogens are also associated with these diseases, such as *Klebsiella* in diabetes, MRSA in intravenous drug abusers, and intracellular pathogens in HIV/AIDS. Iatrogenic immunosuppression is commonly used in chronic inflammatory diseases, such as rheumatoid arthritis and psoriasis. Many of the newer drugs for these conditions are monoclonal antibodies that have immunosuppressive effects. Improved control of these metabolic and immunosuppressive disorders can aid in the host response to infection.

Summary

The principles of medical and surgical management of head and neck infections do not guarantee an ideal outcome. If followed conscientiously, however, these guidelines can reassure the clinician that the standard of care has been met. The first three steps in the process involve evaluation and decision-making. They can be accomplished within the first few minutes of the initial patient encounter. Medical support and surgical therapy logically flow from that initial evaluation. In abscess-forming head and neck infections, initial airway stabilization and early, aggressive surgical drainage of all deep fascial spaces affected by cellulitis or abscess are the keys to reducing the morbidity and potential mortality of these infections. Finally, close clinical and radiographic follow-up are necessary for detection and management of treatment failure after initial therapy.

References

1. Christensen B, Han M, Dillon JK. The cause of cost in the management of odontogenic infections. Part 1: a demographic survey and multivariate analysis. *J Oral Maxillofac Surg.* 2013; 71(12):2058-2067.
2. Christensen B, Han M, Dillon JK. The cause of cost in the management of odontogenic infections. Part 2: multivariate outcome analyses. *J Oral Maxillofac Surg.* 2013;71(12):2068-2076.
3. Williams AC. Ludwig's angina. *Surg Gynecol Obstet.* 1940; 70:140.
4. Williams AC, Guralnick WC. The diagnosis and treatment of Ludwig's angina: a report of twenty cases. *N Engl J Med.* 1943;228:443.
5. Flynn TR, Shanti RM, Hayes C. Severe odontogenic infections. Part 2: Prospective outcomes study. *J Oral Maxillofac Surg.* 2006;64:1104-1113.
6. Flynn TR, Shanti RM, Levi MH, Adamo AK, Kraut RA, Trieger N. Severe odontogenic infections. Part 1: prospective report. *J Oral Maxillofac Surg.* 2006;64(7):1093-1103.
7. Ishinaga H, Otsu K, Sakaida H, et al. Descending necrotizing mediastinitis from deep neck infection. *Eur Arch Otorhinolaryngol.* 2013;270(4):1463-1466.
8. Murray M, Stevens T, Herford A, Roberts J. Lemierre syndrome: two cases requiring surgical intervention. *J Oral Maxillofac Surg.* 2013;71(2):310-315.
9. Desa V, Green R. Cavernous sinus thrombosis: current therapy. *J Oral Maxillofac Surg.* 2012;70(9):2085-2091.
10. da Silva PS, Waisberg DR. Internal carotid artery pseudoaneurysm with life-threatening epistaxis as a complication of deep neck space infection. *Pediatr Emerg Care.* 2011;27(5): 422-424.
11. Wolfe MM, Davis JW, Parks SN. Is surgical airway necessary for airway management in deep neck infections and Ludwig angina? *J Crit Care.* 2011;26(1):11-14.
12. Plaza Mayor G, Martinez-San Millan J, Martinez-Vidal A. Is conservative treatment of deep neck space infections appropriate? *Head Neck.* 2001;23(2):126-133.
13. Shanti RM, Aziz SR. Should we wait for development of an abscess before we perform incision and drainage? *Oral Maxillofac Surg Clin North Am.* 2011;23(4):513-518.
14. Soon SR, Kanagalingam J, Johari S, Yuen HW. Head and neck cancers masquerading as deep neck abscess. *Singapore Med J.* 2012;53(12):840-842.
15. Miller WD, Furst IM, Sandor GK, Keller MA. A prospective, blinded comparison of clinical examination and computed tomography in deep neck infections. *Laryngoscope.* 1999;109(11): 1873-1879.
16. Endicott JN, Nelson RJ, Saraceno CA. Diagnosis and management decisions in infections of the deep fascial spaces of the head and neck utilizing computerized tomography. *Laryngoscope.* 1982;92:630-633.
17. Kirse DJ, Roberson DW. Surgical management of retropharyngeal space infections in children. *Laryngoscope.* 2001;111(8):1413-1422.
18. Chi TH, Tsao YH, Yuan CH. Influences of patient age on deep neck infection: clinical etiology and treatment outcome. *Otolaryngol Head Neck Surg.* 2014;151(4):586-590.
19. Chang JS, Yoo KH, Yoon SH, et al. Odontogenic infection involving the secondary fascial space in diabetic and non-diabetic patients: a clinical comparative study. *J Korean Assoc Oral Maxillofac Surg.* 2013;39(4):175-181.
20. Carey JW, Dodson TB. Hospital course of HIV-positive patients with odontogenic infections. *Oral Surg Oral Med Oral Pathol Oral Radiol Endod.* 2001;91(1):23-27.
21. Miller EJ Jr, Dodson TB. The risk of serious odontogenic infections in HIV-positive patients: a pilot study. *Oral Surg Oral Med Oral Pathol Oral Radiol Endod.* 1998;86(4):406-409.
22. Corsten MJ, Shamji FM, Odell PF, et al. Optimal treatment of descending necrotising mediastinitis. *Thorax.* 1997;52(8):702-708. doi:10.1136/thx.52.8.702.
23. Freeman RK, Vallières E, Verrier ED, Karmy-Jones R, Wood DE. Descending necrotizing mediastinitis: an analysis of the effects of serial surgical debridement on patient mortality. *J Thorac Cardiovasc Surg.* 2000;119(2):260-267. doi:10.1016/S0022-5223(00)70181-4.

8

Principles of Antibiotic Therapy for Head, Neck, and Orofacial Infections

THOMAS R. FLYNN AND RABIE M. SHANTI

The Golden Age of antibiotics is over. Penicillin, introduced clinically in the 1940s, was the first wonder drug. Within 2 years, *Staphylococcus aureus,* the champion bacteria of antibiotic resistance, had developed penicillin-resistant strains. Less than a century later, this *Staphylococcus* and far too many other bacteria, fungi, and viruses are becoming resistant to virtually every antibiotic that humans have been able to devise. The relationship of humans, microbes, and antibiotics has changed; it has new guiding principles that we must learn to be able to survive as a species. This chapter will attempt to elucidate some of those evolving principles as they relate to head and neck infections.

The Principles of Antibiotic Therapy

We are now able to articulate several guiding principles of antibiotic therapy, which are listed in Box 8-1. These principles will certainly evolve as our knowledge increases, yet they can serve as a starting point for a new approach to the wise use of antibiotics by head and neck surgeons in the current era of increasing antibiotic resistance, the declining systemic reserve of our aging population, ever more complicated antibiotic drug interactions with our patients' concurrent medications, and increasing costs of care.

Principle 1: Surgery to Remove the Cause and Establish Drainage is Primary; Antibiotics are Adjunctive Treatment

The most important and overriding principle that we have relearned in recent years is that surgical treatment, along with protection of the airway, is primary in the management of head and neck infections. In 1940, Ashbel Williams of Boston City Hospital presented a series of 37 patients with Ludwig's angina, of whom 54% died, mostly from airway compromise or overwhelming sepsis.[1] Only 3 years later, Drs. Williams and Walter Guralnick published a series of 20 cases of Ludwig's angina in which the mortality was reduced to 10%.[2] They had changed their treatment protocol from expectant observation for the development of airway compromise or a fluctuant abscess to initial airway stabilization with endotracheal intubation or tracheotomy followed immediately by aggressive open surgical drainage of all infected anatomic spaces. This dramatic reduction in the mortality of then-dreaded Ludwig angina was achieved before penicillin was available to civilians. Since the 1940s, the use of antibiotics and advances in medical therapy have further reduced the mortality of Ludwig's angina to less than 4%.[3,4] As bacterial resistance to antibiotics increases, head and neck surgeons will be able to rely on medical therapy less and will be forced to return to surgery as the primary management of head and neck infections. Surgery is primary; antibiotics are adjunctive.

The management of infectious diseases has two cardinal strategies: source control and antibacterial chemotherapy. Source control refers to the physical removal of infected material, including pus, necrotic tissue, bacterial colonies and vegetations, and foreign bodies. Generally, source control is accomplished surgically, but it also includes surface debridement and antiseptic application. Antibacterial chemotherapy is the use of antibiotic medications by the topical, enteral, and parenteral routes.

Most head and neck infections are caused by the abscess-forming combination of gram-positive cocci and anaerobes and this region has abundant hard tissues, consisting of teeth and bone, on which biofilms easily form; therefore, source control is paramount in the management of these infections. Biofilms can also form on sheets of soft tissue, such as fascia. In addition, the head and neck is rich with cavities that require free drainage to the external environment to cleanse them of accumulated bacteria and secretions, such as the sinuses, nose, ears, salivary glands, and the lacrimal apparatus. Surgery is often necessary to establish drainage of normal and pathologic cavities in the head and neck.

The standard treatment for patients presenting to an emergency department (ED) with toothache is the prescription of an antibiotic and an analgesic with the advice to see a dentist as soon as possible. The purpose of the antibiotic prescription is to treat or prevent a severe infection, seen as

1. Surgery to remove the cause and establish drainage is primary; antibiotics are adjunctive treatment.
2. Use therapeutic antibiotics only when clinically indicated.
3. Use specific antibiotic therapy as soon as possible, based on culture and sensitivity testing.
4. Follow the guidance of evidence-based recommendations and professional guidelines when they are available.
5. Use the narrowest spectrum empiric antibiotic effective against the most likely pathogens.
6. Use the least toxic indicated antibiotic, considering interaction with concurrent medications.
7. Avoid the use of combination antibiotics, except in specific situations in which they are shown to be necessary.
8. Minimize the duration of antibiotic therapy, as appropriate to the presenting type of infection.
9. Use the most cost-effective appropriate antibiotic.
10. Use prophylactic antibiotics only where proved effective or according to professional guidelines.

swelling. Brennan et al. reported on a clinical trial comparing the incidence of severe infection in patients presenting to an ED with toothache, when they were given antibiotic or placebo.[5] They found an equal incidence of infection in both the placebo and the antibiotic group. The only significant predictors of severe infection were a periapical radiolucency over 1.5 mm in diameter and a filling in the affected tooth. This study suggests that antibiotics do not prevent the spread of infections beyond the teeth, and that the appropriate dental procedure, such as root canal therapy or extraction, is the most important treatment.

In 2019, the American Dental Association published an evidence-based guideline on antibiotic use for management of pulpal and periapical infections.[6] Based on an extensive literature review, an expert panel recommended against the use of antibiotics for these infections, regardless of whether definitive dental treatment, consisting of root canal therapy, extraction, or other interventions, is available. They recommended antibiotic use only when signs of systemic involvement such as fever and malaise are present or in cases in which the risk of progression to systemic involvement is high, such as in the immunocompromised patient.

Principle 2: Use Therapeutic Antibiotics Only When Clinically Indicated

The clinical indications for antibiotic therapy include fever, lymphadenopathy, and indurated or fluctuant swelling. Purulent discharge may not indicate the need for antibiotic therapy, because spontaneous or surgical drainage marks the onset of the chronic stage of infection. At this point, removal of the cause of infection, such as an infected tooth, may provide resolution of the infection without the need for antibiotics.

Inflammation is not always infection. The five cardinal signs of inflammation, redness, swelling, increased temperature, pain, and loss of function, elicit a reflexive association with infection among clinicians, especially in the postoperative situation. Postoperative edema, which is soft, jelly-like in consistency, and only mildly tender, is merely part of the inflammatory response to surgical trauma. Knowledge of the usual time course of the development of postoperative wound infection, at 5 to 7 days after surgery, can help the surgeon to differentiate between the inflammatory response to surgery and postoperative infection.

The clinician must correlate historical findings, such as the history of pain, other symptoms, and prior treatment, with physical examination to arrive at a clinical diagnosis of infection. For example, fever occurring without indurated or fluctuant swelling may be the result of postoperative dehydration or a viral infection. Lymphadenopathy, likewise, can be reactive, and it can persist for a significant duration after resolution of a prior infection.

The clinician's decision on whether to prescribe antibiotics has important implications, not only for the patient, but also for the patient's family and community. It is obvious that when a patient receives an antibiotic, bacteria resistant to that antibiotic will remain in his/her flora. On the other hand, an antibiotic prescription selects for resistant strains, not only in the patient, but also in entire families. In one study, Brook took throat swab cultures of pediatric patients with pharyngitis before and after a 7-day course of penicillin. After treatment, cultures were taken of the patients and their parents and siblings. The oropharyngeal carriage of one or more penicillin-resistant strains rose from 12% to 46% of patients, but also rose to 45% in the other family members. After 3 months, carriage of resistant organisms had declined only to 27%.[7]

In a second study, Brook and Gober performed monthly throat swab cultures on schoolchildren in the Washington, DC for 2 years.[8] The lowest average carriage of penicillin-resistant strains occurred in September (13%), and the highest rate of carriage of one or more penicillin-resistant strains was in April (60%). The most likely explanation of this phenomenon is that as inclement weather and respiratory infections increase during the winter months, increasingly more children are given courses of antibiotics. They pass the resistant strains to each other, even to children who have not received antibiotics. Then, as the weather improves and the children disperse for summer vacation, the carriage of resistant strains starts to decline.[8]

The implication of these two studies is that by prescribing antibiotics, clinicians increase the incidence of antibiotic-resistant strains, not only in their patients, but also in their patients' families and their entire communities, such as schools and workplaces.

There are many false indications for the use of antibiotics, most of them prompted by fear. Sometimes the fear belongs to our patients, when they make statements such as "Doctor, don't you think I need an antibiotic for this?" or "My other doctor always gave me an antibiotic for this," or "Doctor, I always get an infection when I have this done; I need an antibiotic." At other times, the fear arises in the doctor: fear of litigation, prompting defensive medicine maneuvers; or the fear of changing old habits that seem to have served well over the years.

In recent years, our understanding of the pathophysiology of rhinosinusitis has changed. Although acute sinus infections do occur and require antibiotic therapy when unresponsive to conservative treatment, the pathophysiology of chronic rhinosinusitis is now understood to involve inflammatory responses to allergens, pollutants, and the blockage of drainage pathways, in addition to microbes. Inhaled corticosteroids and surgical reestablishment of natural drainage are now used to manage this inflammatory response, thus decreasing the indication for antibiotic administration.

The Council for Appropriate and Rational Antibiotic Therapy, an independent multidisciplinary group of clinicians and scientists, has identified 5 criteria for the accurate use of antibiotic therapy[9]:

1. The use of antibiotic therapy for a given indication is supported by evidence-based results.
2. The therapeutic benefits of each antibiotic should be considered relative to its effectiveness in treating the given infection, based on regional or specific susceptibility and resistance patterns.
3. The safest effective antibiotic should be chosen, while considering that the safety profile of newer medications may not be as well established as those that have been in use for many years.
4. The most cost-effective antibiotic regimen should be chosen, considering that treatment failures and adverse events can outweigh the higher cost of a more effective initial treatment.
5. Drug and duration: Optimal drug selection requires consideration of local resistance patterns, the patient's systemic condition, and the patient's recent antibiotic exposure; the optimal duration of therapy means prescribing the selected drug for the shortest period required for clinical and microbiologic effectiveness.

These 10 principles of antibiotic therapy for head and neck infections aim to incorporate the 5 criteria for the accurate use of antibiotic therapy in their specific practical recommendations.

Principle 3: Use Specific Antibiotic Therapy as Soon as Possible

Specific antibiotic therapy is currently guided by the results of culture and sensitivity testing on specimens taken from an individual patient. Empiric antibiotic therapy is an educated choice of antibiotic based on knowledge of the most likely pathogens for a given clinical presentation.

Conventional culture methods are time-consuming, which can be a significant disadvantage in severe or life-threatening infections. The polymerase chain reaction (PCR)-based techniques commonly used for diagnosis of COVID infection, for example, do not provide results for 48 to 72 hours currently. Newer molecular methods are being developed, however, that may allow the identification of the pathogens causing an infection as well as their antibiotic sensitivity within an hour.

Particularly promising is surface-enhanced Raman spectroscopy (SERS). Although this technique is still in development, SERS-based techniques have been developed which allow the identification of highly antibiotic-resistant pathogens, such as methicillin-resistant *Staphylococcus aureus* (MRSA), *Klebsiella pneumoniae, Acinetobacter baumannii, Escherichia coli,* and vancomycin-resistant enterococci within 1 hour of sampling. SERS techniques are also in development that can rapidly identify bacterial response to antibiotics, indicating susceptibility or resistance.[10]

Antibiotic resistance rates among the head and neck flora are increasing. During the decade of the 1990s, the percentage of odontogenic infection cases yielding one or more penicillin-resistant strains increased from 33% to 55%, as seen in Table 8-1.[11-14]

Similarly, the carriage of clindamycin-resistant strains in head and neck infections has increased to as high as 41%.[15,16] Clindamycin resistance among α-hemolytic streptococci, MRSA and other staphylococci, and *Bacteroides fragilis* isolated from head and neck infections is also mounting.[17] Clindamycin resistance is also increasing in peritonsillar abscess, with 32% of streptococcal isolates, including *Streptococcus pyogenes* (group A β-hemolytic streptococcus) and *Streptococcus anginosus* (a member of the viridans streptococcal group) resistant to clindamycin.[18] Thus, the almost universal effectiveness of the usual empiric antibiotic choices for odontogenic infections is declining.

Antibiotic resistance mechanisms can be divided into four categories: antibiotic inactivation, receptor site modification, membrane pore deletion, and active transport pumps, as shown in Table 8-2. Table 8-2 also lists examples of head and neck pathogens that can carry these resistance mechanisms.

The classic example of antibiotic inactivation is the β-lactamases, which are common among the head and neck flora. The β-lactamases range from simple penicillinases, which can disrupt the penicillin ring, to cephalosporinases, to the multiple potent carbapenemases, which convey high-level resistance to the entire β-lactam class of antibiotics. There are multiple classes of carbapenemases, ranging from

TABLE 8-1　Increasing Penicillin Resistance Rates Among Oral Pathogens

Year	% of Cases PCN Resistant	Country
1991[8]	33	United States
1992[12]	38	Sweden
1995[13]	55	United States
1999[14]	54	United States
2017[15]	63	United States

PCN, Penicillin.

TABLE 8-2 Antibiotic Resistance Mechanisms

Mechanism	Example	Head and Neck Pathogens That May Have This Mechanism
Antibiotic inactivation	β-Lactamases, adenylyl transferases (aminoglycosides)	*Staphylococcus aureus, Staphylococcus epidermidis, Haemophilus influenzae, Prevotella, Porphyromonas, Capnocytophaga, Eikenella, Fusobacterium*
Receptor site modification	PBPs, D-ala-D-ala (vancomycin), DNA gyrase (fluoroquinolones), methylated RNA, (macrolides)	MRSA, *Streptococcus pneumoniae, Streptococcus sanguis*
Membrane pore deletion	Deleted porins in *Klebsiella pneumoniae* and *Escherichia coli* (cephalosporins, imipenem, aztreonam)	*K. pneumoniae, Pseudomonas aeruginosa, Serratia marcescens, E. coli*
Active transport pumps	tet A (tetracyclines), erm (erythromycin), AcrAB-TolC (multiple antibiotics)	*K. pneumoniae, Acinetobacter baumannii, P. aeruginosa, E. coli, Neisseria gonorrhoeae*

MRSA, Methicillin-resistant *Staphylococcus aureus; PBPs,* penicillin-binding proteins.

TABLE 8-3 Antibiotics for Community-Acquired Methicillin-Resistant *Staphylococcus aureus*

Outpatient, Immunocompetent*	Febrile, Immunocompetent	Bacteremia/Sepsis or Endocarditis
TMP-SMX-DS (160 mg bid)[†] Clindamycin (300-450 mg tid)[†]	Vancomycin (IV) or Linezolid (IV)	Vancomycin or Daptomycin (IV) Daptomycin + Ceftaroline (IV) Or Ceftaroline (IV) Or Telavancin (IV)
I&D + Oritavancin (1200 mg × 1) or Dalbavancin (1000 mg × 1, then 500 mg × 1, 7 days later)		Linezolid (IV) [bacteriostatic, not for intravascular infection]

*If abscess, incision and drainage is most important
[†]If unsatisfactory treatment response, switch to vancomycin after 2-3 d.
Abbreviations: *I&D,* Incision and drainage; *TMP-SMX-DS,* trimethoprim–sulfamethoxazole, double strength; *bid,* twice daily; *po,* by mouth; *tid,* 3 times per day; *IV,* intravenously.

extended-spectrum β-lactamases to *K. pneumoniae* carbapenemases, metallo–β-lactamases, and oxacillinases.[19]

Carbapenemases are particularly concerning because they convey resistance to the carbapenems (as well as the penicillins and cephalosporins), which are considered the antibiotics of last resort for highly resistant organisms, including *K. pneumoniae,* a common pathogen in head and neck infections.

The ESKAPE (*Enterococcus faecium, S. aureus, K. pneumoniae, A. baumannii, Pseudomonas aeruginosa,* and *Enterobacter* species) pathogens have increased levels of resistance toward multiple classes of first-line and last-resort antibiotics.[19,20] Members of the ESKAPE group that are found in head and neck, wound, and nosocomial infections include *Staphylococci, Klebsiella, Enterococci, Acinetobacter,* and *E. coli.*

S. aureus strains developed the ability to synthesize penicillinases within 2 years of the introduction of penicillin. The penicillinase-resistant penicillins, such as methicillin, nafcillin, and dicloxacillin are resistant to these early β-lactamases. Adenylyl transferases inactivate the aminoglycosides.

Receptor site modification is seen with altered penicillin-binding proteins, a group of proteins having varying affinities for penicillins. These proteins, also called transpeptidases, are enzymes necessary for cross-linking of peptidoglycan, a necessary component in bacterial cell wall synthesis. Small alterations in the penicillin-binding proteins, encoded for by the *mecA* gene, decrease their affinity for the β-lactam ring of even the penicillinase-resistant penicillins, yet their transpeptidase function remains. The result is commonly referred to as methicillin resistance, and methicillin-resistant *S. aureus* (MRSA) is the most widely known example. However, *Streptococcus pneumoniae* and *Streptococcus sanguis* can also carry the *mecA* gene, conferring high-level penicillin resistance.

Table 8-3 lists the currently recommended antibiotic regimens for community-acquired MRSA infections. It is important to note that incision and drainage, plus removal of the cause, where appropriate, are the most important treatment. This table also takes into account the fact that transmission of the *vanA* gene, conferring vancomycin resistance, has been reported. In vancomycin-resistant *S. aureus* (VRSA), based in each case on sensitivity testing, linezolid, telavancin, and daptomycin, possibly in combination with ceftaroline or oxacillin, have been recommended.

Porins are transmembrane barrel proteins found in bacteria that regulate and enable the passage of larger and charged molecules into the cell. β-Lactam and fluoroquinolone antibiotics pass into gram-negative bacteria via porins, and when the porin-encoding gene is mutated appropriately, these antibiotics are excluded from the cell. *K. pneumoniae* is a head and neck pathogen that can carry this antibiotic-resistance mechanism.

Several species of gram-negative bacteria produce efflux pumps. These are cell-bound proteins that expel antibiotic molecules to the external environment, thus reducing the intracellular concentration of a given antibiotic to sublethal levels. Efflux pumps have other important functions affording antibacterial resistance, including biofilm formation, cell-to-cell communication, pathogenicity, and virulence. The important role of efflux pumps in bacterial resistance also makes efflux pump inhibitors prime candidates for the chemotherapy of resistant bacteria. Current research has identified several efflux pump inhibitors that may have clinical application in the future.[21]

Multidrug-resistant strains of *S. pneumoniae, Enterococcus, Staphylococcus,* and *Hemophilus* are increasingly cultured from head and neck infections. *K. pneumoniae* is also a common pathogen in head and neck infections; *K. pneumoniae* strains have been found to synthesize extended-spectrum β-lactamases, specifically called *K. pneumoniae* carbapenemase and New Delhi metalloproteinase-1, all of which confer high-level antibiotic resistance. Enterococci, resident oropharyngeal flora, have also recently been shown to have transmitted the *vanA* gene, conferring vancomycin resistance to MRSA, generating a new concern: MRSA and VRSA. Highly resistant organisms are being seen with increasing frequency in head and neck infections.

In addition to the use of new and old antibiotics for highly resistant organisms, surgeons must be aware of and rigorously practice the even more important role of other infection control measures in the prevention and management of infection by these organisms. The recent spread of the COVID virus to health care workers has dramatically illustrated that we must not only have personal protective equipment; we must use it correctly. Box 8-2 lists some of the nonantibiotic measures that can help to limit the spread of highly resistant organisms to our patients and among ourselves.

Because antibiotic resistance is increasing among the flora of head and neck infections, "conservative" management of these infections with antibiotics alone has become less effective. Early operative intervention to reduce the infectious burden, remove necrotic tissue, and reestablish normal drainage pathways has therefore increased in clinical necessity. At the same time, obtaining a clinical sample for culture and sensitivity testing as soon as possible in the course of the disease is additional justification for prompt surgical management of head and neck infections.

Principle 4: Use Evidence-Based Medicine and Guidelines When Available

In general, the guidelines offered by professional societies are usually the consensus of a panel of experts, who must make a recommendation often in the absence of convincing and valid scientifically established data. Such guidelines are necessary, given our lack of evidence, yet they fall lower in the ranking of reliable sources of guidance for clinicians.[22]

A prime example of this is the joint recommendations on prevention of late prosthetic joint infection (LPJI) published by the American Academy of Orthopaedics and the American Dental Association in 2003.[23] These were followed by an online advisory from the American Academy of Orthopaedic Surgeons published in 2009, which contradicted the previous guideline. Again in 2012, the American Academy of Orthopaedics and the American Dental Association published joint guidelines that contradicted yet again the guidance offered in 2003 and 2009. The result is much confusion among clinicians and patients alike. In 2015, the American Dental Association independently updated its guidelines to state: "In general, for patients with prosthetic joint implants, prophylactic antibiotics are not recommended prior to dental procedures to prevent prosthetic joint infection." In cases in which the patient had experienced complications with a prosthetic joint, consultation with the patient and the orthopaedic surgeon was recommended.[24]

The evolution of the guidelines published by the groups interested in this topic demonstrates our improving ability to distinguish between causative and confounding variables in clinical questions. Initially, anecdotal temporal proximity and microbiologic findings led clinicians to suspect that invasive dental procedures caused at least some cases of late prosthetic joint infection. Two case control studies from 2010 and 2011 compared the occurrence of LPJI following dental procedures, with and without antibiotic prophylaxis. Both studies found no significant difference in LPJI between these two groups.[25,26] In the study by Skaar et al. there were no culture data available to indicate the likely source of the LPJI, such that nonodontogenic cases could

---

• BOX 8-2 Nonantibiotic Strategies for Highly Resistant Organisms

- HANDWASHING!!!!!
- Isolation and careful aseptic technique
- Limit number of caregivers
- Minimize/remove colonizing sites (devices, such as ventilators, catheters, intravenous lines, external fixators, etc.)
- Minimize patient transport through the facility
- Minimize length of stay in special care units, such as intensive care
- Close temporarily and disinfect entire units

not be separated from those joint infections likely caused by oral pathogens. In the Berbari et al. study, statistical significance was achieved only for LPJI cases caused by all types of bacteria, 58% of which were due to staphylococci.[26] When cases caused by likely oral pathogens were analyzed separately, there was insufficient statistical power to allow any conclusions. The weaknesses of both of these studies did not provide a clear answer to whether dental procedures cause prosthetic joint infection.

Good evidence is still accumulating, however. In 2022, a cohort study of over 9000 prosthetic joints placed in England, where prophylactic antibiotics for invasive dental procedures have never been recommended, found no temporal association between dental procedures that were followed by prosthetic joint infection.[27]

Frequent reevaluation of the available scientific literature in this area is the best way for surgeons to remain aware of current best practices.

Principle 5: Use the Narrowest Spectrum Empiric Antibiotic Effective Against the Most Likely Pathogens

Empiric antibiotic therapy is used, when clinically indicated, before culture and sensitivity test results are available. Given a working knowledge of the most likely pathogens causing various infections of the head and neck, the clinician can select an antibiotic tailored as narrowly as possible to those pathogens, pending the availability of culture and sensitivity results.

Figure 8-1 illustrates a case of medication-related osteonecrosis of the maxilla 4 months after dental extractions in a woman treated with denosumab for metastatic breast cancer. She presented with chronic right maxillary pain and multiple draining sinus tracts in the attached gingiva and alveolar mucosa (Figure 8-1, A). Exposure of the infected necrotic bone identified a gray-black discoloration of

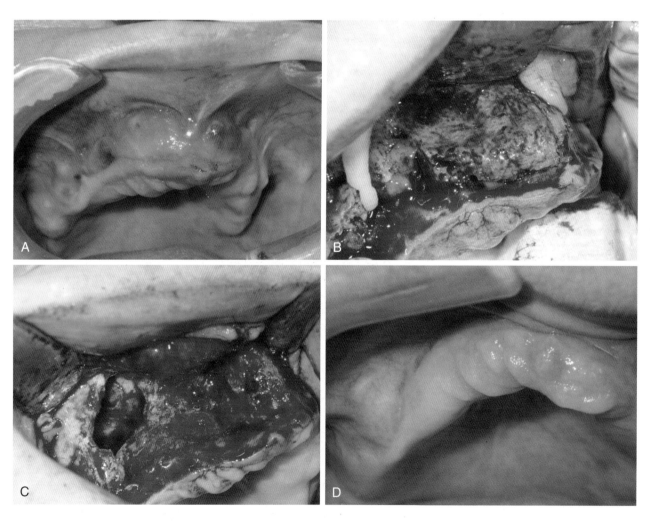

• **Figure 8-1** Medication-related osteonecrosis of the jaws, preceded by therapy with denosumab for metastatic breast cancer. **A,** Inflamed mucosa and multiple sinus tracts draining the right and left anterior maxilla. **B,** Exposure of the maxillary alveolar process, with gray-black discoloration of necrotic bone, suggesting black-pigmented oral anaerobic infection. **C,** Resection of the anterior maxilla, resulting in a large exposure of the maxillary sinus. **D,** Successful healing at 6 months after debridement.

the bone (Figure 8-1, B). Resection of the necrotic bone (Figure 8-1, C) resulted in exposure of the maxillary sinus, with inflamed antral mucosa and suppuration within the sinus. Because of the likelihood of black-pigmented oral anaerobes, such as *Prevotella melaninogenica,* plus the exposure and infection of the maxillary sinus, amoxicillin/clavulanate was chosen as the initial empiric antibiotic. Cultures yielded viridans streptococci and oral gram-negative anaerobes susceptible to amoxicillin/clavulanate. The antibiotic was continued for 6 weeks because of bone infection, resulting in successful closure of the surgical defect, without oroantral fistula, and resolution of pain (Figure 8-1D).

The usual pathogens associated with various head and neck infections and their empiric antibiotics of choice are listed in Table 8-4.

In rhinosinusitis, the infecting pathogens progress from viral to aerobic and then to anaerobic as time progresses, as illustrated in Figure 8-2. Because most acute sinus

TABLE 8-4 | **Major Pathogens of Head and Neck Infections and Their Empiric Antibiotics of Choice**

Type of Infection	Stage	Microorganisms	Empiric Antibiotics of Choice
Acute necrotizing ulcerative gingivitis		*Borellia vincentii* Head and neck anaerobes (Peptostreptococcus, *Prevotella, Porphyromonas, Fusobacterium*)	PCN + metronidazole Clindamycin
Bite wounds	Cat (infection in 80%)	*Pasteurella multocida* *Staphylococcus. aureus* *Streptococcus* *Neisseria* *Moraxella*	Amoxicillin/clavulanate Cefuroxime (avoid cephalexin, dicloxacillin, clindamycin—*P. multocida* resistant)
	Dog (infection in only 5%)	*Pasteurella canis* *S. aureus* *Streptococcus* *Fusobacterium* *Capnocytophaga canimorsus*	Amoxicillin/clavulanate Clindamycin + FQ (adults) Clindamycin + TMP-SMX (children)
	Human	Odontogenic abscess flora (see later) *S. aureus* *Staphylococcus epidermidis* *Corynebacterium*	Amoxicillin/clavulanate (early, not clinically infected) BL/BLI (IV) or cefoxitin (infected) Clindamycin + FQ or TMP-SMX (infected)
Brain abscess	Rhinogenic (arising from contiguous paranasal sinuses)	*Streptococcus* Head and neck anaerobes (*Peptostreptococcus, Prevotella, Porphyromonas, Fusobacterium*) Enterobacteriaceae *S. aureus*	Cefotaxime or ceftriaxone + metronidazole PCN G + metronidazole
Cellulitis, facial (erysipelas)		*Streptococcus* *S. aureus* (including MRSA) *S. pneumoniae*	Vancomycin Daptomycin Linezolid
Cervical lymphadenitis (therapy guided by aspiration for aerobic, anaerobic, and mycobacterial C&S; Gram and acid-fast stains)	Cat-scratch disease	*Bartonella henselae*	Azithromycin No treatment (spontaneous resolution in 2-6 mo)
	Mycobacterial	*Mycobacterium tuberculosis* (scrofula) *Mycobacterium avium* (esp. with HIV) Atypical mycobacteria	Therapy guided by aspiration for aerobic, anaerobic, and mycobacterial C&S; Gram and acid-fast stains
	Nonspecific	GABHS *S. aureus* Anaerobes	Therapy guided by aspiration for aerobic, anaerobic, and mycobacterial C&S; Gram and acid-fast stains
Deep neck abscess (lateral pharyngeal, retropharyngeal, pretracheal, mediastinal spaces)		Odontogenic abscess flora (see below) Necrotizing fasciitis flora (see below) *S. aureus*	Ceftriaxone + metronidazole BL/BLI (IV) Moxifloxacin Carbapenem + vancomycin if necrotizing fasciitis suspected, pending C&S results

Continued

TABLE 8-4	Major Pathogens of Head and Neck Infections and Their Empiric Antibiotics of Choice—cont'd		
Type of Infection	**Stage**	**Microorganisms**	**Empiric Antibiotics of Choice**
Epiglottitis	Adults	GABHS *Haemophilus influenzae* Odontogenic abscess flora (see below)	Cefotaxime or ceftriaxone + vancomycin Levofloxacin + clindamycin (only in life-threatening PCN allergy)
	Children	*H. influenzae* GABHS *S. pneumoniae* *S. aureus* Viruses	Cefotaxime or ceftriaxone + vancomycin Levofloxacin + clindamycin (only in life-threatening PCN allergy)
Fungal infections	Mucosal or disseminated	*Candida* sp.	Caspofungin, micafungin, or anidulafungin Fluconazole or voriconazole Amphotericin B (various preparations) + Flucytosine
	Sinus	*Aspergillus* *Rhizopus (Mucor)*	Itraconazole Liposomal amphotericin B Posaconazole, isavuconazole
	Soft tissue	*Histoplasma* sp. *Blastomyces* sp.	Liposomal amphotericin B Amphotericin B Itraconazole + methylprednisolone
Jugular vein septic thrombophlebitis (Lemierre's syndrome)		*Fusobacterium necrophorum* Other Fusobacteria Odontogenic abscess flora (see later)	BL/BLI (IV) Imipenem Ceftriaxone + metronidazole Clindamycin (Avoid macrolides: Fusobacteria are resistant)
Mastoiditis	Acute, first episode	*S. pneumoniae* *Streptococcus pyogenes* *S. aureus*	C&S before antibiotic treatment Vancomycin + BL/BLI Or vancomycin + ceftazidime
	Chronic or recurrent	*S. pneumoniae* *S. pyogenes* *S. aureus* *Pseudomonas aeruginosa* Anaerobes Fungi	C&S before antibiotic treatment Topical FQ ear drops May need surgical debridement
Necrotizing fasciitis		GABHS Polymicrobial (oral and sinus pathogens in head and neck) *Clostridium* sp. MRSA *Vibrio vulnificus* *Aeromonas* spp. *Klebsiella* spp.	Carbapenem + vancomycin, pending C&S results
Odontogenic cellulitis/abscess		*Streptococcus* viridans group (esp. *intermedius*, *anginosus*, and *constellatus*) Head and neck anaerobes (*Peptostreptococcus, Prevotella, Porphyromonas, Fusobacterium*)	BL/BLI Clindamycin Moxifloxacin
Osteomyelitis of the jaws	Acute	Odontogenic abscess flora (see earlier) *S. aureus* and skin flora in trauma *Salmonella* in hemoglobinopathy (e.g., sickle cell disease)	C&S before antibiotic treatment BL/BLI Clindamycin Moxifloxacin Vancomycin FQ in hemoglobinopathy
	Chronic	*Actinomyces* sp.	Ampicillin Penicillin Doxycycline Ceftriaxone Clindamycin Macrolides

TABLE 8-4   Major Pathogens of Head and Neck Infections and Their Empiric Antibiotics of Choice—cont'd

Type of Infection	Stage	Microorganisms	Empiric Antibiotics of Choice
Otitis media	Acute	Viruses *S. pneumoniae* *H. influenzae* *Moraxella catarrhalis*	If no antibiotics in past month: Amoxicillin or amoxicillin/clavulanate If recent antibiotics: Amoxicillin/clavulanate Ceftriaxone, cefdinir, cefpodoxime, cefprozil, or cefuroxime
	Treatment failure after 3 days: (consider tympanocentesis)	Resistant *S. pneumoniae* likely	If no antibiotics in past month before past 3 days: Amoxicillin/clavulanate high dose Cefuroxime, cefdinir, cefpodoxime, or cefprozil If prior antibiotics in past month: Levofloxacin
Parotitis	"Cold" (nontender)	Granulomatous disease (mycobacterial, sarcoidosis, Sjögren's syndrome) Parotid hypertrophy (diabetes, cirrhosis, HIV) Neoplastic (40% malignant) Drugs (iodides, etc.)	Therapy guided by aspiration for aerobic, anaerobic, and mycobacterial C&S; Gram and acid-fast stains
	"Hot" (red, tender, inflamed)	*S. aureus* GABHS *Streptococcus* viridans group (esp. *intermedius, anginosus,* and *constellatus*) Head and neck anaerobes (*Peptostreptococcus, Prevotella, Porphyromonas, Fusobacterium*)	Therapy guided by aspiration for aerobic, anaerobic, and mycobacterial C&S; Gram and acid-fast stains
Pharyngitis/tonsillitis	Exudative/diffuse erythema	GABHS Viruses Streptococci *Fusobacterium* *Neisseria gonorrhoeae*	PCN V Cefdinir or cefpodoxime Amoxicillin/clavulanate Clindamycin For gonorrhea: ceftriaxone + azithromycin
	Membranous pharyngitis	*Corynebacterium diphtheriae*	Erythromycin or PCN G + diphtheria toxoid vaccine
	Peritonsillar abscess	*Fusobacterium necrophorum* GABHS *Streptococcus*	BL/BLI (IV) Ceftriaxone + metronidazole Clindamycin (Avoid macrolides: Fusobacteria are resistant)
	Vesiculo-ulcerative	Coxsackie virus Enteroviruses Herpes simplex	For herpes simplex only: acyclovir In HIV: famciclovir or valacyclovir
Rhinosinusitis	Acute (antibiotics only for fever, severe pain, purulent discharge; symptoms >10 d; failed antibiotic treatment)	*S. pneumoniae* *H. influenzae* *M. catarrhalis* Head and neck anaerobes (*Peptostreptococcus, Prevotella, Porphyromonas, Fusobacterium*) GABHS Viruses *S. aureus*	Amoxicillin or Amoxicillin/clavulanate Clindamycin Cefpodoxime Levofloxacin (adults only) Doxycycline (adults only)
	Chronic	Head and neck anaerobes	Otolaryngology consultation
	Fungal (esp. in diabetes)	*Aspergillus* *Rhizopus* sp. *(Mucor)*	Itraconazole Liposomal amphotericin B Posaconazole, isavuconazole

Continued

TABLE 8-4	Major Pathogens of Head and Neck Infections and Their Empiric Antibiotics of Choice—cont'd		
Type of Infection	**Stage**	**Microorganisms**	**Empiric Antibiotics of Choice**
	Nosocomial (esp. if intubated)	Enterobacteriaceae (esp. *Pseudomonas, Acinotobacter, Escherichia coli*) *S. aureus* *Candida* sp.	Remove nasoendotracheal tube C&S by sinus aspiration Carbapenem + vancomcyin Ceftazidime or cefepime + vancomycin Itraconazole or fluconazole for *Candida*, other yeasts

BL/BLI, β-Lactam antibiotic plus β-lactamase inhibitor; *C&S,* culture and sensitivity testing; *FQ,* fluoroquinolone; *GABHS,* group A β-hemolytic streptococci; *HIV,* human immunodeficiency virus; *IV,* intravenously; *PCN,* penicillin G or V; *MRSA,* methicillin-resistant *Staphylococcus aureus; TMP-SMX,* trimethoprim–sulfamethoxazole.

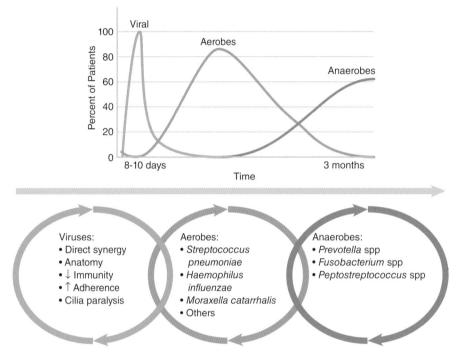

• **Figure 8-2** Pathogens associated with sinusitis over time. (Reprinted with permission of the American Thoracic Society. Copyright © 2024 American Thoracic Society. All rights reserved. From Brook I. Microbiology of sinusitis. *Proc Am Thorac Soc.* 2011 Mar;8(1):90-100. The American Journal of Respiratory and Critical Care Medicine is an official journal of the American Thoracic Society.)

infections early in their course are caused by viruses, antibacterial chemotherapy is generally withheld unless fever, facial swelling, purulent nasal discharge, and severe pain are present at 7 to 10 days after onset. The most common pathogens in acute bacterial rhinosinusitis are *S. pneumoniae, Hemophilus influenzae, S. pyogenes,* and *Moraxella catarrhalis.* By and large, high-dose amoxicillin/clavulanate has been shown to be effective against these respiratory pathogens, and it affects the gut flora to a much lesser extent than other effective antibiotics.

For this reason, among others, the practice guidelines of the American Academy of Otolaryngology–Head and Neck Surgery Foundation recommend amoxicillin-clavulanate as the first-line antibiotic in adults and children at low risk for antibiotic-resistant organisms in acute sinusitis.[28]

The American College of Physicians and the Centers for Disease Control and Prevention recommend antibiotic therapy for acute rhinosinusitis when symptoms persist for more than 10 days without clinical improvement, if fever greater than 39°C, purulent nasal discharge, or facial pain lasts for 3 or more days, or when the symptoms of a typical viral illness worsen 5 days or more after an initial period of improvement. Further, these guidelines recommend doxycycline or levofloxacin or moxifloxacin in penicillin allergy.[29]

Initial use of first-line antibiotics rather than second-line ones reduces antibiotic resistance and toxicity in general. On the other hand, an initial prescription of doxycycline or a fluoroquinolone, for example, to a patient with acute sinusitis may unnecessarily alter the gastrointestinal flora. Cefixime or clindamycin may unnecessarily target head and neck anaerobic bacteria. Also, the cephalosporins in general favor the growth of enterococci in the body, and these organisms have a propensity to pass antibiotic resistance genes to other species. They reside in the oropharynx. Further, clindamycin, among other antibiotics, can favor superinfection by *Clostridioides difficile,* resulting in antibiotic-associated colitis.

In addition to increasing environmental selection pressure for antibiotic-resistant bacterial strains, the use of broad-spectrum antibiotics often increases pharmacologic toxicity. For example, doxycycline can cause photosensitivity, permanent dental staining in developing children, and hepatotoxicity. The fluoroquinolones can prolong the electrocardiographic QT interval, which predisposes to torsades de pointes, a polymorphic ventricular tachycardia that can be fatal. The risk of torsades is increased yet further in the presence of multiple other drugs, including the selective serotonin reuptake inhibitors (SSRIs), commonly used for depression.

Broader spectrum antibiotics are generally more expensive as well. The cost of a 1-week prescription for amoxicillin/clavulanate 875 mg orally twice daily at a nationwide pharmacy chain is approximately $119, but the cost of linezolid 600 mg twice daily for 1 week is more than 15 times greater.

For these reasons, using the narrowest spectrum effective antibiotic decreases the unwanted side effects of selection for antibiotic-resistant organisms, pharmacologic toxicity, and cost.

Principle 6: Use the Least Toxic Antibiotic, Considering Drug Interactions

Even though the penicillins can be considered the oldest family of antibiotics, they are among the least toxic, and yet among the most effective, especially for head and neck pathogens. Although the incidence of fatal anaphylactic shock is 0.002% with penicillins, much of this risk can be eliminated by obtaining a careful medical history.[30] Other rare toxicities of the penicillins include thrombocytopenia and suppression of other blood-forming elements, serum sickness, erythema multiforme, and Stevens-Johnson syndrome.

Many patients report they are allergic to penicillin but the incidence of severe reactions is declining over time, most likely due to less frequent use of parenteral penicillins. Risk stratification of penicillin allergy based on the patient's history may allow evaluation of the penicillin allergy. The evaluation methods range from a challenge dose of oral amoxicillin when the history suggests low risk. When the history indicates moderate risk, penicillin skin testing may be indicated. Penicillin skin testing has a negative predictive value that exceeds 95% and approaches 100% when combined with amoxicillin challenge. Evaluation of a history of penicillin allergy before deciding not to use penicillin or other β-lactam antibiotics is an important tool for antimicrobial stewardship.[31]

Table 8-5 lists the antibiotics commonly used for head and neck infections and their salient pharmacologic characteristics. The relative toxicities of the major antibiotic families can be generally ranked in the following order of severity: cephalosporins, penicillins, lincosamides (clindamycin), macrolides (erythromycins), linezolid, carbapenems, glycopeptides (vancomycin), and aminoglycosides.

The cephalosporins are generally well-tolerated by the gastrointestinal tract and have a significantly lower incidence of allergic reactions than their beta-lactam cousins, the penicillins. The lincosamides, of which clindamycin is the most commonly used member, are well tolerated in general, except for gastrointestinal discomfort and antibiotic-associated colitis. The macrolides, in general, are plagued by gastrointestinal intolerance and interactions with multiple drugs, in particular those that compete with the macrolides for the liver microsomal enzyme, CYP3A4. Linezolid is a member of a new family of peptide antibiotics, which is well-tolerated except for increased sensitivity to epinephrine, serotonergic drugs such as the SSRIs and monoamine oxidase inhibitors, which can result in a serotonin syndrome, manifested as confusion, sweating, fever, and tremors. The carbapenem antibiotics, such as imipenem, meropenem, and ertapenem, can cause seizures, toxic epidermal reactions such as erythema multiforme and Stevens-Johnson syndrome, and myelosuppression. The glycopeptides, such as vancomycin and teicoplanin, are nephrotoxic and ototoxic, requiring careful monitoring of antibiotic blood levels during therapy. The aminoglycosides, such as gentamicin, are also neurotoxic, nephrotoxic, and ototoxic, plus they can increase or prolong neuromuscular blockade and can cause agranulocytosis and toxic epidermal reactions.

Within antibiotic families, some antibiotics are safer than others, while having at least equal effectiveness. For example, among the cephalosporins, ceftriaxone and ceftazidime both cross the blood-brain barrier, which is not common among the cephalosporins. On the other hand, ceftriaxone has been associated with sludging of the bile salts, whereas ceftazidime has not. Among the macrolides, both erythromycin and clarithromycin have multiple interactions with other drugs that also are metabolized by CYP3A4. Generally, these interactions result in an increased serum level of the other drug, causing toxicity from the other drug. The best examples of this are seizures caused by elevated theophylline levels and bleeding caused by elevated warfarin levels during macrolide administration. On the other hand, azithromycin is not metabolized by CYP3A4, and therefore has far fewer drug interactions than the other macrolide antibiotics. Among the carbapenems, imipenem can cause seizures in doses at high, but therapeutic, levels whereas meropenem is less likely to cause seizures at therapeutic levels.

Our understanding of antibiotic-associated colitis (now called *Clostridioides difficile* infection [CDI]) was significantly advanced by the identification of the causative exotoxin, synthesized by *C. difficile.* Although many antibiotics have been associated with this complication, cephalosporins, fluoroquinolones, clindamycin, and amoxicillin/clavulanate have been most characteristically associated with it. It is important to recognize the profile of the patient likely to experience this complication; the risk factors are listed in Box 8-3. The clinical manifestations of CDI include five or more bloody or mucoid stools per day, abdominal cramping, and fever. On colonoscopy, sloughing of the colonic mucosa is seen. Enzyme immunoassays and PCR tests are now available for the direct detection of *C. difficile* toxins A and B. The cytotoxicity assay for CDI is the gold standard diagnostic test, but its use is limited because it is time-consuming and expensive.

TABLE 8-5 Pharmacology of Commonly Used Antibiotics in Head and Neck Infection

Antibiotic	Spectrum	Dosage (po unless stated)	Mode of Action	Side Effects	Comments
Penicillin V	Oral streptococci Oral anaerobes Resistant: Staphylococcus Enteric flora Bacteroides fragilis	500 mg qid Children: 25-75 mg/kg/day	Bactericidal. Interferes with cell wall synthesis of bacteria in their growth phase.	Allergy—may cause anaphylactic shock (0.05%) Rare GI disturbances Superinfection by resistant bacteria may occur. Rash in 3% of patients. Serum sickness in 4%.	Produces lower blood levels than IV PCN G. Excreted by kidneys. Administer before meals.
Amoxicillin (Semisynthetic penicillin)	Oral streptococci Oral anaerobes Resistant: Actinomyces Staphylococci Pseudomonas sp.	500 mg tid, 875 mg bid Children: 20-45 mg per kg/day	Bactericidal. Interferes with cell wall synthesis of bacteria in their growth phase.	Allergy – may cause anaphylactic shock Most common cause of antibiotic-associated colitis Diarrhea in 10% of patients.	Less effective against oral streps than PCN V; more effective against oral anaerobes.
Amoxicillin + clavulanic acid (Augmentin)	Oral Streptococcus Oral anaerobes Resistant: Actinomyces Staphylococcus Enteric gram-negative rods Haemophilus influenzae	500 mg/125 mg tid; 875 mg/125 mg bid Children: 25-45 mg/kg/day	Bactericidal. Interferes with cell wall synthesis of bacteria in their growth phase. Clavulanic acid inhibits penicillinase made by staphs and some gram-negative rods.	Allergy may cause anaphylactic shock. Common cause of antibiotic-associated colitis. Diarrhea in 9% of patients; less frequent with bid dosing (less clavulanate).	Not effective against MRSA. Improved coverage for Staphylococcus, oral anaerobes, and enteric flora.
Azithromycin (Zithromax)	Some oral streptococci Atypical pathogens in HIV + patients Resistant: Most Staphylococci Bacteroides fragilis Fusobacterium	500 mg on day 1, then 250 mg/d for days 2-5 Children: 12 mg/kg on day 1, then 6 mg/kg/day for days 2-5	Bactericidal or bacteriostatic Interferes with protein synthesis during growth phase. Active uptake of the antibiotic by phagocytes may improve coverage over in vitro data.	GI upset: Less common than with other macrolides. Prolongs QT interval. Fewer drug interactions than with other macrolides.	Fewer drug interactions than with the other macrolides; concentrates in phagocytes at up to 15× concentration in serum.
Clindamycin (Cleocin)	Oral streptococci Some Staphylococci Anaerobes Resistant: Enteric flora Eikenella corrodens	150-450 mg qid Children: 10-25 mg per kg/d	Bactericidal or bacteriostatic. Interferes with protein synthesis.	Common cause of Clostridioides difficile colitis.	Does not cross blood-brain barrier. Some streptococci are becoming resistant.
Cephalexin (Keflex first-generation cephalosporin)	Streptococci Resistant: Oral anaerobes Enteric flora B. fragilis	500-800 mg qid Children: 25-50 mg per kg/d	Bactericidal. Interferes with cell wall synthesis of bacteria in their growth phase.	Allergy: May cross-react with those who have had an anaphylactoid reaction to penicillins.	Does not cross blood-brain barrier in a predictable fashion.
Cefdinir (Omnicef—third-generation cephalosporin)	Streptococci Oral anaerobes Resistant: Staphylococci	300 mg bid Children: 14 mg/kg/d	Bactericidal. Interferes with cell wall synthesis of bacteria in their growth phase.	Allergy: may cross-react with those who have had an anaphylactoid reaction to penicillins.	Does not cross blood-brain barrier in a predictable fashion.

Drug	Organisms / Resistant	Dosage	Mechanism	Adverse Reactions	Notes
Ceftriaxone (Rocephin—third-generation cephalosporin)	Streptococci, Oral anaerobes; Resistant: Staphylococci	Parenteral only: 1-2 g qd; Children: 50 mg/kg/d	Bactericidal. Interferes with cell wall synthesis of bacteria in their growth phase.	Allergy: may cross-react with those that have had an anaphylactoid reaction to penicillins. Sludging of bile-salts.	Crosses blood-brain barrier.
Metronidazole (Flagyl)	Obligate anaerobes only; Resistant: All facultative and aerobic bacteria	500 mg qid; Children >1 yr: 30-50 mg/kg/d in 3 doses	Bactericidal. Interferes with folic acid metabolism.	Metallic taste Antabuse-like effect Carcinogenic in rats: use only when indicated.	Crosses blood-brain barrier. Can be used with other antibiotics.
Moxifloxacin (Avelox)	Oral streps and anaerobes, E. corrodens Actinomyces, B. fragilis, Staphylococcus, including some MRSA, most enteric flora; Resistant: Enterococci, Pseudomonas aeruginosa	400 mg qd; Children: DO NOT USE; Pregnancy: DO NOT USE	Bactericidal. Interferes with DNA synthesis.	Possible ↑QT interval, especially if used with quinidine, procainamide, amiodarone, sotalol, other drugs, or if hypokalemic.	Chondrotoxic in pregnancy and children. May cause Achilles tendon rupture. Mental clouding and decreased energy common.
Linezolid (Zyvox)	MRSA Streptococci Vancomycin-resistant enterococci; Resistant: Enterobacteriaceae	600 mg bid; Children: 30 mg/kg/d in 3 doses	Bactericidal to streptococci; Bacteriostatic to staphylococci, enterococci. Interferes with protein synthesis.	Epinephrine hypersensitivity; bone marrow suppression; serotonin syndrome; Stevens-Johnson syndrome; seizures.	Weekly CBCs for monitoring; monitor BP for hypertension; may be toxic to fetus (insufficient data).
Imipenem/Cilastatin (Primaxin)	Staphylococci Streptococci Anaerobes Enterobacteriaceae; Resistant: ESBL Klebsiella	500 mg–1 g IV q6-8h; Children: 60-100 mg/kg/d in 4 doses	Bactericidal. Interferes with cell wall synthesis of bacteria in their growth phase.	Allergy: May cross-react with those that have had an anaphylactoid reaction to penicillins; seizures at high doses; bone marrow suppression; hepatotoxicity.	Seizures less likely with meropenem. Cilastatin inhibits renal excretion of imipenem.
Vancomycin (Vancocin)	Staphylococci, including MRSA Streptococci Enterococci; Resistant: Gram-negative bacteria	15-20 mg/kg IV. 2 8-12h; Children: 60-80 mg/kg in 3-4 does Dosage adjustment in elderly and renal failure	Bactericidal. Inhibits cell wall and RNA synthesis.	Nephrotoxic, neurotoxic, and ototoxic, especially in combination with aminoglycosides; flushing and hypotension with rapid infusion; tissue necrosis if infiltrated.	Pregnancy risk in animals; monitor peak and trough serum levels.
Gentamicin	Streptococci Enterobacteriaceae	1-1.7 mg/kg IM/IV q8h; Children: 2.5 mg/kg IV/IM q8h	Bactericidal. Inhibits protein synthesis at 30S ribosome.	Nephrotoxic, neurotoxic, and ototoxic. Neuromuscular blockade, especially with other neuromuscular blockers.	Adjust dosage according to peak and trough serum levels. Nephrotoxic, neurotoxic, and ototoxic to fetus.

bid, Twice daily; BP, blood pressure; CBC, complete blood count; ESBL, extended-spectrum β-lactamase; GI, gastrointestinal; HIV, human immunodeficiency virus; IM, intramuscular; IV, intravenous; kg, kilograms; mg, milligrams; MRSA, methicillin-resistant Staphylococcus aureus; PCN, penicillin; po, by mouth; qd, once daily; sp., species; tid, three times per day; TMP-SMX-DS, trimethoprim/sulfamethoxazole, double strength; X, times.

• BOX 8-3 **Risk Factors for *Clostridioides difficile* Colitis**

- Prolonged antibiotic therapy
- Gastrointestinal surgery
- Hospitalized patient
- Female
- Inflammatory bowel disease
- Cancer chemotherapy
- Renal disease

Fidaxomicin has considerably more effectiveness in the antibiotic management of recurrent CDI than metronidazole or vancomycin. Thus it is now the initial treatment of choice per the Infectious Diseases Society of America and the European Society of Clinical Microbiology and Infectious Diseases. Fecal microbiota transplant has shown promise. Concerns have arisen because of the possibility of transmission of SARS-COVID and reported cases of transmission of highly virulent strains of *E. coli*. Fecal microbiota transplant, however, is accepted for treatment of second or subsequent recurrence of nonsevere CDI and for severe recurrent or refractory cases in which surgery is not advisable.[32]

There is a subset of *C. difficile* colitis, 1 to 3% of cases, called fulminant *C. difficile* colitis or toxic megacolon, which manifests as a sudden onset of acute abdomen with elevated white blood cell count over 18,000 cells/mm³, high fever, and hemodynamic instability. The risk factors for this condition include age over 70 years, prior CDI, and use of antiperistaltic medications.[33] Early diagnosis and treatment of fulminant *C. difficile* colitis are essential to minimize mortality, and early surgical intervention (within 48 hours) should be used in patients who are unresponsive to medical therapy or if multiple organ failure or a bowel perforation develops. The most commonly used surgical procedure is a total abdominal colectomy, although the mortality rate remains high, at 40% or more. A newer procedure, diverting loop ileostomy with colonic lavage may reduce mortality into the 20% range.[34]

There has been considerable controversy over the potential for various antibiotics to interfere with the effectiveness of oral contraceptives, with little new information presenting since the 1980s. Rifampin, primarily used for tuberculosis, has the strongest anecdotal association with unwanted pregnancy.[35] Other monitoring studies have associated the penicillins, tetracyclines, and cotrimoxazole with breakthrough bleeding and unwanted pregnancy.[36] The speculated cause for this association is competition between estrogen and the antibiotics for the hepatic microsomal drug metabolism processes. As a practical matter, clinicians should continue to advise their patients taking oral contraceptives to use a backup birth control method for the remainder of the menstrual cycle following the end of an antibiotic regimen.

Table 8-6 lists the pregnancy risk categories assigned by the U.S. Food and Drug Administration (FDA) to selected antibiotics, as well as those antibiotics with special risks in children.

Antibiotic-drug interaction with concurrent medications is increasing in frequency as our patient population ages and is treated with an ever-increasing number of medications for acute and chronic conditions. Certain families of antibiotics, especially because of their metabolism by the liver microsomal enzyme system, are more prone to drug interactions than others. The antibiotic families most associated with interactions are the macrolides, the fluoroquinolones, and the azole antifungal drugs, such as fluconazole and ketoconazole. Table 8-7 lists some of the interactions between these antibiotics and other drugs. The overall pattern of these interactions is that the serum level of the other drug is increased, resulting in an increased therapeutic effect of the other drug, or its expected toxic overdose reactions.

However, antibiotics that are metabolized in the liver microsomal enzyme system, especially by CYP3A4, such as the macrolides and the fluoroquinolones, when combined with a broad range of drugs, such as the SSRIs, amiodarone, and other antibiotics such as pentamidine and the macrolides can prolong the QT interval as seen on the electrocardiogram. This predisposes to and can cause torsades de pointes, which can rapidly degenerate into ventricular fibrillation.

Therefore, selection of the least toxic effective antibiotic can minimize toxicities and drug interactions, which appear likely to increase, given the systemic compromise and multiple medications often seen in our aging population.

Principle 7: Use Combination Antibiotics Only When Necessary

For most head and neck infections, even though they are polymicrobial, a single antibiotic usually can be selected that is effective against the most likely pathogens. On the other hand, combinations of antibiotics may be indicated in severe infections of unknown cause, in polymicrobial infections for which no single antibiotic is effective against all of the pathogens, and to prevent the emergence of resistance to a single antibiotic.

Combining multiple antibiotics can increase toxicities and costs, select for resistant organisms, and cause antagonistic interactions between the antibiotics. For example, vancomycin has minimal renal toxicity when used alone. In combination with an aminoglycoside, such as gentamicin, renal toxicity is significantly increased.

A classic example of mutual antibiotic antagonism is the combination of a bactericidal with a bacteriostatic antibiotic. In general, the bactericidal antibiotics are effective during the rapid growth and cellular division phases of the bacterial life cycle, often by interfering with cell wall synthesis; thus, their action is antagonized by antibiotics that suppress rapid bacterial growth. Most antibiotics that interfere with protein synthesis slow bacterial growth without a killing effect. Thus, combining a protein synthesis inhibitor, such as a macrolide, with a cell wall synthesis inhibitor, such as a penicillin or cephalosporin, has a net bacteriostatic effect. Table 8-8 lists bactericidal and bacteriostatic antibiotics.

TABLE 8-6   Pregnancy and Pediatric Risk Categories of Selected Antibiotics

Antibiotic	Pregnancy Risk Category	Pregnancy Risk	Antibiotic	Pregnancy Risk Category	Pregnancy Risk
Penicillins			**Antianaerobics**		
Penicillin G and V	B	A = Studies in pregnant women; no risk	Clindamycin	B	
			Metronidazole	B	
Ampicillin	B	B = Animal studies no risk; human	Fluoroquinolones		Avoid under age 18 in children
Amoxicillin	B	Studies inadequate; OR animal	Ciprofloxacin	C	Chondrotoxic in growing rats
Amoxicillin/ clavulanate	B	Toxicity; but human studies no risk	Moxifloxacin	C	Chondrotoxic in growing rats
Ticarcillin/ clavulanate	B	C = Animal studies show toxicity; human studies inadequate	**Aminoglycosides**		
			Gentamicin	D	Ototoxicity in human fetuses
Cephalosporins			**Antifungals**		
Cephalexin	B	Benefit may outweigh risk	Fluconazole	D	Teratogenic at high doses
Cefazolin	B	D = Evidence of human risk	Itraconazole	C	Teratogenic at high doses
Cefuroxime	B	Benefit may outweigh risk	Voriconazole	D	Teratogenic at high doses
Cefdinir	B	X = Fetal abnormalities in humans	Caspofungin	C	Fetal toxicity in animals
Cefotaxime	B	Risk outweighs benefit	Amphotericin B preparations	B	
Carbapenems			**Other**		
			Vancomycin	C	Potential ototoxicity in human fetuses
Imipenem	C	Dose adjustment required	Daptomycin	B	
Meropenem	B	Spontaneous abortions in monkeys	Tetracyclines	D	Intrinsic dental staining; avoid in children under 12
Macrolides			Doxycycline	D	Intrinsic dental staining; avoid in children under 12
Erythromycin	B				
Clarithromycin	C	Increased risk of miscarriage	Linezolid	C	Fetal toxicity in rodents
Azithromycin	B	Fetal defects in mice and monkeys	Trimethoprim/sulfamethoxazole	C	Increased risk of cleft palate

There are a few well-established clinical situations, however, in which antibiotic combinations have been shown to be more effective than single antibiotic therapy.

A penicillin, such as ampicillin, and an aminoglycoside, such as gentamicin, have long been used in streptococcal endocarditis. Although the aminoglycosides are protein synthesis inhibitors, they are bactericidal, as are the penicillins. A 2-week course of this combination is as effective as

4 weeks of a penicillin only, and relapse is less frequent.[37] Further, a recent meta-analysis was able to identify no difference in antibiotic resistance rates between β-lactam monotherapy and an aminoglycoside/β-lactam combination on the development of antimicrobial resistance among initially susceptible isolates.[38]

In invasive streptococcal infections, which can lead to streptococcal toxic shock and some forms of necrotizing

TABLE 8-7 Selected Antibiotic Interactions With Other Drugs

Antibiotic	Second Drug	Adverse Effects	Mechanism
Erythromycin, clarithromycin, ketoconazole, itraconazole	Theophylline	Seizures, dysrhythmias	Antibiotic inhibits cytochrome P450 metabolism of second drug; ketoconazole not implicated
	Cisapride	Dysrhythmias (torsades de pointes)	Antibiotic inhibits cytochrome P450 metabolism of second drug
	Alfentanil	↑ Respiratory depression	Antibiotic inhibits cytochrome P450 metabolism of second drug; ketoconazole not implicated
	Bromocriptine	↑ CNS effects, hypotension	Antibiotic inhibits cytochrome P450 metabolism of second drug
	Carbamazepine	Ataxia, vertigo, drowsiness	Antibiotic inhibits cytochrome P450 metabolism of second drug
	Cyclosporine	↑ Immunosuppression and nephrotoxicity	Antibiotic inhibits cytochrome P450 metabolism of second drug
	Felodipine possibly other calcium channel blockers	Hypotension, tachycardia, edema	Antibiotic inhibits cytochrome P450 metabolism of second drug
	Methylprednisolone prednisone	↑ Immunosuppression	Antibiotic inhibits cytochrome P450 metabolism of second drug
	Lovastatin possibly other statins	Muscle pain, rhabdomyolosis	Antibiotic inhibits cytochrome P450 metabolism of second drug
	Triazolam oral midazolam	↑ Sedative depth and duration	Antibiotic inhibits cytochrome P450 metabolism of second drug
	Disopyramide	Dysrhythmias	Antibiotic inhibits cytochrome P450 metabolism of second drug
Erythromycin	Clindamycin	↓ Antibiotic effect	Mutual antagonism
Erythromycin tetracyclines	Digoxin	Digitalis toxicity, dysrhythmias, visual disturbances, hypersalivation	Antibiotic kills *Eubacterium lentum,* which metabolizes digoxin in the gut
Erythromycin, clarithromycin, metronidazole	Warfarin anisindione	↑ Anticoagulation	Antibiotic interferes with metabolism of the second drug
Tetracycline, cefamandole, cefotetan, cefoperazone, sulfonamides, aminoglycosides	Warfarin anisindione	↑ Anticoagulation	Antibiotic kills gut flora that synthesize vitamin K, which antagonizes the second drug; poor vitamin K intake a factor
Metronidazole, cephalosporins	Alcohol Ritonavir	Flushing, headache, palpitations, nausea	Antibiotic inhibits acetaldehyde dehydrogenase, causing accumulation of acetaldehyde; ritonavir preparations contain alcohol
Metronidazole	Disulfiram	Acute toxic psychosis	
Metronidazole, tetracyclines	Lithium	Lithium toxicity: confusion, ataxia, kidney damage	Antibiotic inhibits lithium excretion by kidney; tetracycline interaction not well established
Tetracyclines, fluoroquinolones	Divalent and trivalent cations (dairy, antacids, vitamins) Didanosine	↓ Absorption of antibiotic	Second drug interferes with absorption of antibiotic; didanosine is formulated with calcium carbonate and magnesium hydroxide buffers
Clindamycin, aminoglycosides, tetracyclines, bacitracin	Neuromuscular blocking agents	↑ Depth and duration of paralysis	Additive effect because of inherent minor neuromuscular blocking effect of the antibiotic; seen with clindamycin in the presence of low pseudocholinesterase levels and abnormal liver function tests

TABLE 8-7 Selected Antibiotic Interactions With Other Drugs—cont'd

Antibiotic	Second Drug	Adverse Effects	Mechanism
Clindamycin	Erythromycin	↓ Antibiotic effect	Mutual antagonism
Penicillins, cephalosporins, metronidazole, erythromycin, clarithromycin, tetracyclines, rifampin	Estrogen- and progestin-containing oral contraceptives	Contraceptive failure	Interference with enterohepatic recirculation of estrogen caused by killing of gut flora; rifampin is the only antibiotic in which this has been clinically proven
Ampicillin, amoxicillin	Allopurinol	Rash	Unknown, possibly because of hyperuricemia in patients taking allopurinol
Cephalosporins	Aminoglycosides	↑ Nephrotoxicity	Additive or potentiating effect
Trimethoprim–sulfamethoxazole	Thiazide diuretics	Purpura, bleeding in elderly patients	Thrombocytopenia
Vancomycin	Aminoglycosides	↑ Renal toxicity	Additive effect
Fluoroquinolones, sulfonamides, chloramphenicol, fluconazole, itraconazole	Oral hypoglycemic agents	Hypoglycemia	Antibiotic displaces second drug from plasma proteins
Ciprofloxacin, sulfonamides, chloramphenicol, fluconazole, ketoconazole, itraconazole	Phenytoin	↑ Serum level of phenytoin, confusion, delirium	Interference with phenytoin metabolism
Sulfonamides	Methotrexate	↑ Methotrexate concentration	Antibiotic displaces methotrexate from plasma proteins

Note: This list of antibiotic-drug interactions is only partial and selected according to the interests of oral and maxillofacial surgeons. Drug prescribers remain responsible to ascertain the complete drug interactions of any medications they may prescribe.

TABLE 8-8 Bactericidal and Bacteriostatic Antibiotics

Bactericidal	Bacteriostatic
β-Lactams	Macrolides
Penicillins	Erythromycin
Cephalosporins	Clarithromycin
Carbapenems	Azithromycin
Monobactams	Clindamycin
Aminoglycosides	Tetracyclines
Glycopeptides	Doxycycline
Vancomycin	Tigecycline
Telavancin	Sulfa antibiotics
Metronidazole	
Fluoroquinolones	
Ciprofloxacin	
Moxifloxacin	
Daptomycin	

of the bacterial exotoxins responsible for toxic shock is increased. Although penicillin may be effective in the rapid growth phase of the streptococci, clindamycin can inhibit the synthesis of the bacterial exotoxins, such as streptococcal pyrogenic exotoxin B (SpeB), that appear to be responsible for many of the clinical manifestations of streptococcal toxic shock syndrome. This is an example of the synergy of two antibiotics that target different sites within the same organism.

A severe, aggressive head and neck infection, necrotizing fasciitis, "flesh-eating bacteria infection," can be caused by five categories of bacteria that are susceptible to varying antibiotics, as detailed in Figure 8-3. Until the causative bacteria have been identified in culture, the surgeon must use an antibiotic combination that will kill all the potential pathogens. When the surgeon is promptly able to deescalate the antibiotic regimen based on specific culture results, selection of antibiotic-resistant strains, drug toxicities and interactions, and the costs of care are reduced.

As an exception to the general rule, certain bacteria undergo relatively frequent mutations responsible for antibiotic resistance. For these specific organisms, combining two antibiotics that have independent bactericidal mechanisms may have a synergistic effect in preventing the emergence of resistant strains. Specifically, if the frequency of mutation conferring resistance to the first antibiotic is 10^{-6}, and it is

fasciitis, streptococcal toxin synthesis and release is decreased when a penicillin is combined with clindamycin. This may be due to the phenomenon of quorum sensing among the group A β-hemolytic streptococci *(S. pyogenes)*. As the concentration of streptococci in a location reaches the maximum census that can be supported, the colony is able to slow down its growth rate. At the same time, synthesis

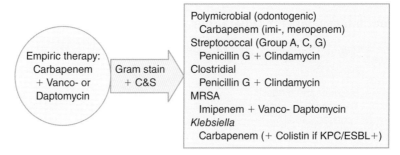

• **Figure 8-3** Empiric antibiotics of choice in necrotizing fasciitis. *ESBL,* Extended-spectrum β-lactamase; *imi-* imipenem; *KPC, Klebsiella pneumoniae* carbapenemase; *MRSA,* methicillin-resistant *Staphylococcus aureus; Vanco-,* vancomycin.

10^{-7} to a second antibiotic, the probability of both of those mutations occurring simultaneously is 10^{-13}. This strategy is used in combination therapy for staphylococcal osteomyelitis (vancomycin or linezolid plus a third- or fourth-generation cephalosporin), prosthetic valve endocarditis (vancomycin, rifampin, and gentamicin), and tuberculosis (isoniazid, rifampin, pyrazinamide, and ethambutol).

Principle 8: Minimize the Duration of Antibiotic Therapy

Reducing the duration of antibiotic administration to the shortest period that provides clinical and microbiologic effectiveness provides several advantages. These include reduced potential for adverse effects, better patient compliance with the prescribed regimen, decreased promotion of antibiotic resistance, and lower costs.

Clinicians used to think that short courses of antibiotic therapy invited the survival of antibiotic-resistant strains of bacteria, yet the opposite appears to be true. Short-term, high-dose courses of oral β-lactam antibiotics have been shown to result in pharyngeal carriage of fewer residual antibiotic-resistant strains of *S. pneumoniae* in schoolchildren, than longer courses (>5 days) and lower-dose regimens.[39]

In odontogenic infections, two randomized clinical trials comparing 3- to 4-day antibiotic courses with 7- to 10-day courses found no difference in clinical effectiveness between the groups, as long as the appropriate dental/surgical treatment was performed, such as incision and drainage and extraction or root canal treatment.[40,41] However, these studies did not provide convincing evidence that antibiotic resistance was lower in the short regimen group than in the long regimen group. Another study by Feres et al., however, found that amoxicillin resistance returned to baseline by 90 days after antibiotic exposure.[42]

Nonetheless, the duration of antibiotic therapy will vary with the type of infection encountered. In osteomyelitis, probably because of the decreased vascular supply of bone, plus the bacterial propensity to form biofilms on calcified surfaces, much longer antibiotic courses are required, to prevent recrudescence of the infection. Further, the

TABLE 8-9	Recommended Duration of Antibiotic Therapy
Type of Infection	**Duration of Antibiotic (assuming appropriate surgery)**
Odontogenic abscess/cellulitis	3-4 d
Sinusitis	Children: 10-14 d Adults: 5-7 d
Otitis media	<2 years old: 10 d >2 years old: 7 d Adults (first episode): 5-7 d Adults (recurrent): 5-10 d
Cellulitis, facial (erysipelas)	10 d
Pharyngitis due to GABHS (strep throat)	Benzathine penicillin IM: 1 dose Cefdinir or cefpodoxime: 5 d Penicillin V: 10 d
Pharyngitis due to *Neisseria gonorrhoeae*	Ceftriaxone or azithromycin: 1 dose Doxycycline: 7 d
Pharyngitis due to Coxsackie virus	10 d
Diphtheria	14 d
Osteomyelitis	42 d (until ESR or CRP normalizes*)
Actinomycosis	42 d (soft tissue) to 180 d (osteomyelitis)
Brain abscess	Until resolution on CT imaging

*Using normalization of laboratory tests as a treatment endpoint in osteomyelitis of the jaws is controversial.
CRP, C-reactive protein; *CT,* Computerized tomographic scan; *ESR,* erythrocyte sedimentation rate; *GABHS,* group A β-hemolytic streptococci; *IM,* intramuscular.

formation of biofilm on calcified bony surfaces often necessitates surgical debridement of the involved bone.

Table 8-9 lists the current recommendations for duration of antibiotic therapy for various types of head and neck infections.

Principle 9: Use the Most Cost-Effective Antibiotic

In our profit-driven health care system, there can be significant sales pressure placed on clinicians by pharmaceutical companies to use newer drugs whose patent protection has not expired. Since the 1999 revised guidance from the FDA, which allowed direct consumer advertising by pharmaceutical companies, patients may also request their physicians to use the latest, most frequently advertised drug.[43]

On the other hand, well-performed clinical trials very often demonstrate that older drugs, including antibiotics, are at least as effective as their newer comparators. Thus, once the more important criteria of effectiveness and safety have been met, it is wise for the clinician to select the antibiotic that costs less than its alternatives. The comparative costs of oral and intravenous antibiotics commonly used in head and neck infections are listed in Tables 8-10 and 8-11. For orally administered antibiotics, amoxicillin is the reference drug to which the other antibiotics are compared in the cost ratio in the last column of Table 8-10. For intravenous antibiotics, clindamycin is the reference drug in the last column of Table 8-11, because it is among the least expensive of the commonly used antibiotics in head and neck infections when given intravenously.

A special factor in the cost of intravenous antibiotics is the cost of administration, which includes the intravenous administration sets, nursing and pharmacy labor, and other factors. Those costs are conservatively estimated at $4.00 per dose, which makes the frequency of dosing a very significant cost factor. Thus, an expensive drug that is given only once per day can be significantly less costly overall than one given 4 or 6 times per day. For this reason, cefotaxime administered once per day, for example, is much less expensive per day than penicillin G, which is given 6 times per day.

In osteomyelitis of the jaws, a recent study found that the commonly recommended 6-week course of intravenous antibiotics was no more successful than a 6-week course of oral antibiotics, consisting of twice-daily amoxicillin clavulanate with a mid-day dose of amoxicillin in nonallergic patients. Appropriate surgical debridement was performed in all cases. The advantages of oral therapy versus intravenous therapy included a 94% reduction in antibiotic cost, as well as avoidance of the complications of peripherally inserted central catheters, which occur in 30% of cases.[44]

Principle 10: Use Prophylactic Antibiotics Only Where Proved Effective or According to Professional Guidelines

All too often, clinicians respond to the pressures of defensive medicine and patient expectations in prescribing prophylactic antibiotics. Yet, the reliable scientific evidence illuminating this treatment decision is mounting.

Prophylactic antibiotics have been proved effective in ablative head and neck cancer surgery, orthognathic surgery, and third molar surgery. The American Heart Association has periodically convened a panel of experts to present consensus guidelines on the use of prophylactic antibiotics for certain dental and urogenital procedures. Such guidelines are often necessary because ethical considerations prohibit the design of experimental studies that would conclusively answer these questions.

Until recently, the scientific support for and against the use of prophylactic antibiotics for mandibular third molar surgery was insufficient to allow surgeons to draw conclusions on its use. Therefore, surgeons relied on their judgment, training, and experience in choosing whether to use prophylactic antibiotics for prevention of surgical site infection in third molar surgery.

However, in recent years, first-level evidence, consisting of meta-analyses and randomized controlled clinical trials, have indicated that a prophylactic antibiotic started shortly (≤ 2 hours) before surgery significantly decreases the rate of surgical site infection after mandibular third molar removal.[45,46] The validity of these results was confirmed in a recent systematic review and meta-analysis by Lodi et al.[47] The highest quality evidence available strongly indicates that a preoperative antibiotic is effective in preventing postoperative infection after third molar removal.

In dental implantology, the role of prophylactic antibiotics in preventing implant failure is not clear. Four randomized clinical trials comparing dental implant procedures with and without a prophylactic antibiotic have found a trend toward a greater implant success rate in the antibiotic prophylaxis group, but without statistical significance. However, when a meta-analysis was applied to these studies, a statistically significant advantage in dental implant survival was found when 1 to 2 g of amoxicillin was given preoperatively, with a number needed to treat of 33. This means that 33 patients had to be treated with an antibiotic to prevent 1 patient from suffering early implant loss. The effectiveness of continuing the antibiotic postoperatively in this review was not clear; in addition, a preoperative chlorhexidine oral rinse was used in all of the included clinical trials.[48] Recent meta-analyses have confirmed the benefit of preoperative antibiotic prophylaxis for dental implant survival,[49,50] but the benefit may not be significant when uncomplicated dental implant placement is performed for healthy patients.[51]

Antibiotic prophylaxis in orthognathic surgery, especially by the transoral approach, has long been advocated. Zijderveld et al. performed a randomized clinical trial comparing preoperative intravenous amoxicillin-clavulanate, cefuroxime, and placebo in preventing postoperative infection in orthognathic surgery. The infection rate exceeded 50% in the placebo group and was below 20% in the two antibiotic groups, a statistically significant difference.[52] In 2011, Danda and Ravi performed a meta-analysis comparing perioperative antibiotic prophylaxis with extended term antibiotic prophylaxis in orthognathic surgery.[53] The postoperative infection rate in the perioperative antibiotic group was significantly higher (11%) versus the extended postoperative antibiotic group (4%), with a number needed to

TABLE 8-10	Costs of Oral Antibiotic Therapy			
Antibiotic	**Usual Dose (mg)***	**Usual Interval (h)**	**1-Week Retail Cost ($)[†]**	**Amoxicillin Cost Ratio[‡]**
Penicillins				
Amoxicillin	500	8	11.99	1.00
Penicillin V	500	6	18.79	1.57
Augmentin	875	12	118.99	9.92
Augmentin XR (1000 mg ×2)	2000	12	61.99	5.17
Dicloxacillin	500	6	37.39	3.12
Cephalosporins (Generation)				
Cephalexin caps (first)	500	6	26.29	2.19
Cefadroxil (first)	500	12	37.09	3.09
Cefuroxime (second)	500	8	67.59	5.64
Cefaclor ER (generic)	500	12	264.99	22.10
Cefdinir (third) (300 mg X2)	600	24	61.59	5.14
Erythromycins				
Erythromycin base	500	6	503.99	42.03
Clarithromycin (Biaxin XL)	500	24	46.19	3.85
Azithromycin (Zithromax)	250	12	86.59	7.22
Fidoxamicin (Dificid)	200	12	3,687.99	307.59
Antianaerobic				
Clindamycin (generic)	150	6	28.99	2.42
Clindamycin (2 T generic)	300	6	89.59	7.47
Clindamycin (generic)	300	6	89.59	7.47
Metronidazole	500	6	29.59	2.47
Other				
Trimethoprim–sulfamethoxazole	160/800	12	11.99	1.00
Vancomycin	125	6	726.99	60.63
Ciprofloxacin	500	12	20.09	1.68
Moxifloxacin (Avelox)	400	24	118.99	9.92
Doxycycline	100	12	56.59	4.72
Linezolid (Zyvox)	600	12	1,868.99	155.88

Notes

*Usual doses and intervals are for moderate infections and are not to be considered prescriptive.
[†]Amoxicillin cost ratio = Retail cost of antibiotic for 1 wk/retail cost of amoxicillin for 1 wk.
[‡]Retail cost/1 wk = Retail price charged for a 1 wk prescription at a large national pharmacy chain.
Courtesy Nerissa Aguas, RPh.

treat of 13. The maximum benefit in preventing infection appeared to be when the antibiotic was continued for 2 days postoperatively. These studies are high-level evidence that antibiotic prophylaxis is effective in orthognathic surgery.

Postoperative wound infection in clean-contaminated head and neck oncologic surgery requiring an incision through mucosa has been reported to be between 24% and 45% of cases. The following risk factors have been identified: tobacco consumption, presence of metastatic lymph nodes, immediate flap reconstruction, antimicrobial prophylaxis exceeding 48 hours[54]; preoperative hemoglobulin less than 10.5 g/dl, reconstruction with a free flap or pectoris major myocutaneous flap during the operation[55]; and post-laryngectomy tracheostoma.[56]

TABLE 8-11	Costs of Intravenous Antibiotic Therapy					
Antibiotic	Usual Dose	Usual Interval (h)	Pharmacy Cost per Dose ($)*	Total Cost for 24 Hours ($)	Total Cost for 7 Days ($)	Clindamycin Cost Ratio
Penicillins						
Penicillin G	2 m.u.**	4	13.19	103.13	721.89	3.11
Ampicillin	1 g	6	8.33	49.32	345.24	1.49
Unasyn	3 g	6	19.46	93.84	656.88	2.83
Oxacillin	2 g	6	28.90	131.60	921.20	3.97
Ticarcillin	3 g	4	12.37	98.25	687.72	2.97
Timentin	3 g	4	16.00	120.00	840.00	3.62
Cephalosporins (Generation)						
Cefazolin (first)	1 g	8	3.65	22.95	160.65	0.69
Cefotetan (second)	1 g	12	4.80	17.60	123.20	0.53
Cefuroxime (second)	1.5 g	8	6.56	31.69	221.81	0.96
Ceftazidime (third)	2 g	8	12.62	49.86	349.02	1.50
Ceftriaxone (third)	1 g	24	4.18	8.18	57.26	0.25
Cefepime (fourth)	2 g	12	51.10	110.19	771.34	3.33
Monobactam						
Aztreonam	1 g	8	39.54	130.62	914.34	3.94
Carbapenem						
Imipenem-cilastatin	0.5 g	6	41.26	181.04	1,267.28	5.46
Meropenem	1 g	8	78.19	246.57	1,725.99	7.44
Penicillin Allergy						
Erythromycin	1 g	6	21.66	102.64	718.48	3.10
Azithromycin	0.5 g	24	13.44	17.44	122.08	0.53
Vancomycin	0.5 g	6	3.82	31.28	218.96	0.94
Vancomycin	1.0 g	12	7.42	22.84	159.88	0.69
Antianaerobic						
Clindamycin	0.9 g	8	7.04	33.13	231.91	1.00
Metronidazole	0.5 g	6	2.50	26.00	182.00	0.78
Other						
Doxycycline	0.1 gm	12	18.55	45.10	315.70	1.36
Levofloxacin†	750 mg	24	58.16	62.16	435.12	1.88
Moxifloxacin†	400 mg	24	42.00	46.00	322.00	1.39
Linezolid	600 mg	12	120.11	248.22	1,737.54	7.49

*Total cost of therapy includes $1.00 for infusion materials and $3.00 labor cost, per dose. Penicillin cost ratio = 24 h. Cost of antibiotic/24-h cost of penicillin G. Usual doses and intervals are for moderate infections and are not to be considered prescriptive.
**m.u., Million units
†IV Fluoroquinolones are for NPO patients only due to excellent oral absorption.

Although an older study found a benefit from a prolonged postoperative antibiotic regimen in head and neck oncologic surgery,[57] more recent studies indicate that a 1-day antibiotic course is equally effective as 3-day courses.[58,59] In fact, Lotfi et al. observed a significantly increased rate of wound infection when antibiotic prophylaxis exceeded 48 hours duration.[54] Callender found that ampicillin-sulbactam was more effective than clindamycin in preventing postoperative wound infection in this type of case, and that gram-negative infection was lower in the ampicillin-sulbactam group.[60]

Further, in a recent review of antibiotic prophylaxis for adult oncologic head and neck surgery, Koshkareva and

Johnson reported that independent of antibiotic regimen, there is no significant difference in 1-day versus 3- to 5-day courses. Postoperative infection rates ranged from 10% with cefotaxime to 3.4% with clindamycin. Intermediate results were achieved with clindamycin-gentamicin, cefoperazone, cefazolin, and ampicillin-sulbactam.[61]

There are several other types of head and neck surgery in which the use of antibiotics has been reviewed, and the results are equivocal at best. In tonsillectomy, antibiotics seem to reduce fever, but not bleeding or postoperative pain. However, the limitations of the studies that find reduced postoperative fever cannot afford reliable conclusions that justify the increased risk of antibiotic complications, such as allergic reactions and gastrointestinal upset.[62]

There are no studies that provide adequate guidance on the use of prophylactic antibiotics in clean contaminated ear surgery.[63]

In chronic suppurative otitis media, middle ear infection is complicated by the drainage of pus through a perforated tympanic membrane. A systematic review of topical antibiotic drops compared with systemic antibiotics included nine randomized controlled trials of varying quality. Over a relatively short follow-up period, when the selected outcome was drying of the ear suppuration, fluoroquinolone antibiotic drops such as ciprofloxacin were superior to oral or injected antibiotics of the fluoroquinolone or other antibiotic families.[64]

There is only one well-designed study of chronic rhinosinusitis that compares systemic antibiotics with a placebo. In 64 patients, roxithromycin (which is not available in the United States) was only marginally and insignificantly more effective than placebo, with a short-term follow-up.[65] High-quality studies of the effectiveness of various antibiotics in treating chronic rhinosinusitis may be helpful, but the pathophysiology of this condition may involve the inflammatory response to pollutants, allergens, and bacterial contamination to a greater extent than primary infection.

Admittedly, there are other types of surgery for which the scientific evidence is not determinative, yet the community of surgeons appears to think prophylactic antibiotics are justified. A good example is bone grafting in clean-contaminated head and neck surgery.

Modern clinicians must stay abreast of developments in the use of prophylactic antibiotics and adjust their treatment patterns as new evidence becomes available.

New Antibiotics and Antimicrobial Strategies in Development

The development of antibiotic drugs was one of the most significant medical advances of the last century. After the discovery of penicillin in the 1928 by Alexander Fleming, new antibiotic families were discovered during each following decade until the 1980s, when an apparent discovery gap was encountered. The enormous costs of drug development inhibited for-profit corporations from undertaking this

often Sisyphean task, especially when antibiotics are taken only episodically, as compared to the life-long need for medications that treat chronic diseases, such as diabetes and cardiovascular conditions. In 1969, the U.S. Surgeon General stated, "We could close the book on infectious diseases." Since then, highly antibiotic-resistant organisms, such as the ESKAPE group have caused refractory disease and death among ever wider segments of our population.[19,20] Public health factors in this mounting problem include unnecessary antibiotic prescriptions, use of antibiotics in animal agriculture to enhance growth rates and combat unsanitary conditions, uncontrolled dispensing of antibiotics without a prescription in some countries, and widespread lack of sanitation in some developing countries.[66] Nowadays, highly resistant microbes can travel around the globe at the speed of commercial airliners.

Fortunately, a surprising number of new antibiotics are currently in the development pipeline. New members of the quinolones, tetracyclines, oxazolidinones, glycopeptides, and cephalosporins with enhanced antimicrobial or pharmacologic properties are undergoing clinical testing. Of special interest to those treating head and neck infections are promising new β-lactamase inhibitors, used in combination with new and old β-lactam antibiotics, such as ceftolozane-tazobactam, avibactam in combination with ceftazidime, ceftaroline or aztreonam, and with carbapenems.

Cefiderocol is a new cephalosporin that resists all of the classes of carbapenemase, making it effective against most ESKAPE group pathogens. Its clinical use will likely be restricted to the most critical cases, however, to maintain its effectiveness against these highly resistant organisms for as long as possible.[67]

Multiple fluoroquinolones are in development, and they have promise in both gram-positive and gram-negative infections. Delafloxacin (Baxdela) was approved in 2017. It has a safety advantage, as compared to the other fluoroquinolones, because it does not prolong the QT interval, which can lead to dysrhythmias. Nemonoxacin is close to clinical approval and is especially effective against gram-positive bacteria, including MRSA. Finafloxacin has demonstrated 2- to 256-fold increased activity in acidic environments, such as urine and abscesses. In such conditions, it has shown promise against the gram-negative *A. baumannii*, a highly resistant bacterium found in complex wounds, particularly in the blast wounds seen in military casualties. It is currently approved for acute otitis externa. JNJ-Q2 and ozenoxacin reportedly have equipotent activity against DNA gyrase and topoisomerase IV, the two enzyme targets of the fluoroquinolones, as well as reduced efflux out of bacterial cells. These properties hold the promise of reduced propensity for bacterial resistance, because they involve three separate metabolic sites of bactericidal effectiveness.[68]

Tetracycline antibiotics have long been used, but widespread resistance mechanisms have arisen through expression of tetracycline-specific efflux pumps and by ribosomal modifications that prevent tetracycline binding. Tigecycline is a currently available parenteral-only tetracycline effective against a broad range of gram-positive and gram-negative bacteria, including *A. baumannii. Pseudomonas* and *Proteus* species are resistant, however. Tigecycline now has a black box warning because in meta-analyses, all-cause mortality was higher than with comparator drugs. Several new tetracyclines appear to be able to evade efflux pumps while binding effectively to their ribosomal site of action, including omadacycline and eravacycline. They are primarily used against gram-negative bacteria.

Linezolid (Zyvox) was the first available oxazolidinone, a family of peptide antibiotics effective against gram-positive bacteria. Recently, linezolid resistance has been discovered in clinical isolates. New oxazolidinone analogs are in development that may expand the spectrum, overcome resistance, and improve safety. Tedizolid (Sivextro), a second-generation oxazolidinone, has improved potency, decreased resistance, shorter dosing regimens, and a broader spectrum of activity over the first-generation agents. Contezolid is in development.

Dalbavancin and oritavancin are two new glycopeptides (vancomycin family) that have significant advantages over vancomycin because they both have long half-lives and can be dosed at long intervals. Dalbavancin's half-life of 258 hours, allows treatment with two doses, and oritavancin, with a half-life of 393 hours, allows treatment with a single dose.

The ketolides, semisynthetic derivatives of erythromycin, have had a promising but troubled history in development. Telithromycin (Ketek) was the first antibiotic of this class to be approved for clinical use. Its indications have been sharply curtailed because of hepatotoxicity, visual deficits, and exacerbation of myasthenia gravis. Solithromycin is undergoing additional phase III trials because of potential hepatotoxicity.

The cyclic lipodepsipeptides include daptomycin (Cubicin), which is approved for the treatment of complicated soft tissue infections caused by gram-positive bacteria, including MRSA, *S. pyogenes,* and enterococci. Resistance to daptomycin, with cross-resistance to vancomycin in *S. aureus,* has been reported among staphylococci and enterococci.

In the intermediate and long term, entirely new pharmacologic categories that target bacterial pathways not previously exploited would be most beneficial.

One of the strategies for combating antibiotic resistance is the use of adjuvant drugs in combination with existing antibiotics that increase or restore their effectiveness against resistant organisms.

β-Lactamase inhibitors (BLIs) have been in clinical use for some time. New classes of BLIs are under development, however, that are chemically unrelated to those in current clinical use. Avibactam, used in combination with aztreonam and ceftaroline, is the first clinically available member of the diazabicyclooctane class of BLIs. Relebactam, in combination with imipenem-cilastatin, has recently been approved for clinical use in the United States. The boronic acids are a new class of BLIs under development.[69]

Eight different efflux pump inhibitors are under development. These compounds may reduce the bacterial cell's ability to excrete antibiotic compounds, thus increasing the antibiotic's concentration within the bacterial cell to lethal levels.[21]

Other antibiotic adjuvant categories are under development. Some compounds are designed to alter the bacterial cell membrane to enhance its permeability to antibiotics, independent of the efflux pump mechanism. Other compounds target bacterial sulfur metabolism and the synthesis of quorum-sensing compounds, decreasing the ability of bacteria to synthesize toxins and other virulence factors. This would allow antibiotics and the immune system to attack infecting bacteria unimpeded.[69]

Such a new category of antibiotic is the pleuromutilins. These diterpene antibiotics inhibit bacterial protein synthesis by selectively binding to prokaryotic ribosomes with no effect on eukaryotic protein synthesis. Although these compounds have encountered difficulties with clinical synthesis and stability, their unique mechanism of action prevents cross-resistance with currently available antibiotics. Retapamulin was the first pleuromutilin approved for human indications as a topical antibiotic in 2007. Lefamulin (Xenleta) is effective against gram-positive bacteria, including *S. pneumoniae,* viridans group streptococci, *Moraxella catarrhalis, E. faecium,* and MRSA. Its primary current indication is community-acquired bacterial pneumonia.[68]

Bacteriophages are viruses that can kill bacteria. They were used historically in eastern Europe and Russia, and are still approved in Georgia and Russia, especially for highly resistant bacteria. Because their mode of action is very specific to bacteria, bacteriophages appear to have a few side effects on humans. On the other hand, mixtures of bacteriophages often must be used because each phage is strain-specific. Bacteriophages appear to be able to penetrate biofilms, which would be a very useful property in head and neck infections such as osteomyelitis, implant-related infections, caries, and periodontal disease. There are many obstacles to the widespread clinical use of phages, however, including the potential for the viruses to evolve, the need for banking and mixing of phage virus strains, absorption, and distribution to the site of infection.[72]

Many of the investigational agents discussed here are primarily active against gram-positive pathogens. Even though vancomycin has proven over time to be quite effective against MRSA, for example, the prowess of *S. aureus* at developing antibiotic resistance mechanisms should spur even more development. Further, some of these agents have distinct advantages, such as the glycopeptides oritavancin and dalbavancin, which may provide single-dose therapy for some infections. Tedizolid is 4 to 16 times more potent against gram-positive bacteria than linezolid. Among the fluoroquinolones, delafloxacin, JNJ-Q2, and ozenoxacin have the promise of reduced resistance propensities when used for otherwise resistant staphylococci and streptococci.

Antimicrobial Stewardship Programs

Many hospitals and some clinics have instituted antibiotic stewardship programs, whose policies range from restricting certain antibiotics to use only by approval from an infectious diseases consultant, to the establishment of antibiotic prescription and usage care pathways and clinical oversight committees, to computer-based restrictions on the duration of antibiotic administration orders, and prompt deescalation of broad-spectrum antibiotic therapy after culture and sensitivity results become available.[71] Some hospitals, in order to decrease the selection pressure for antibiotic-resistant enterococci, have restricted the use of antibiotics that select for enterococci, such as the cephalosporins, with significant reduction in enterococcal infections over the ensuing months. Thus, rotation of use among different antibiotic families may become a useful tool in combating antibiotic resistance.

The Infectious Diseases Society of America has published guidelines for the establishment of antimicrobial stewardship programs in hospitals.[72]

A simple, yet important step toward the more rational and accurate use of antibiotics is close clinical follow-up. Guidelines published by the American College of Physicians, the American Academy of Otolaryngology–Head and Neck Surgery (AAOHNS), and the American Dental Association recommend clinical reevaluation at 3 to 7 days after prescribing an antibiotic.[6,28]

As an example, for acute bacterial rhinosinusitis (ABRS), the AAOHNS recommends that the antibiotic prescriber "should reassess the patient to confirm ABRS, exclude other causes of illness, and detect complications if the patient worsens or fails to improve with the initial management option by 7 days after diagnosis or worsens during the initial management."[28] The American Dental Association's guidelines include the following statement: "Clinicians should reevaluate or follow up with their patient after 3 days to assess if there is resolution of systemic signs and symptoms. If the patient's signs and symptoms begin to resolve, clinicians should instruct the patient to discontinue antibiotics 24 hours after complete resolution, irrespective of reevaluation after 3 days."[6]

Summary

In this chapter, the principles of antibiotic therapy for head and neck infection have been discussed. As clinicians, we can do our part in minimizing the emergence of antibiotic-resistant bacteria, while optimizing our patient care, by following the 10 principles described here.

References

1. Williams AC. Ludwig's angina. *Surg Gynecol Obstet.* 1940; 70:140.
2. Williams AC, Guralnick WC. The diagnosis and treatment of Ludwig's angina: a report of twenty cases. *N Engl J Med.* 1943;228:443.
3. Hought RT, Fitzgerald BE, Latta JE, Zallen RD. Ludwig's angina: report of two cases and review of the literature from 1945 to January 1979. *J Oral Surg.* 1980;38:849-855.
4. Wang LF, Kuo WR, Tsai SM, Huang KJ. Characterizations of life-threatening deep cervical space infections: a review of one hundred ninety-six cases. *Am J Otol.* 2003;24:111-117.
5. Brennan MT, Runyon MS, Batts JJ, et al. Odontogenic signs and symptoms as predictors of odontogenic infection: a clinical trial. *J Am Dent Assoc.* 2006;137(1):62-66.
6. Lockhart PB, Tampi MP, Abt E, et al. Evidence-based clinical practice guideline on antibiotic use for the urgent management of pulpal- and periapical-related dental pain and intraoral swelling: a report from the American Dental Association. *JADA.* 2019;150(11):906-921.
7. Brook I. Emergence and persistence of beta-lactamase-producing bacteria in the oropharynx following penicillin treatment. *Arch Otolaryngol Head Neck Surg.* 1988;114(6):667-670.
8. Brook I, Gober AE. Monthly changes in the rate of recovery of penicillin-resistant organisms from children. *Pediatr Infect Dis J.* 1997;16(2):255-257.
9. Slama TG, Amin A, Brunton SA, et al. A clinician's guide to the appropriate and accurate use of antibiotics: the Council for Appropriate and Rational Antibiotic Therapy (CARAT) criteria. *Am J Med.* 2005;118(7A):1S-6S.
10. Hassanain WA, Johnson CL, Faulds K, et al. Recent advances in antibiotic resistance diagnosis using SERS: focus on the "Big 5" challenges. *Analyst.* 2022;147(21):4674-4700.
11. Brook I, Frazier EH, Gher ME. Aerobic and anaerobic microbiology of periapical abscess. *Oral Microbiol Immunol.* 1991;6(2):123-125.
12. von Konow L, Köndell PA, Nord CE, Heimdahl A. Clindamycin versus phenoxymethylpenicillin in the treatment of acute orofacial infections. *Eur J Clin Microbiol Infect Dis.* 1992;11(12):1129-1135.
13. Lewis MA, Parkhurst CL, Douglas CW, et al. Prevalence of penicillin resistant bacteria in acute suppurative oral infection. *J Antimicrob Chemother.* 1995;35(6):785-791.
14. Flynn TR, Shanti RM, Levy M, Adamo, AK, Kraut RA, Trieger N. Severe odontogenic infections, part one: prospective report. *J Oral Maxillofac Surg.* 2006;64:1093-1103.
15. Kim MK, Chuang SK, August M. Antibiotic resistance in severe orofacial infections. *J Oral Maxillofac Surg.* 2017;75(5):962-968.
16. Sabino MC, Lunos S, Zadroga R, Svoboda L. Emerging trends in antibiotic management of deep fascial space infections of the head and neck. *J Oral Maxillofac Surg.* 2018;76:e34-e35.
17. Border M, Lin SI, Coke D. Increased incidence of clindamycin-resistance in head and neck infections within oral and maxillofacial surgery. *J Oral Maxillofac Surg.* 2018;75:e379-e380.
18. Sowerby LJ, Hussain Z, Husein M. The epidemiology, antibiotic resistance and post-discharge course of peritonsillar abscesses in London, Ontario. *J Otolaryngol Head Neck Surg.* 2013;42:5. Available at: https://doi.10.1186/1916-0216-42-5.
19. Halat DH, Moubareck CA. The current burden of carbapenemases: review of significant properties and dissemination among gram-negative bacteria. *Antibiotics (Basel).* 2020;9(4):186. Available at: https://doi.10.3390/antibiotics9040186.
20. Denissen J, Reyneke B, Waso-Reyneke M, Havenga B. Prevalence of ESKAPE pathogens in the environment: antibiotic resistance status, community-acquired infection and risk to human health. *Int J Hyg Environ Health.* 2022;244:114006.
21. Compagne N, Vieira Da Cruz A, Müller RT, et al. Update on the discovery of efflux pump inhibitors against critical priority gram-negative bacteria. *Antibiotics.* 2023;12:180. Available at: https://doi.org/10.3390/antibiotics12010180.
22. Wilson W, Taubert KA, Gewitz M, et al. Prevention of infective endocarditis: guidelines from the American Heart Association—a

guideline from the American Heart Association Rheumatic Fever, Endocarditis, and Kawasaki Disease Committee, Council on Cardiovascular Disease in the Young, and the Council on Clinical Cardiology, Council on Cardiovascular Surgery and Anesthesia, and the Quality of Care and Outcomes Research Interdisciplinary Working Group. *Circulation*. 2007;116:1736-1754.

23. American Dental Association, American Academy of Orthopaedic Surgeons. Advisory statement: antibiotic prophylaxis for dental patients with total joint replacements. *JADA*. 2003;134:895-899.

24. Sollecito TP, Abt E, Lockhart PB, Truelove E. The use of prophylactic antibiotics prior to dental procedures in patients with prosthetic joints: evidence-based clinical practice guideline for dental practitioners—a report of the American Dental Association Council on Scientific Affairs. *JADA*. 2015;146(1):11-16.

25. Skaar DD, O'Connor H, Hodges JS, Michalowicz BS. Dental procedures and subsequent prosthetic joint infections: findings from the Medicare current beneficiary survey. *JADA*. 2011;142: 1343-1351.

26. Berbari EF, Osmon DR, Carr A, et al. Dental procedures as risk factors for prosthetic hip or knee infection: a hospital-based prospective case-control study. *Clin Infect Dis*. 2010;50:8-16.

27. Thornhill MH, Crum A, Nicholl J. Analysis of prosthetic joint infections following invasive dental procedures in England. *JAMA Netw Open*. 2022;5(1):e2142987. Available at: https://doi.org/10.1001/jamanetworkopen.2021.42987.

28. Rosenfeld RM, Piccirillo JF, Chandrasekhar SS, Brook I. Clinical practice guideline (update): adult sinusitis. *Otolaryngol Head Neck Surg*. 2015;152(suppl 2):S1-S39. Available at: http://doi.org/10.1177/0194599815572097.

29. Harris AM, Hicks LA, Qaseem A. Appropriate antibiotic use for acute respiratory tract infection in adults: advice for high-value care from the American College of Physicians and the Centers for Disease Control and Prevention. *Ann Intern Med*. 2016;164:425-434. Available at: http://doi.org/10.7326/M15-1840.

30. Neugut AI, Ghatak AT, Miller RL. Anaphylaxis in the United States: an investigation into its epidemiology. *Arch Intern Med*. 2001;161:15-21.

31. Shenoy ES, Macy E, Rowe T, Blumenthal KG. Evaluation and management of penicillin allergy: a review. *JAMA*. 2019;321(2): 188-199. Available at: http://doi.org/10.1001/jama.2018.19283.

32. Bishop EJ, Tiruvoipati R. Management of *Clostridioides difficile* infection in adults and challenges in clinical practice: review and comparison of current IDSA/SHEA, ESCMID and ASID guidelines. *J Antimicrob Chemother*. 2023;78:21-30. Available at: https://doi.org/10.1093/jac/dkac404.

33. Girotra M, Kumar V, Khan JM, et al. Clinical predictors of fulminant colitis in patients with *Clostridium difficile* infection. *Saudi J Gastroenterol*. 2012;18(2):133-139. Available at: http://doi.org/10.4103/1319-3767.93820.

34. Kazanowski M, Smolarek S, Kinnarney F, Grzebieniak Z. *Clostridium difficile*: epidemiology, diagnostic and therapeutic possibilities—a systematic review. *Tech Coloproctol*. 2014;18(3): 223-232. Available at: http://doi.org/10.1007/s10151-013-1081-0.

35. Back DJ, Grimmer SF, Orme ML, Proudlove C, Mann RD, Breckenridge AM. Evaluation of Committee on Safety of Medicines yellow card reports on oral contraceptive-drug interactions with anticonvulsants and antibiotics. *Br J Clin Pharmacol*. 1988;25(5):527-532.

36. Drug interaction with oral contraceptive steroids. *Br Med J*. 1980;281(6233):93-94.

37. Baddour LM, Wilson WR, Bayer AS, et al. Infective endocarditis: diagnosis, antimicrobial therapy, and management of complications—a statement for healthcare professionals from the Committee on Rheumatic Fever, Endocarditis, and Kawasaki Disease, Council on Cardiovascular Disease in the Young, and the Councils on Clinical Cardiology, Stroke, and Cardiovascular Surgery and Anesthesia, American Heart Association. *Circulation*. 2005;111(23):e394-e434

38. Bliziotis IA, Samonis G, Vardakas KZ, Chrysanthopoulou S, Falagas ME. Effect of aminoglycoside and beta-lactam combination therapy versus beta-lactam monotherapy on the emergence of antimicrobial resistance: a meta-analysis of randomized, controlled trials. *Clin Infect Dis*. 2005;41(2):149-158.

39. Guillemot D, Carbon C, Balkau B, et al. Low dosage and long treatment duration of beta-lactam: risk factors for carriage of penicillin-resistant *Streptococcus pneumoniae*. *JAMA*. 1998;279:365-370.

40. Lewis MA, McGowan DA, MacFarlane TW. Short course high-dosage amoxicillin in the treatment of acute dento-alveolar abscess. *Br Dent J*. 1986;161(8):299-302.

41. Chardin H, Yasukawa K, Nouacer N, et al. Reduced susceptibility to amoxicillin of oral streptococci following amoxicillin exposure. *J Med Microbiol*. 2009;58(Pt 8):1092-1097.

42. Feres M, Haffajee AD, Allard K, et al. Antibiotic resistance of subgingival species during and after antibiotic therapy. *J Clin Periodontol*. 2002;29:724-735.

43. Greene JA, Herzberg D. Hidden in plain sight marketing prescription drugs to consumers in the twentieth century. *Am J Public Health*. 2010;100(5):793-803. Available at: https://doi.org/10.2105/AJPH.2009.181255.

44. Lim R, Mills C, Burke AB, et al. Are oral antibiotics an effective alternative to intravenous antibiotics in treatment of osteomyelitis of the jaw? *J Oral Maxillofac Surg*. 2021;79:1882-1890.

45. Halpern LR, Dodson TB. Does prophylactic administration of systemic antibiotics prevent postoperative inflammatory complications after third molar surgery? *J Oral Maxillofac Surg*. 2007;65:177-185.

46. Ren YF, Malmstrom HS. Effectiveness of antibiotic prophylaxis in third molar surgery: a meta-analysis of randomized controlled clinical trials. *J Oral Maxillofac Surg*. 2007;65:1909-1921.

47. Lodi G, Azzi L, Varoni EM, et al. Antibiotics to prevent complications following tooth extractions. *Cochrane Database Syst Rev*. 2021;2(2):CD003811. Available at: https://doi.org/10.1002/14651858.CD003811.pub3.

48. Sharaf B, Dodson TB. Does the use of prophylactic antibiotics decrease implant failure? *Oral Maxillofac Surg Clin North Am*. 2011;23(4):547-550.

49. Jain A, Rai A, Singh A, Taneja S. Efficacy of preoperative antibiotics in prevention of dental implant failure: a meta-analysis of randomized controlled trials. *Oral Maxillofac Surg*. 2020;24(4):469-475. Available at: https://doi.org/10.1007/s10006-020-00872-5.

50. Kim AS, Abdelhay N, Levin L, et al. Antibiotic prophylaxis for implant placement: a systematic review of effects on reduction of implant failure. *Br Dent J*. 2020;228(12):943-951. Available at: https://doi.org/10.1038/s41415-020-1649-9.

51. Khouly I, Braun RS, Chambrone L. Antibiotic prophylaxis may not be indicated for prevention of dental implant infections in healthy patients: a systematic review and meta-analysis. *Clin Oral Investig*. 2019;23(4):1525-1553. Available at: https://doi.org/10.1007/s00784-018-2762-x.

52. Zijderveld SA, Smeele LE. Preoperative antibiotic prophylaxis in orthognathic surgery: a randomized, double-blind, and placebo-controlled clinical study. *J Oral Maxillofac Surg*. 1999;57:1403.

53. Danda AK, Ravi P. Effectiveness of postoperative antibiotics in orthognathic surgery: a meta-analysis. *J Oral Maxillofac Surg*. 2011;69:2650-2656.

54. Lotfi CJ, Cavalcanti R de C, Costa e Silva AM, et al. Risk factors for surgical-site infections in head and neck cancer surgery. *Otolaryngol Head Neck Surg.* 2008;138(1):74-80. Available at: https://doi.org/10.1016/j.otohns.2007.09.018.

55. Liu SA, Tung KC, Shiao JY, Chiu YT. Preliminary report of associated factors in wound infection after major head and neck neoplasm operations: does the duration of prophylactic antibiotic matter? *J Laryngol Otol.* 2008;122(4):403-408.

56. Penel N, Fournier C, Lefebvre D, Lefebvre JL. Multivariate analysis of risk factors for wound infection in head and neck squamous cell carcinoma surgery with opening of mucosa: study of 260 surgical procedures. *Oral Oncol.* 2005;41(3):294-303.

57. Johnson JT, Myers EN, Thearle PB, Sigler BA, Schramm VL Jr. Antimicrobial prophylaxis for contaminated head and neck surgery. *Laryngoscope.* 1984;94(1):46-51.

58. Liu SA, Tung KC, Shiao JY, Chiu YT. Preliminary report of associated factors in wound infection after major head and neck neoplasm operations: does the duration of prophylactic antibiotic matter? *J Laryngol Otol.* 2008;122(4):403-408.

59. Righi M, Manfredi R, Farneti G, Pasquini E, Cenacchi V. Short-term versus long-term antimicrobial prophylaxis in oncologic head and neck surgery. *Head Neck.* 1996;18(5):399-404.

60. Callender DL. Antibiotic prophylaxis in head and neck oncologic surgery: the role of gram-negative coverage. *Int J Antimicrob Agents.* 1999;12(suppl 1):S21-S25; discussion S26-S27.

61. Koshkareva YA, Johnson JT. What is the perioperative antibiotic prophylaxis in adult oncologic head and neck surgery? *Laryngoscope.* 2014;124:1055-1056.

62. Dhiwakar M, Clement WA, Supriya M, McKerrow W. Antibiotics to reduce post-tonsillectomy morbidity. *Cochrane Database Syst Rev.* 2012;(12):CD005607. Available at: https://doi.org/10.1002/14651858.CD005607.pub4.

63. Verschuur HP, de Wever WW, van Benthem PP. Antibiotic prophylaxis in clean and clean-contaminated ear surgery. *Cochrane Database Syst Rev.* 2004;(3):CD003996. Available at: https://doi.org/10.1002/14651858.CD003996.pub2.

64. Macfadyen CA, Acuin JM, Gamble CL. Systemic antibiotics versus topical treatments for chronically discharging ears with underlying eardrum perforations. *Cochrane Database Syst Rev.* 2006;(1):CD005608. Available at: https://doi.org/10.1002/14651858.CD005608.

65. Piromchai P, Thanaviratananich S, Laopaiboon M. Systemic antibiotics for chronic rhinosinusitis without nasal polyps in adults. *Cochrane Database Syst Rev.* 2011;(5):CD008233. Available at: https://doi.org/10.1002/14651858.CD008233.pub2.

66. Gulberg E, Cao S, Berg OG, Ilba C. Selection of resistant bacteria at very low antibiotic concentrations. *PLoS Pathog.* 2011;7(7):e1002158. Available at: https://doi.org/10.1371/journal.ppat.1002158.

67. Maseda E, Suárez de la Rica A. The role of cefiderocol in clinical practice. *Rev Esp Quimioter.* 2022;35(suppl 2):39-44.

78. Shi Z, Zhang J, Tian L, et al. A comprehensive overview of the antibiotics approved in the last two decades: retrospects and prospects. *Molecules.* 2023;28:1762. Available at: https://doi.org/10.3390/molecules28041762.

69. Annunziato G. Strategies to overcome antimicrobial resistance (AMR) making use of non-essential target inhibitors: a review. *Int J Mol Sci.* 2019;20:5844. Available at: https://doi.org/10.3390/ijms20235844.

70. Verbeken G, Pirnay JP, Lavigne R, et al. Call for a dedicated European legal framework for bacteriophage therapy. *Arch Immunol Ther Exp (Warsz).* 2014;62(2):117-129. Available at: https://doi.org/10.1007/s00005-014-0269-y.

71. Leuthner KD, Doern GV. Antimicrobial stewardship programs. *J Clin Microbiol.* 2013;51(12):3916-3920. Available at: https://doi.org/10.1128/JCM.01751-13.

72. Barlam TF, Cosgrove SE, Abbo LM, MacDougall C. Implementing an antibiotic stewardship program: guidelines by the Infectious Diseases Society of America and the Society for Healthcare Epidemiology of America. *Clin Infect Dis.* 2016;62(10):e51-e77.

9

Antimicrobial Pharmacology for Head, Neck, and Orofacial Nonbacterial Infections

STEVEN HALEPAS, TYLER T. BOYNTON, AND ELIE M. FERNEINI

This chapter focuses on the pharmacology, spectrum, and clinical applications of antimicrobial drugs in the management of nonbacterial infections of the head and neck, specifically antifungal and antiviral agents.

Antifungals

Fungal cells differ from mammalian cells in that they have cell walls that are composed of chitin, glucans, mannans, and glycoproteins. Both mammalian and fungal cells have cell membranes; however, they differ in their lipid composition. Mammalian cells have a cholesterol-rich cell membrane, whereas fungal cells have a membrane that is primarily composed of ergosterol. Despite these differences, fungi are metabolically like mammalian cells and offer few pathogen-specific targets.[1]

Antifungal agents used to treat fungal infections can be classified based on their site of action (intracellular, cell membrane, and cell wall) (Figure 9-1). The principal classes of drugs used in fungal head and neck infections are the azole and polyene antifungals. These agents target the ergosterol-rich cell membrane. The azoles prevent the synthesis of ergosterol by inhibiting 14-α-sterol demethylase, a cytochrome P-450–dependent enzyme.[2] The azoles' inhibition of CYP-450–dependent enzymes in membranes is not limited to fungal membranes and can cause drug–drug interactions because of inhibition of mammalian CYP enzymes. Azoles have some important drug interactions with terfenadine (Seldane) and loratadine (Claritin). Levels of these drugs tend to increase in patients concurrently taking azole agents.[3] Multiple toxicities are associated with antifungal agents (Figure 9-2). Appropriate knowledge of these common toxicities improves patient management.

Azoles

The two main classes of azoles are the imidazoles, which contain two nitrogen molecules in the azole ring (clotrimazole,

miconazole, and ketoconazole), and the triazoles, which contain three (itraconazole, fluconazole, voriconazole, and posaconazole) (Table 9-1). The imidazoles, with the exception of ketoconazole, are used for treating superficial fungal infections, whereas the triazoles have a broader spectrum and are used for treating more serious systemic fungal infections in immunocompromised and immunodeficient patients.

Imidazoles

Clotrimazole is available as a 1% topical solution used for tinea versicolor or as a 10-mg troche used for oral thrush. The troches contain sugar and may promote caries if used in excess; otherwise, they are nontoxic. They must be completely dissolved because any swallowed troche provides no benefit. The typical dosage for the treatment of oral candidiasis is four to five troches per day for 10 to 14 days. Miconazole is available as a 50-mg tablet for the treatment of oropharyngeal candidiasis. The tablet is taken once daily and should be placed into the buccal vestibule.

Ketoconazole is used for the treatment of the following systemic fungal infections: candidiasis, chronic mucocutaneous candidiasis, oral thrush, blastomycosis, coccidioidomycosis, histoplasmosis, chromomycosis, and paracoccidioidomycosis. It is only available in the oral form in 200-mg tablets. These tablets are taken once daily (with a maximum daily dose of 800 mg in severe fungal disease).[4] The absorption of ketoconazole is affected by gastric acidity and food. The drug should not be taken with food, and drugs that reduce gastric acidity may impair absorption. Ketoconazole poorly penetrates the cerebrospinal fluid (CSF), eye, urine, and saliva because of its high affinity and degree of protein binding. Common side effects include decreased libido and gynecomastia, particularly at higher doses.[3] Additionally, adrenal suppression has been reported.[5] Other side effects include fatigue, rash, and nausea. Hepatitis is a rare complication of ketoconazole use.

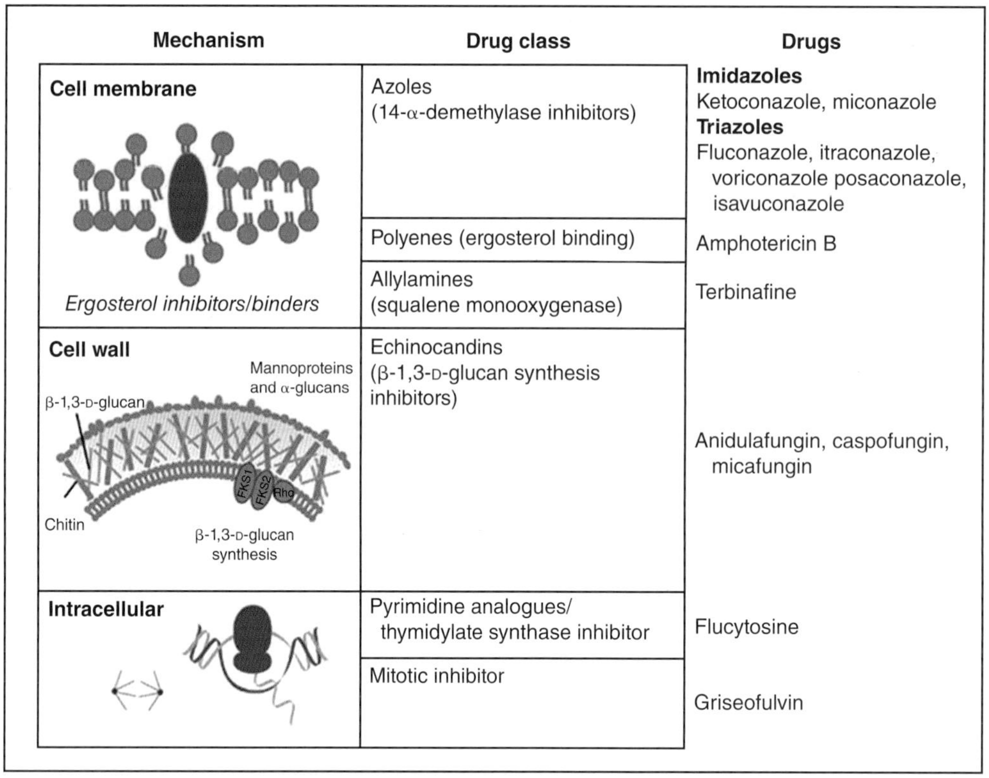

Mechanism
Drug class
Drugs
Cell membrane
Azoles (14-α-demethylase inhibitors)
Imidazoles
Ketoconazole, miconazole
Triazoles
Fluconazole, itraconazole, voriconazole posaconazole, isavuconazole
Polyenes (ergosterol binding)
Amphotericin B
Allylamines (squalene monooxygenase)
Terbinafine
Ergosterol inhibitors/binders
Cell wall
Mannoproteins and α-glucans
β-1,3-D-glucan
Chitin
β-1,3-D-glucan synthesis
FKS1
FKS2
Rho
Echinocandins (β-1,3-D-glucan synthesis inhibitors)
Anidulafungin, caspofungin, micafungin
Intracellular
Pyrimidine analogues/ thymidylate synthase inhibitor
Flucytosine
Mitotic inhibitor
Griseofulvin

• **Figure 9-1** Sites of Action and Mechanisms of Systemic Antifungal Agents. (From Lewis RE. Current concepts in antifungal pharmacology. *Mayo Clin Proc*. 2011;86:806.)

Hepatic
All azoles
Amphotericin B
5-FC
Echinocandins
Renal toxicity
Amphotericin B
Cyclodextrins possibly toxic (IV voriconazole)
CNS
Voriconazole
Photopsia
Voriconazole
Cutaneous
Rash (all antifungal agents)
Photosensitivity/malignancy? (voriconazole)
GI
Itraconazole
Posaconazole
5-FC
Cardiac
Cardiomyopathy (itraconazole)
QTc prolongation (all azoles, especially with drug interactions)
Infusion reactions
Amphotericin B
Echinocandins
Bone marrow suppression
5-FC
Amphotericin B (anemia associated with decreased epoetin production)

• **Figure 9-2** Common Toxicities of Antifungal Agents. *CNS,* Central nervous system; *5-FC,* 5-fluorocytosine; *GI,* gastrointestinal; *IV,* intravenous. (From Lewis RE. Current concepts in antifungal pharmacology. *Mayo Clin Proc*. 2011;86:806.)

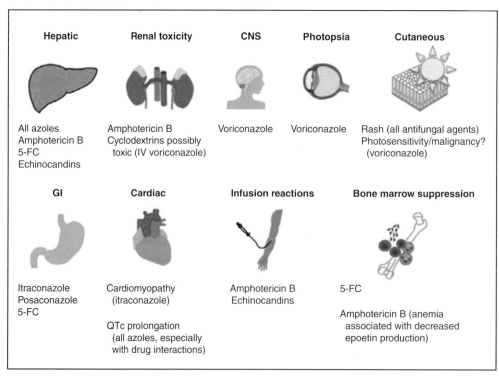

TABLE 9-1   Azole Antifungal Agents

Generic	U.S. Trade Name(s)	Chemical Structure	U.S. Formulations	Clinical Use
Ketoconazole	Nizoral		200-mg oral tablet 2% cream 2% dandruff shampoo	Systemic and superficial mycoses
Itraconazole	Sporanox		100-mg oral capsule 10-mg/mL oral solution	Systemic and superficial mycoses
Fluconazole	Diflucan		50-, 100-, 150-, and 200-mg oral tablets 10- and 40-mg/mL oral suspension 2-mg/mL sterile IV solution	Systemic and superficial mycoses
Clotrimazole	Mycelex Mycelex-G Lotrimin Gyne-Lotrimin Fungoid		1% cream, lotion, solution, tincture, vaginal cream 500-mg vaginal tablet 10-mg oral troche	Superficial mycoses

From Sheehan DJ, Hitchcock CA, Sibley CM. Current and emerging azole antifungal agents. *Clin Microbiol Rev.* 1999;12:41.

Triazoles

Fluconazole is the most versatile of the azole antifungal drugs. It is available in oral and intravenous formulations and does not require the action of gastric acid for absorption. It is not highly protein bound, allowing wide distribution among body compartments.[6] Its long serum half-life allows once-daily dosing of 100 mg for minor infections, and up to 400- to 800-mg daily dosing for serious infections.[7] Fluconazole has greater than 90% oral bioavailability and has fewer side effects and drug interactions than the other azoles. It is used for the treatment of oropharyngeal candidiasis and cryptococcal meningitis. However, it lacks activity against *Aspergillus* species and other opportunistic fungal species such as *Mucorales* and *Fusarium*.[1] The azoles are most frequently used in the management of mucocutaneous candidiasis.[8] Fluconazole is more effective than ketoconazole and clotrimazole troches for thrush in immunocompromised patients.

Itraconazole is available in both oral and intravenous formulations. It has a wide spectrum of activity against many yeasts, dimorphic fungi, and *Aspergillus* species.[9] It can be administered as a 100-mg capsule taken once daily, with a maximum dosage of 400 mg/day. Doses greater than 200 mg do not appear to increase serum levels; thus, it must be given in separate doses if used for severe infection requiring a daily dose of 400 mg. For less serious infections, a total daily dose of 100 to 200 mg is usually adequate.[10] Itraconazole, like ketoconazole, is not well distributed to areas such as the CSF, eye, and urine.[7,11] Intravenous itraconazole offers a less toxic alternative for patients with deep fungal infections who are unable to take amphotericin B.[12] Side effects of itraconazole are less severe than those of ketoconazole, and those of fluconazole are even more minor. Side effects of itraconazole include nausea, fatigue, rash, and hepatitis. Table 9-2 compares three of the most commonly used azoles: ketoconazole, itraconazole, and fluconazole.

Voriconazole and posaconazole are broader-spectrum triazoles that were introduced in 2002 and 2006, respectively. They were a significant development for the treatment of fungal infections in severely immunocompromised patients. Voriconazole is used for the treatment of esophageal candidiasis, invasive pulmonary aspergillosis, and serious fungal infections caused by *Scedosporium apiospermum* and *Fusarium* species. Posaconazole is useful for patients who have oropharyngeal candidiasis refractory to itraconazole, fluconazole, or both. In addition, it is used for prophylaxis against invasive *Aspergillus* and *Candida* infections in children 13 years of age and older who are severely immunocompromised.[13,14] Although these drugs have a greater spectrum of

TABLE 9-2 Clinically Important Features of Some Azoles

Feature	Ketoconazole	Itraconazole	Fluconazole
Formulation	200-mg tablets	100-mg capsules	50-, 100-, 150-, 200-mg tablets 2 mg/mL IV solution 50-mg or 200-mg/5 mL suspension
Absorption	Requires acid; decreased with antacids, omeprazole, histamine$_2$ blockers, sucralfate	Requires acid; decreased with antacids, omeprazole, histamine$_2$ blockers, sucralfate	Excellent; not affected by antacids, omeprazole, histamine$_2$ blockers, sucralfate
Distribution	Minimal in CSF, eye, and other sites	Minimal in CSF, eye, and other sites	Excellent in CSF, eye, and other sites
Protein binding	High (~99%)	High (~99%)	Low (~10%)
Metabolism	Almost entirely hepatic	Almost entirely hepatic	Minimal hepatic metabolism
Excretion in urine	Little unchanged drug in urine	Little unchanged drug in urine	>80% excreted by kidneys
Reduction of dose in renal failure	Not necessary	Not necessary	20-50 mL/min ↓ by 50% <20 mL/min ↓ by 75% Hemodialysis: administer dose after dialysis
Dosing regimen	Once-daily dosing	Once daily for 200 mg; twice daily if higher dose required	Once-daily dosing
Usual daily dose	200-800 mg	100-400 mg	100-800 mg

CSF, Cerebrospinal fluid.
From Johnson JT, Yu VL. *Infectious Diseases and Antimicrobial Therapy of Ears, Nose, and Throat.* Philadelphia: Saunders; 1997.

activity, their use is limited by their pharmacokinetic variability and drug interactions.[15]

Polyenes

Two drugs are part of the polyene drug class: amphotericin B and nystatin. The polyenes directly bind ergosterol, causing a conformational change in the structure of the cell membrane leading to leakage of intracellular contents.[16]

Amphotericin B

Amphotericin B was one of the earliest antifungal agents on the U.S. market (Figure 9-3). Developed in 1955, it remains the most effective agent for treating a broad range

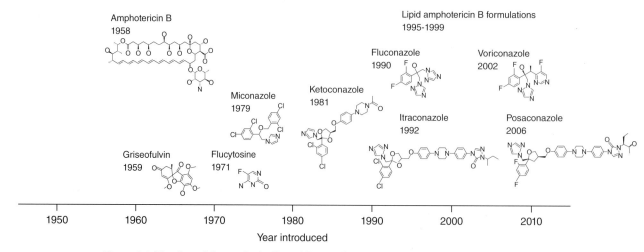

• **Figure 9-3** Timeline of Systemic Antifungal Drugs. (From Lewis RE. Current concepts in antifungal pharmacology. *Mayo Clin Proc.* 2011;86:806.)

of systemic fungal infections.[17] It has antifungal activity against *Candida* species; dermatophytes; filamentous fungi-like *Aspergillus, Rhizopus,* and *Mucor* species; and dimorphic endemic mycoses.[3] It is the treatment of choice for life-threatening mycotic infections.[18,19] In the head and neck, amphotericin B is used most commonly for severe sinusitis, cavernous sinus thrombosis, orbital apex syndrome, and otitis externa caused by fungal organisms.[20] Flucytosine is typically given in conjunction with amphotericin B for cryptococcal meningitis and serious candidal infections.[21,22]

Amphotericin B binds sterols in cell membranes with a higher affinity toward ergosterol than mammalian cholesterol. As the concentration of the drug increases in organs such as the kidney, it begins to bind cholesterol in mammalian membranes, leading to nephrotoxicity. The amphotericin B dosing regimen is complex, and assistance from an infectious disease specialist or others with regular experience using this drug may be indicated. The drug is given intravenously, and titration from a low to a therapeutic dose is performed over several days while renal function is monitored. Amphotericin B directly stimulates mononuclear phagocytic cells to release proinflammatory cytokines, which leads to nausea and vomiting, rigors, and fever during administration.[23] Veins used for infusion are irritated, and phlebitis is common. Anemia occurs while the drug is in use but reverses once the drug is discontinued. Different forms of amphotericin B are available (Abelcet, Amphotec, AmBisome) and were created to reduce the toxic side effects. These new formulations use lipid complexes or lipid encapsulation to diminish the toxicity of the parent compound.[22,24]

Nystatin

Nystatin is helpful as topical therapy for mild to moderate mucocutaneous candidiasis. Nystatin is available as a suspension (100,000 units/mL) and pastilles (200,000 units each). The suspension is administered in a swish-and-swallow format four times a day and also can be used for soaking dental prostheses. The pastilles should be dissolved in the mouth until gone and are taken one or two at a time 4 or 5 times per day for 10 to 14 days. Nystatin is nontoxic and usually effective during use, but relapses after therapy are common.[25,26]

Echinocandins

The echinocandins are the only agents that target the fungal cell wall by inhibiting the synthesis of β-1,3-d-glucan polymers.[27] This leads to instability of the cell and eventual cell lysis. Mammalian cells do not have cell walls; this is a very effective target and avoids direct human cell toxicity. The echinocandins are fungicidal against most *Candida* species and fungistatic against *Aspergillus* species. However, they do not have activity against Zygomycetes, *Cryptococcus neoformans,* or *Fusarium* species.[28] Caspofungin, micafungin, and anidulafungin are echinocandins that are available as intravenous preparations. Caspofungin is used for the treatment of esophageal candidiasis and invasive aspergillosis in patients who are refractory to or intolerant of other therapies. Micafungin and anidulafungin are used for the treatment of candidemia, disseminated candidiasis, esophageal candidiasis, and other invasive *Candida* infections. These medications are administered intravenously once daily and have very few drug interactions.

Pyrimidine Analogues

Flucytosine is used to treat serious systemic infections caused by *Candida* and *Cryptococcus,* and it is often used in conjunction with an azole agent. It exhibits its effects via inhibition of intracellular enzymes. Once it is taken up by fungal cells, it is converted into 5-fluorouracil (5-FU), which is further converted to metabolites that inhibit fungal RNA and DNA synthesis.[29] Flucytosine is available as 250- and 500-mg capsules; the drug is administered every 6 to 12 hours for a total of 100 mg/kg/day. If the creatinine clearance decreases to critical levels, the total daily dose should be reduced with guidance from infectious disease specialists. The bone marrow suppression caused by flucytosine usually reverses once the drug is discontinued. Side effects include nausea, vomiting, hepatotoxicity, and rashes. Peak and trough levels should be monitored.[29]

Antifungal agents provide antimicrobial coverage for fungal head and neck infections. They have a wide spectrum of action (Figure 9-4). Selecting the proper agent based on culture and sensitivity will lead to an accurate and speedy resolution of the infection.

Antivirals

Most viral infections in immunocompetent patients are self-limiting, and antiviral agents are unnecessary. The goals of therapy are to decrease the severity of the infection as well as reduce the rate of transmission of the virus. In immunocompromised patients, viral infections can be devastating or even fatal. Antiviral agents can be used preemptively, prophylactically, or when there is overt disease.[30]

Oral and facial surgeons are often the first health care providers to treat patients who show oral manifestations of systemic viral infections. It is essential to have a general knowledge of viral infections as well as the antiviral agents used to treat them. These include (1) human herpesviruses (HHVs), (2) human papillomaviruses (HPVs), (3) enteroviruses, (4) hepatitis virus, and (5) human immunodeficiency virus (HIV). With the exception of HIV, there are three major groups of viruses that are targets of antiviral therapy. These include herpes, hepatitis, and influenza viruses. Many of these viral infections require the expertise of an infectious disease specialist, but it is important to be familiar with common antiviral treatments (Table 9-3). Current strategies for HIV-1 antiretrovirals include starting with two nucleoside reverse transcriptase inhibitors (NRTIs)—tenofovir alafenamide or tenofovir disoproxil fumarate plus emtricitabine

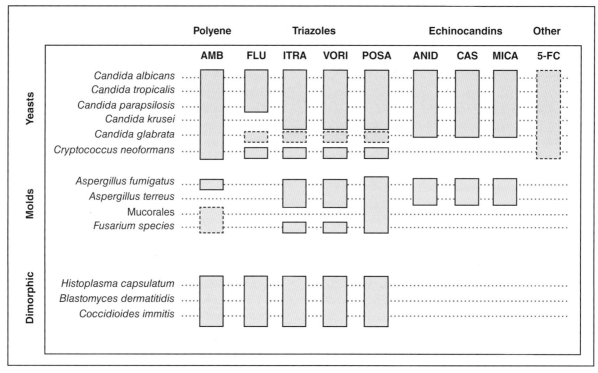

• **Figure 9-4** Spectrum of Action of Systemic Antifungal Agents. *AMB,* amphotericin B; *ANID,* anidulafungin; *CAS,* caspofungin; *5-FC,* 5-fluorocytosine; *FLU,* fluconazole; *ITRA,* itraconazole; *MICA,* miconazole; *POSA,* posaconazole; *VORI,* voriconazole. (From Lewis RE. Current concepts in antifungal pharmacology. *Mayo Clin Proc.* 2011;86:806.)

TABLE 9-3 Antiviral Drugs

Antiviral Drugs	Molecule	Mechanism of Action	Treatment	Properties

Acyclovir		Acyclovir is converted by viral thymidine kinase to acyclovir monophosphate, which is then converted by host cell kinases to acyclovir triphosphate to inhibit viral DNA polymerase.	• Herpes simplex
			• Varicella-zoster
			• Epstein-Barr
			• Cytomegalovirus
				• Oral bioavailability: 15-30%
				• Peak plasma concentration: 1-2 h
				• Half-life:
				  • Neonates: 4 h
				  • Children/adults: 3 h

Valacyclovir		Acyclo-GTP, the active triphosphate metabolite of acyclovir, is a very potent inhibitor of viral DNA replication. Acyclo-GTP competitively inhibits and inactivates the viral DNA polymerase.	• Herpes simplex • Varicella-zoster • Epstein-Barr • Cytomegalovirus	• Oral bioavailability is 55% • Half-life: 1-2 h
Ganciclovir		Inhibition of the replication of viral DNA by ganciclovir-5'-triphosphate (ganciclovir-TP). This inhibition includes a selective and potent inhibition of the viral DNA polymerase.	• Cytomegalovirus	• Oral bioavailability: 8-9% • Plasma half-life: 2.5 h • Intracellular half-life: 12 h

TABLE 9-3   Antiviral Drugs—cont'd

Antiviral Drugs	Molecule	Mechanism of Action	Treatment	Properties
Penciclovir	Penciclovir	Within a virally infected cell, a viral thymidine kinase adds a phosphate group to the penciclovir molecule; this is the rate-limiting step in the activation of penciclovir. Cellular (human) kinases then add two more phosphate groups, producing the active penciclovir triphosphate. This activated form inhibits viral DNA polymerase, thus impairing the ability of the virus to replicate within the cell.	• Herpes simplex	• Poor oral bioavailability— used as a topical
Famciclovir		Prodrug of penciclovir	• Herpes simplex • Varicella-zoster	• Oral Bioavailability: 75% • Plasma half-Life: 2 h • Intracellular half-life: 7-20 h
Foscarnet		Structural mimic of the anion pyrophosphate that selectively inhibits the pyrophosphate binding site on viral DNA polymerases at concentrations that do not affect human DNA polymerases.	• Cytomegalovirus • Herpes simplex • Varicella-zoster • Human herpesvirus 9 • Human immunodeficiency virus type 1	• Poor oral bioavailability • Plasma half-life: 6 h
Ribavirin		It is a guanosine (ribonucleic) analog used to stop viral RNA synthesis and viral mRNA capping, thus, it is a nucleoside analog. Ribavirin is a prodrug, which when metabolized resembles purine RNA nucleotides. In this form, it interferes with RNA metabolism required for viral replication.	• Respiratory syncytial virus • Parainfluenza • Influenza A and B • Measles • Hantavirus • Hepatitis C virus	• Bioavailability: 64% • Half-life: 43 h
Lamivudine		Analog of cytidine. It is phosphorylated to active metabolites that compete for incorporation into viral DNA. They inhibit the HIV reverse transcriptase enzyme competitively and act as a chain terminator of DNA synthesis. The lack of a 3'-OH group in the incorporated nucleoside analog prevents the formation of the 5' to 3' phosphodiester linkage essential for DNA chain elongation, and therefore, the viral DNA growth is terminated.	• Hepatitis B • Human immunodeficiency type 1	• Bioavailability: 86% • Half-life: 5-7 h

continued

TABLE 9-3	Antiviral Drugs—cont'd				

Antiviral Drugs	Molecule	Mechanism of Action	Treatment	Properties
Amantadine	NH$_2$	Amantadine targets the influenza A M2 ion channel protein. The M2 protein's function is to allow the intracellular virus to replicate (M2 also functions as a proton channel for hydrogen ions to cross into the vesicle), and exocytose newly formed viral proteins to the extracellular space (viral shedding). By blocking the M2 channel, the virus is unable to replicate because of impaired replication, protein synthesis, and exocytosis.	• Influenza A	• Bioavailability: 86-90% • Half-life: 10-31 h
Rimantadine	H$_2$N	Rimantadine inhibits influenza activity by binding to amino acids in the M2 transmembrane channel and blocking proton transport across the M2 channel. Rimantadine is thought to inhibit influenza's viral replication, possibly by preventing the uncoating of the virus's protective shells, which are the envelope and capsid.	• Influenza A	• Bioavailability: >90% • Half-life: 25-35 h
Interferon alfa		Induction of cellular enzymes that interfere with viral protein synthesis.	• Hepatitis B • Hepatitis C • Human herpesvirus 8 • Papillomavirus	• Poor oral bioavailability • Half-life: 2-3 h

(FTC) or lamivudine (3TC)—with a fully active drug that has a high resistance barrier, such as dolutegravir (DTG), boosted darunavir (BIII), or bictegravir (CIII).[31] Highly active antiretroviral therapy (HAART) requires three or more drugs targeting inhibiting viral replication, and although the management of HIV is outside the scope of this discussion, there can be overlap between many of the antiviral drugs with use for other viruses. Antiretroviral drugs include nucleoside reverse transcriptase inhibitors, nucleotide reverse transcriptase inhibitors, nonnucleoside reverse transcriptase inhibitors, protease inhibitors, and fusion inhibitors. General antivirals include nucleoside/nucleotide analogs, pyrimidines, antisense drugs, and interferon-α.

Interferons

Interferons (IFNs) are a group of signaling proteins that are produced by host cells in response to invasion by pathogens. These glycoproteins are made commercially in bacteria by recombinant DNA techniques. They have antiviral activity because of the induction of cellular enzymes that interfere with the synthesis of viral proteins.[30] The three major classes of interferons are α, β, and γ. IFN-α is given parenterally and is used to treat hepatitis B, hepatitis C, HPV, and HHV-8 (Kaposi's sarcoma). Common side effects include flulike symptoms, neuropsychiatric disorders, neurologic disturbances, and myelosuppression.

Pyrophosphate Analog

Foscarnet is a pyrophosphate analog that selectively inhibits the pyrophosphate binding site on virus-specific DNA polymerases. It is used for the treatment of acyclovir-resistant mucocutaneous herpes simplex and varicella-zoster virus infections in immunocompromised patients. It is also approved for the use of cytomegalovirus retinitis in patients with acquired immunodeficiency syndrome (AIDS).[32] Foscarnet is not orally bioavailable and can only be given intravenously. Common side effects include nephrotoxicity, hypocalcemia, myelosuppression, and nausea.

Nucleoside Analogs

Lamivudine is a nucleoside analog of cytosine. It inhibits hepatitis B DNA polymerase and HIV reverse transcriptase. It is approved for use in combination with other antiretroviral drugs for the treatment of HIV-1 infection or as monotherapy to treat chronic hepatitis B infection.[30] It was the first drug to be used as an alternative to IFN-α for the treatment of chronic hepatitis B.[33] Lamivudine has high oral bioavailability and a long half-life, making once-daily dosing convenient for patients. Ribavirin is a guanosine analog that inhibits the activity of the enzyme-dependent RNA polymerase. It is used in the treatment of chronic hepatitis C infection and for respiratory syncytial virus (RSV) infection.

Acyclovir, valacyclovir, ganciclovir, penciclovir, and famciclovir are acyclic analogs of guanine deoxyribose; valacyclovir and famciclovir are prodrugs that are biotransformed to penciclovir and acyclovir, respectively.[34] These antivirals inhibit viral DNA replication and are therefore effective agents in treating HHV. There are eight HHVs that cause a variety of clinical conditions (Table 9-4).

TABLE 9-4   Features of Herpesvirus Infections of Humans

Virus	Seroprevalence in the United States		Typical Primary Infections	Infection in the Compromised Host	Association With Human Cancers	Common Treatments
	Healthy Children	Healthy Adults				
Neurotropic						
HSV-1	20-40%	50-70%	Gingivostomatitis, keratoconjunctivitis, cutaneous herpes, genital herpes, encephalitis	Gingivostomatitis, keratoconjunctivitis, cutaneous herpes, esophagitis, pneumonitis, hepatitis	None	PO ACV, FAM, VAL, IV ACV, PCV
HSV-2	0-5%	20-50%	Genital herpes, cutaneous herpes, gingivostomatitis, meningoencephalitis, neonatal herpes	Genital herpes, cutaneous herpes, disseminated infection	?	PO VAL, FAM, ACV or IV ACV
VZV	50-75%	85-95%	Varicella	Disseminated infection	None	None, PO ACV, or IV ACV
Lymphotropic						
HCMV	10-30%	40-70%	Mononucleosis, hepatitis, congenital cytomegalic inclusion disease	Hepatitis, retinitis, pneumonitis, encephalitis, colitis, polyradiculopathy	None	None, GCV, FOS
EBV	10-30%	80-95%	Mononucleosis, hepatitis, encephalitis	Polyclonal and monoclonal lymphoproliferative syndromes, oral hairy leukoplakia	African-type Burkitt's, lymphoma, CNS lymphoma, and other lymphomas; nasopharyngeal carcinoma, leiomyosarcoma	None, steroids in selected cases
HHV-6	80-100%	60-100%	Roseola infantum, fever and otitis media, encephalitis	Pneumonitis? Encephalitis?	Rare B-cell lymphomas?	None
HHV-7	40-80%	60-100%	Roseola infantum?	None	None	
HHV-8	<3%?	<3%?	?	Kaposi's sarcoma?	Kaposi's sarcoma, multicentric Castleman's disease, primary effusion lymphoma	Radiation, cytotoxic drugs, IFN-α, ?GCV

ACV, Acyclovir; *EBV,* Epstein-Barr virus; *FAM,* famciclovir; *FOS,* foscarnet; *GCV,* ganciclovir; *HCMV,* human cytomegalovirus; *HHV,* human herpesvirus; *HSV,* herpes simplex virus; *IFN-α,* interferon-α; *IV,* intravenous; *PCV,* penciclovir; *PO,* oral; *VAL,* valacyclovir; *VZV,* varicella zoster virus.
From Coen DM, Schaffer PA. Antiherpesvirus drugs: a promising spectrum of new drugs and drug targets. *Nat Rev Drug Disc.* 2003;2:279.

Because these drugs are highly selective for viral DNA, they do not harm human cells. Their low protein binding improves distribution to the CSF, saliva, and other fluid compartments. Oral absorption is low, and therefore the intravenous form of these drugs is necessary for serious infections. The toxicity of these agents is low, although reversible encephalopathy or nephropathy occurs rarely.[34] Viruses in their latent stage are not affected; therefore, these antiviral agents do not eradicate viruses.

Herpes Simplex Virus

Oral and facial surgeons often treat patients with recurrent herpes simplex virus (HSV-1) infections that affect the oral and perioral tissues. These infections sometimes are severe, or patients are bothered by frequent recurrences or a fear of spreading the virus to others.[33] In these circumstances, some clinicians prescribe antiviral agents to speed the resolution of lesions or prevent outbreaks of herpetic lesions.[25,35-37]

Primary or recurrent orolabial herpes is managed with oral acyclovir (200 to 400 mg 5 times a day) or valacyclovir (1000 mg 3 times a day). To be effective, these drugs must be used within the first 3 days of initial symptoms. Topical acyclovir decreases viral shedding but does not significantly hasten the resolution of herpetic lesions. Prophylactic use of acyclovir and valacyclovir frequently prevents outbreaks but is not curative. Resistance to acyclovir does occur, and a dose of 400 mg twice a day reduces recurrences by approximately 50%. Suppression of herpes during periods of therapeutic immunosuppression is achieved using intravenous acyclovir (250 mg/m^2 over 8 hours).[38] Table 9-5 highlights the major antiviral agents used in the management of head and neck infections.

TABLE 9-5	Antiviral Drugs
Generic (Trade Name)	**Suggested Dosage (days)***
Systemic	
Acyclovir (Zovirax)	400 mg 3 × daily (7)
Famciclovir (Famvir)	125 mg 1 × daily (5)
Valacyclovir (Valtrex)	500 mg 2 × daily (5)
Topical	
Acyclovir (Zovirax)	5% ointment
Penciclovir (Denavir)	1% cream
Docosanol (Abreva)	10% cream (over-the-counter)

Apply topical medications to oral lesions at least four times daily.
*Dosage levels are adjusted according to clinical severity and response. For severe infection: acyclovir 5-10 mg/kg IV q8h for 7-10 days, famciclovir 500 mg tid, or valacyclovir 1000-2000 mg bid. For acyclovir-resistant cases: foscarnet (Foscavir) 40-60 mg/kg IV q8h for 7-10 days, or cidofovir (Vistide) 5 mg/kg.
From Silverman S, Miller CS. Diagnosis and treatment of viral infections. *Oral Maxillofac Surg Clin North Am.* 2003;15:79-89.

COVID-19 and Associated Conditions

Coronaviruses are enveloped, nonsegmented, positive sense, RNA viruses that usually cause a mild cold or flulike symptoms.[39-41] Three β-coronaviruses have been attributed to severe acute respiratory syndromes in 2002, 2012, and in 2019. Since December 2019, the novel strain severe acute respiratory syndrome coronavirus 2 (SARS-CoV-2), the virus responsible for COVID-19, has caused a global pandemic. Although this virus is primarily a respiratory disease and outside the scope of this review, it does have some oral manifestations in a specific pediatric population. An association has been identified between COVID-19 and multisystem inflammatory syndrome in children (MIS-C).[42-46]

MIS-C is defined by a disease in patients under the age of 21 with fevers, elevated inflammatory markers, and clinical evidence of severe illness of two or more organ systems. Although not all patients with MIS-C are expected to have the same signs and symptoms, clinical features may include fatigue, rash, oropharyngeal erythema, cardiac abnormalities, and dilation of conjunctival blood vessels.[47] MIS-C shares many similarities with Kawasaki's disease (KD), and specifically oral mucosal changes. KD is well known to be associated with a strawberry tongue.[48] Strawberry tongue describes a hyperplastic appearance of the fungiform papilla set against either a white (white strawberry tongue) or erythematous (red strawberry tongue) background. Many of MIS-C patients have oral mucosal changes, including swelling, redness, or cracking of the labial mucosa, while only a small population have documented strawberry tongue.[49] Diagnosis of KD requires the presence of fever lasting for more than 5 days with at least four of the following five physical examination findings: conjunctival injection, oral mucous membrane changes (including erythema of the lip vermilion and labial mucosa, erythema of the oral and oropharyngeal mucosa, and strawberry tongue), peripheral extremity changes (erythema, edema), polymorphous rash, or cervical lymphadenopathy.[50] Although treatment for KD and MIS-C are supportive and medications to suppress inflammation, including immunoglobulins and aspirin, treatment of the offending agent is also important.

COVID-19 treatment has progressed rapidly over the course of the pandemic. In addition to rapid testing, an mRNA vaccine has proven invaluable in controlling the spread. Some antivirals have been approved by the Centers for Disease Control and Prevention and U.S. Food and Drug Administration, such as nirmatrelvir with ritonavir, remdesivir and molnupiravir. Nirmatrelvir with ritonavir is a drug that received emergency authorization for the treatment of adults and children 12 years and older weighing at least 40 kg with current mild to moderate COVID-19 with high risk of progression.[51] It is prescribed as 450 mg of nirmatrelvir and 100 mg of ritonavir twice a day for 5 days or a lower dose for patients with kidney disease. Nirmatrelvir is a medication that is a 3C-protease inhibitor. Ritonavir is a protease inhibitor and has been used in combination with other medications to treat viral infections such as hepatitis

C and HIV/AIDS. Remdesivir is a nucleotide prodrug of an adenosine analog. This binds to the viral RNA- dependent RNA polymerase to inhibit viral replication. General dosing is 200 mg on day one followed by 100 mg daily for 4 additional days.[52] Molnupiravir is a prodrug of a synthetic nucleoside derivative and introduces copying errors during viral replication; it is 800 mg dosed twice a day for 5 days.[53] COVID-19 has wreaked havoc across the globe, and many of these medications have been developed and deployed quickly. It is likely that as humanity begins to contain this virus, the treatment strategies may change and become more targeted to the virus' replication.

Monkeypox

Monkeypox is a zoonotic infection caused by the Monkeypox virus. It is a double-stranded DNA virus belonging to the Orthopoxvirus genus and the poxvirus family.[54] This virus was contained to certain regions in Africa, with transient outbreaks outside of the region from international travel or exotic pets. An outbreak occurred in May of 2022 in the United States and other international areas. More than 85,000 cases were reported in 100 countries, with 30,000 in the United States mainly targeting the homosexual or bisexual patient population.[55]

Patients with Monkeypox infection will often report fever, fatigue, and influenza-like symptoms such as headaches, muscle aches, and swollen, painful lymph nodes. Most notably, patients will develop a pustular rash involving the skin. Although not every patient has oral mucosal involvement, it has been documented to predate skin findings. The lesions are typically on the midline of the anterior aspect of the tongue.[56] Monkeypox infection can spread from person to person by close contact with an infected individual. Transmission may occur via direct contact with the rash, respiratory secretions, or fomites that have previously encountered an infected individual. Vertical transmission from infected mother to fetus through the placenta also has been documented. The virus is generally self-limiting. Treating the underlying condition is treatment for the oral manifestation, and this can include antivirals such as tecovirimat, brincidofovir, cidofovir, and vaccinia immune globulin intravenous.[57]

REFERENCES

1. Lewis RE. Current concepts in antifungal pharmacology. *Mayo Clin Proc.* 2011;86(8):805-817.
2. Sheehan DJ, Hitchcock CA, Sibley CM. Current and emerging azole antifungal agents. *Clin Microbiol Rev.* 1999;12(1):40-79.
3. Kauffman CA, Carver PL. Antifungal agents in the 1990s. Current status and future developments. *Drugs.* 1997;53(4):539-549. doi:10.2165/00003495-199753040-00001.
4. Van Tyle JH. Ketoconazole: Mechanism of action, spectrum of activity, pharmacokinetics, drug interactions, adverse reactions and therapeutic use. *Pharmacotherapy.* 1984;4(6):343-373.
5. Khosla S, Wolfson JS, Demerjian Z, Godine JE. Adrenal crisis in the setting of high-dose ketoconazole therapy. *Arch Intern Med.* 1989;149(4):802-804.
6. Brammer KW, Farrow PR, Faulkner JK. Pharmacokinetics and tissue penetration of fluconazole in humans. *Rev Infect Dis.* 1990;12(suppl 3):S318-S326.
7. Martin MV. The use of fluconazole and itraconazole in the treatment of Candida albicans infections: a review. *J Antimicrob Chemother.* 1999;44(4):429-437.
8. Bodey GP. Azole antifungal agents. *Clin Infect Dis.* 1992;14(suppl 1):S161-S169.
9. Wilks D, Farrington M, Rubenstein D. Fungi. In: *The Infectious Diseases Manual.* 2nd ed. Malden, MA: Blackwell Science; 2008.
10. Grant SM, Clissold SP. Itraconazole: a review of its pharmacodynamic and pharmacokinetic properties, and therapeutic use in superficial and systemic mycoses. *Drugs.* 1989;37(3):310-344.
11. De Beule K, Van Gestel J. Pharmacology of itraconazole. *Drugs.* 2001;61(suppl 1):27-37.
12. Slain D, Rogers PD, Cleary JD, Chapman SW. Intravenous itraconazole. *Ann Pharmacother.* 2001;35(6):720-729.
13. Wingard JR, Carter SL, Walsh TJ, et al. Randomized, double-blind trial of fluconazole versus voriconazole for prevention of invasive fungal infection after allogeneic hematopoietic cell transplantation. *Blood.* 2010;116(24):5111-5118.
14. Cornely OA, Maertens J, Winston DJ, et al. Posaconazole vs. fluconazole or itraconazole prophylaxis in patients with neutropenia. *N Engl J Med.* 2007;356(4):348-359.
15. Girmenia C. New generation azole antifungals in clinical investigation. *Expert Opin Investig Drugs.* 2009;18(9):1279-1295.
16. Brajtburg J, Powderly WG, Kobayashi GS, Medoff G. Amphotericin B: current understanding of mechanisms of action. *Antimicrob Agents Chemother.* 1990;34(2):183-188.
17. Cleary JD, Rogers PD, Chapman SW. Variability in polyene content and cellular toxicity among deoxycholate amphotericin B formulations. *Pharmacotherapy.* 2003;23(5):572-578.
18. Lortholary O, Denning DW, Dupont B. Endemic mycoses: a treatment update. *J Antimicrob Chemother.* 1999;43(3):321-331.
19. Skiada A, Lass-Floerl C, Klimko N, Ibrahim A, Roilides E, Petrikkos G. Challenges in the diagnosis and treatment of mucormycosis. *Med Mycol.* 2018;56(suppl 1):93-101.
20. Gallis HA, Drew RH, Pickard WW. Amphotericin B: 30 years of clinical experience. *Rev Infect Dis.* 1990;12(2):308-329.
21. Medoff G, Kobayashi GS. Strategies in the treatment of systemic fungal infections. *N Engl J Med.* 1980;302(3):145-155.
22. Terrell CL, Hughes CE. Antifungal agents used for deep-seated mycotic infections. *Mayo Clin Proc.* 1992;67(1):69-91.
23. Rogers PD, Jenkins JK, Chapman SW, Ndebele K, Chapman BA, Cleary JD. Amphotericin B activation of human genes encoding for cytokines. *J Infect Dis.* 1998;178(6):1726-1733.
24. Bishara J, Weinberger M, Lin AY, Pitlik S. Amphotericin B—not so terrible. *Ann Pharmacother.* 2001;35(3):308-310.
25. Fleischman J. Topical and systemic antifungal and antiviral agents. In: Newman MG, van Winkelhoff AJ, eds. *Antibiotic and Antimicrobial Use in Dental Practice.* 2nd ed. Chicago: Quintessence; 2001.
26. Lyu X, Zhao C, Yan ZM, Hua H. Efficacy of nystatin for the treatment of oral candidiasis: a systematic review and meta-analysis. *Drug Des Devel Ther.* 2016;10:1161-1171.
27. Eschenauer G, Depestel DD, Carver PL. Comparison of echinocandin antifungals. *Ther Clin Risk Manag.* 2007;3(1):71-97.
28. Denning DW. Echinocandin antifungal drugs. *Lancet.* 2003;362(9390):1142-1151.

29. Vermes A, Guchelaar HJ, Dankert J. Flucytosine: a review of its pharmacology, clinical indications, pharmacokinetics, toxicity and drug interactions. *J Antimicrob Chemother*. 2000;46(2):171-179.

30. Balfour HH Jr. Antiviral drugs. *N Engl J Med*. 1999;340(16): 1255-1268.

31. Saag MS, Gandhi RT, Hoy JF, et al. Antiretroviral drugs for treatment and prevention of HIV infection in adults: 2020 recommendations of the International Antiviral Society–USA Panel. *JAMA*. 2020;324(16):1651-1669.

32. Chrisp P, Clissold SP. Foscarnet: a review of its antiviral activity, pharmacokinetic properties and therapeutic use in immunocompromised patients with cytomegalovirus retinitis. *Drugs*. 1991;41(1):104-129.

33. Dienstag JL, Schiff ER, Wright TL, et al. Lamivudine as initial treatment for chronic hepatitis B in the United States. *N Engl J Med*. 1999;341(17):1256-1263.

34. Acosta EP, Fletcher CV. Valacyclovir. *Ann Pharmacother*. 1997;31(2):185-191.

35. Esmann J. The many challenges of facial herpes simplex virus infection. *J Antimicrob Chemother*. 2001;47(suppl T1):17-27.

36. Rooney JF, Straus SE, Mannix ML, et al. Oral acyclovir to suppress frequently recurrent herpes labialis: a double-blind, placebo-controlled trial. *Ann Intern Med*. 1993;118(4):268-272.

37. Whitley RJ, Gnann JW Jr. Acyclovir: a decade later. *N Engl J Med*. 1992;327(11):782-789.

38. Michelle R. Salvaggio, John W. Gnann. drugs for herpesvirus infecitons. In: Cohen, JF, Poderly, W, Opal, S eds. *Infectious Disease*. 4th ed. St. Louis: Mosby; 2017:1309-1317.e1.

39. Weiss SR, Navas-Martin S. Coronavirus pathogenesis and the emerging pathogen severe acute respiratory syndrome coronavirus. *Microbiol Mol Biol Rev*. 2005;69(4):635-664.

40. Woo PCY, Lau SKP, Huang Y, Yuen KY. Coronavirus diversity, phylogeny and interspecies jumping. *Exp Biol Med*. 2009; 234(10):1117-1127.

41. Sutton D, Fuchs K, D'Alton M, Goffman D. Universal screening for SARS-CoV-2 in women admitted for delivery. *N Engl J Med*. 2020;382(22):2163-2164.

42. Riphagen S, Gomez X, Gonzalez-Martinez C, Wilkinson N, Theocharis P. Hyperinflammatory shock in children during COVID-19 pandemic. *Lancet*. 2020;395(10237):1607-1608.

43. Feldstein LR, Rose EB, Horwitz SM, et al. Multisystem inflammatory syndrome in U.S. children and adolescents. *N Engl J Med*. 2020;383(4):334-346.

44. Belhadjer Z, Méot M, Bajolle F, et al. Acute heart failure in multisystem inflammatory syndrome in children (MIS-C) in the context of global SARS-CoV-2 pandemic. *Circulation*. 2020; 142(5):429-436.

45. Chiotos K, Bassiri H, Behrens EM, et al. Multisystem inflammatory syndrome in children during the COVID-19 pandemic: a case series. *J Pediatric Infect Dis Soc*. 2020;13(9):393-398.

46. Toubiana J, Poirault C, Corsia A, et al. Kawasaki-like multisystem inflammatory syndrome in children during the covid-19 pandemic in Paris, France: prospective observational study. *BMJ*. 2020;369:m2094.

47. Rowley AH. Understanding SARS-CoV-2-related multisystem inflammatory syndrome in children. *Nat Rev Immunol*. 2020; 20(8):453-454.

48. Chang LY, Lu CY, Shao PL, et al. Viral infections associated with Kawasaki disease. *J Formos Med Assoc*. 2014;113(3): 148-154.

49. Halepas S, Lee KC, Myers A, Yoon RK, Chung W, Peters SM. Oral manifestations of COVID-2019-related multisystem inflammatory syndrome in children: a review of 47 pediatric patients. *J Am Dent Assoc*. 2021;152(3):202-208.

50. Kawasaki T. [Acute febrile mucocutaneous syndrome with lymphoid involvement with specific desquamation of the fingers and toes in children]. *Arerugi*. 1967;16(3):178-222.

51. Lam C, Patel P. Nirmatrelvir/ritonavir. In: *StatPearls*. Treasure Island, FL: StatPearls Publishing; 2022.

52. Goldman JD, Lye DCB, Hui DS, et al. Remdesivir for 5 or 10 days in patients with severe Covid-19. *N Engl J Med*. 2020;383(19):1827-1837.

53. Pourkarim F, Pourtaghi-Anvarian S, Rezaee H. Molnupiravir: a new candidate for COVID-19 treatment. *Pharmacol Res Perspect*. 2022;10(1):e00909.

54. Brown K, Leggat PA. Human Monkeypox: current state of knowledge and implications for the future. *Trop Med Infect Dis*. 2016;1(1):8.

55. Kumar S, Subramaniam G, Karuppanan K. Human monkeypox outbreak in 2022. *J Med Virol*. 2023;95(1):e27894.

56. Peters SM, Hill NB, Halepas S. Oral manifestations of Monkeypox: a report of 2 cases. *J Oral Maxillofac Surg*. 2022;80(11): 1836-1840.

57. Rizk JG, Lippi G, Henry BM, Forthal DN, Rizk Y. Prevention and treatment of Monkeypox. *Drugs*. 2022;82(9):957-963.

PART 2

Infections of the Head and Neck

10

Infections of the Facial Skin and Scalp

ALI BANKI, SARAH M. STANO, FRANK M. CASTIGLIONE JR, AND CINDY HOFFMAN

The primary and most important function of the epidermal tissues is to act as a barrier from potential infectious organisms. When this barrier is broken, the underlying soft tissue can become infected, resulting in significant morbidity and sometimes mortality. Although facial soft tissues are resilient and resist infection, several diseases can occur when the infectious organisms colonize and spread.

Anatomy of Facial Skin, Fascia, and Muscle

The skin is the largest organ in the body; it has two distinct layers with associated appendages. When these layers are interrupted, infections can develop. In addition to warding off infection, the skin is important in temperature and fluid regulation and sensorineural function.

The outer layer of the skin, the epidermis, rests on a basement membrane and contains germinal cells in the basal layer of the skin. These cells give rise to keratinocytes, the primary cell type that makes up the epidermis, and are important in producing keratin with an overlying stratum corneum. Other cells that can be found within the epidermis include melanocytes, which give rise to melanin, Langerhans cells, which are antigen-presenting cells and Merkel cells, which are mechanoreceptors. Langerhans cells serve as a first line of defense against foreign pathogens and infections. It should be noted that there are no blood vessels, nerves, or lymphatics in the epidermis.

The inner mesoderm layer of the skin, the dermis, lies just below the basement membrane of the epidermis. It is divided into papillary, mid, and reticular regions, which contain collagen and elastin fibers. There are many appendages within the dermis, including hair follicles, eccrine and apocrine sweat glands, sebaceous glands, and nerve endings.

The arterial supply to the skin arises from a flat plexus of vessels located in the superficial fascia near the junction with the dermis. Blood flow is controlled by smooth muscle function around the endothelium of the blood vessels, and the profusion of blood helps regulate skin temperature. Venules and lymphatics are also present.

The fascia, which is fibrous connective tissue, is in superficial, deep, and subserous locations in many areas of the body. However, there is no deep fascia in the maxillofacial region. The facial muscles lay deep to the superficial fascia and are superficial to the underlying periosteum.

Pathophysiology of Soft Tissue Infections

The most important factor in preventing skin infections is the overall integrity of the skin and adjacent soft tissues. When there is an interruption in skin integrity, resident and transient bacteria can invade tissues. There are both endogenous and exogenous factors that affect the skin integrity. Exogenous factors include topical medications, irritant and allergen exposures, climate control, and improper skin care. Endogenous factors include age, genetics, and skin disorders, such as atopic dermatitis, diabetes, psoriasis, and ichthyosis.[1] Incisions, wounds, or disease can also disrupt the epithelium, allowing bacteria to invade the tissue. However, the skin has numerous mechanisms to stop the invasion of bacteria, including an acidic barrier, humoral immunity, and local adaptive immunity.

The development of skin infections depends on the nature of the bacteria and the environment that allows bacteria to grow. Studies have shown that 2×10^9 bacteria/mL are needed to produce an infection. When there are foreign materials on the skin, such as dirt or suture material, the inoculum size to cause an infection is lowered.

The acidic pH of the outer stratum corneum is termed the *acid mantle;* it is important for both the formation of the skin permeability barrier and antimicrobial defense. The sebum, sweat secretion, and stratum corneum maintain the normal skin pH at 4.1 to 5.9, with the average being 4.7.[2,3] The formation of the barrier involves numerous pH-dependent enzymes, including phospholipases, sphingomyelinases and β-glucocerebrosidase. These enzymes optimally function in an acidic pH to synthesize ceramides and create the lamellar arrangement of the skin barrier lipids.[4] Additionally, the acidic pH inhibits the colonization of pathogens while promoting the growth of normal skin flora.[3]

Epidermal antimicrobial peptides (AMPs) and Langerhans cells are the most prominent factors in the defense against bacteria. These AMPs are produced by keratinocytes, granulocytes, sebocytes, or sweat glands. There are two major classes of dermal peptides that express antibacterial activity—cathelicidins and B-defensins. There is an inverse relationship between the severity of disease and the level of AMP production.[5]

Local immunity depends primarily on the vascularity of the tissue. Because of the rich blood supply of the head and neck, skin infections are less common than in more dependent areas, such as the back and lower extremities. Other considerations regarding the reduced infection rate of the head and neck relate to the pathogenicity of the local flora, the likelihood of an area of skin to be injured, and the concentration of local bacteria.

Manifestations of Soft Tissue Infections

Several terms are used to describe soft tissue lesions. Primary skin lesions, which develop as a direct result of the disease, and secondary skin lesions, which develop from the primary lesion or as a consequence of the patient's actions. Primary lesions include macules, papules, plaques, vesicles/bullae, pustules, and nodules. Secondary lesions include scale, crust, and ulcers.

A *macule* is a flat, circumscribed area of skin that is less than 1 cm in size. In infectious processes, macules usually are red because of vasodilation or blue-black because of tissue infarction. A *papule* is a raised, solid lesion less than 1 cm in diameter. A *plaque* is a raised, solid lesion that is greater than 1 cm in diameter. Several infections manifest as maculopapular eruptions—for example, scarlet fever. Vesicles (<0.5 cm) and bullae (>0.5 cm) are elevated, fluid-filled lesions usually containing serum. These may be intraepidermal or subepidermal. Vesicles and bullae can be seen in herpes and bullous impetigo. A *pustule* is a vesicle containing purulent material, which can be seen in folliculitis and acne.

A *crust* is produced by the rupture of a vesicle or pustule. An *ulcer* is an area in which a break in the continuity of the epithelium exists because of tissue destruction. Scales develop as desquamation of epidermal keratin cells accumulate and may sometimes be shed or scraped off in thin sheets, as seen in Kawasaki's disease and scarlet fever.

Subcutaneous manifestations of infection are less specific than cutaneous signs. *Cellulitis* represents an area of redness and tenderness of the dermal and subcutaneous tissues, often secondary to streptococcal or staphylococcal infection. A *nodule* is a solid lesion caused by swelling and accumulation of cells within the dermal and subcutaneous tissue. Such lesions are often seen in granulomatous infections and acne. An *abscess* is a localized accumulation of purulent material within the epidermis and subcutaneous tissue. *Gangrene* refers to death of a body tissue after compromised blood flow or bacterial infection. The process can involve the subcutaneous tissue, fascia, and muscle. The diminished blood flow in areas of gangrene can cause a bluish-black discoloration. *Crepitus* can occur when there is gas accumulation within the tissues, a pathognomonic sign for necrotizing fasciitis. *Lymphadenitis* develops when there is swelling and tenderness in the tissues around the lymph nodes within regional zones of drainage of a primary infection.

Identification of the nature of the infectious agent that causes these lesions can be difficult with skin examination alone. Culture and sensitivity, as well as a biopsy, may be necessary to establish the nature of the infecting organism.

Acne

Acne vulgaris is a disorder of the pilosebaceous glands of the head, neck, and trunk. It is characterized by obstruction of the hormonally stimulated sebaceous gland ducts with sebum and keratin. As the surface is occluded with oil, *Cutibacterium acnes* proliferates. This bacterium produces lipase that hydrolyzes the sebum to form a free fatty acid within the follicle. This process creates an inflammatory response characterized by papules and cysts (Figures 10-1 and 10-2).[6,7]

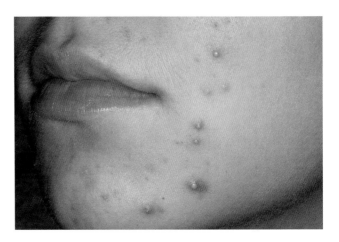

• **Figure 10-1** Mild Acne with Papules, Pustules, and Comedones. (From Habif TP. *Clinical Dermatology: A Color Guide to Diagnosis and Therapy.* 5th ed. St. Louis: Elsevier; 2010.)

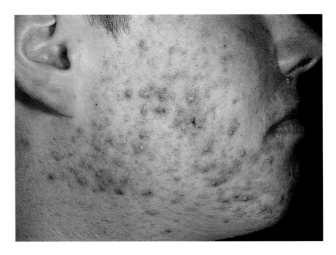

• **Figure 10-2** Severe Acne with Papules, Nodules, and Cysts Covers the Entire Face. Scarring is extensive. (From Habif TP. *Clinical Dermatology: A Color Guide to Diagnosis and Therapy.* 5th ed. St. Louis: Elsevier; 2010.)

Clinical Presentation and Diagnosis

Acne is often a disorder of adolescents and young adults, although it can persist well into adulthood. It is often due to overstimulation of the oil glands and may be associated with hormonal abnormalities in women (polycystic ovarian syndrome)[8] and emotional stress.[9] Other factors that can trigger acne include medications such as glucocorticoids, lithium, phenytoin, isoniazid, and halogens such as bromides and iodides. In addition, photodamage and occupational exposures (to machine and cutting oils) can trigger acne. Acne fulminans is a severe nodulocystic form of acne with systemic manifestation that requires treatment with oral steroids followed by isotretinoin. Acne conglobata is similar to acne fulminans but lacks the systemic manifestations.

There are several acne-associated syndromes, including SAPHO syndrome, PAPA, and PASH. SAPHO syndrome (i.e., chronic recurrent multifocal osteomyelitis) is characterized by *s*ynovitis, *a*cne, *p*ustulosis, *h*yperostosis, and *o*steitis. It is more common in children and young adults. PAPA is caused by an autosomal dominant mutation in CD2-binding protein, characterized by the triad of *p*yogenic *a*rthritis, *p*yoderma gangrenosum, and *a*cne conglobate. PASH (*p*yoderma gangrenosum, *a*cne, *s*uppurative *h*idradenitis) and PAPASH (*p*yogenic *a*rthritis, *p*yoderma gangrenosum, *a*cne and *s*uppurative *h*idradenitis) share a mechanism similar to that of PAPA. In all three there is an overactive innate immune system, causing an increase in interleukin-1 (IL-1) and a neutrophil-rich cutaneous inflammation.

The differential diagnosis of acne vulgaris includes perioral dermatitis, folliculitis, rosacea, and eosinophilic pustular folliculitis.

Treatment

Treatment has improved over the past few decades. The mainstay of treatment involves the use of topical retinoids such as tretinoin, adapalene, trifarotene, and tazarotene. Retinoids dissolve the comedones and reduce inflammation.[10] Benzoyl peroxides are used, alone or in combination with topical antibiotics (e.g., clindamycin, erythromycin), to reduce the inflammation around the lesions; they also inhibit the emergence of bacterial resistance. Topical clascoterone, an antiandrogen, can be helpful in hormonally driven acne. Topical dapsone and azelaic acid also have been used with improvement.

Systemic tetracyclines (including doxycycline) have been the mainstay of oral medication over the years, although erythromycin and trimethoprim-sulfamethoxazole (TMP-SMX) have also been used. Tetracycline is contraindicated in children 8 years of age and younger, because it can cause permanent yellow-gray horizontal staining of their teeth. Of note, there has been increasing resistance of *C. acnes* to antibiotics.[11] Resistance to retinoids and benzoyl peroxides have not been noted, although these agents might not be effective topically in cystic acne. Systemic spironolactone, although not approved by the U.S. Food and Drug Administration

(FDA), is useful in hormonally driven acne. It is generally thought to be safe; however, it may cause hyperkalemia (which may worsen when taking it with medications such as trimethoprim) and breast enlargement in men (for whom it is not helpful in acne). Despite the effect on potassium, routine blood monitoring is not currently recommended.[12]

Systemic isotretinoin can be used for chronic cystic acne that has not cleared with first- and second-line treatments. Its response is often remarkable; it works by decreasing sebum formation, reducing colonization of *C. acnes,* and reversing the retention of follicular keratin in the pilosebaceous unit. However, systemic isotretinoin has multiple side effects, including xerosis, photosensitivity, possible changes in night vision, birth defects (if used during pregnancy), psychiatric disturbances, alopecia, cheilitis, pseudotumor cerebri, hypertriglyceridemia, and liver enzyme abnormalities. The course of treatment is often 3 to 5 months, with an average cumulative dose of 120 to 150 mg/kg.

Finally, acne cysts may be injected with an intralesional steroid, incised and drained, or even excised. In addition, it is important to address infected cysts on the "danger triangle of the face." The danger triangle of the face consists of the area from the corners of the mouth to the bridge of the nose. If the skin barrier is disrupted, it can lead to an extremely rare but serious retrograde infection into the cavernous sinus and brain. A midline dermoid cyst with deep underlying sinus tract should be considered if the patient has a long-standing cyst on the glabella and nose since childhood.

Folliculitis

Folliculitis involves an infection characterized by papules, pustules, or deeper nodules centered around a hair follicle. It can be superficial or deep and can produce chronic inflammation, scarring, or alopecia.

Clinical Presentation

Follicular-centered papules and pustules, often with a rim of erythema, can be seen on the hair-bearing areas of the face, scalp, and neck. On occasion, the lesions coalesce and form abscesses, draining sinuses, or a larger group of infected hair follicles called *carbuncles.* On the face, the folliculitis can arise from disruption of the hair follicle by trauma, such as shaving. In the beard area, this is called *folliculitis barbae* or *sycosis barbae.* In addition, folliculitis can be aggravated in the face by epilating agents or depilatories. There also may be occupational factors, such as exposures to oils or chemicals such as halogens (e.g., chloracne; see Acne), which induce folliculitis on the face or scalp.

In the scalp, the folliculitis can extend to form a dissecting cellulitis: perifolliculitis capitis abscedens et suffodiens. This condition may be seen in association with acne vulgaris or a folliculitis tetrad syndrome of acne conglobata, hidradenitis suppurativa, dissecting cellulitis, and pilonidal cysts. In addition, there may be scarring alopecia and keloid formation. On the neck, the chronic folliculitis is often called *acne keloidalis* nuchae. The cause involves different bacteria, including *Staphylococcus aureus,* and colonization of the nares may be a factor in causing the infection. Folliculitis also can be caused by gram-negative bacteria such as *Klebsiella* and *Pseudomonas* species, which can be seen in "hot tub folliculitis." Mixed flora, including *C. acnes* (which is also causative in acne vulgaris), also may cause folliculitis. Yeast, such as *Malassezia* species and mites *(Demodex folliculorum),* can cause folliculitis.

In human immunodeficiency virus (HIV)-infected individuals, folliculitis can occur and is diagnostic of eosinophilic folliculitis. Clinically, there are groups of itchy urticarial papules and occasional pustules on the scalp, face, neck, and trunk. These papules are sometimes seen in the setting of peripheral eosinophilia. Histopathologically, there are collections of lymphocytes and eosinophils around the follicular infundibulum. In addition, there may be elevated immunoglobulin E (IgE) levels and peripheral eosinophilia.[13]

Diagnosis

The diagnosis can be confirmed by the clinical appearance of papules or pustules around hair follicles on the scalp or face. Bacterial culture can be useful in determining the causative agent and appropriate treatment of the eruption.

Treatment

Common treatment options include oral tetracycline, doxycycline, erythromycin, clindamycin, and topical agents such as benzyl peroxides and retinoic acid. Although some lesions may resolve spontaneously, warm compresses and topical antibiotics such as mupirocin, clindamycin, or erythromycin solution also may be helpful. Bacterial culture is also important to rule out methicillin-resistant *S. aureus* (MRSA). Of note, MRSA is becoming more common, especially in the nose. In cases in which a culture is positive for MRSA, applying mupirocin ointment to the nasal vestibule, chlorohexidine rinses on the body, and bleach baths can be helpful to eliminate the infection; however, it is important to avoid contact with the eyes and ears. Bleach baths can be taken 1 or 2 times per week with ½ cup of bleach in a ¼-filled tub for 10 minutes in a well-ventilated room.

Pseudomonas folliculitis, which is often caused by contaminated water from a hot tub or swimming pool exposure, is often self-limited and clears spontaneously. If severe, it can be treated with ciprofloxacin or quinolone antibiotics.[14]

Malassezia folliculitis can be treated with mild shampoo or an antidandruff shampoo containing antifungal agents such as ketoconazole or ciclopirox. In addition, isotretinoin can be helpful with chronic folliculitis, presumably by altering the follicular size of the pilosebaceous unit. This affects the microenvironment, making it less favorable for the overgrowth of *C. acnes.* It also reduces comedogenesis by reducing sebum production and has antiinflammatory properties. Individual lesions may respond to intervention with an intralesional steroid injection.

Demodex folliculitis can be treated with topical therapies, including metronidazole-based creams, ivermectin, sulfur-based creams, and benzoyl peroxide. Additionally, oral therapies can be helpful, including tetracyclines and oral metronidazole.

Finally, topical treatment with antibacterial cleansers, such as triclosan or chlorhexidine, may be useful in reducing folliculitis. For men, growing a beard is often helpful. Shaving techniques, such as shaving in one direction and in the direction of the hair follicle, using a protective shaving cream such as a gel-based soap, or using a hair clipper, can lessen the outbreaks of folliculitis barbae.

Anthrax

Anthrax is a rare illness caused by the gram-positive, aerobic bacteria *Bacillus anthracis.* The organism exists in soil and on animals, but it has received much attention as a potential bioterrorism agent. This was highlighted in 2001. This infection otherwise is rare, although it may be seen in individuals who handle animal hides.

Although anthrax is not a contagious disease, it is contracted as three major syndromes: cutaneous, inhalation, and alimentary tract anthrax. The usual infection is by contact with *B. anthracis* spores via open wounds, the mucosa of the gastrointestinal tract, or inhalation.[15,16]

Clinical Course

The cutaneous form of anthrax is the most common form of the disease. It manifests as small pruritic papules that develop at the site of cutaneous abrasions 1 to 13 days after contact with the spores. The papule then enlarges and forms a vesicle with edema before ulceration occurs from the release of toxins by the spores. The ulceration develops a black necrotic and depressed eschar. The spores often vegetate and multiply because the spore capsule has antiphagocytic properties.

Regional lymphadenopathy is present. There may be systemic symptoms with cutaneous lesions, including fever and headache. However, if the disease is treated early in its course with antibiotics, the symptoms often resolve. Without treatment, the mortality rate of cutaneous anthrax may be as high as 20%.

The gastrointestinal form of anthrax is much more serious; it can progress to life-threatening symptoms if not treated promptly. It can develop from eating raw or undercooked food from animals that are infected with *B. anthracis.* This disease can affect both the lower gastrointestinal tract and the pharynx. There may be nausea, vomiting, anorexia, and fever, with abdominal pain and bloody diarrhea. The fatality rate of alimentary tract anthrax ranges from 4 to 60%.[17,18] The oropharyngeal form of anthrax is characterized by oral lesions that are edematous initially and then progress to necrotic ulcers with a pseudomembrane covering. There may be cervical lymphadenopathy, pharyngitis, and fever.

The pulmonary form of anthrax develops when the *B. anthracis* spores are inhaled. The incubation period can vary from 1 to 43 days and can result in 90% mortality rate if left untreated. The spores can spread rapidly through the pulmonary tissue and destroy lung parenchyma.[19]

Diagnosis

Diagnosis of cutaneous or oropharyngeal lesions may be through Gram stain, culture, and polymerase chain reaction testing. Similar testing can be done on pleural effusion, stool, rectal, or ascites fluid. In addition, blood cultures and acute and convalescent serum samples may be diagnostic. More than 50% of patients with systemic anthrax may have meningitis; therefore, lumbar puncture is advised for all patients who have systemic anthrax, unless otherwise contraindicated.[20]

Treatment

Penicillin G has been the historic treatment of choice for infection with anthrax spores. Naturally occurring strains also may be sensitive to fluoroquinolones, chloramphenicol, tetracycline, erythromycin, and streptomycin. It is, however, not susceptible to cephalosporins or TMP-SMX. Bacterial resistance can emerge during treatment with β-lactam–resistant organisms.[21,22]

Anthrax antitoxin is available through the Centers for Disease Control and Prevention (CDC) and is advised for those who have systemic disease. In addition, raxibacumab (a monoclonal antibody) has shown to be effective for inhalation anthrax, and the CDC should be consulted regarding its use.[23] Intravenous fluids, ventilatory assistance, and supportive treatment are important for nondermatologic disease.

Cellulitis and Erysipelas

Cellulitis refers to an acute spreading infection involving the skin and subcutaneous tissues. The most common causative agents are group A streptococci and *S. aureus*. In addition, in the immunocompromised patient, there may be other infectious agents such as *Pseudomonas* species and other gram-negative bacteria.

Clinical Presentation

Cellulitis often manifests with redness, edema, and tenderness of the affected tissues. The clinical lesions are often warm and are associated with lymphangitis. Cellulitis can affect any part of the body; however, the most common location is unilaterally on the legs and feet. Cellulitis is often accompanied by systemic complaints such as fever, malaise, pain, tenderness, and lymphadenopathy. Microscopically, it involves the deeper dermis and subcutaneous fat.

Erysipelas is more superficial and generally more raised than cellulitis, with well-demarcated borders (Figure 10-3).

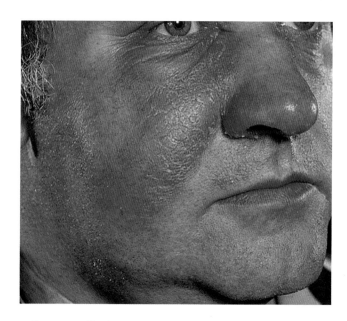

• **Figure 10-3** Erysipelas. Streptococcal cellulitis. The acute phase with intense erythema. (From Gawkrodger D, Ardern-Jones MR. *Dermatology: An Illustrated Colour Text.* 5th ed. Edinburgh: Churchill Livingstone; 2012.)

The most common locations for erysipelas are the legs and face. Microscopically, it involves the upper dermis and superficial lymphatics and is often due to *Streptococcus pyogenes*, which is a β-hemolytic group A *Streptococcus*. In addition, group B streptococcus may be causative.[24]

Erysipelas was initially described as having a butterfly-like distribution on the face, with the rash caused by production of exotoxin rather than the *Streptococcus* itself. The infection does not involve the deeper subcutaneous tissues, although there may be associated edema of the tissue.

Cellulitis, in contrast, has plaques that are not as well defined as in erysipelas and may have a deeper, more indurated component with associated lymphangitis. The patient may be toxic in either infection. Cellulitis in the scalp can produce nodules and draining abscesses and is termed *dissecting cellulitis*. Cellulitis may be recurrent in many cases. In a study of 209 cases of cellulitis, recurrences were observed in 17% of patients; among 143 patients with erysipelas, 29% had recurrent infection.

Wells' syndrome (eosinophilic cellulitis) manifests similarly to bacterial cellulitis and erysipelas, making it difficult to differentiate these diseases. In Wells' syndrome, recurrent indurated cellulitis-plaques are seen on the extremities and trunk. Malaise and eosinophilia are commonly associated findings. Interstitial eosinophils with flame figures will be seen on histologic examination.

Sweet's syndrome (acute febrile neutrophilic dermatosis) also can be difficult to differentiate from cellulitis. Sweet's syndrome is characterized by an abrupt onset of tender and/or burning "juicy" papules most commonly on the head, neck, and upper extremities. Systemic manifestations, such as fever, arthralgia, and leukocytosis are commonly seen. Although the pathogenesis has not been fully elucidated, there are several known triggers, including streptococcal and yersiniosis infections, cancers (e.g., acute myelogenous leukemia), inflammatory bowel disease (Crohn's disease and ulcerative colitis), and medications (minocycline, granulocyte colony-stimulating factor [G-CSF], granulocyte-macrophage CSF [GM-CSF], TMP-SMX, and oral contraceptive pills).

Diagnosis

The diagnosis is made by the appearance of erythematous, warm, advancing plaques, often with pain, fever, edema, or lymphangitis.

The lesions are not to be confused with what is termed *pseudocellulitis,* which may, for example, be due to viral infections such as herpes simplex or, more commonly, herpes zoster, arthropod reactions, erythema migrans, fixed drug eruptions, panniculitis, and angioedema. These entities can have prominent redness, heat, and edema, although the presence of a primary vesicle is more typical of a viral infection than of a bacterial cellulitis. Other diagnostic considerations include an acute contact dermatitis, which may be red and edematous. The presence of vesicles, with occasionally linear morphology and itching, rather than pain or fever, is often helpful to differentiate this.

It is even more important to differentiate an acute eczematous dermatitis that has become secondarily infected. In this situation, there may be associated fever and lymphadenopathy that would not otherwise be present with an allergic contact dermatitis. Additionally, unlike an acute eczematous dermatitis, cellulitis is rarely seen bilaterally. Culturing of the skin lesions themselves, or sometimes the nasopharynx, is helpful in identifying the causative agent. These results would help confirm the correct therapeutic options.

Treatment Options

The usual treatment of cellulitis includes antibiotics, both oral and intravenous. The majority of staphylococcal and streptococcal cellulitis cases are sensitive to many antibiotics, including cephalosporins, erythromycin, clindamycin, and amoxicillin-clavulanic acid. However, with the advent of MRSA, antibiotics such as oral doxycycline, TMP-SMX, or intravenous vancomycin may be necessary. In the setting of drainage or exudate, treatment for possible MRSA infections is appropriate.[25] In addition, there may be symptomatic relief from open wet dressings and topical therapy, such as mupirocin ointment.[26] In recurrent cellulitis or erysipelas, prophylactic continuous antibiotic therapy may be useful to prevent further outbreaks. Penicillin V (250 mg bid) can reduce the frequency of recurrent infections.[27,28,29]

Streptococcal Infections

Scarlet Fever

Scarlet fever, which is also known as *scarlatina,* can be due to either a primary acute systemic infection by strains

of *S. pyogenes* or a secondary response to localized streptococcal infections, such as a streptococcal pharyngitis or impetigo. The rash is generally caused by a delayed hypersensitivity reaction to the erythrogenic toxin usually produced by type A, B, or C streptococcal infection.[24,28,30]

Clinical Presentation

A rash appears 2 to 4 days after the symptoms of streptococcal infection and is characterized by a diffuse erythema that blanches with pressure and causes flushing of the facial region with circumoral pallor. There are multiple 1- to 2-mm papules that have small, punctate elevations diffusely over the skin surface, producing a sandpaper-like texture. The exanthem rapidly expands to cover the entire trunk and then undergoes desquamation after 4 to 5 days. The rash is often more intense in the body folds, the antecubital fossa and axillary folds, and may form pink or red hemorrhagic transverse lines known as the Pastia sign. The palms and soles are often affected by the rash. Additionally, there may be an enanthem with edema, redness, and petechiae on the soft palate. The tongue may have a white coating that then resolves, leading to a red "strawberry tongue" with swollen papillae (Figure 10-4). It then progresses over a few days to a beefy red "raspberry" tongue.

Diagnosis

The diagnosis of scarlet fever is based on the characteristic rash and enanthem after pharyngitis or a systemic flulike illness, a positive throat culture for streptococcus, or increasing antistreptomycin O antibodies.

The differential diagnosis of a strawberry tongue includes toxic shock syndrome, which is a life-threatening illness characterized by high fever and toxemia owing to *S. aureus* or the toxins of group A *Streptococcus.* This condition often

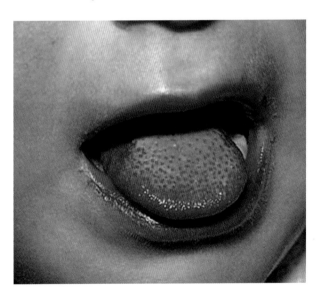

• **Figure 10-4** Portions of the White Coat Remain in the Center, but the Remainder of the Tongue is Red with Engorged Papillae ("Strawberry Tongue"). (From Zitelli BJ, McIntire SC, Nowalk AJ. *Zitelli and Davis' Atlas of Pediatric Physical Diagnosis.* 6th ed. Philadelphia: Saunders; 2012.)

has a diffuse macular erythroderma without the punctate papules of scarlet fever. In addition, a strawberry tongue may be seen in Kawasaki's disease, also known as *mucocutaneous lymph node syndrome*. The cause of this autoimmune condition is not known, but it may be infectious. It should be noted that although there may be an infectious cause, Kawasaki's disease is not thought to be contagious. In addition to a strawberry tongue, there may be a red rash on the trunk without the sandpaper papules, and there may be more prominent cracking of the lips and cervical adenopathy of at least 15 mm. In addition, there is often involvement of the palms and soles with swelling and redness.

Treatment

Scarlet fever may be treated with the appropriate antibiotics to control the streptococcal infection. It is important to recognize this condition, because untreated streptococcal pharyngitis can progress to acute rheumatic fever, shock or multiple organ failure, and poststreptococcal glomerulonephritis.[31] In addition, there may be suppurative tonsillopharyngeal cellulitis or abscess, sinusitis, otitis media, or necrotizing fasciitis.

Necrotizing Fasciitis

Necrotizing fasciitis is an aggressive necrosis of subcutaneous fat and fascia associated with high mortality and morbidity. The disease usually affects the trunk and extremities, but it also can be seen in the maxillofacial region. Early recognition and aggressive treatment with intravenous antibiotics, fluid resuscitation, and surgical debridement, are essential in treating this life-threatening condition.[32-34]

Clinical Features and Presentation

At first, the affected area becomes red, tender, and edematous. The initial stage could resemble cellulitis. The area changes to a dusky gray color as the disease progresses. Anesthesia might ensue as the cutaneous nerve endings are being destroyed, and a malodorous smell is common as the fascia and fat become necrotic. The tissue becomes tense and wooden, and hemorrhagic bullae formation is common at this stage. Gas can form between the fascia and the overlying skin. Eventually, frank gangrene can occur with sloughing of the skin, thereby exposing necrotic subcutaneous fat and fascia (Figure 10-5).

Systemic manifestations of this condition can include fever, tachycardia, sepsis, shock, hemolysis, and intravascular volume depletion. The patient can appear jaundiced and anemic as a result of hemolysis caused by the bacteria.[33]

Pathogenesis

Group A streptococci account for 10% of infections, but other organisms have been reported, including, but not limited to, *Klebsiella*, *Bacteroides* species, *Clostridium*

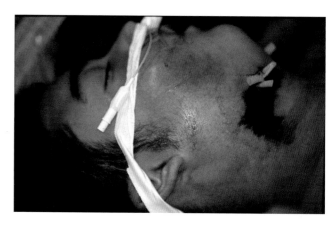

• **Figure 10-5** Necrotizing Fasciitis of the Face. (From Hupp JR, Ellis E, Tucker MR. *Contemporary Oral and Maxillofacial Surgery*. 6th ed. St. Louis: Mosby; 2014. Courtesy Dr. Robert Ord, Department of Oral and Maxillofacial Surgery, Baltimore College of Dental Surgery, University of Maryland, Baltimore.)

species, *Escherichia coli*, *S. aureus*, *Pseudomonas aeruginosa*, and *Haemophilus influenzae*.

Some of the predisposing factors for this condition include an immunocompromised host, diabetes, peripheral vascular disease, and alcoholism. Necrotizing fasciitis usually occurs after trauma or surgery when fascia is being exposed to the organisms.[35]

Diagnosis

The diagnosis is based on clinical grounds; however, computed tomography (CT) or magnetic resonance imaging (MRI) can help determine the depth of tissue involvement. Swab sampling of necrotic tissue for culturing, blood culture, and Gram staining also may be helpful. Frozen section biopsy of the tissue also can be a valuable tool for the early diagnosis of this condition. Blood chemistries, including, but not limited to, complete metabolic panel, complete blood count, electrolytes, and calcium, urea, and creatinine levels might be useful in determining the extent of systemic involvement.[36]

Treatment

High-dose intravenous antibiotics to cover streptococci, staphylococci, and gram-negative bacteria, as well as some of the anaerobes, must be initiated and continued until the culture and sensitivity results are finalized. Intravenous access with a central venous line helps with the determination of intravascular volume status and rapid fluid administration.

Surgical debridement of the affected tissue, including resection of necrotic tissue and packing the area with gauze, is essential. Daily debridement is sometimes necessary to remove all necrotic tissue. Hyperbaric oxygen, although controversial in the treatment of this condition, has been thought to be beneficial in some cases.[33,37,38]

Lyme Disease

Lyme disease is a tick-transmitted infection caused by *Borrelia* species. It usually manifests as an annular erythematous lesion (erythema migrans). Lyme disease could have detrimental neurologic, cardiac, and arthritic sequelae if early diagnosis is delayed and proper antibiotics are not initiated.[32,39]

Clinical Features and Presentation

The clinical presentation can be divided into an early-localized phase, an early-disseminated phase, and chronic disease. The lesions tend to occur on the trunk, legs, groin, axillae, and, on rare occasions, face.

Early Localized Phase

The most recognized early manifestation of Lyme disease is erythema migrans, which manifests as an annular red patch with central clearing or with a red patch at the center (bull's-eye appearance [Figure 10-6]). The lesion will appear at the site of the tick bite, 3 to 30 days after the patient gets infected and can last up to 6 weeks. It will then gradually expand, reaching up to 30 cm. Approximately 80% of patients infected with Lyme disease will develop erythema migrans. During the early phase, patients also experience constitutional symptoms of malaise, fever, arthralgia, lymphadenopathy, headache, and conjunctivitis.

Early Disseminated Phase

Some patients experience a diffuse form of the disease, ranging from 2 to 100 annular red patches. These lesions usually emerge days to weeks after the original erythema migrans lesion and are much smaller in size. Of the patients who are left untreated, approximately 60% experience arthritis; 10% experience neurologic sequelae, including facial nerve palsy; and 5% have cardiac manifestations, including atrioventricular block and pericarditis.

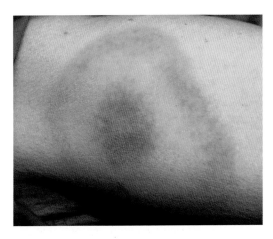

• **Figure 10-6** Erythema Migrans Rash (Bull's-Eye Appearance). (Courtesy Centers for Disease Control and Prevention, Atlanta, GA.)

Chronic Disease

Some of the manifestations of chronic disease include encephalopathy, encephalomyelitis, neuropathy, chronic arthritis, and acrodermatitis chronica atrophicans (bluish-red diffuse patches of skin with underlying atrophy), usually seen in Europe.

Pathogenesis

The main culprit is *Borrelia burgdorferi,* a spirochete that is usually transmitted by various families of Ixodidae ticks. *Ixodes scapularis* is the main tick in the Northeast and Midwest areas of the United States. In Europe, *Borrelia garinii* and *Borrelia afzelii* are the main spirochetes and are transmitted by the tick *Ixodes ricinus.*

Diagnosis

The diagnosis is made mainly by the clinical presentation of erythema migrans rash occurring with some of the constitutional symptoms. The enzyme-linked immunosorbent assay (ELISA) and Western blot tests (detecting IgM antibodies against the *Borrelia* antigen) can be useful; however, these tests are usually positive 3 to 6 weeks after the initial infection and therefore are not of great diagnostic value in early infections. Sometimes tissue biopsy of the erythema migrans can isolate *Borrelia* organisms as well.[33]

Treatment

Early localized disease usually responds well with a dose of doxycycline 100 mg twice a day for 10 to 14 days.[40] Patients with early disseminated disease or mild chronic disease with cranial nerve palsy and second-degree heart block also respond well to doxycycline 100 mg twice a day for 14 to 28 days. For pregnant women, amoxicillin 500 mg three times a day for 14 days or cefuroxime 500 mg twice a day for 14 days is sufficient for early-localized disease.[33,39] According to the CDC guidelines, for younger than age of 8, amoxicillin 50 mg/kg orally divided into 3 doses for 14 days, doxycycline 4.4 mg/kg divided into two doses for up to 14 days, or cefuroxime 30 mg/kg per day divided into 2 doses for 14 days is appropriate for early-localized disease.[40]

Facial palsy is treated with doxycycline for both adults and children. In adults, doxycycline 100 mg twice per day for 14 to 21 days is appropriate. In children, 4.4 mg/kg divided into 2 doses should be given for 12 to 21 days.[41]

Actinomycosis

Actinomyces israelii is an anaerobic gram-positive bacterium that causes purulent abscesses and sinus tract formation. This organism can affect the cervicofacial and pulmonary/thoracic areas and gastrointestinal and female reproductive tracts. This section focuses on cervicofacial actinomycosis, which represents the majority of infections caused by this organism.

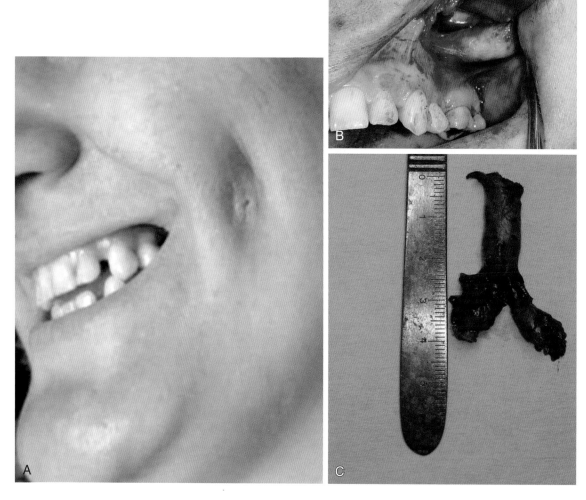

• **Figure 10-7 A,** View of the extraoral termination of actinomycotic sinus tract. Note the shallow depression with cheek motion. **B,** Intraoral view of the dissected sinus tract. Note the unusual thickness of the sinus tract. **C,** Macroscopic view of the resected sinus tract. (From Göçmen G, Varol A, Göker K, et al. Actinomycosis: report of a case with a persistent extraoral sinus tract. *Oral Surg Oral Med Oral Pathol Oral Radiolo Endod.* 2011;112[6]:e121-e123.)

Clinical Features and Presentation

In cervicofacial actinomycosis, patients present with a hard swelling associated with the jaw. As the swelling progresses, a bluish discoloration of the skin appears. Over time, a fistulous abscess forms within the hard swelling and sinus tracts develop (Figure 10-7). A yellowish purulent material is usually discharged from these sinuses.

Pathogenesis

Actinomyces israelii, an anaerobic, gram-positive, non–acid fast filamentous bacterium is the causative agent. This organism is part of the natural flora of the mouth. The main factor for infection in the cervicofacial region is usually regional trauma or injury (e.g., dental procedures) in a patient with poor hygiene or who is immunocompromised.

Cervicofacial actinomycosis mainly affects the soft tissues and rarely originates or localizes in the bone.[32]

Diagnosis

Clinical presentation of hard swelling in the maxillofacial region, as well as microscopic examination and culture, should help make a definite diagnosis.[42] Microscopic examination of purulent discharge usually demonstrates sulfur granules. On hematoxylin-eosin stain, these granules appear as an eosinophilic branching network at the periphery, with collections of basophilic actinomycosis at the center.

The organism can also grow in an anaerobic condition (e.g., beef infusion glucose agar) within 5 to 7 days. However, culturing this organism can be difficult; therefore, direct microscopy or Gram stain showing a long filamentous gram-positive organism is very useful.[32,33]

Treatment

Surgical management and correct dose and duration of antibiotic treatment are the key to management of this condition. Penicillin has remained the standard of treatment for cervicofacial actinomycosis. Penicillin G intravenously 10 to 20 million units/day for 2 to 6 weeks followed by several months of oral penicillin V 2 to 4 g/day is usually effective. Several other antibiotics have proven to be good alternatives for penicillin-allergic patients. These include minocycline, clindamycin, and erythromycin. Surgical management, including drainage of purulent material and surgical excision of sinus tracts, is sometimes necessary in addition to the use of antibiotic treatment.[43]

Tinea Faciei and Tinea Capitis

Fungal infections of the skin can occur on many areas, including the scalp, body, groin, hands, and feet. Superficial or dermatophyte infections involving the face are less common. The causative organisms include *Epidermophyton, Trichophyton,* and *Microsporum* species.[44] On the hair-bearing areas of the face and mustache, it is termed *tinea barbae.* On the scalp, it is termed *tinea capitis.*

These dermatophytes release keratinases that invade the stratum corneum and promote inflammatory reactions. The infection with zoophilic fungi, such as *Microsporum canis,* promotes more severe reactions than do anthropophilic infections.[45]

Tinea Faciei

The clinical presentation of tinea faciei is often characterized by red scaly superficial plaques. The plaques are classically annular with scale at the perimeter (Figure 10-8). The differential of tinea faciei includes eczematous dermatitis, seborrheic dermatitis, lupus erythematosus, granuloma fasciale, granuloma annulare, and sarcoidosis.[46]

On occasion, the lesions can become pustular or nodular, particularly within the hair-bearing areas, and can be spread by shaving or trauma. In addition, there may be associated local adenopathy. Conditions such as Majocchi granuloma develop when the dermatophyte invades the dermal and subcutaneous tissue via penetration of hair follicles.[47,48]

Tinea Capitis

Tinea capitis most commonly occurs in children aged 3 to 7 but can be seen in immunocompromised adults. In the United States the most common organism is *Trichophyton tonsurans* and worldwide is *M. canis.* Affected individuals will often present with numerous scaly patches of alopecia and black dots, which are due to broken hairs. There may be associated cervical lymphadenopathy.

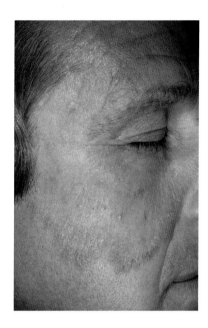

• **Figure 10-8** Facial Tinea. The active border is sharply defined. The initial diagnosis was eczema. (From Habif TP. *Clinical Dermatology: A Color Guide to Diagnosis and Therapy.* 5th ed. St. Louis: Elsevier; 2010.)

A kerion is a more severe inflammatory form of tinea capitis. It is usually caused by a zoophilic species of dermatophytes and will manifest with painful, erythematous, and boggy plaques associated with pustules and alopecia. The alopecia is often permanent.

Favus is a rare chronic inflammatory infection that is caused by *Trichophyton schoenleinii.* Clinically, there will be scutula (yellow-brown, crusted lesions) around the base of the hair follicle leading to alopecia. It is more commonly seen in areas with poor hygiene and malnutrition.

Diagnosis

The diagnosis is confirmed by potassium hydroxide examination. Keratinocytes are obtained by scraping the perimeter of the plaques, mounting the scale on a glass slide with 10% potassium hydroxide solution, and then heating, which demonstrates the dermatophyte within the keratinous scale. Dimethyl sulfoxide can be added and does not require heating. In addition, staining with dye-like chlorazol/black E or Parker blue-black stain can identify tinea.

Fungal cultures with Sabouraud medium are also helpful in diagnosis and to identify the nature of the dermatophyte, although they may take 3 to 4 weeks. Dermatophyte test medium is a rapid medium that relies on color change from yellow to red to diagnose a dermatophyte.

Treatment

The dermatitis can usually be treated with topical antifungals, such as imidazoles, ciclopirox, or allylamine antifungals. If topical antifungal therapy does not work, and particularly for the deeper granulomatous lesions or in tinea barbae, systemic agents such as terbinafine,[48] itraconazole, or griseofulvin may be required. Treatment duration is generally 3 to 4 weeks, either topically or with systemic therapy. Tinea capitis requires systemic treatment for at least 4 weeks, because topical treatments cannot penetrate deep enough into the hair follicle. Griseofulvin is more effective against *Microsporum* species, whereas terbinafine is more effective for infections with *Trichophyton* species. All members of a household should be screened for tinea capitis.

Herpes Simplex Virus Type I Infection

Herpes simplex virus (HSV) infections may be categorized as primary, nonprimary, or recurrent. In a primary infection, the patient develops lesions without preexisting antibodies to either HSV-1 or HSV-2. A nonprimary HSV infection occurs when a patient develops lesions for the first time with preexisting antibodies. A recurrent infection refers to the reactivation of a previously dormant HSV lesion. These lesions may be sexually or nonsexually acquired.

The HSV type 1 (HSV-1) is also known as herpes labialis when it is inoculated into the mucosal surface of the lips. It can also infect other areas of the body, including the eye and scalp. The immunocompromised patient may develop devastating central nervous system infection, hepatitis, or pneumonitis. In addition, HSV-1 gingivostomatitis often can occur in children before the age of 5 years and can be associated with fever, painful oral lesions, and secondary dehydration.[49,50]

Clinical Presentation

Primary Infection

When the virus is inoculated into the mucosal surface or other areas of the skin, the virus enters the epidermis, dermis, and then the sensory and autonomic nerve endings. The initial lesions become vesicles that are clustered on a red base with associated inflammation. In the mouth, the oral lesions may coalesce to form punched-out, painful oral ulcerations. There may be fever and malaise associated with the initial infection, although subsequent outbreaks are frequently without systemic symptoms.

The lesions usually last for 10 to 14 days, although this can be shortened using antiviral drugs (discussed later). The initial infection is often severe; however, recurrent infection may be asymptomatic. It is estimated that 20 to 25% of patients have HSV-1 antibodies, and that 10 to 20% of patients with HSV-2 antibodies have a history of either oral or genital infections.[51] Transmission can occur because of viral shedding from infected areas. Sometimes the shedding lasts for days after apparent clearing of the clinical lesions.

Recurrent Infections

After initial inoculation of the HSV virus, the virus remains latent along the nerve ganglia and can reactivate later. This reactivation can be triggered by multiple factors, including sunlight, emotional or physical stress, menstrual cycles, and

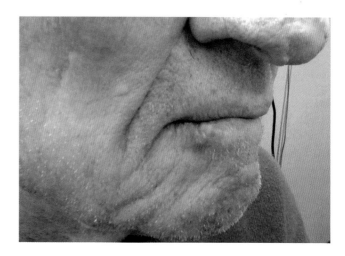

• **Figure 10-9** Herpes Simplex Virus, Right Lower Lip. (Courtesy David Suhocki.)

immunodeficiency. Dental trauma, as with extraction of a tooth in a trigeminal distribution, can also trigger a recurrence.[52]

Before a recurrence of lesions, there may be a prodrome of itching, burning, or tingling. The symptoms may be present for several hours to 2 days before the eruption develops. The patterns and frequency of recurrence vary among patients. There may be triggering factors such as sunlight, illness, or menstrual cycles that can produce a similar pattern within the same patient. Recurrent episodes are generally milder than the primary outbreaks, with less in the way of constitutional signs and lymphadenopathy with a speedier resolution of lesions, usually within 1 week (Figure 10-9).

Diagnosis

Herpes simplex infections can be diagnosed with various methods. Viral culture is common, but it can take several days to obtain a result. DNA polymerase testing is more sensitive and sometimes more accessible.[52] Skin biopsy, serologic testing, or immunofluorescence tests are also useful. A Tzanck preparation done by scraping the roof of an active blister is often performed in the office; it measures the presence of multinucleated viral giant cells, although this method is less sensitive based on the age of the lesions.

The differential diagnosis of HSV gingivostomatitis includes aphthous ulcers, hand-foot-and-mouth disease, oral candidiasis, Stevens-Johnson syndrome, erythema multiforme, or Behçet's syndrome. Herpes labialis may be confused with impetigo or contact dermatitis.

Treatment

Primary Infections

Prompt treatment of primary HSV infections is important. Treatment within the first 72 hours of developing lesions decreases the viral shedding and duration needed for antiviral therapy, decreased pain, and faster healing of lesions.[53] Constitutional symptoms are also lessened relative to placebo.[54]

TABLE 10-1 Treatment Options for Primary Gingivostomatitis

Medication	Dose	Duration
Acyclovir	400 mg 3 times daily or 200 mg 5 times daily	7 to 10 days
Famciclovir	250 mg 3 times daily or 500 mg 2 times daily	7 to 10 days
Valacyclovir	1000 mg 2 times daily	7 to 10 days

Treatment agents include acyclovir, famciclovir, and valacyclovir. The dosing frequency varies between these medications, but all are effective in shortening the duration of the outbreak. Famciclovir, which is the precursor oral form of penciclovir, shows increased bioavailability and a longer half-life than acyclovir does; therefore, the dosing can be less frequent. Table 10-1 reviews the updated guidelines for a primary gingivostomatitis.[55]

Supportive care is important for herpes simplex gingivostomatitis, with particular attention required to avoid dehydration. Topical treatment with diphenhydramine, viscous lidocaine, or benzocaine has been used with some improvement, but the risks of toxicities may outweigh their benefit. In particular, lidocaine can predispose a child to aspiration if the area is numb and can cause difficulty swallowing, including secretions with subsequent choking. Topical benzocaine can induce methemoglobinemia; therefore, it is not recommended before the age of 2 years.[56] Rinsing with saline can be helpful and soothing for the lesions, and topical aluminum/magnesium hydroxide antacid preparations or hydroxypropyl cellulose film can be protective of the oral mucosa.

Recurrent Infections

The treatment for recurrent infections depends on the severity of the symptoms, the frequency of recurrences, and patient preference. If the patient has minimal symptoms and few outbreaks, treatment may not be necessary. However, for patients who have bothersome symptoms and numerous outbreaks, treatment can be helpful to decrease the length of infection and should be given at the onset of prodromal symptoms or development of vesicles. Table 10-2 reviews treatment guidelines for HSV1.[55]

TABLE 10-2 Episodic Treatment Options for Herpes Simplex Virus Type I Infection

Medication	Dose	Duration
Acyclovir	400 mg 3 times daily	5 days
Famciclovir	750 mg 2 times daily Or 1500 mg single dose	750 mg for 1 day
Valacyclovir	2000 mg 2 times daily	1 day

TABLE 10-3 Treatment Options for Chronic Suppressive Therapy for Herpes Simplex Virus Type 1 Infection

Medication	Dose	Duration
Acyclovir	400 mg 2 times daily	Daily
Valacyclovir	500 mg daily	Daily

The need for continuous suppressive therapy should be reevaluated on a yearly basis.

Chronic suppressive therapy is often used for patients who have six or more episodes per year or recurrence that are associated with severe pain or disfiguring lesions. Table 10-3 reviews chronic suppressive therapy HSV1.[55]

Herpes Zoster

Varicella-zoster virus (VZV) causes both chickenpox and herpes zoster. Primary infection with VZV can cause chickenpox, characterized by vesicles in various stages of development on the face, trunk, and extremities. Varicella is often associated with fever, malaise, and other constitutional symptoms, such as headache and cough. Rarely, there may be complications of meningitis and pneumonia.

Herpes zoster, which is also known as *shingles,* is represented by a similar vesicular eruption that occurs along a dermatome. It frequently occurs among individuals who have had varicella in the past, and it is sometimes triggered as the VZV cell-mediated immunity wanes. It is estimated that 32% of the U.S. population will develop zoster during their lifetime.[57]

Age is the most common risk factor in herpes zoster with the increase because of the waning of cell-mediated immunity in patients older than 50 years. Immunocompromised patients are at more risk, including transplant patients,[58] patients receiving chemotherapy, or HIV-infected patients.[59] These patients also have a higher incidence of recurrent zoster, which in immunocompetent patients can occur in 1 to 3% of individuals.

Clinical Presentation

The clinical presentation of shingles is a unilateral rash with painful lesions and may involve more than two or three adjacent dermatomes. The eruption starts as red papules that then coalesce into grouped vesicles and sometimes hemorrhagic or pustular lesions. The lesions are often painful and sometimes itchy. They may heal with pain in the dermatomal distribution called postherpetic neuralgia (PHN). The risks for developing PHN include age, immunosuppression, diabetes, and severe pain during zoster outbreak.[60,61]

Herpes zoster often represents the reactivation of a latent VZV, which resides in the nerve ganglia. The pain often can be severe, and the virus may sometimes have devastating results when in areas of the eye, known as *herpes zoster ophthalmicus.* In this situation,[62] VZV can be reactivated

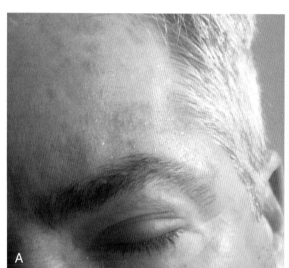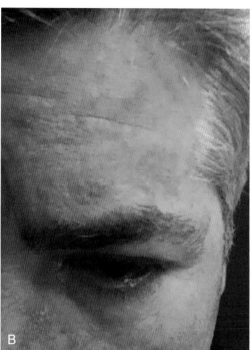

• **Figure 10-10** A and B, Patient with Left Herpes Zoster Ophthalmicus. (Courtesy Dr. Elie M. Ferneini.)

within the trigeminal ganglion, and the patient may develop conjunctivitis, episcleritis, keratitis, or iritis (Figure 10-10). If the virus progresses to involve the cornea, there may be loss of vision. One prognostic factor that can indicate impending ocular involvement is Hutchinson's sign, which is involvement of the tip of the nose; this is part of the nasociliary branch of the ophthalmic nerve.

If herpes zoster involves the eighth nerve, there may be vesicles around the ear and complications such as facial paresis, vertigo, and deafness (known as *Ramsay Hunt syndrome*).[63] There may also be effects on taste and lacrimation. The eruption is due to reactivation of the virus in the geniculate ganglion; it may also involve cranial nerves V, IX, and X.[64] Although it may respond to antiviral treatment, the damage may be permanent.[65]

Diagnosis

The diagnosis of VZV is based on the presentation of vesicles within a dermatomal distribution. Pain may often precede the appearance of the cutaneous lesions on the head or neck by hours or several days. It can be triggered by local trauma, such as dental work, and many cases of herpes zoster on the head and neck usually follow craniofacial trauma.[66] The diagnosis can be confirmed with a Tzanck preparation, which may reveal multinucleated viral giant cells when the blister roof is debrided or scraped.

Treatment

Therapeutically, the treatment involves antiviral therapy with acyclovir, valacyclovir, or famciclovir. It is important to

Table 10-4	Treatment Options for Varicella-Zoster Virus	
Medication	Dose	Duration
Acyclovir	800 mg 5 times daily	7 days
Famciclovir	500 mg 3 times daily	7 days
Valacyclovir	1000 mg 3 times daily	7 days

initiate treatment within the first 48 to 72 hours to enhance the antiviral effect. The dosing is higher than for HSV. Valacyclovir and famciclovir are more convenient with less frequent dosing and may have somewhat lesser gastrointestinal side effects. The overall efficacy of these drugs, however, is comparable (Table 10-4).[67,68,69] In herpes zoster ophthalmicus, topical steroid drops also can be used in addition to oral therapy to reduce the inflammation, episcleritis, and keratitis—corneal involvement that occurs in up to two thirds of patients. In addition, iritis can occur in 40% of patients with dysfunction of the pupillary response.[62,70]

In herpes zoster virus (HZV), secondary infection may need to be ruled out by bacterial culture and sensitivity, in the event of increased purulent drainage or associated inflammation. Treatment with an antibiotic for secondary impetiginization, which often includes streptococcal or staphylococcal organisms, is important.

One of the more devastating effects of HZV is the development of PHN, which occurs in 10 to 15% of patients, half of whom are older than 60 years. As a result, vaccination with a HZV is often recommended. This live attenuated VZV vaccine has been shown to reduce the incidence of herpes zoster and PHN. Some data indicate that the vaccine may reduce herpes zoster and PHN in adults between 50 and 59 years old. It is possible for herpes zoster to occur more than once in the same individual; therefore, the vaccine is often recommended even for those who have a history of previous zoster.

The incidence and severity of PHN is greater in those older than 60 years, and antiviral therapy is often given to individuals within the first 72 hours of symptoms to lessen the severity of the outbreak. Glucocorticoids, such as prednisone, have been used with acyclovir to lessen the degree of pain and to hasten the resolution of VZV. A recent study, however, did not demonstrate any appreciable difference with acyclovir alone versus acyclovir with systemic steroids.[71,72] In fact, the potential for secondary bacterial infection when taking glucocorticoids outweighs its benefit.

There have been several treatments for PHN, including tricyclic antidepressants, which inhibit the reuptake of norepinephrine and serotonin in the central nervous system. Amitriptyline was shown to be more effective than a placebo or lorazepam for pain relief in one study. Pain medication, including opioids and nonsteroidal antiinflammatory drugs, are sometimes used, as are topical lidocaine or topical capsaicin. The latter, derived biochemically from hot pepper, interferes with substance P, a pain neurotransmitter. It can cause some burning, stinging, and redness, but may be of some benefit with pain reduction.

Anticonvulsant medications such as gabapentin and pregabalin are also used to treat PHN. Studies show some modest improvement in pain reduction with these medications, although the potential for side effects, including dizziness, dry mouth, weight gain, and somnolence, can sometimes limit their usefulness.[73]

Finally, the shingles vaccine, Shringrix, is a recombinant zoster vaccine that is recommended for adults 50 years and older (two doses) and adults 19 years and older who are immunocompromised (two doses). In adults aged 50 to 69 years, Shringrix was 97% effective at preventing shingles and 91% effective in preventing PHN. In adults 70 years and older it was 91% effective against shingles and 89% against PHN. In immunocompromised adults, Shringrix was 68 to 91% effective at preventing shingles.[74] Immunity lasts for 7 years.[74]

Impetigo

Impetigo is a superficial skin infection, usually caused by *S. aureus* and less commonly group A *S. pyogenes*. It is the most common cause of bacterial infection in children. The two clinical forms of this disease are bullous and nonbullous.[75]

Clinical Presentation

Nonbullous impetigo is the most common form of impetigo, accounting for 70% of cases. It usually presents

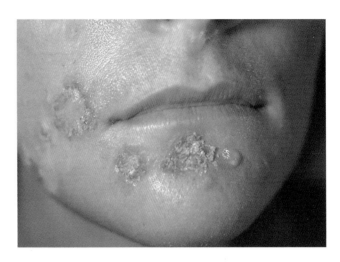

• **Figure 10-11** Nonbullous Impetigo on the Face. (From Cordoro KM, Ganz JE. Training room management of medical conditions: sports dermatology. *Clin Sports Med.* 2005;24[3]:565-598.)

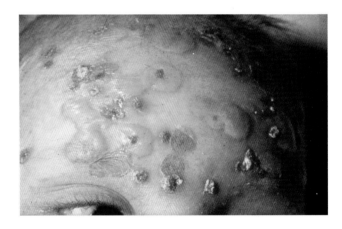

• **Figure 10-12** Bullous Impetigo. (From Bennett JE, Dolin R, Blaser MJ. *Mandell, Douglas, and Bennett's Principles and Practice of Infectious Diseases.* 8th ed. Philadelphia: Saunders; 2015.)

with vesicles, bullae, and pustules that rupture, releasing yellowish fluid that dries up easily. This leaves a honey-colored crusted area that is the hallmark of the disease (Figure 10-11).[32,33]

Bullous impetigo manifests as flaccid bullae or mostly as shallow erosions with peripheral collarette of scale (Figure 10-12). In this entity, there are no thick crusts and no surrounding erythema. It usually manifests in the neonatal period and less commonly in children.[39]

Pathogenesis

Impetigo occurs usually after a minor injury, trauma, insect bite, or laceration. The most common agent is *S. aureus,* which accounts for 50 to 70% of cases. Nasal carriers of *S. aureus* are at a higher risk for recurrent infections. The other less common pathogen is group A β-hemolytic *Streptococcus.* At the cellular level, bullous impetigo results from the exfoliative toxin of *S. aureus,* which binds to desmoglein-1 (a desmosomal protein that joins cells to one another) at the granular level of epidermis, leading to acantholysis (loss of intercellular connection) and blister formation.[33,39]

Diagnosis

The diagnosis is primarily based on clinical grounds. However, bacterial culture of exudates could be positive. White blood cell counts are also sometimes elevated in impetigo.

Treatment

In healthy individuals with limited disease, topical mupirocin ointment is an effective first-line treatment. For widespread infections, oral antibiotics, including penicillin, β-lactamase–resistant penicillin, macrolides, and cephalosporins are treatment options. With an emergence of MRSA, recalcitrant cases that do not respond to treatment should have culture and sensitivity testing so that an appropriate antibiotic can be selected. Additionally, for nasal carriers of *S. aureus* who will get recurrent infections, nasal application of mupirocin can be highly effective.

If effectively treated, the disease usually runs a benign, self-limited process. In 2 to 5% of cases of nonbullous impetigo caused by *S. pyogenes,* acute poststreptococcal glomerulonephritis (APSG) can occur. The important predisposing factors are *S. pyogenes* serotypes 1, 4, 12, 25, and 49. The early treatment with antibiotics will not prevent occurrence of APSG in this group of patients. There is no association between impetigo and rheumatic fever.[33,39,75]

Molluscum Contagiosum

Molluscum contagiosum (MC) is a self-limited viral infection caused by the poxvirus family. It is the most common infection in humans. The condition can be transmitted by skin-to-skin contact and autoinoculation. It usually affects children, sexually active adults, and immunocompromised (e.g., AIDS) patients.

Clinical Features and Presentation

MC usually presents as 1- to 2-mm flesh-colored, shiny, dome-shaped papules (Figure 10-13). Most of the lesions have a central umbilication that can be best observed by magnification or when lesions get frozen with liquid nitrogen. During the course of the disease, the papules become redder and central umbilication becomes more obvious. The lesions that are untreated last about 9 months before resolving.[76]

In children, lesions tend to number from a few to several dozen and usually affect the face, trunk, and extremities. In adults, MC is a sexually transmitted disease and lesions tend to be more common in the lower abdomen, thighs, and penile shaft.[77,78]

In HIV patients, lesions occur when patients have been diagnosed with AIDS and have T cell counts of less than 100. In these individuals, lesions tend to occur on the face

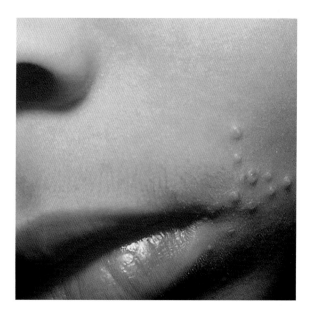

• **Figure 10-13** Child with Facial Molluscum Contagiosum. (From Zitelli BJ, McIntire SC, Norwalk AJ. *Zitelli and Davis' Atlas of Pediatric Physical Diagnosis.* 6th ed. Philadelphia: Saunders; 2012.)

and genitalia. The presentation could be the typical dome-shaped umbilicated papules as well as large lesions greater than 1 cm. Involvement of the oral mucosa implies AIDS with a T cell count of less than 50.[79]

Pathogenesis

MC virus (MCV), a DNA virus, is a member of the poxvirus family. There are MCV 1 to 4 serotypes, but MCV 1 induces the majority of the infections in children. The disease is transmitted by skin-to-skin contact, by autoinoculation, and during sexual activity, and it also occurs in immunocompromised hosts including AIDS patients.[76-78]

Diagnosis

Diagnosis is usually based on the clinical presentation. Biopsy of the specimen can be helpful to confirm the diagnosis. The histologic evaluation has characteristic intracytoplasmic viral inclusion bodies known as molluscum bodies or Henderson-Paterson bodies within the infected keratinocytes.[76,79]

Treatment

Treatment varies depending on the location, age, and immune status of the patient. Lesions usually resolve spontaneously in healthy hosts, and because there is a risk of scarring with treatment, no intervention sometimes is the best course.

Children should be educated on the risk of transmission with autoinoculation and direct contact with MC. The treatment options for children is based on the location, number of lesions, and risk and benefits of treatment.

Curettage is one of the treatment options. It could cause scarring, and it may be traumatic for patients; therefore, an anesthetic is required before the procedure. It is usually not recommended for the pediatric patient.

Topical treatment modalities include tretinoin cream, salicylic acid gel 12%, topical cantharidin (although the FDA has not approved it for use in the United States), imiquimod, and 40% silver nitrate paste. Most of these topical agents will induce redness, irritation, scar formation, and changes in the skin color; therefore, parents of pediatric patients should be aware of the possible side effects before treatment.

Cryotherapy is another treatment option that is very effective, but it has side effects of pain, redness, hypopigmentation/hyperpigmentation, blister formation, and rarely scarring. Patients most likely need several treatments before lesions resolve.

In patients with AIDS, both imiquimod and topical cidofovir 3% (competitive inhibitor of DNA polymerase) have been shown to be effective. However, most of the MC lesions usually resolve after improvement of immune status.[79-81]

References

1. Del Rosso J, Zeichner J, Alexis A, Cohen D, Berson D. Understanding the epidermal barrier in healthy and compromised skin: clinically relevant information for the dermatology practitioner: proceedings of an expert panel roundtable meeting. *J Clin Aesthet Dermatol*. 2016;9(4 suppl 1):S2-S8.
2. Lambers H, Piessens S, Bloem A, Pronk H, Finkel P. Natural skin surface pH is on average below 5, which is beneficial for its resident flora. *Int J Cosmet Sci*. 2006;28:359-370. Available at: https://doi.org/10.1111/j.1467-2494.2006.00344.x.
3. Proksch E. pH in nature, humans and skin. *J Dermatol*. 2018;45:1044-1052. Available at: https://doi.org/10.1111/1346-8138.14489.
4. Schmid-Wendtner MH, Korting HC. The pH of the skin surface and its impact on the barrier function. *Skin Pharmacol Physiol*. 2006; 19(6):296-302. Available at: https://doi.org/10.1159/000094670.
5. Schittek B, Paulmann M, Senyürek I, et al. The role of antimicrobial peptides in human skin and in skin infectious diseases. *Infect Disord Drug Targets*. 2008;8:135-143.
6. Goulden V, Clark SM, Cunliffe WJ. Post-adolescent acne: a review of clinical features. *Br J Dermatol*. 1997;136:66-70.
7. Jeremy AH, Holland DB, Roberts SG, et al. Inflammatory events are involved in acne lesion initiation. *J Invest Dermatol*. 2003;121:20-27.
8. Timpatanapong P, Rojanasakul A. Hormonal profiles and prevalence of polycystic ovary syndrome in women with acne. *J Dermatol*. 1997;24:223-229.
9. Yosipovitch G, Tang M, Dawn AG, et al. Study of psychological stress, sebum production and acne vulgaris in adolescents. *Acta Derm Venereol*. 2007;87:135-139.
10. Leyden JJ, Shalita A, Thiboutot D, et al. Topical retinoids in inflammatory acne: a retrospective, investigator-blinded, vehicle-controlled, photographic assessment. *Clin Ther*. 2005;27:216-224.
11. Ross JI, Snelling AM, Eady EA, et al. Phenotypic and genotypic characterization of antibiotic-resistant *Propionibacterium acnes* isolated from acne patients attending dermatology clinics in Europe, the U.S.A., Japan and Australia. *Br J Dermatol*. 2001;144:339-346.
12. Plovanich M, Weng QY, Mostaghimi A. Low usefulness of potassium monitoring among healthy young women taking spironolactone for acne. *JAMA Dermatol*. 2015;151(9):941. Available at: https://doi.org/10.1001/jamadermatol.2015.34.
13. Basarab T, Russell Jones R. HIV-associated eosinophilic folliculitis: case report and review of the literature. *Br J Dermatol*. 1996; 134:499-503.
14. Ratnam S, Hogan K, March SB, et al. Whirlpool-associated folliculitis caused by *Pseudomonas aeruginosa*: report of an outbreak and review. *J Clin Microbiol*. 1986;23:655-659.
15. Brachman P, Kaufmann A. Anthrax. In: Evans A, Brachman P, eds. *Bacterial Infections of Humans: Epidemiology and Control*. 3rd ed. New York: Plenum Publishing; 1998:95.
16. Carucci JA, McGovern TW, Norton SA, et al. Cutaneous anthrax management algorithm. *J Am Acad Dermatol*. 2002;47:766-769.
17. Meselson M, Guillemin J, Hugh-Jones M, et al. The Sverdlovsk anthrax outbreak of 1979. *Science*. 1994;266:1202-1208.
18. Beatty ME, Ashford DA, Griffin PM, et al. Gastrointestinal anthrax: review of the literature. *Arch Intern Med*. 2003;163:2527-2531.
19. Sirisanthana T, Navacharoen N, Tharavichitkul P, et al. Outbreak of oral-oropharyngeal anthrax: an unusual manifestation of human infection with *Bacillus anthracis*. *Am J Trop Med Hyg*. 1984;33:144-150.
20. Hoffmaster AR, Meyer RF, Bowen MD, et al. Evaluation and validation of a real-time polymerase chain reaction assay for rapid identification of *Bacillus anthracis*. *Emerg Infect Dis*. 2002;8: 1178-1182.
21. Hendricks KA, Wright ME, Shadomy SV, et al. Centers for Disease Control and Prevention expert panel meetings on prevention and treatment of anthrax in adults. *Emerg Infect Dis*. 2014;20:e130687.
22. Bradley JS, Peacock G, Krug SE, et al. Pediatric anthrax clinical management. *Pediatrics*. 2014;133:1411-1436.
23. U.S. Food and Drug Administration. Raxibacumab prescribing information. Available at: https://www.accessdata.fda.gov/drugsatfda_docs/label/2012/125349s000lbl.pdf. Accessed August 27, 2015.
24. Bisno AL, Stevens DL. Streptococcal infections of skin and soft tissues. *N Engl J Med*. 1996;334:240-245.
25. Moran GJ, Krishnadasan A, Gorwitz RJ, et al. Methicillin-resistant *S. aureus* infections among patients in the emergency department. *N Engl J Med*. 2006;355:666-674.
26. Liu C, Bayer A, Cosgrove SE, et al. Clinical practice guidelines by the Infectious Diseases Society of America for the treatment of methicillin-resistant *Staphylococcus aureus* infections in adults and children. *Clin Infect Dis*. 2011;52:e18.
27. Jorup-Rönström C, Britton S. Recurrent erysipelas: predisposing factors and costs of prophylaxis. *Infection*. 1987;15:105-106.
28. Stevens DL. Invasive group A streptococcus infections. *Clin Infect Dis*. 1992;14:2-11.
29. Ong BS, Dotel R, Ngian VJJ. Recurrent cellulitis: who is at risk and how effective is antibiotic prophylaxis? *Int J Gen Med*. 2022;15:6561-6572. doi:10.2147/IJGM.S326459.
30. Begovac J, Kuzmanović N, Bejuk D. Comparison of clinical characteristics of group A streptococcal bacteremia in children and adults. *Clin Infect Dis*. 1996;23:97.
31. Stevens DL, Tanner MH, Winship J, et al. Severe group A streptococcal infections associated with a toxic shock-like syndrome and scarlet fever toxin A. *N Engl J Med*. 1989;321:1-7.

32. Halpern AV, Heymann WR. Bacterial diseases. In: Bolognia JL, Jorizzo JL, Rapini RP, et al., eds. *Dermatology.* 2nd ed. St. Louis: Mosby Elsevier; 2009:1085-1086.

33. Bacterial infections. In: James WD, Berger TG, Elston DM, eds. *Andrew's Diseases of the Skin Clinical Dermatology.* 10th ed. Philadelphia: Saunders Elsevier; 2006:261-262.

34. Krespi RP, Lawson W, Blaugrund SM, et al. Massive necrotizing infections of the neck. *Head Neck Surg.* 1981;3:475-481.

35. Rapoport Y, Himelfarb MZ, Zikk D, et al. Cervical necrotizing fasciitis of odontogenic origin. *Oral Surg.* 1991;72:15-18.

36. Stamenkovic I, Lew PE. Early recognition of potentially fatal necrotizing fasciitis. *N Engl J Med.* 1984;310:1689-1693.

37. Mladenov A, Diehl K, Müller O, et al. Outcome of necrotizing fasciitis and Fournier's gangrene with and without hyperbaric oxygen therapy: a retrospective analysis over 10 years. *World J Emerg Surg.* 2022;17:43. Available at: https://doi.org/10.1186/s13017-022-00448-6.

38. Roser SM, Chow AW, Brady FA. Necrotizing fasciitis. *J Oral Surg.* 1977;35:730-732.

39. Bacterial, mycobacterial, and protozoal infections of the skin. In: Paller AS, Mancini AJ, eds. *Hurwitz Clinical Pediatric Dermatology.* 4th ed. Philadelphia: Elsevier Saunders; 2011:341.

40. Centers for Disease Control and Prevention. Erythema migrans rash treatment guidelines. Available at: https://www.cdc.gov/lyme/treatment/erythema-migrans-rash.html.

41. Centers for Disease Control and Prevention. Neurologic Lyme disease treatment guidelines. Available at: https://www.cdc.gov/lyme/treatment/NeurologicLyme.html.

42. Lerner PI. The lumpy jaw. *Infect Dis Clin North Am.* 1988;2:203-220.

43. Blume JE. Actinomycosis. In: Lebwohl MG, Heyman WR, Berth-Jones J, et al., eds. *Treatment of Skin Disease.* 3rd ed. St. Louis: Saunders Elsevier; 2009:21-23.

44. Atzori L, Aste N, Aste N, et al. Tinea faciei due to *Microsporum canis* in children: a survey of 46 cases in the District of Cagliari (Italy). *Pediatr Dermatol.* 2012;29:409-413.

45. Belhadjali H, Aounallah A, Youssef M, et al. Tinea faciei, under-recognized because clinically misleading: 14 cases [in French]. *Presse Med.* 2009;38:1230-1234.

46. Meymandi S, Wiseman MC, Crawford RI. Tinea faciei mimicking cutaneous lupus erythematosus: a histopathologic case report. *J Am Acad Dermatol.* 2003;48(suppl 2):S7-S8.

47. Smith KJ, Neafie RC, Skelton HG III, et al. Majocchi's granuloma. *J Cutan Pathol.* 1991;18:28-35.

48. Tanuma H, Doi M, Nishiyama S, et al. A case of tinea barbae successfully treated with terbinafine. *Mycoses.* 1998;41:77-81.

49. Annunziato PW, Gershon A. Herpes simplex virus infections. *Pediatr Rev.* 1996;17:415-423.

50. Kolokotronis A, Doumas S. Herpes simplex virus infection, with particular reference to the progression and complications of primary herpetic gingivostomatitis. *Clin Microbiol Infect.* 2006;12:202-211.

51. Johnson RE, Nahmias AJ, Magder LS, et al. A seroepidemiologic survey of the prevalence of herpes simplex virus type 2 infection in the United States. *N Engl J Med.* 1989;321:7-12.

52. Spruance SL, Overall JC Jr, Kern ER, et al. The natural history of recurrent herpes simplex labialis: implications for antiviral therapy. *N Engl J Med.* 1977;297:69-75.

53. Cernik C, Gallina K, Brodell RT. The treatment of herpes simplex infections: an evidence-based review. *Arch Intern Med.* 2008;168:1137-1144.

54. Amir J, Harel L, Smetana Z, et al. Treatment of herpes simplex gingivostomatitis with acyclovir in children: a randomised double blind placebo controlled study. *BMJ.* 1997;314:1800-1803.

55. Wald A, Johnston C. Treatment and prevention of herpes simplex virus type 1 in immunocompetent adolescents and adults. In: Post TW, ed. Waltham, MA: UpToDate. Accessed March 1, 2023.

56. So TY, Farrington E. Topical benzocaine-induced methemoglobinemia in the pediatric population. *J Pediatr Health Care.* 2008;22:335-339.

57. Harpaz R, Ortega-Sanchez IR, Seward JF, Advisory Committee on Immunization Practices, Centers for Disease Control and Prevention. Prevention of herpes zoster: recommendations of the Advisory Committee on Immunization Practices (ACIP). *MMWR Recom Rep.* 2008;57:1-30.

58. Carby M, Jones A, Burke M, et al. Varicella infection after heart and lung transplantation: a single-center experience. *J Heart Lung Transplant.* 2007;26:399.

59. Buchbinder SP, Katz MH, Hessol NA, et al. Herpes zoster and human immunodeficiency virus infection. *J Infect Dis.* 1992;166:1153.

60. Gruver C, Guthmiller KB. Postherpetic neuralgia. In: *StatPearls* [Internet]. Treasure Island, FL: StatPearls Publishing; 2023.

61. Choo PW, Galil K, Donahue JG, et al. Risk factors for postherpetic neuralgia. *Arch Intern Med.* 1997;157:1217-1224.

62. Pavan-Langston D. Herpes zoster ophthalmicus. *Neurology.* 1995;45:S50-S51.

63. Adour KK. Otological complications of herpes zoster. *Ann Neurol.* 1994;35(suppl):S62-S64.

64. Furuta Y, Takasu T, Fukuda S, et al. Detection of varicella-zoster virus DNA in human geniculate ganglia by polymerase chain reaction. *J Infect Dis.* 1992;166:1157-1159.

65. Robillard RB, Hilsinger RL Jr, Adour KK. Ramsay Hunt facial paralysis: clinical analyses of 185 patients. *Otolaryngol Head Neck Surg.* 1986;95:292-297.

66. Zhang JX, Joesoef RM, Bialek S, et al. Association of physical trauma with risk of herpes zoster among Medicare beneficiaries in the United States. *J Infect Dis.* 2013;207:1007-1011.

67. Shafran SD, Tyring SK, Ashton R, et al. Once, twice, or three times daily famciclovir compared with aciclovir for the oral treatment of herpes zoster in immunocompetent adults: a randomized, multicenter, double-blind clinical trial. *J Clin Virol.* 2004;29:248-253.

68. Dworkin RH, Johnson RW, Breuer J, et al. Recommendations for the management of herpes zoster. *Clin Infect Dis.* 2007;44(suppl 1):S1-26. doi:10.1086/510206.

69. Gnann Jr JW. Chapter 65: Antiviral therapy of varicella-zoster virus infections. In: Arvin A, Campadelli-Fiume G, Mocarski E, et al., eds. *Human Herpesviruses: Biology, Therapy, and Immunoprophylaxis.* Cambridge: Cambridge University Press; 2007. Available at: https://www.ncbi.nlm.nih.gov/books/NBK47401/.

70. Tyring SK, Beutner KR, Tucker BA, et al. Antiviral therapy for herpes zoster: randomized, controlled clinical trial of valacyclovir and famciclovir therapy in immunocompetent patients 50 years and older. *Arch Fam Med.* 2000;9:863-869.

71. Wood MJ, Johnson RW, McKenrick MW, et al. A randomized trial of acyclovir for 7 days or 21 days with and without prednisolone for treatment of acute herpes zoster. *N Engl J Med.* 1994;330:896-900.

72. Han Y, Zhang J, Chen N, He L, Zhou M, Zhu C. Corticosteroids for preventing postherpetic neuralgia. *Cochrane Database Syst Rev.* 2013;28(3):CD005582. Available at: https://doi.org/10.1002/14651858.CD005582.pub4.

73. Moore RA, Wiffen PJ, Derry S, et al. Gabapentin for chronic neuropathic pain and fibromyalgia in adults. *Cochrane Database Syst Rev.* 2011;16(3):CD007938.

74. Centers for Disease Control and Prevention. Shingrix vacation guidelines. Available at: https://www.cdc.gov/vaccines/vpd/shingles/public/shingrix/index.html.

75. Burd R, Sladden M. Impetigo. In: Lebwohl MG, Heyman WR, Berth-Jones J, et al., eds. *Treatment of Skin Disease*. 3rd ed. Philadelphia: Saunders; 2010;327-329.

76. Mancini AJ, Shani-Adir A. Other viral diseases. In: Bolognia JL, Jorizzo JL, Rapini RP, et al., eds. *Dermatology*. 2nd ed. St. Louis: Mosby Elsevier; 2008:1229-1232.

77. Viral diseases of the skin. In: Paller AS, Mancini AJ, eds. *Hurwitz Clinical Pediatric Dermatology*. 4th ed. Philadelphia: Elsevier Saunders; 2012:362-365.

78. Viral diseases. In: James WD, Berger TG, Elston DM, eds. *Andrew's Diseases of the Skin Clinical Dermatology*. 10th ed. Philadelphia: Saunders Elsevier; 2006:394-396.

79. Viral infections. In: Habif TP, Campbell JL, Chapman MS, et al., eds. *Skin Disease Diagnosis and Treatment*. 2nd ed. St. Louis: Elsevier Mosby; 2004:194-197.

80. Gordon PM, Benton EC. Molluscum contagiosum. In: Lebwohl MG, Heyman WR, Berth-Jones J, et al., eds. *Treatment of Skin Disease*. 3rd ed. Philadelphia: Saunders Elsevier; 2009:442-445.

81. Wu JJ, Huang DB, Tyring SK. Dermatologic virology. In: Hall JC, ed. *Sauer's Manual of Skin Diseases*. 9th ed. Philadelphia: Lippincott Williams and Wilkins; 2006:230-232.

11

Brain and Meningeal Infections*

HILAL A. KANAAN AND JAMES R. HUPP

The brain and its covering tissues are a complex organ that controls bodily functions, including thought, motor activity, the basic senses, and processes that regulate the body. Anything that affects the health of the brain and meninges jeopardizes a person's well-being and even the person's life. Infections of the brain and/or meninges are particularly threatening because of their ability to quickly spread and disrupt brain functions. Thus, the need to rapidly diagnose and effectively treat infections of this part of the body are critical. As is true in other parts of the head and neck, the brain and meninges are highly vascularized, which can be helpful in the brain's ability to resist infection but can also provide pathways for infection in other parts of the body to spread to the brain. This chapter covers the pathophysiology and management of brain and meningeal infections.

Meningitis

Meningitis, by definition, is a chronic or acute inflammation of the meninges. When of infectious origin, it is the most common form of brain/meningeal infection. The two most common causes of infected meninges are pneumococcus (Figure 11-1) and meningococcus (Figure 11-2) meningitis. Bacterial meningitis can be a complication of a neurosurgical procedure. Factors increasing the risk for meningitis after neurosurgery include cerebrospinal fluid (CSF) leakage, clean-contaminated or dirty wounds, operative time longer than 4 hours, emergency surgery, and reoperations.[1] Many of the classic organisms that infect patients include gram-negative bacteria (*Escherichia coli*, *Klebsiella pneumoniae*, *Pseudomonas* species, *Acinetobacter* species). Gram-positive bacteria causing postsurgical meningitis include *Staphylococcus aureus* and *Staphylococcus pneumoniae*, coagulase-negative staphylococci, and group B *Streptococcus*.[2] The possibility of postoperative bacterial meningitis makes it important to administer antibiotic prophylaxis. Neurosurgeons frequently order intravenous cloxacillin or amikacin to be administered at induction and continue for 24 hours after the completion of surgery. The CSF leak rather than the brain surgery itself is considered to be the reason for the postoperative infection.[3] Fever or a delayed postsurgical recovery of normal brain function should trigger a workup for bacterial meningitis. Other nonclassic signs or symptoms after open brain surgery may occur, especially those with diabetes mellitus or other conditions that may compromise the immune system, so meningitis should be kept in the differential diagnosis.

Community-acquired meningitis manifests differently than postsurgical meningitis. The cardinal signs and symptoms are severe headache, neck rigidity, fever, and impaired consciousness. In the patient suspected of having community-acquired meningitis a lumbar puncture (LP) is indicated to help differentiate between viral versus bacterial infections. In bacterial meningitis, typically the opening pressure is elevated (>180 mm H_2O), white blood cell count (WBC) is elevated (10 to 10,000 cells/μL), percentage of neutrophils is increased ($>80\%$), protein is increased (100 to 500 mg/dL), glucose is decreased (<40 mg/dL), and CSF-to–serum glucose ratio is below 0.4. CSF findings in patients with viral meningitis, in contrast, include moderately increased WBCs (25 to 500 cells/μL of CSF lymphocytes), normal or slightly increased elevated protein (20 to 80 mg/dL), normal glucose concentration, and a negative Gram stain.[4]

Empiric treatment for postneurosurgical meningitis should include ceftazidime, which covers *Pseudomonas aeruginosa* and other gram-negative bacteria, and vancomycin, for *S. aureus* and other gram-positive bacteria.[5] Once CSF cultures and Gram staining have been done, antibiotics can be more precisely determined. Imaging should be performed after the LP and antibiotic administration has begun. Imaging should be performed in the neurosurgical patient who develops meningitis to help determine the possible bacterial point of entry. Furthermore, both neurosurgical and non-neurosurgical patients who develop hydrocephalus require surgical intervention. As the infection is being treated, a ventriculostomy should be placed; also, once the infection has resolved, a ventriculoperitoneal shunt should be done if natural drainage does not return.[6]

Having a high index of suspicion for meningitis after neurosurgery is critical because a failure to make the diagnosis often leads to serious complications or death. These long-term complications include sensorineural hearing loss, intellectual

*The authors gratefully acknowledge the original contributions to this chapter by Dr. Ryan A. Zengou of Joliet, Illinois, United States.

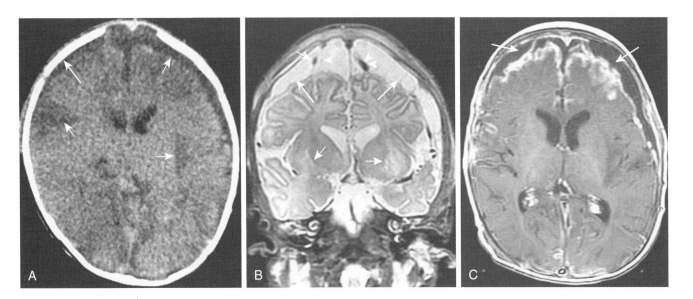

• **Figure 11-1** Pneumococcal Meningitis. Computed tomography scan **(A)** and coronal T2-weighted **(B)** and gadolinium-enhanced T1-weighted **(C)** MR images demonstrate enhancing subdural collections (**A** to **C,** *top long and short arrows*), venous thromboses (**B,** *top short arrows and arrowheads*), and infarctions (**A** and **B,** *bottom short arrows*). (From Blickman JG, Parker BR, Barnes PD. *Pediatric Radiology: The Requisites.* 3rd ed. Philadelphia: Mosby; 2007.)

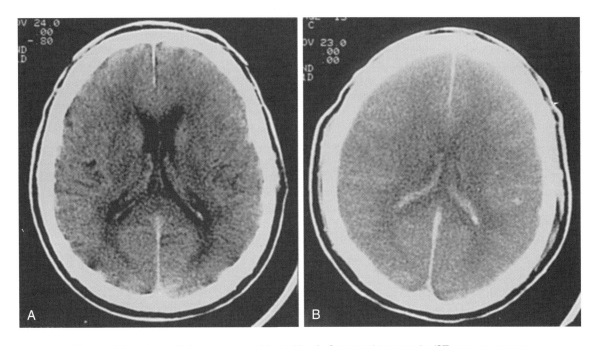

• **Figure 11-2** Patient with Pneumococcal Meningitis. **A,** Computed tomography (CT) scan on presentation reveals moderate cortical atrophy. **B,** CT scan 3 days later reveals diffuse swelling of the cerebral hemispheres bilaterally, with effacement of the ventricular system. (From Bennett JE, Dolin R, Blaser MJ. *Mandell, Douglas, and Bennett's Principles and Practice of Infectious Diseases.* 8th ed. Philadelphia: Saunders; 2015.)

impairment, seizure activity cerebral edema, and cranial nerve palsies.[7] Thus, one must recognize the signs and symptoms of meningitis and begin immediate treatment.

Intracranial Subdural Empyema

An intracranial subdural empyema (the terms *subdural abscess* or *suppuration* have been used in the past) is a loculated accumulation of purulence located between the arachnoid and dura mater. The condition is serious and can be life-threatening, especially if not promptly diagnosed and properly treated. Intracranial subdural empyemas (ISEs) can arise after cranial surgery, open skull fractures, or penetrating injury, or as a result of hematomas or effusions that become infected. A large percentage of patients suffering an ISE have ear or paranasal sinus infections that spread to the subdural space.

The most common organisms associated with an ISE are streptococci, staphylococci, *Haemophilus influenzae*, *Streptococcus pneumoniae*, and other gram-negative bacteria. Empyemas associated with the paranasal sinuses are frequently the result of anerobic and microaerophilic streptococci spreading by valveless diploic veins of Breschet. Infections after open cranial surgery are typically the result of *S. aureus*.

ISE can manifest asymptomatically but usually have the typical signs and symptoms of an infection in the central nervous system (CNS). These include fever, headache, nausea and vomiting, seizures, focal neurologic deficits, and changes in mental status. There may also be signs of meningeal irritation and/or intracranial pressure (Cushing's triad of bradycardia, bradypnea, and hypertension). A neurologic examination may reveal contralateral hemiplegia, cranial nerve palsies, anisocoria, and papilledema. The existence of an otitis or sinusitis should heighten the suspicion of ISE.

On computed tomography (CT) imaging an ISE will appear as a hypodense area over the cerebral hemisphere or along the falx. There may also be a mass effect with a midline shift. The imaging study of choice is an MRI with gadolinium enhancement, with a crescent-shaped or elliptical area of hypodensity on T1-weighted images appearing under the skull or next to the falx cerebri. Laboratory studies will tend to be consistent with the presence of an acute infection. Although sometimes considered, blood cultures are usually negative because of the capsulation of ISE. Spinal puncture is not recommended because it is not useful diagnostically and can cause serious complications because of an elevated intracranial pressure.

Intravenous antibiotic treatment started very early in the course of the disease may be successful, but in more advanced cases multiple burr holes or a craniotomy are needed to establish drainage. Pus should be sent for a rapid Gram-stain to direct initial antibiotic choices until culture and sensitivity studies have revealed the causative organism(s). After drainage and lavage, antibiotic decisions should be guided by infectious disease specialists and antibiotics are usually needed for 3 to 6 weeks. If seizures appear, antiseizure medications also may be necessary.

Encephalitis

Encephalitis represents diffuse inflammation of brain parenchyma causing clinical evidence of brain dysfunction. It is frequently due to a viral infection.[8] The distinguishing feature of encephalitis in comparison to meningitis or cerebritis is the presence of brain impairment with encephalitis. The initial symptoms of encephalitis are fever, headache, altered level of consciousness, and other signs of cerebral dysfunction.[9] If the affected individual shows signs of meningismus (headache, nuchal rigidity, photophobia), the infection has likely spread to the meninges. If the encephalitic infection also involves the meninges, the process is called meningoencephalitis. Common viral causes of encephalitis are herpes simplex virus (HSV-1 and 2), human herpesvirus

(HHV-6 being the most common), varicella-zoster virus (VZV), Epstein-Barr virus (EBV), and cytomegalovirus (CMV). Bacteria known to sometimes cause encephalitis include *Rickettsia*, *Ehrlichia*, and *Borrelia burgdorferi*. Encephalitis also may be the result of infection by fungi, protozoa, or parasites.[9]

A careful medical history and physical examination are necessary to determine the etiologic pathogens that have caused the clinical picture. Bacteria causes of encephalitis often manifest suddenly, whereas viral encephalitis commonly manifests in a more insidious manner. If there is a clinical picture of encephalitis along with cranial nerve damage, listeriosis should be strongly considered.[10] In patients presenting with encephalitis along with a cerebellar syndrome, the patient should be tested for VZV[11] (Figure 11-3). Encephalitis in the presence of respiratory problems make consideration of possible tuberculosis (TB), mycoplasma, or adenovirus infection.[10] Other important clues to the causative agent include season of the year (e.g., mosquito season suggests arboviruses), geography (e.g., being in a western state such as California or Arizona may indicate West Nile virus),[12] and animal exposure (e.g., an animal bite can lead to suspicion of rabies). A physical examination can help differentiate the cause of encephalitis. The coexistence of parotitis suggests mumps, vesicles in a dermatomal pattern suggests VZV, and flaccid paralysis evolving into encephalitis suggests West Nile virus.[13] Determining the cause of the encephalitis is necessary to provide proper treatment.

Initial testing in patients with suspected encephalitis includes a complete blood cell count, complete metabolic profile, coagulation studies, blood cultures, LP (for CSF for glucose, protein, and culture), HSV polymerase chain reaction (PCR), electroencephalogram (EEG), and magnetic resonance imaging (MRI) or CT with and without contrast.[8] Imaging can also help determine the cause of encephalitis such as with HSV encephalitis that often begins in the anterior part of the temporal lobe and extends to the inferior orbital cortex, the cingulate gyrus, and the insula.[10]

Care for encephalitis should be targeted at the causative agent; however, sometimes patients with acute viral encephalitis empirically receive acyclovir to treat herpes simplex viral encephalitis until diagnostic testing (imaging and PCR of the CSF) proves a different cause.[14] For most other causes, care is mostly supportive.[14] General supportive care includes management of elevated intracranial pressure with intravenous mannitol and/or steroids, anticonvulsants if seizures are occurring, and correction of fluid and electrolyte imbalances.[15]

Serious complications of encephalitis include increased intracranial pressure, cerebral venous thrombosis, cerebral infarction, syndrome of inappropriate antidiuretic hormone (SIADH), and disseminated intravascular coagulation, requiring intensive care unit monitoring. Long-term sequelae of encephalitis include behavioral and speech disorders, poor concentration, and memory loss.[14]

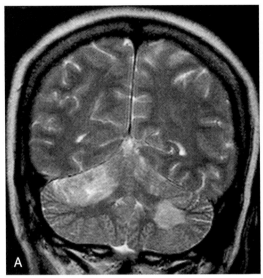
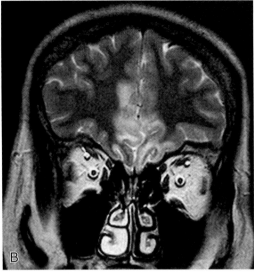

• **Figure 11-3** Varicella-Zoster Virus Encephalitis. Coronal T2-weighted images passing through occipital **(A)** and frontal **(B)** lobes show cortical gray and subcortical white matter involvement of cerebellum and frontal lobes. (From Bulakbasi N, Kocaoglu M. Central nervous system infections of herpesvirus family. *Neuroimag Clin North Am.* 2008;18[1]:53-84.)

Rhombencephalitis

Rhombencephalitis (RE) refers to an inflammatory disease of the rhombencephalon (hindbrain). It is usually due to an infection, but an autoimmune disorder or paraneoplastic syndrome also can be the cause. Three quarters of cases first appear with a cranial nerve palsy. RE also can cause cerebellar ataxia and an altered level of consciousness.

Listeria monocytogenes (Figure 11-4) is the most frequent infectious cause of RE. Listerial RE usually affects immunocompetent patients, manifesting with prodromal headache, nausea, vomiting, fever, and malaise lasting for 1 to 15 days, leading to brainstem dysfunction. This presents with unilateral cranial nerve deficiency (CN VII most commonly), and is often accompanied by ipsilateral long tract signs, cerebellar deficits, and respiratory failure. Serial CSF cultures are the most specific diagnostic test. MRI signs of RE consist of increased signal intensity in the rhombencephalon and upper cervical cord, with some cases also showing ring-enhancing abscesses on T2-weighted and fluid attenuation inversion recovery (FLAIR) sequences. Administration of antibiotics early in the clinical course helps reduce the mortality rate of 20 and 30%; 55% of recovered patients will continue to have neurologic sequelae.

Viral causes of RE include enterovirus 71 (EV71) and, less commonly, HSV. Epidemics of EV71 have occurred regularly in the Asian-Pacific and, more recently, in European countries. Patients with EV71, typically children and adolescents, present with RE, hand-foot-and-mouth disease, and pulmonary edema. Neurologic signs and symptoms include myoclonic jerks, tremors, ataxia, CN palsies, coma, and, eventually, respiratory failure. Patients with HSV present with neuro-ophthalmologic symptoms and other CN deficits, with occasional cases

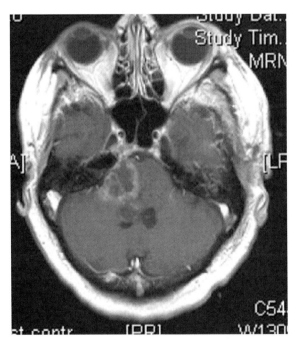

• **Figure 11-4** Magnetic Resonance Image of a Patient with *Listeria Monocytogenes* Rhombencephalitis. Patient's symptoms included facial numbness, peripheral facial weakness, and rapid obtundation. (From Pruitt AA. Neurologic infectious disease emergencies. *Neuro Clin.* 2012;30[1]:129-159.)

showing inflammation of the temporal and/or frontal lobes. The diagnosis is made with CSF analysis, MRI, and virus isolation, if possible. There is no well-accepted therapy for EV71, although there is anecdotal support for the use of IV immunoglobulin. For HSV, treatment with acyclovir reduces mortality.

Cerebritis

Cerebritis is an area of brain parenchyma with poorly demarcated acute inflammation accompanied by increased local vascular permeability. Without intervention, these pockets of disease progress to brain abscesses in 10 to 15 days. There are two stages of cerebritis. The first stage is characterized by neutrophil accumulation, edema, and tissue necrosis; the second stage shows an accumulation of lymphocytes and macrophages. A fibrous wall forms walling off an abscess cavity.

There are three routes of infection leading to cerebritis. First, accounting for 25 to 50% of cases, is the spread of an infection from a pericranial nidus such as the middle ear, paranasal sinus, or the mouth. The second, occurring in 15 to 30% of cases, is hematogenous spread from a distant infectious source. Direct exposure of brain parenchyma from trauma or surgery is the third source of infection causing cerebritis, accounting for 8 to 19% of cases. *Streptococcus* is cultured in 70% of the bacterial brain abscesses. Other bacterial causes depend on location of origin. Brain abscesses (covered more completely in the next section) are more common in men than women and occur most often in elderly or pediatric male patients. Symptoms of brain abscesses are nonspecific and include headache and severe pain near the lesion, with focal neurologic deficiency and fever seen in about 50% of patients. MRI is preferred to CT for diagnosis because it is especially sensitive for picking up early cerebritis. Cerebritis is treated with appropriate antibiotics. Surgical drainage is commonly indicated once cerebritis has progressed to the abscess stage.

Brain Abscess

A brain abscess is a collection of purulence located within the brain parenchyma (Figure 11-5). They most commonly

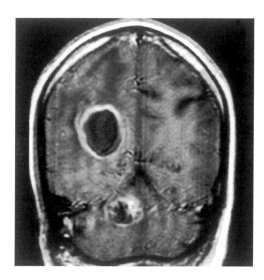

• **Figure 11-5** Brain Abscess of Invasive Aspergillosis with Ring Enhancement and Extensive Edema. (From Bennett JE, Dolin R, Blaser MJ. *Mandell, Douglas, and Bennett's Principles and Practice of Infectious Diseases.* 8th ed. Philadelphia: Saunders; 2015.)

arise from contiguous spread from a sinus abscess, otitis media, or a dental infection.[16] They can also be derived by hematogenous spread from chronic pulmonary infections, intraabdominal infection, or endocarditis.[16] Contamination after surgery or trauma also can occur, but is less common. Patients who are immunocompromised, have pulmonary arteriovenous malformations, or have congenital heart malformations are predisposed to brain abscesses.[6] These abscesses develop from a later stage of cerebritis and white matter edema that eventually encapsulates into the abscess. The causal pathogen depends on the infectious source. For patients with paranasal sinus infections, and lung infections or those with congenital cardiac malformations, *Streptococcus* species are the most likely cause. Viridans streptococci and *S. aureus* are the most common causes in patients with bacterial endocarditis. In patients with penetrating head trauma or a recent neurosurgical intervention, *S. aureus, Streptococcus* species, *P. aeruginosa,* and *Enterobacter* are the most common causes of brain abscesses. Brain abscesses tend to manifest in the first three decades of life.[17]

Although there are a variety of presentations for brain abscesses, the classic one is a patient with an isolated mass syndrome with signs of intracranial hypertension (headache, nausea, vomiting), seizures, and progressive neurologic deficit. The pain typically localizes to the side of the abscess and can be either sudden or gradual in onset. Frontal lobe abscesses, however, can present with no signs or symptoms early in their development. Abscesses in the cerebellum may cause cranial-nerve palsy, gait disorder, or hydrocephalus with headache or altered mental status.[18] Importantly, cardinal signs of infections, such as fever, are not consistently present in patients with brain abscesses.

Brain CT with contrast is a valuable initial diagnostic tool, providing rapid data showing the location, size, number of abscesses, and mass effects, shifts, and the presence of intraventricular rupture.[17] Although contrast-enhanced MRI can be more sensitive, it is not as helpful in the acute setting. Classically, the CT of a patient with a brain abscess shows a thick and diffuse ring-enhancing lesion(s) after contrast injection.[17] Yet, in the early cerebritis stage of the infection, it may only show an irregular area of low density that demonstrates poor enhancement following contrast injection.[19] In addition, once the abscess has matured and becomes encapsulated, the contrast studies will likely show a thin ring, which may or may not have uniform thickness. Early use of CT has dramatically lowered the mortality of this of brain abscesses.

Once a brain abscess has been identified, antibiotics should be started promptly along with neurosurgical intervention. If the disease is severe and the patient is clinically unstable, or surgery cannot be performed in a few hours antibiotics should be given empirically.[16] If the causal organism is unknown, all abscesses greater than 1 cm in diameter should be aspirated to determine the causal organism to help guide medical treatment.[16] If the causal organism is known, treatment depends on the size and extent of the lesion. Small abscesses (lesions <2.5 cm) and lesions in the cerebritis phase tend to respond well to medical therapy alone (i.e., appropriate antibiotics and symptom management).[20] In the face of multiple abscesses, the largest one should be aspirated and antibiotics should be subsequently administered along with weekly CT scans to monitor the size of the abscess.[20] Craniotomy and excision also should be done for abscesses that continue to grow after 2 weeks of antibiotic therapy, that fail to shrink after 3 to 4 weeks of antibiotics, that are larger than 2.5 cm on presentation, that are multiloculated on presentation, or that are large with significant mass effect.[16,17] Also, excision of all cerebellar abscesses is recommended. In either situation, total excision of the abscess is not required; however, it should be considered in those that are superficial, are not located in eloquent brain tissue, and/or are caused by fungi or TB.[16]

Neurocysticercosis

Neurocysticercosis (Figure 11-6) is an infection of the brain parenchyma caused by the larval form of *Taenia solium*. It is the most common parasitic infection of the CNS, affecting approximately 2.5 million people worldwide. It is most prevalent in the northern coast of Africa, India, and southern Africa.[21] It is acquired by ingesting eggs of *T. solium* shed in the stool of a human tapeworm carrier, such as pork, although people who do not eat pork can auto-infect themselves through ano-oral contamination. After ingesting

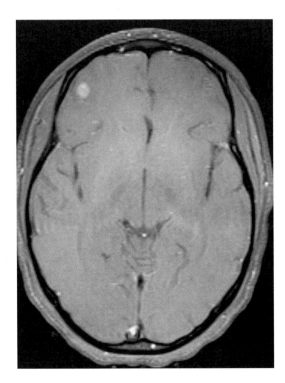

• **Figure 11-6** Neurocysticercosis in a 13-Year-Old Immigrant from Africa. Patient presented with seizures. Fairly homogeneous solid enhancement identified in the right frontal lobe on a postcontrast spin echo T1-weighted image. (From Dahmoush HM, Vossough A, Roberts TPL. Pediatric high-field magnetic resonance imaging. *Neuroimag Clin North Am.* 2012;22[2]:297-313.)

the cysts, the embryos can spread hematogenously to various areas of the body and form cysts. Depending on where the cysts are located in the brain, there are different presenting symptoms. In general, if the cysts are located in the brain parenchyma, patients present with seizures and headache, while patients with extraparenchymal cysts present with signs of elevated intracranial pressure or hydrocephalus along with altered mental status.[22] To confirm clinical suspicion of the disease, imaging and serodiagnosis are used. With respect to imaging, CT provides the best detection of parenchymal calcification, although MRI is most sensitive for detecting cysts in the ventricles.[23] For a serodiagnosis, the most reliable immunologic test that is currently available is the enzyme-linked immunoelectrotransfer blot (EITB), which can detect antibodies to *T. solium* cysts.[22] Treatment consists of albendazole or praziquantel, and possibly seizure medications if the patient presents with seizures.[22] Surgery is reserved for patients with complicated disease. Endoscopic procedures are used to remove free intraventricular cysts. If endoscopic efforts are not successful, ventriculoperitoneal (VP) shunts are the treatment of choice in patients with obstruction of the ventricular system and hydrocephalus. Additionally, large cysts with scolex in the interior should be completely removed.[6]

Prion Diseases

Prion diseases are rare and unusual, due to the fact that the causal pathogen is an abnormal, mutated form of a cellular protein that resists proteolysis. On interacting with normal proteins, this abnormal protein can induce a conformation change that propagates the formation of more abnormal proteins. This, combined with their resistance to proteolysis, causes an accumulation of prion proteins in neurons. Although the underlying mechanisms are not completely elucidated, this eventually leads to neuronal death. These diseases are known for having incubation periods upward of several decades.

Kuru, a form of prion disease endemic to Papua New Guinea, is thought to be transmitted from person to person through now-ceased practices of ritual cannibalism. New cases have been identified as recently as 2004; they are thought to have had over a 50-year incubation period. Kuru occurs in well-defined stages. The early stage is characterized by tremors, ataxia, and postural instability. The sedentary stage follows, with a loss of ambulation from worsening of symptoms, and the appearance of involuntary movements. Dementia occurs in the late stage of the disease, and patients usually die from pneumonia 9 to 24 months after onset.

Creutzfeldt-Jakob disease (CJD), another form of prion disease, occurs in several forms. The iatrogenic form, discussed here, has occurred after a variety of procedures, such as administration of human pituitary hormones from cadaveric origins, dural graft transplants, liver transplants, and the use of contaminated neurosurgical instruments or deep implantation electrodes. Iatrogenic transmission of CJD is thought to be under control currently; however, cases still occur and, similar to kuru, are likely to be due to very long incubation periods. CJD classically manifests with rapid, progressive mental deterioration and myoclonus. Brain biopsy is the gold standard for diagnosis. Unfortunately, there is no known effective treatment, and death occurs within a year of symptom onset.

Progressive Multifocal Leukoencephalopathy

Progressive multifocal leukoencephalopathy (PML) (Figure 11-7), an opportunistic infection, involves demyelination of the CNS instigated by a reactivation (asymptomatic primary infection occurring in childhood) of the polyomavirus JC (JC virus). In severely immunocompromised individuals, the virus can reactivate and spread to the CNS, where it causes an infection characterized by lysis of oligodendrocytes. The prevalence of PML in the population with HIV/AIDS is estimated at 5%. PML classically manifests with subacute neurologic deficits such as altered mental status, neuro-ophthalmologic symptoms, hemiparesis, ataxia, and occasionally seizures. Neuroimaging results will appear with multifocal lesions spread across multiple vascular territories, without contrast enhancement or mass effect. Despite being considered the gold standard of diagnosis, brain biopsy carries significant morbidity and mortality in these populations.

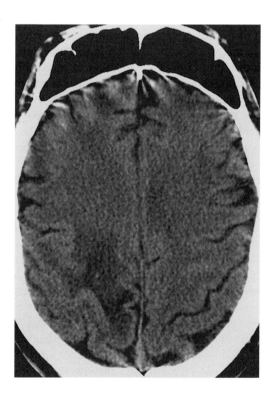

• **Figure 11-7** Computed Tomography Appearance Showing a Hypodense Lesion Typical of Progressive Multifocal Leukoencephalopathy Involving the Subcortical White Matter in the Right Posterior Frontal Lobe. The overlying cortex is not involved and there is no mass effect. (From Shah R, Bag AK, Chapman PR, et al. Imaging manifestations of progressive multifocal leukoencephalopathy. *Clin Radiol.* 2010;65[6]:431-439.)

Taking context and presentation into account, a reliable diagnosis often can be made with CSF analysis. No definitive treatment approach exists for PML. The main goal of treatment is to restore immunocompetency.

Immunosuppression-Related Infections

Toxoplasmic Encephalitis

Toxoplasma gondii is an intracellular protozoan parasite that can be present asymptomatically in immunocompetent patients. Infection is often acquired through ingestion of food and water that are contaminated with oocysts shed by cats or by eating undercooked or raw meat containing tissue cysts. In immunocompromised people, the parasite can reactivate and lead to infection, which most commonly manifests as cerebral abscesses. Toxoplasmic abscesses are characterized by a necrotic center with surrounding inflammation.[10] The clinical course of neurocysticercosis can range from an insidious course developing over a few weeks to acute confusional state with or without focal neurologic deficits.[24] Other manifestations of this disease process include cranial nerve disturbances, sensory abnormalities, movement disorders, and cerebellar signs.[24]

It is important to screen for *T. gondii* in patients with newly diagnosed HIV because toxoplasmic encephalitis is commonly observed in patients who have a latent infection with *T. gondii*.[25] If a patient with newly diagnosed HIV tests positive for *Toxoplasma* immunoglobulin G (IgG) and there is a CD4 count of less than 100 cells/μL, the patient should be started on trimethoprim-sulfamethoxazole (TMP-SMX) prophylaxis. In patients with toxoplasmic encephalitis, an "eccentric target sign" is seen on postcontrast T1-weighted imaging, although a "concentric target sign" with areas of hyperintensity and hypointensity on T2-weighted imaging is more specific for cerebral toxoplasmosis.[26] Often, these lesions show evidence of edema. Although definitive diagnosis requires a brain biopsy, it has been shown that the combination of oral sulfadiazine and pyrimethamine is effective when the clinical picture (CD4 cell count <100, seropositivity for *T. gondii* IgG antibody, patient has not been receiving effective prophylaxis for *Toxoplasma*) and imaging suggest infection with *T. gondii*.[27] If the patient does not improve with treatment, a brain biopsy should be performed to rule out CNS lymphoma.[27]

Cytomegalovirus Encephalitis

HIV-associated CMV is an uncommon complication of late-stage AIDS that has decreased in incidence because of the institution of highly active antiretroviral therapy (HAART). This disease process often occurs in patients with a CD4 count below 100 cells/mm^3 and results from hematogenous spread of CMV.[28] People are often infected in an immunocompetent state; once the host becomes immunocompromised, such as in AIDS, the virus becomes reactivated. CMV infection can lead to multiple CNS manifestations. It can cause focal parenchymal necrosis, microglial nodules of the gray or white matter, or ventriculoencephalitis, with focal or diffuse destruction of the ependymal lining and periventricular tissue.[29] Patients with CNS disease tend to present with an altered mental status that may be confused with HIV dementia. The diagnosis of CMV encephalitis requires detection of pp65 antigen in leukocytes and can be further confirmed with CSF analysis showing an elevated protein level and mononuclear leukocytosis, as well as PCR of CMV present in the CSF.[30-32] A CT or MRI of the cerebral hemisphere and brainstem showing encephalitis or ventriculitis helps to confirm the diagnosis. Once the diagnosis of CMV encephalitis has been made, patients should be started on an aggressive course of ganciclovir or foscarnet because the prognosis of the disease is only about 50%, even with antiretroviral therapy.[32]

Tuberculous Meningitis

TB is a mycobacterial infection that continues to increase in incidence globally. Although there are three categories of CNS TB (tuberculous meningitis, intracranial tuberculoma, and spinal tuberculous arachnoiditis), the most severe extrapulmonary manifestation of TB is tuberculous meningitis, which has a high mortality rate and leaves many of the survivors with chronic neurologic sequelae.[33] There are multiple ways in which TB may reach the meninges. In one model, a tuberculous focus may form in the meninges, subpial, or subependymal region of the brain and later rupture into the subarachnoid space or ventricular system, leading to meningitis.[34] In another model, the meninges may be secondarily involved as a result of rupture of a tuberculoma into a vessel in the subarachnoid space.[34] Once the tuberculous focus has reached the subarachnoid space, it forms a thick, gelatinous, inflammatory exudate, which can lead to hydrocephalus, cerebral infarction, or, in rare cases, abscesses. Patients with tuberculous meningitis can present in one of three stages. During stage I, patients are lucid and have no focal neurologic signs. Patients in stage II exhibit lethargy and confusion and may show mild focal neurologic signs such as cranial nerve palsy or hemiparesis. Finally, in stage III, patients present with delirium, stupor, coma, seizures, multiple cranial nerve palsies, and/or dense hemiplegia.[35] Often the course of tuberculous meningitis is chronic. Because it does not usually manifest with the classic meningitis picture, there should be a high index of suspicion in certain patient populations, such as those that are immunocompromised. It is important for this infectious process to be recognized early because clinical outcome is greatly dependent on the stage at which treatment is started. Diagnosis of TB includes both an analysis of the CSF and radiologic testing. CSF analysis consists of culture and sensitivity for *Mycobacterium tuberculosis*. Contrast-enhanced MRI is the superior imaging technique in evaluating patients with tuberculous meningitis. It can show meningeal thickening of the peripontine, perimesencephalic cisterns and sylvian fissures. Meningeal thickening is often accompanied by dilation of the third and lateral ventricles.[34] Treatment of the disease requires four-drug therapy: isoniazid, rifampin, pyrazinamide, and a fluoroquinolone (either moxifloxacin or levofloxacin).[33] Patients with hydrocephalus may require surgical decompression of the ventricular system.[6]

Cryptococcal Meningitis

Cryptococcus is an encapsulated saprophytic yeast that is spread by aerosolized spores, which can disseminate to the CNS, leading to meningitis. *Cryptococcus neoformans* causes meningitis in immunocompromised people as a result of impaired cell-mediated immunity. Cryptococcal meningitis is particularly prevalent in Southeast Asia and East Africa.[36] Patients usually present with subacute headache, fever, malaise, and altered mental status of several weeks duration. Notably, the "classic" features of meningitis (e.g., neck stiffness) are not as prevalent.[37] Ocular symptoms, such as papilledema and uveitis with multifocal chorioretinitis, are relatively common signs of cryptococcal meningitis.[37] The diagnosis of cryptococcal meningitis is done with India ink preparations of CSF and cryptococcal antigen testing of the blood.[36] Radiologic confirmation of the disease is not necessary but is useful in detecting the complications of the disease. Flucytosine and amphotericin B remain the mainstay of induction therapy for immunocompromised patients.[38] Furthermore, aggressive management of raised CSF pressure associated with this infection is an important part of management and usually requires serial LP and occasionally placement of a shunt.[38] Because of the poor prognosis, prevention programs are vital to the management of immunocompromised patients who are at risk for contracting this organism. One prevention program aims to treat patients with asymptomatic antigenemia, while another program aims at treating all patients who have a CD4 count of below 100 cells/μL with fluconazole.[38] Unfortunately, both programs have shown varying efficacy and the search for an effective prevention program remains elusive.

References

1. Srinivas D, Veena Kumari HB, Somanna S, et al. The incidence of postoperative meningitis in neurosurgery: an institutional experience. *Neurol India.* 2011;59(2):195.
2. Morris A, Low DE. Nosocomial bacterial meningitis, including central nervous system shunt infections. *Infect Dis Clin North Am.* 1999;13(3):735-750.
3. Korinek AM, Baugnon T, Golmard JL, et al. Risk factors for adult nosocomial meningitis after craniotomy role of antibiotic prophylaxis. Neurosurgery. 2006;58(7):126–133.
4. Longo DL, Harrison TR Harrison's Principles of Internal Medicine. New York: McGraw-Hill Education; 2022. 21st ed.
5. Weisfelt M, Van De Beek D, Spanjaard L, et al. Nosocomial bacterial meningitis in adults: a prospective series of 50 cases. *J Hosp Infect.* 2007;66(1):71-78.

6. Heth JA. Neurosurgical aspects of central nervous system infections. *Neuroimag Clin North Am*. 2012;22(4):791-799.

7. Pfister HW, Feiden W, Einhaupl KM. Spectrum of complications during bacterial meningitis in adults: results of a prospective clinical study. *Arch Neurol*. 1993;50(6):575-581.

8. Simon DW, Da Silva YS, Zuccoli G, et al. Acute encephalitis. *Crit Care Clin*. 2013;29(2):259-277.

9. Bloch KC, Glaser C. Diagnostic approaches for patients with suspected encephalitis. *Curr Infect Dis Rep*. 2007;9(4):315-322.

10. Sarrazin JL, Bonneville F, Martin-Blondel G. Brain infections. *Diag Intervent Imag*. 2012;93(6):473-490.

11. Whitley RJ. Viral encephalitis. *N Engl J Med*. 1990;323(4):242-250.

12. Hayes EB, Komar N, Nasci RS, et al. Epidemiology and transmission dynamics of West Nile virus disease. *Emerg Infect Dis*. 2005;11(8):1167-1173.

13. Gray TJ, Webb CE. A review of the epidemiological and clinical aspects of West Nile virus. *Int J Gen Med*. 2014;7:193-203.

14. Chaudhuri A. Diagnosis and treatment of viral encephalitis. *Postgrad Med J*. 2002;78(924):575-583.

15. Kennedy PGE. Viral encephalitis. *J Neurol*. 2005;252(3):268-272.

16. Brouwer MC, Tunkel AR, McKhann GM, et al. Brain abscess. *N Engl J Med*. 2014;317(18):1756-1758.

17. Quintana LM. Brain abscess: aspiration versus excision. *World Neurosurg*. 2011;76(5):388-389.

18. Shaw MD, Russell JA. Cerebellar abscess. a review of 47 cases. *J Neurol Neurosurg Psych*. 1975;38(5):429-435.

19. Britt RH, Dieter R, Enzmann DR. Clinical stages of human brain abscesses on serial CT scans after contrast infusion. *J Neurosurg*. 1983;59(6):972-989.

20. Moorthy RK, Rajshekar V. Management of brain abscess: an overview. *Neurosurg Focus*. 2008;24:1-6.

21. Zymberg ST. Neurocysticercosis. *World Neurosurg*. 2013;79(2):S24.e5-S24.e8.

22. Coyle CM, Tanowitz HB. Diagnosis and treatment of neurocysticercosis. *Interdiscip Perspect Infect Dis*. 2009;2009:1-9.

23. Sehgal R, Goyal K, Mewara A. Neurocysticercosis: a disease of neglect. *Tropic Parasitol*. 2013;3(2):106.

24. Montoya JG, Liesenfeld O. Toxoplasmosis. *Lancet*. 2004;363(9425):1965-1976.

25. Yan J, Huang B, Liu G, et al. Meta-analysis of prevention and treatment of toxoplasmic encephalitis in HIV-infected patients. *Acta Tropica*. 2013;127(3):236-244.

26. Mahadevan A, Ramalingaiah AH, Parthasarathy S, et al. Neuropathological correlate of the "concentric target sign" in MRI of HIV-associated cerebral toxoplasmosis. *J Magnet Res Imag*. 2013;38(2):488-495.

27. Luft BJ, Hafner R, Korzun AH, et al. Toxoplasmic encephalitis in patients with the acquired immunodeficiency syndrome. *N Engl J Med*. 1993;329(14):995-1000.

28. Springer KL, Weinberg A. Cytomegalovirus infection in the era of HAART: fewer reactivations and more immunity. *J Antimicrob Chemo*. 2004;54(3):582-586.

29. Arribas JR, Storce GA, Clifford DB, et al. Cytomegalovirus encephalitis. *Ann Intern Med*. 1996;125(7):577.

30. Debiasi RL, Kleinschmidt-Demasters BK, Weinberg A, et al. Use of PCR for the diagnosis of herpesvirus infections of the central nervous system. *J Clin Virol*. 2002;25:5-11.

31. Castagnola E, Cappelli B, Erba D, et al. Cytomegalovirus infection after bone marrow transplantation in children. *Hum Immunol*. 2004;65(5):416-422.

32. Kirubakaran SI. Update: cytomegalovirus infection in HIV-infected patients: a review. *Clin Microbiol News*. 2004;26(18):137-144.

33. Van T, Farrrar J. Tuberculous meningitis. *J Epidemiologic Comm Health*. 2013;8:195-196.

34. Patkar D, Narang J, Yanamandala R, et al. Central nervous system tuberculosis. *Neuroimag Clin North Am*. 2012;22(4):677-705.

35. Kent SJ, Crowe SM, Yung A, et al. Tuberculous meningitis: a 30-year review. *Clin Infect Dis*. 1993;7(6):987-994.

36. Bicanic T, Harrison TS. Cryptococcal meningitis. *Br Med Bull*. 2005;72(1):99-118.

37. Sloan DJ, Parris V. Cryptococcal meningitis: epidemiology and therapeutic options. *Clin Epidemiol*. 2014;6:169-182.

38. Jarvis JN, Dromer F, Harrison TS, et al. Managing cryptococcosis in the immunocompromised host. *Curr Opin Infect Dis*. 2008;21(6):596-603.

12
Orbital Infections

KATHERINE ZAMECKI-VEDDER

Orbital infections are among the most serious of all infections of the face. This is due to the possibility of the infectious process affecting the critical sense of vision, as well as to the close proximity to, and ease of spread, of the infection to the central nervous system (CNS). This chapter will discuss the cause, diagnosis, and management of infections of the orbit. Primary emphasis will be on bacterial infection, with some mention made of fungal infections affecting the orbit.

Bacterial Orbital Cellulitis

Of all the infectious processes involving the orbit, bacterial infection is by far the most common variety encountered clinically. Bacterial infection involving the tissues posterior to the orbital septum is categorized as orbital cellulitis. Orbital cellulitis should be differentiated from preseptal cellulitis, which is a superficial infection limited to the eyelids and arising most commonly from skin infection (e.g., a secondarily infected hordeolum, insect bite), penetrating trauma (e.g., surgery), or foreign body. A patient with preseptal cellulitis may have significant erythema, edema and induration of the eyelids, and mechanical ptosis, but will have a white and quiet eye with full ocular motility. In contrast, orbital cellulitis involves the retroseptal structures and will often result in chemosis (fluid accumulation under the conjunctiva), ophthalmoplegia, axial or nonaxial proptosis, and elevated orbital and/or intraocular pressure (Figures 12-1 and 12-2). Patients will typically have more pain and will appear more toxic.

Orbital cellulitis requires urgent attention because it can lead to blindness, significant morbidity, or death if untreated or undertreated. It must be recognized and treated early with appropriate antibiotic therapy, typically in a hospital setting and with close monitoring for involvement of the visual system.

Most cases of orbital cellulitis arise from an endogenous source, such as the adjacent paranasal sinuses, with the ethmoid sinuses being the most commonly involved. Infection also can occur secondary to trauma (including surgical trauma),[1,2] acute dacryocystitis (Figures 12-3 and 12-4), extension of a dental abscess, intraorbital foreign body, and metastatic seeding from an underlying septicemia. There are several reasons why infection can spread readily to the orbit. These include the paper-thin lamina papyracea separating the orbit from the adjacent ethmoid sinuses and anastomosis of the ophthalmic venous system with that of the facial, pterygoid, and cranial venous systems. In addition, the orbit lacks lymphatic tissue by which to drain infectious material. Only a minority of cases of orbital cellulitis develop an intraorbital abscess, but this is a feared complication and always requires surgical drainage (Figures 12-5 and 12-6). An abscess should always be considered if the patient is failing to improve on appropriate antibiotic therapy. Identification on an abscess requires orbital imaging with contrast.

A subperiosteal abscess (SPA) can be a complication of orbital cellulitis in children and adults. It occurs most commonly in the setting of acute bacterial sinusitis. SPA is seen more commonly in the pediatric population, most likely because of the thicker, more elastic nature of the periosteum in the pediatric orbit. When purulent material from the adjacent sinuses (most commonly the ethmoids) traverses the thin lamina papyracea, it will accumulate in the potential space under the periosteum, causing a characteristic convex, enhancing opacity on orbital imaging (Figure 12-7). SPA occurs in approximately 15% of cases of pediatric orbital cellulitis and can result in various visual sequelae in 15% to 30% of these patients.[3] It is most common along the medial orbital wall and will result in nonaxial proptosis and impaired gaze toward the side of the abscess (e.g., adduction deficit because of more medial SPA).

The microbiology of SPA may depend on the age of the patient, as demonstrated by Harris in his multiple retrospective reviews of immunocompetent patients with SPA.[4-7] Patients younger than 9 years more often have monomicrobial infections and often have negative culture results. Patients older than 9 years often have polymicrobial infections and anaerobic organisms on culture. This is thought to explain why younger children may respond better to conservative management with intravenous antibiotics alone. Harris' 2015 updated review of the microbiology of surgically drained SPA showed an increase in all of the following microbes: methicillin-resistant *Staphylococcus aureus* (MRSA), *S. aureus, Staphylococcus anginosus,* and group A β-hemolytic *Streptococcus,* compared to the microbiologic findings of the originally studied cohort of patients from

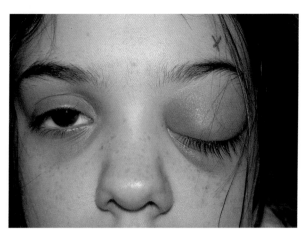

• **Figure 12-1** Left Orbital Cellulitis with Significant Erythema and Edema of the Eyelids. There is mechanical ptosis.

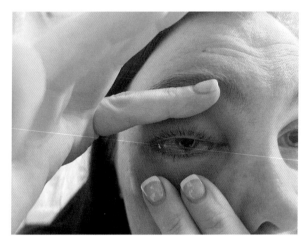

• **Figure 12-2** Right Orbital Cellulitis Demonstrating Diffuse Conjunctival Chemosis.

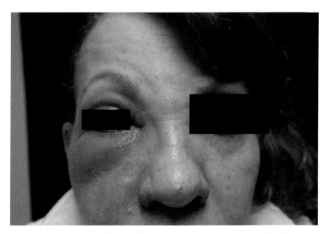

• **Figure 12-3** Clinical Color Photograph of a Patient with Right Orbital Cellulitis Secondary to Acute Dacryocystitis. Note the significant induration, erythema and edema of the periocular tissues. There is mechanical ptosis of the right upper eyelid.

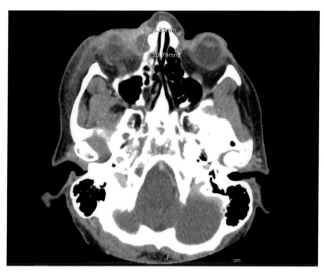

• **Figure 12-4** Axial Contrast-Enhanced CT Image Demonstrating a Well-Circumscribed, Enhancing Lesion in the Right Lacrimal Sac Fossa, Consistent with an Abscess.

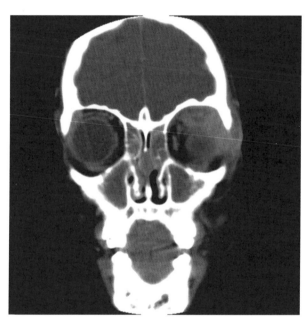

• **Figure 12-5** Coronal Computed Tomographic Scan with Contrast Showing a Loculated, Enhancing Mass in the Superior Orbit Consistent with an Abscess.

1977 to 1992.[7] These findings, however, did not alter the triage and management paradigm for SPA (discussed later) established in 1994.

Management of SPA should be guided by factors such as size of the abscess, location within the orbit, anticipated microbiology based on age of the patient and history, and visual status of the patient.[5] Management strategies fall into three categories: expectant observation, urgent (within 24 hours) surgical drainage, and emergent (as soon as possible) surgical drainage.[4-7] If the abscess is small, along the medial orbital wall, and occurring in a patient younger than 9 years and there is no visual compromise, broad-spectrum intravenous antibiotics with close observation often may be adequate therapy. Some of these patients may still require surgical intervention. Prompt surgical drainage should be considered if and when there is visual deterioration (e.g., development of a relative afferent pupillary defect, decreased vision, decreased color vision), the patient fails to improve on the appropriate antibiotic therapy, or the patient worsens

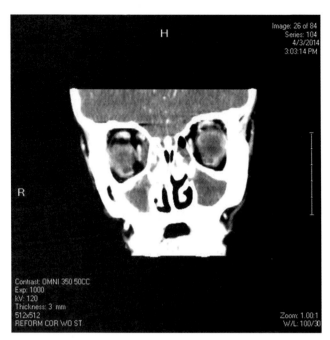

• **Figure 12-6** Coronal Computed Tomographic Scan with Contrast Showing a Subperiosteal Abscess Along the Right Medial Orbital Wall. Note the significant opacification of the bilateral maxillary and ethmoid sinuses.

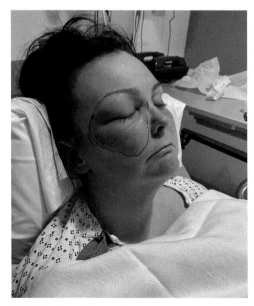

• **Figure 12-7** An Area of Induration.

clinically. If the abscess is large, the source of infection (e.g., dental origin) or age of the patient suggests a polymicrobial anaerobic infection, presence of gas on computed tomography (CT) images suggests anaerobic cause, there is evidence of frontal sinusitis, the abscess is not along the medial orbital wall, there is evidence of chronic sinus disease (e.g., polyps), the abscess has reaccumulated after prior surgical drainage, or there is any evidence on examination of visual compromise, urgent surgical drainage is necessary to minimize permanent visual complications and other potentially devastating complications. Surgical drainage can be accomplished endoscopically or by external incision. The

technique used will be dictated by the location of the abscess and the patient's underlying anatomy. A retrospective chart review from 2011 by Dewan et al[8] found that for abscesses larger than 2 cm in greatest diameter, combined abscess and sinus drainage led to no abscess reaccumulation and shorter hospitalization (as opposed to abscess drainage alone).

There are no universally accepted guidelines regarding treatment, and each case must be approached independently. Some small children with SPA will require surgical drainage. Likewise, some older children may respond to conservative management. Recognition of the typically less aggressive nature of the infection in children younger than 9 years and this group's general success with medical management alone, is critical in reducing the morbidity associated with unnecessary surgery. What remains most important is the prompt and accurate recognition of any visual compromise or other serious complications, such as intracranial spread. A case-by-case and cooperative approach among ophthalmologists, otolaryngologists, and sometimes neurosurgeons is often necessary.

Microbiology

The most common causative organisms in orbital cellulitis are *Staphylococcus* and *Streptococcus* species. Less common causative agents include *H. influenzae* type B (HiB), *Pseudomonas, Klebsiella, Enterococcus, Peptostreptococcus, Fusobacterium,* and *Bacteroides* species.[9-12] Since the advent of the HiB vaccine in 1985, *H. influenzae* has gone from being the most common causative pathogen in pediatric orbital cellulitis to an infrequent cause.[13] With recent expanded use of *Streptococcus pneumoniae* vaccination in children, a similar downtrend may be observed for this organism.

In recent years, there has been an increased incidence of orbital cellulitis cases caused by MRSA.[14-17] In a retrospective review of pediatric orbital cellulitis cases, 36% of positive cultures yielded MRSA.[12] The rising incidence of a variety of MRSA infections is of public health concern because of the limited number of effective antibiotics presently available. MRSA periocular infections also may have a poorer outcome. Rutar et al[17] reported a case of bilateral blindness resulting from orbital cellulitis caused by community-acquired MRSA. In a small retrospective review of 15 cases of culture-positive MRSA orbital cellulitis, Mathias et al[18] found that eyelid swelling was the predominant presenting sign, there was a low incidence of concomitant paranasal sinus disease (17% in the pediatric group, 22% in the adult group), there was a high percentage of lacrimal gland abscesses in the pediatric group (typically a rare finding in orbital cellulitis), 27% of cases demonstrated multiple orbital abscesses, and 27% of patients had a final visual acuity of light perception or worse.[18] This was a small, retrospective study and larger studies are needed, but the authors concluded that MRSA orbital cellulitis should be suspected when there is a lack of associated paranasal sinus disease, there is a lack of antecedent trauma or upper respiratory tract infection, and there are multiple orbital abscesses. Treatment consists of appropriate antibiotic coverage and surgical intervention for the abscesses.

Rarely, group A β-hemolytic *Streptococcus* can cause necrotizing fasciitis of the periocular area. Necrotizing fasciitis of the head and neck region is rare (accounting for 10% of cases) but can result in significant morbidity, including blindness.[19] Infection can occur in healthy or chronically ill patients and after minor trauma or surgery. Necrotizing fasciitis of the eyelids is even less common and has a mortality of 10%.[20] It can involve the bilateral periocular area, and it has been described as occurring after blepharoplasty and dacryocystorhinostomy.[20] Elner et al[21] describe seven cases of periocular necrotizing fasciitis; six of the patients developed blindness in one eye. The most common reason for loss of vision was central retinal artery occlusion. Necrotizing fasciitis should be suspected when there is rapid spread of infection and cyanosis of the tissues. Patients usually need systemic monitoring because of the high level of concomitant septic shock. Treatment is with systemic antibiotic treatment and surgical debridement. The amount of debridement will depend on the level of involvement by the infection. Sometimes multiple sessions of debridement are necessary. Hyperbaric oxygen therapy may play a role, although it is not the standard of care. In serious periocular infection, treatment may involve orbital exenteration.

Atypical organisms such as *Mycobacterium tuberculosis* should be suspected in immunocompromised patients with a clinical history suggestive of extrapulmonary tuberculosis.

Examination

The examination of the patient with orbital cellulitis is critically important in deciding severity of infection, level of concern for negative sequelae, and treatment. Patients with orbital cellulitis are often systemically ill with fever and an elevated white blood cell count. Blood culture results may be positive. A thorough history may reveal the possible source of infection. Many patients will have a history of a recent upper respiratory tract infection or active sinus disease symptoms. Vital signs, such as heart rate, blood pressure, and temperature, should be evaluated. A neurologic examination may be indicated.

Ophthalmic examination should consist of measurement of visual acuity, evaluation of ocular rotations, assessment for an afferent pupillary defect, assessment for proptosis, color vision evaluation (in each eye individually), intraocular pressure measurement, palpation of the globe to assess for ease (or lack thereof) to retropulsion, palpation of the periocular tissue (to assess for fluctuant mass) and a dilated fundus with careful examination of the optic nerve. Proptosis can be measured with an exophthalmometer. If the equipment is not available, the patient can be asked to tilt his or her head back and the amount of globe projection can be assessed and any asymmetry noted. A difference of more than 2 mm between the two eyes is atypical. It is best to consult the ophthalmology service to follow the patient closely. Any signs of possible optic nerve compromise, such as decreased vision, presence of a relative afferent pupillary defect, decreased color vision, or optic nerve swelling,

demand aggressive treatment with emergency surgical intervention. Aggressive treatment is also warranted in cases of orbital compartment syndrome, orbital apex syndrome, and cavernous sinus thrombosis, because these complications can result in significant morbidity and even possible mortality. Examinations should be performed from every few hours to once daily, depending on the clinical situation and level of concern. It is helpful for the same examiner to examine the patient serially so that improvement or deterioration can readily be observed. Examiners should document specific objective examination findings that can be clearly followed. External photographs can be helpful. It is helpful for the patient to keep his or her head elevated most of the time to avoid exacerbating any orbital or periorbital edema that could be interpreted as clinical worsening. Marking the perimeter of tissue erythema and/or edema with a marking pen can be useful in monitoring for spread of infection in the soft tissue.

Imaging should be obtained in every patient to confirm the diagnosis and to assess the extent of disease in the orbit and paranasal sinuses. Imaging is of critical importance if the clinical examination suggests an abscess, if there is uncertainty about the diagnosis and possible suspicion for a different orbital process (i.e., idiopathic orbital inflammation, tumor), or if a patient is continuing to worsen despite appropriate antibiotic therapy. In the latter case, there should be a high suspicion for an orbital abscess. Contrast-enhanced CT of the orbits and sinuses with 3-mm cuts is the preferred imaging modality. An abscess will be radiopaque on CT with an area of enhancement and possible air-fluid level. Magnetic resonance imaging (MRI) with gadolinium and fat suppression should be obtained if there is a need to image the cavernous sinus or intracranial structures or if no abscess was found on CT but clinical suspicion remains high.[22] If there is a concern about radiation exposure with CT in a young child, MRI can be obtained. MRI using diffusion-weighted imaging has recently been demonstrated as effective in identifying an abscess.[23] The advantage of diffusion-weighted imaging is that it does not require contrast administration and has a rapid acquisition time. Imaging also can help to differentiate orbital cellulitis from other inflammatory conditions of the orbit if clinical examination alone is not sufficient to tell them apart. The clinical examination should always be relied on more heavily than the radiologic examination. Radiologic evidence of disease resolution might not reflect clinical improvement and can make management decision-making difficult, especially if surgical intervention or oral corticosteroid therapy is being considered.

Treatment

Before the antibiotic era, 17% of patients with orbital cellulitis died from meningitis and 20% of patients went blind. Today, prompt treatment with broad-spectrum intravenous antibiotics and close observation makes these unfortunate sequelae a rarity. The chosen antibiotic should have good

CNS penetration in case of intracranial spread of infection. If anaerobic organisms or drug-resistant organisms (e.g., MRSA) are suggested, appropriate antibiotics should be chosen. Blood cultures may be completed; if the results are positive, they can help with streamlining antibiotic therapy. Blood cultures may not need to be used routinely, because they seem to be of low yield, especially in the pediatric population.[12] If blood is to be drawn for cultures, it is best to draw blood before initiating intravenous antibiotics. Doing so will maximize the chance of a positive culture result. A consultation with an infectious disease specialist is highly recommended, especially in atypical cases such as an immunocompromised patient or an atypical organism. Intravenous antibiotics are typically continued until the patient defervesces and it is clear that the orbital cellulitis is improving. With clinical improvement, there should be improvement in periorbital and ocular edema, improvement in ocular motility, and decreased pain. Return of appetite and improvement in general appearance is often a good indicator of improvement in children with subperiosteal abscess.[24] The patient then can be switched to oral antibiotics and discharged home. Antibiotic treatment for 2 to 3 weeks is typical.

If an orbital abscess is identified, it requires urgent surgical drainage to decrease the chance for the development of any negative sequelae. Intraoperative cultures should be taken to help further tailor antibiotic treatment. An SPA can be initially treated with intravenous antibiotics and with the patient being followed closely (see discussion of SPA). Any sign of clinical decompensation will require surgical drainage as well. An orbital compartment syndrome may require decompression with a lateral canthotomy and inferior cantholysis to relieve intraorbital pressure. Evaluation of the sinuses and correction of any underlying structural abnormality that may predispose the patient to recurrent sinusitis should be identified and corrected by an otolaryngologist.

There has been increased interest in the role of adjunct corticosteroids in the treatment of the significant orbital inflammation that often accompanies orbital cellulitis. It is known that significant and prolonged inflammation can lead to complications. A small, prospective, randomized, comparative clinical trial by Pushker et al[25] from India compared patients with orbital cellulitis treated with broad-spectrum intravenous antibiotics with and without oral corticosteroids. Corticosteroids were started after patients demonstrated a clinical response to antibiotic therapy. Patients treated with adjuvant oral corticosteroids had statistically significantly less ptosis, proptosis, and extraocular motility deficit at 3 months. These patients also achieved better vision more rapidly and had faster resolution of ocular and orbital edema and pain. Final visual outcome was the same in the two groups. These authors advocate for judicious use of oral corticosteroids in orbital cellulitis and recommend further exploration of the subject. Yen et al[26] in their small, retrospective study found that intravenous corticosteroids given early in the treatment of pediatric subperiosteal abscess had no adverse effects. More patients not treated initially with intravenous corticosteroids required outpatient intravenous antibiotic therapy, but patients in both groups had eventual resolution of the abscess. Unfortunately, the retrospective and small nature of the study severely limits its power. Going forward, randomized controlled, prospective studies are needed to demonstrate whether and when adjunct corticosteroids should be started, at what dose, and for how long.

The eye and adnexa may require supportive care during the orbital infection. If there is proptosis resulting in lagophthalmos, frequent lubrication to minimize the effects of corneal exposure should be initiated. If exposure keratopathy is significant and vision is threatened, a temporary tarsorrhaphy may be required. This can be done at the bedside with local anesthetic. If a surgical procedure is not possible, moisture goggles can be used. If there is significant inflammation of the conjunctiva, topical antibiotic–corticosteroid drops can be administered. Emollients may be necessary for any skin breakdown.

Complications

Complications arising from orbital cellulitis can be classified as visual or neurologic. Both can be potentially devastating to the patient, but luckily are rare.

Visual loss by a variety of mechanisms and to a varying degree occurs in approximately 11% of patients with orbital cellulitis.[27] Visual complications range from corneal exposure owing to proptosis and lagophthalmos to optic nerve compression from an abscess with loss of vision. An orbital "compartment syndrome" can occur secondary to edema and inflammation that accompany an infection; this can lead to optic nerve compression, elevated intraocular pressure, and ischemia to the extraocular muscles and globe. There can be inflammation-related occlusion of intraocular or orbital vasculature resulting in profound loss of vision. Rarely, infection spreads intraocularly and causes an acute endophthalmitis, a condition with a very poor visual prognosis. An orbital apex syndrome can occur when inflammatory or infectious material infiltrates or compresses the apex of the orbit and results in visual loss, ophthalmoplegia, and sensory deficits because of involvement of branches of the trigeminal nerve.

Neurologic complications include meningitis, intracranial abscess, cavernous sinus thrombosis, and secondary complications resulting from CNS spread. CNS involvement can occur because of thrombophlebitis, direct transmission of infection through orbital bony dehiscences or osteomyelitis.[28] Meningitis has been reported to occur in 1.9% of patients with orbital cellulitis receiving antibiotic therapy.[29] Patients may exhibit altered mental status, fever, lethargy, a stiff neck, and possibly focal neurologic signs. Meningitis is usually treated medically. Intracranial abscess formation occurs in approximately 3% of patients with orbital cellulitis (or sinusitis) and nearly always requires neurosurgical intervention.[30] As previously mentioned, a subperiosteal abscess along the orbital roof can increase the risk for intracranial spread and should be monitored appropriately. Cavernous sinus thrombosis, a complication occurring in 19.2% of patients with orbital cellulitis, manifests with unilateral proptosis, ophthalmoplegia, and multiple cranial nerve palsies.[25] Involvement of the contra-lateral cavernous sinus can occur rapidly, and meningeal signs are often present. Cavernous sinus thrombosis can be differentiated from orbital apex syndrome by the direct involvement of the optic nerve seen in the latter condition.

Fungal Orbital Cellulitis

Fungal infections of the orbit are uncommon and usually arise secondarily to involve the orbit in the setting of nasal, sinus, and skull base infection. This is a potentially devastating type of infection with a high mortality rate and usually occurs in immunocompromised patients. Aspergillosis, however, can affect immunocompetent patients. Tadros et al[31] noted a significant increase in the incidence of acute invasive fungal rhinosinusitis among patients convalescing from COVID-19 infection. This may be explained by reduction in innate immunity, underlying immunologic compromise (e.g., diabetes mellitus) and common use of systemic corticosteroids in the management of post COVID-19 infection symptoms and inflammation. Common fungal organisms include aspergillus and those from the *Mucor* genus. Primary fungal orbital infection can be seen secondary to a penetrating orbital foreign body. Treatment includes intravenous antifungal therapy and surgical debridement. Especially with mucormycosis, which is an especially aggressive organism, debridement may need to include exenteration to decrease the chance for further spread of infection. Unfortunately, no clear guidelines exist as to when to exenterate or not, and each patient should be managed on a case-by-case basis.[32]

References

1. Strul S, McCracken MS, Cunin K. Orbital cellulitis and intraconal abscess formation after strabismus surgery in an adult patient. *J AAPOS*. 2014;18:82-84.
2. Dhrami-Gavazi E, Lee W, Garg A, et al. Bilateral orbital abscesses after strabismus surgery. *Ophthal Plast Reconstr Surg*. 2015;31(6):e141-e142.
3. Rahbar R, Robson CD, Petersen RA, et al. Management of orbital subperiosteal abscess in children. *Arch Otolaryngol Head Neck Surg*. 2001;127:281-286.
4. Harris GJ. Subperiosteal abscess of the orbit: age as a factor in the bacteriology and response to treatment. *Ophthalmology*. 1994;101:585-595.
5. Garcia GH, Harris GJ. Criteria for nonsurgical management of subperiosteal abscess of the orbit: analysis of outcomes 1988-1998. *Ophthalmology*. 2000;107:1454-1458.
6. Harris GJ. Subperiosteal abscess of the orbit: older children and adults require aggressive treatment. *Ophthalmic Plast Reconstr Surg*. 2001;17:395-397.
7. Liao JC, Harris GJ. Subperiosteal abscess of the orbit. *Ophthalmology*. 2015;122:639-647.
8. Dewan MA, Meyer DR, Wladis EJ. Orbital cellulitis with subperiosteal abscess: demographic and management outcomes. *Ophthalmic Plast Reconstr Surg*. 2011;27(5):330-332.
9. Brook I. Microbiology and antimicrobial treatment of orbital and intracranial complications of sinusitis in children and their management. *Int J Pediatr Otorhinolaryngol*. 2009;73:1183-1186.
10. Botting AM, McIntosh D, Mahadevan M. Paediatric pre and postseptal periorbital infections are different disease: a retrospective review of 262 cases. *Int J Pediatr Otorhinolaryngol*. 2008;72:377-383.
11. Liao S, Durand ML, Cunningham MJ. Sinogenic orbital and subperiosteal abscesses: microbiology and methicillin-resistant *Staphylococcus aureus* incidence. *Otolaryngol Head Neck Surg*. 2010;143:392-396.
12. McKinley SH, Yen MT, Miller AM, et al. Microbiology of pediatric orbital cellulitis. *Am J Ophthalmol*. 2007;144:497-458.
13. Barone SR, Aiuto LT. Periorbital and orbital cellulitis in the *Haemophilus influenzae* vaccine era. *J Pediatr Ophthalmol Strabismus*. 1997;34:293-296.
14. Shome D, Jain V, Natarajan S, et al. Community-acquired methicillin-resistant *Staphylococcus aureus* (CAMRSA): a rare cause of fulminant orbital cellulitis. *Orbit*. 2008;27:179-181.
15. Miller A, Castanes M, Yen M, et al. Infantile orbital cellulitis [letter]. *Ophthalmology*. 2008;115:594.
16. Vazan DF, Kodsi SR. Community-acquired methicillin-resistant *Staphylococcus aureus* orbital cellulitis in a non-immunocompromised child. *J AAPOS*. 2008;12:205-206.
17. Rutar T, Zwick OM, Cockerham KP, et al. Bilateral blindness from orbital cellulitis caused by community-acquired methicillin-resistant *Staphylococcus aureus*. *Am J Ophthalmol*. 2005;140:740-742.
18. Mathias MT, Horsley MB, Mawn LA, et al. Atypical presentations of orbital cellulitis caused by methicillin-resistant *Staphylococcus aureus*. *Ophthalmology*. 2012;119:1238-1243.
19. Childers BJ, Potyondy LD, Nachreiner E, et al. Necrotizing fasciitis: a fourteen-year retrospective study of 163 consecutive patients. *Am Surg*. 2002;68:109-116.
20. Bilyk JR. Periocular infection. *Curr Opin Ophthalmol*. 2007;18:414-423.
21. Elner VM, Demirici H, Nerad JA, et al. Periocular necrotizing fasciitis with visual loss: pathogenesis and treatment. *Ophthalmology*. 2006;113:2338-2352.
22. McIntosh D, Mahadevan M. Failure of contrast enhanced computed tomography scans to identify an orbital abscess: the benefit of magnetic resonance imaging. *J Laryngol Otol*. 2008;122:639-640.
23. Sepahdari AR, Aakalu VK, Kapur R, et al. MRI of orbital cellulitis and orbital abscess: the role of diffusion-weighted imaging. *Am J Roentgenol*. 2009;193:W244-W250.
24. Greenberg MF, Pollard ZF. Nonsurgical management of subperiosteal abscess of the orbit [letter]. *Ophthalmology*. 2001;108:1167-1168.
25. Pushker N, Tejwani LK, Bajaj MS, et al. Role of oral corticosteroids in orbital cellulitis. *Am J Ophthalmol*. 2013;156:178-183.
26. Yen MT, Yen KG. Effect of corticosteroids in the acute management of pediatric orbital cellulitis with subperiosteal abscess. *Ophthalmic Plast Reconstr Surg*. 2005;21:363-367.
27. Patt BS, Manning SC. Blindness resulting from orbital complications of sinusitis. *Otolaryngol Head Neck Surg*. 1991;104:789-795.
28. Hartstein ME, Steinvurzel MD, Cohn CP. Intracranial abscess as a complication of subperiosteal abscess of the orbit. *Ophthalmol Plast Reconstr Surg*. 2001;17:398-403.
29. Kloeck CE, Rubin PAD. Role of inflammation in orbital cellulitis. *Int Ophthalmol Clin*. 2006;46:57-68.
30. Lerner DN, Choi SS, Zalzal GH, et al. Intracranial complications of sinusitis in childhood. *Ann Otol Rhinol Laryngol*. 1995;104:288-293.
31. Tadros D, Tomoum MO, Shafik HB, et al. Orbital complications of acute invasive fungal rhinosinusitis: a new challenge in COVID-19 convalescent patients. *Clin Ophthalmol*. 2022;16:4011–4019.
32. Hargrove RN, Wesley RE, Klippenstein KA, et al. Indications for orbital exenteration in mucormycosis. Ophthalmic Plast Reconstr Surg. 2006;22:286–291.

13

Infections of the Ear and Mastoid

ALEXA J. KACIN, REGAN C. MANAYAN, AND JAMES G. NAPLES

Infections of the ear and mastoid encompass a broad category of infections. Acute ear infections can be broken down into infections of the external ear (acute otitis externa [AOE]) and acute infections of the middle ear (acute otitis media [AOM]). Acute middle ear infections are among the most common causes of bacterial infection, especially in children.[1-3] They are also the most common cause of antibiotic prescriptions in children in the United States.[4-6] When AOM extends from the middle ear into the mastoid cavity, it results in acute mastoiditis, the most common complication of AOM.[7,8] AOE occurs in children and adults. It is often an uncomplicated infection; however, in immunocompromised or diabetic patients, it can have serious sequelae.

Diagnosis is often based on clinical findings for these infections; however, radiology plays an adjunct role in diagnosing AOM by confirming extension of infection to the mastoid and assessing for intracranial complications.[9,10] There is also a role for different types of imaging in assessing AOE complications.[11]

The most common bacterial organisms responsible for AOM and mastoiditis are *Streptococcus pneumoniae, Moraxella catarrhalis,* and *Haemophilus influenzae.*[12,13] However, since the advent of the pneumococcal conjugate vaccine (PCV), the microbiology of these acute middle ear and mastoid infections continue to demonstrate a decreasing incidence of *S. pneumoniae.*[12-15] AOE treatment has been unaffected by vaccinations. *Pseudomonas aeruginosa,* along with *Staphylococcus aureus,* are the organisms commonly linked with this infection.[16]

Treatment modalities vary based on the type of infection and degree of extension of disease. Some guidelines suggest that uncomplicated AOM in children older than 2 years old may not need any treatment, but rather a period of observation.[17-19] When there is concern for complications of AOM or AOE, such as acute mastoiditis, antibiotic therapy is indicated, but the changing pathogens of AOM have complicated the discussion on antibiotic options. Not only is medical management an option for acute ear infections and mastoiditis but there also is a definitive role for surgical and procedural management as well.[20]

Complications of acute ear infections and mastoiditis can be life threatening because of the proximity to the intracranial space. Complications of external ear infections are often self-limited, but mortality was not infrequent before the advent of appropriate antibiotic therapy. In AOM and mastoiditis, the complications can be divided into intracranial and extracranial complications. Neurologic complications can occur and progress rapidly if not addressed.

It is not feasible to discuss all types of ear infections in a single chapter. The focus here will be on acute infections. Chronic middle ear infections and cholesteatoma are different topics altogether and will not be covered. There is little published literature on AOM and mastoiditis in adults; therefore, much of the discussion is based on the pediatric population. AOM and AOE will be discussed separately because they are two independent processes. There will be a brief introduction to relevant anatomy of the ear and mastoid followed by the epidemiology of each type of infection. The focus will then be on the pathophysiology and the organisms causing each type of infection. The role of radiology will be discussed, but it should be emphasized that an adequate physical examination is essential, and this should be supplemented with imaging, not replaced by it. Finally, treatment options—both medical and surgical—along with complications will be discussed, with emphasis on mastoiditis as a complication of AOM. The goal of this chapter is to outline the cause, pathologic processes, diagnosis, and management of AOM and AOE.

Anatomy

The anatomy of the ear and mastoid is complex and often confusing.[21] One logical way to approach this complexity is from the outside in, starting with the external ear, followed by the middle ear, and finally the mastoid cavity (Figure 13-1).

The external anatomy of the ear consists of a number of cartilaginous ridges. The external auditory canal (EAC) begins laterally at the external auditory meatus and extends to the tympanic membrane (TM). It is 2.5 cm in length and consists of a lateral cartilaginous portion and a medial bony portion. The skin overlying the cartilaginous portion contains sebaceous and apocrine glands with hair follicles, whereas the medial bony portion consists of overlying skin without hair or glands. Its blood supply is the posterior auricular and superficial

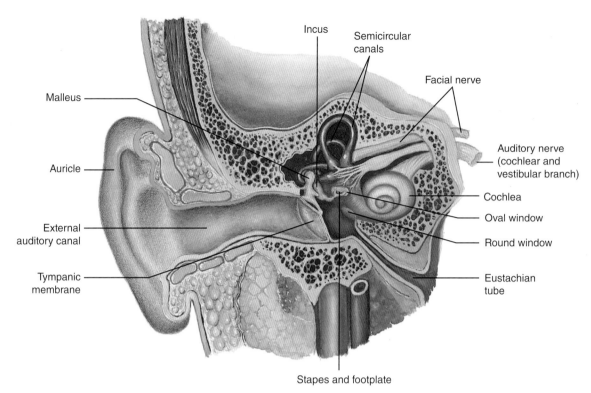

• **Figure 13-1** Anatomy of the External and Middle Ear. (From Ball JW, Seidel HM, Dains JE, et al. *Mosby's Guide to Physical Examination*. 7th ed. St Louis: Mosby; 2011.)

temporal arteries from the external carotid. The external ear lymphatic drainage varies by location. The anterior and superior part of the EAC and the tragus are drained by the preauricular nodes. The concha and antihelix are drained posteriorly into the mastoid lymph nodes. The inferior EAC and helix drain to the infraauricular nodes.

The middle ear can be divided into three distinct spaces: the mesotympanum, the hypotympanum, and the epitympanum. The mesotympanum is bounded medially by the TM, anteriorly by the eustachian tube, and posteriorly by the facial nerve. Inferiorly the mesotympanum extends to the inferior annulus of the TM. The hypotympanum is bounded inferiorly by the jugular bulb and inferomedially by the cochlea and superiorly by the mesotympanum. Finally, the epitympanum consists of the ossicular chain, its ligaments, and associated mucosal folds. The lateral border is the scutum, and the posterior border is the aditus before entry into the mastoid cavity. Medially and inferiorly the epitympanum is bounded by the lateral semicircular canal and fossa incudis, respectively. The arterial supply to the middle ear is via branches of the internal and external carotid. From the internal maxillary branch of the external carotid, the anterior tympanic and deep auricular arteries supply the middle ear. From the middle meningeal branch of the internal carotid are the superior petrosal and the superior tympanic artery. The lymphatic drainage of the external ear is complex, with multiple lymphatic pathways, with the most common drainage pattern being to the cervical level II, preauricular and postauricular lymph nodes.[22]

When considering middle ear infections, it is important to remember that the mastoid is an extension of the middle ear. It is a pneumatized region of the temporal bone that communicates directly with the middle ear via the aditus ad antrum. The medial border consists of the semicircular canals and the vestibule, and laterally it is bound by Körner's septum, which is the thin bony segment separating the squamous and petrous part of the temporal bone. The degree of pneumatization is clinically relevant because it is often an indicator of a patient's ability to aerate his or her middle ear.

Acute Otitis Media

Epidemiology

The incidence of acute ear infections and mastoiditis varies based on the age of the patient. AOM is more likely to occur in young children because of a more horizontal position of the eustachian tube. As development occurs, it assumes a more vertical position, which allows for better aeration of the middle ear. AOM is particularly common in children between the ages of 6 and 24 months and is the most common bacterial infection of childhood.[1,2,23-25] In the post-PCV era, Kaur et al. reported by 1 year of age 23% of children experience one or more episodes of AOM and by 3 years of age 60% had one or more episodes.[12] Male children, children who attend day care, and children with siblings have been shown to be at increased risk for infection.[12,24,26-28] The PCV was first introduced in the United

States in 2000, covering seven serotypes of the organism (PCV-7). Since the introduction of PCV-7, multiple versions of this vaccine have been produced that cover more serotypes. The most recent version being PCV-15 or PCV-20 introduced in 2021.[29] There is also a polysaccharide vaccine (PSV-23), which is recommended for adults older than 65 years. The proportion of *S. pneumoniae* isolates continues to be lower than reported in the pre-PCV7 era. However, one study indicates that in recent years pneumococcal isolates from AOM isolates in children exhibited reduced susceptibility to penicillin, cephalosporins, and fluoroquinolones, with the new strains having a different profile of resistance compared to those in the pre-PCV13 era.[12] There had been a downward trend in health care costs related to AOM since the updated PCV-13 vaccine was introduced.[30] However, a more recent study suggests no appreciable changes in the health care costs related to AOM from 2008 to 2014 in the United States.[6] The incidence of AOM in adults has decreased compared with that in children, and the reason for the decline is mostly anatomic.[31]

Pathophysiology

Acute middle ear infections are caused by a dysfunction of the eustachian tube, which connects the nasopharynx to the middle ear. The normal middle ear is sterile and aerated by a normally functioning eustachian tube that opens with contraction of the tensor and levator veli palatini muscles. When there is edema or inflammation of the eustachian tube—commonly caused by preceding upper respiratory infection (URI)—the normal mechanism of aerating the middle ear is disrupted. There is a negative pressure in the middle ear, and organisms from the nasopharyngeal secretions are refluxed into the middle ear. This creates an environment ideal for bacterial organism growth and AOM.[3,32] A preceding URI also induces damage to the respiratory mucosal epithelium that prevents normal mucociliary clearance of the middle ear into the nasopharynx.[3,25] In children with a more horizontal eustachian tube, this is especially problematic. It should be noted that eustachian tube dysfunction can be caused by a variety of other pathologic conditions, such as cleft lip or palate, nasopharyngeal mass, allergy, or reflux.[33,34]

Microbiology

The bacterial organism most often responsible for AOM has traditionally been *S. pneumoniae*. Other species associated with AOM are *H. influenzae, M. catarrhalis,* and *S. aureus.*[12,13] Since the advent of the pneumococcal vaccine, there has been a shift in the microbiology of AOM. The incidence of *S. pneumoniae* has declined (15 to 25% of bacterial isolates from the middle ear fluid of children), whereas newer data suggest that nontypeable *H. influenzae* is now the dominant strain of organism associated with AOM (50 to 60% of bacterial isolages from the middle ear fluid of children), with relative increases in *M. catarrhalis.*[12,15,35-37] There also has

been a trend toward more virulent strains of *S. pneumoniae,* with the most common AOM effusion isolates being serotypes 35B, 23B, and 15B/C between 2015 and 2019 (Figure 13-2).[38] The organism responsible for AOM can be determined only by tympanocentesis, but this is rarely necessary because it would be unlikely to affect management. Studies examining complications of AOM, such as mastoiditis, have shown similar trends in the microbiology of the disease; however, recent studies report continued infections with *S. pneumoniae* in the postvaccine era.[39] Although some studies suggest the vaccine has not reduced the number of patients who get mastoiditis, and the organisms are showing trends toward antibiotic resistance,[40,41] another conducted out of Israel showed a decline in the incidence of AM in the post-PCV era.[42] The role of viruses alone causing AOM directly is unclear. The implication is that it predisposes to bacterial infection, but isolates of viruses have not been reported and have little clinical significance.

Diagnosis

AOM is a clinical diagnosis, and otoscopy is essential for a full evaluation of the middle ear and TM. It is not possible to diagnose AOM without evaluating the TM. Symptoms include new-onset otalgia (<48 hours), which typically causes fever and irritability and interrupts sleep.[3,25,43] History usually indicates a preceding URI. On otoscopy, one should look for bulging of the TM, erythema of the TM, otorrhea, and the presence of middle ear fluid or purulence (Figure 13-3).[17,20] If pneumatic otoscopy is available, there will be decreased mobility of the TM because of the middle ear infection. If otorrhea is present, TM perforation should be suspected. The sensitivity and specificity of clinical signs can be difficult to interpret in the pediatric population and even more so in infants. Overall, ear pain, rubbing of the ear, excessive crying, and vomiting were shown to be the most common.[25,26,44] Although ear pain has been cited as the most common presenting symptom, only 50 to 60% of children with AOM complain of pain, underscoring the importance of physical examination in diagnosis.[25,45] Hearing will be decreased in the affected ear during acute infections because of the fluid present in the middle ear; however, it is not often tested in the acute setting. Persistent fluid after a bout of otitis media is possible. Thus, unresolved AOM should be evaluated with audiometry and tympanometry. Persistent serous fluid without signs of acute infection is termed otitis media with effusion (OME), which is distinct from AOM. When the serous fluid is present for 3 or more months on otoscopy this is defined as chronic OME.

Medical

Treatment

The medical treatment of AOM with oral antibiotics has been a source of considerable controversy. Guidelines were

	Serotypes (*N*= 492)	Healthy visits NP (*N*= 492) Isolate # (%)	AOM visits NP (*N*= 209) # (%)	MEF taps (*N*= 98) # (%)	AOM follow-up visits NP (*N*= 34) # (%)
Non-vaccine-type serotypes	35B	90 (18.3)	44 (21.1)	22 (22.4)	4 (11.8)
	23B	88 (17.9)	19 (9.1)	11 (11.2)	2 (5.9)
	15B/C	63 (12.8)	33 (15.8)	18 (18.4)	6 (14.7)
	15A	34 (6.9)	13 (6.2)	6 (6.1)	2 (5.9)
	21	32 (6.5)	16 (7.7)	8 (8.2)	–
	23A	27 (5.5)	12 (5.7)	5 (5.1)	2 (5.9)
	35F	21 (4.3)	3 (1.4)	1 (1.0)	–
	11A	20 (4.1)	8 (3.8)	2 (2.0)	2 (5.9)
	NT	11 (2.2)	2 (1.0)	–	1 (2.9)
	10	10 (2.0)	3 (1.4)	3 (3.1)	1 (2.9)
	22F	10 (2.0)	6 (2.9)	3 (3.1)	–
	16F	9 (1.8)	4 (1.9)	3 (3.1)	–
	11C	6 (1.2)	5 (2.4)	3 (3.1)	–
	9 (A, L, or N)	5 (1.0)	2 (1.0)	–	–
	6C	5 (1.0)	2 (1.0)	–	–
	31	5 (1.0)	3 (1.4)	–	2 (5.9)
	38	4 (0.8)	3 (1.4)	–	–
	7 (B or C)	4 (0.8)	2 (1.0)	–	–
	11B	3 (0.6)	–	–	–
	33F	3 (0.6)	7 (3.3)	5 (5.1)	–
	Other	8 (1.6)	7 (3.3)	1 (1.0)	–
Vaccine types	19F	13 (2.6)	7 (3.3)	3 (3.1)	–
	19A	9 (1.8)	3 (1.4)	3 (3.1)	3 (8.8)
	3	8 (1.6)	3 (1.4)	3 (3.1)	
	9 V	–	1 (0.5)	–	–
	4	–	1 (0.5)	–	–
	6A	–	–	–	1 (2.9)
	6B	3 (0.6)	–	–	–
	23F	1 (0.2)	–	–	–

• **Figure 13-2** *Spn* Serotype Distribution from Healthy, AOM, and Follow-Up Visits. Dynamic changes in otopathogens colonizing the nasopharynx and causing acute otitis media in children after 13-valent (PCV-13) pneumococcal conjugate vaccination during 2015-2019. (Kaur R, Fuji N, Pichichero ME. Dynamic changes in otopathogens colonizing the nasopharynx and causing acute otitis media in children after 13-valent (PCV13) pneumococcal conjugate vaccination during 2015-2019. *Eur J Clin Microbiol Infect Dis.* 2022;41[1]:37-44. https://doi.org/10.1007/s10096-021-04324-0.)

established in the pediatric population to help reduce the use of antibiotics in an era of concern for increasing antibiotic resistance. The guideline accounts for age, severity of symptoms, and certainty of diagnosis when considering treatment options.[17] For children 6 months to 23 months of age with unilateral AOM and less severe symptoms (mild otalgia for <48 hours, temperature <39°C) observation is a reasonable option if close follow-up is certain for any worsening symptoms. If the infection in this age group is severe (i.e., body temperature >39°C, severe otalgia, otalgia for at least 48 hours), treatment with antibiotics is recommended. For children younger than 2 years with bilateral AOM without severe signs or symptoms antibiotic therapy should be initiated. Allowing a period of observation for children 6 months to 2 years of age with a certain diagnosis is a change from the previous guidelines released in 2004, which recommended definitive antibiotic therapy. This change is supported by evidence on the safety of

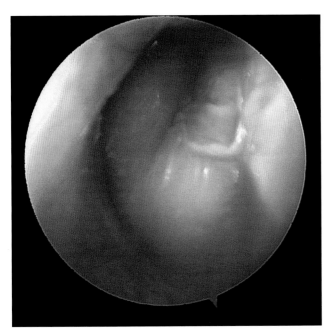

• **Figure 13-3** Otoscopic View of the Ear. Note the presence of a bulging tympanic membrane and purulence in the middle ear. (From Lambert E, Soham R. Otitis media and ear tubes. *Pediatr Clin North Am.* 2013;60:809-826.)

observation or delayed prescribing in children.[1,2,46] Despite the introduction of this guideline, adherence to it varies and poor compliance rates are noted when it comes to observation of an AOM.[47] It should be noted that despite the guideline recommending an observation period, some studies indicate that when compared with placebo, antibiotics reduce the need for additional treatments and promote improvement in symptoms.[1,2]

If antimicrobial therapy is initiated, the currently accepted first-line therapy is high-dose amoxicillin (80 to 90 mg/kg/day). This therapy provides good coverage against *S. pneumoniae*, a common AOM pathogen, and ensures appropriate dose delivery to the middle ear.[1] *H. influenzae* and *M. catarrhalis* produce β-lactamase; therefore, the efficacy of amoxicillin alone is reduced, but not zero. Amoxicillin alone can be used as empiric therapy; however, the addition of a β-lactamase inhibitor is warranted when these pathogens are suggested.[25,33] These organisms are more likely to occur in patients with increasing risk factors for AOM.[24] Current guidelines recommend that amoxicillin-clavulanate should be used as an agent if amoxicillin was used within the last month because of risk of colonization with β-lactamase organisms.[17] Notably, a recent study suggests regular dose amoxicillin-clavulanate as the preferred treatment given the combination of increasing *H. influenzae*–related AOM with a decrease in penicillin-resistant *S. pneumoniae*.[36] However, the recommendation is not currently in alignment with the latest treatment guidelines released by the American Academy of Pediatrics and American Academy of Family Physicians in 2013.

Cephalosporin antibiotics can be used as an alternative to amoxicillin. Cefdinir or cefuroxime are often used. Intramuscular ceftriaxone is also a reasonable alternative to amoxicillin, and requires at least 2 to 3 doses and follow-up for injection. Macrolide antibiotics have been studied and found to be effective, but when compared with amoxicillin-clavulanate, they have a significant clinical failure rate.[33,43] Recently, a retrospective cohort study analyzed the efficacy of amoxicillin versus other antibiotic agents (amoxicillin-clavulanate, cefdinir, and azithromycin) with combined failure and recurrence rates being low for all agents at less than 12%, but lowest for amoxicillin at less than 1.7%.[48] One other option for antibiotic therapy is clindamycin, which does not provide adequate coverage for *H. influenzae* and *M. catarrhalis,* but it can be used in conjunction with cephalosporins to provide good microbial coverage.[33]

In patients who have continued signs of infection despite appropriate antibiotic therapy, clinical treatment failure should be considered. If this is the case, tympanocentesis and culture are a reasonable next step. This procedure is routinely performed in the otolaryngologist's office in compliant patients, but it carries risk to the TM and middle ear. The role of myringotomy does not appear to be superior to antibiotics alone.[25,49]

Surgical

The role of surgery in AOM is somewhat limited in uncomplicated cases. Tympanostomy tubes are placed to maintain patency of the TM so that the middle ear can drain and the negative middle ear pressure is relieved. It is performed in the operating room for children and in the office for adults. The indications for tympanostomy tubes have been a source of debate. Recurrent AOM is defined as three episodes of AOM in 6 months or four episodes in the last 12 months, with at least one of those episodes occurring in the immediately preceding 6 months.[50] Current guidelines recommend against placing tympanostomy tubes in children with recurrent AOM who do not show evidence of effusion in either ear at the time of evaluation.[20] If middle ear effusion is present, a tympanostomy tube should be placed. In certain populations, such as patients with cochlear implant, AOM can be a more serious problem and urgent drainage of middle ear purulence should be considered. The observation period does not apply to this population because of the risk for serious, potentially life-threatening complications.[51]

Mastoiditis: A Complication of Acute Otitis Media

AOM can spread beyond the borders of the middle ear, creating complications. There are a variety of ways in which spread of the infection from the middle ear and the mastoid, and spread of the infection beyond the confines of the mastoid, can have serious consequences because of adjacent intracranial contents. Anatomic spread is common, but it can also spread directly through bony erosion or thrombophlebitis.[10] If AOM becomes sufficiently severe, it can spread to the mastoid air cells through the aditus ad antrum. If there is blockage of the aditus because of mucus and exudates from the middle ear, it creates continued inflammation in the mastoid. Acidosis ensues with ischemia, thus causing bony resorption and breakdown of the septa of the air cells. Acute mastoiditis is the result.[8,10,52]

Acute mastoiditis is a disease of young children, most often because children develop AOM more frequently. The incidence of acute mastoiditis has decreased rapidly since the preantibiotic era of the first half of the twentieth century. Some reports indicate a 50% decline in admissions for AOM and 80% in the number of mastoidectomies performed since the introduction of sulfonamines.[52] There is conflicting evidence regarding the incidence of acute mastoiditis in the post-PCV era. Some reports indicate an increase in cases with rationale being the change in algorithm that withholds antibiotic treatment for some patients with AOM or possibly the increasing virulence of organisms since the introduction of PCV-7.[10,53,54] King et al conducted a study analyzing the trends of mastoiditis between 2000 and 2012 and found that rates increased from 2000 to 2006, but then decreased from 2006 to 2012.[55] Regardless of the conflicting studies, acute mastoiditis is a diagnosis that cannot be overlooked because of the life-threatening nature of the complications.

Mastoiditis, like AOM and AOE, is a clinical diagnosis. It has been demonstrated that acute mastoiditis can be diagnosed without the use of computed tomography (CT) or magnetic resonance imaging (MRI) in many cases;[56] however, this is controversial. The classic presentation of mastoiditis is with otalgia, fever, postauricular swelling, and mastoid tenderness (Figure 13-4).[7] Pain was the most frequent symptom, with persistent fever being the second most common in one study.[52] The clinician should suspect mastoiditis in the setting of an AOM with clinical signs of mastoiditis. It is important to note that mastoiditis can occur in the setting of adequate AOM treatment, thus masking the effects of mastoiditis.[8] The TM is commonly hyperemic and bulging with middle ear purulence. The TM also may be normal. Therefore, clinical suspicion is often necessary to make this diagnosis.

A CT scan will typically show breakdown of the bony septa within the mastoid and opacification and fluid within the mastoid air cells (Figure 13-5). CT scanning is often available to evaluate for complications of mastoiditis. The utility of imaging lies in identification of these complications.[9,10] MRI should also be ordered if intracranial extension is suspected, because it will give more information regarding the soft tissues of the cranial contents. Patients can have intracranial complications with little symptomatology; therefore, there should be a low threshold to order imaging if mastoiditis is suspected. Ultimately, imaging should be ordered to evaluate for suspected complications, no clinical response to intravenous antibiotics, or an abnormal result from a neurologic examination.[7]

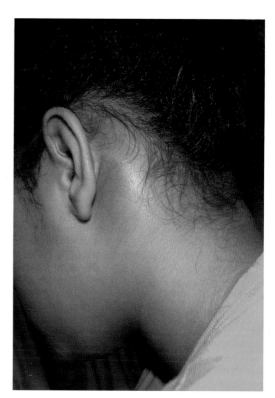

• **Figure 13-4** Acute Mastoiditis with Erythema and Swelling Behind the Affected Ear. (From Neslon D, Jeanmonod R. Bezold abscess: a rare complication of mastoiditis. *Am J Emerg Med.* 2013;31:1626.e3-1626.e4.)

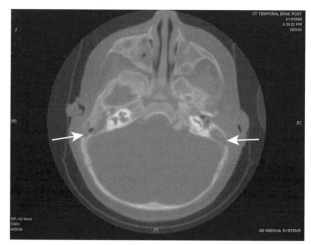

• **Figure 13-5** Coalescent Mastoiditis Demonstrated on Computed Tomographic Scan. There is fluid extending from the middle ears into the mastoid air cells bilaterally with breakdown of bony trabeculae *(arrows)*. (From Alwedyani E, AlSanosi A. Bilateral simultaneous acute coalescent mastoiditis: a rare complication. *Inter J Pediatr Otorhinolaryngol.* 2011;6:226-228.)

Management of Mastoiditis

Historically, the management of mastoiditis was surgical. Currently, with potent intravenous antibiotic therapy, it is becoming more amenable to conservative medical treatment with myringotomy, without the need for mastoidectomy. Myringotomy with antibiotics is regarded as the first-line therapy by many, and has been shown to be adequate in patients with uncomplicated mastoiditis.[7,8,57-60] It should be noted that just as different age groups present differently with acute mastoiditis, it is thought that the different age groups also respond differently to treatments. Young children often respond more quickly to IV antibiotics, whereas older patients are more likely to require surgical drainage.[7] There are a variety of adequate antibiotics for treatment of acute mastoiditis, and because it is generally an extension of an AOM, the pathogens are similar. Medical management of acute mastoiditis varies in terms of antibiotic choice and duration among providers (even within a single institute), but generally, initial antibiotic treatment should be administered parenterally and then transitioned to orally as appropriate for a total of 3 weeks. First-line antibiotics include those in the penicillin or cephalosporin class (ampicillin-sulbactam or ceftriaxone).[61] Geva et al. reported frequent use of amoxicillin-clavulanate and cefuroxime.[8] If one is not responding to antibiotics after approximately 48 hours, surgical intervention should be considered, and if possible, cultures should be taken at that time if they were not taken during myringotomy.

In the era preceding IV antibiotics, acute mastoiditis was a common complication of AOM, and up to 2% to 6% of patients developed intracranial complications of mastoiditis.[62,63] Thus, operative intervention and mastoidectomy was a common procedure for this disease. The use of this procedure declined with the introduction of antibiotics.[52] In general, surgical procedures are required for complications of acute mastoiditis, whether intracranial or extracranial. Another indication is failure to improve with antibiotics and myringotomy tube placement.[63] The procedure to be performed depends on the complication. Imaging is also necessary before operative intervention is undertaken because it helps to define the extent of disease and can confirm extracranial or intracranial complication.[9,10] If there is exteriorization of the abscess, incision and drainage is indicated, whereas intracranial or neurologic complications require mastoidectomy with or without a ventilating tube.[63] Neurosurgical intervention may also be necessary if there is any concern for intracranial abscess.

Other Complications of Acute Otitis Media and Mastoiditis

In AOM, life-threatening complications can occur that are associated with spread of infection to the adjacent structures. The infection can spread into the cranium and surrounding structures or it can spread out to the overlying soft tissue. These are best classified as intracranial and extracranial complications. Each complication will be discussed here.

Intracranial

Meningitis
Meningitis is the most common intracranial complication of AOM and mastoiditis. The route of spread is either via hematogenous seeding or direct extension through the bony portions of the temporal bone. Diagnosis is suspected on

clinical grounds, and imaging is used to rule out other causes of similar symptoms. Imaging will show dural enhancement and thickening.[10] Treatment with IV antibiotics and steroids is necessary. Steroids help to decrease neurologic and auditory complications.[64,65]

Lateral or Sigmoid Sinus Thrombosis
When AOM or mastoiditis extends through the bony aspects of the temporal bone, a thrombophlebitis of the surrounding dural sinuses occurs. This predisposes to thrombus and potentially serious complications and should be suspected in patients who have mastoiditis and a "picket fence" pattern of fevers with associated headaches. Imaging shows a filling defect on CT (Figure 13-6) with contrast and a flow void within the affected dural sinus on MRI. Managing this complication is controversial, and there is no consensus regarding whether the sinus should be managed surgically during a mastoidectomy. Ligation of the affected sinus is also something that should be considered if there is concern for propagation of septic emboli; however, this is not routine.[64] Anticoagulation is also a consideration. One group reviewing a 12-year experience in treating otogenic sigmoid sinus thrombosis found anticoagulants are safe if correctly administered and may prevent extension of the thrombus.[66]

Epidural Abscess or Brain Abscess
Continued extension of the infection through surrounding bony structures can create coalescence of infection that results in abscess formation. The degree of abscess extension

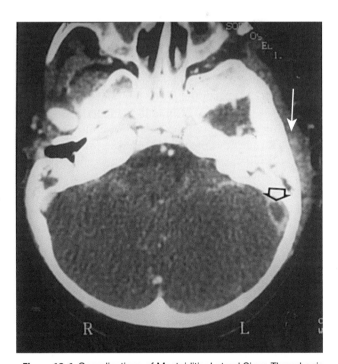

• **Figure 13-6** Complications of Mastoiditis: Lateral Sinus Thrombosis and Subperiosteal Abscess. There is a flow void of the dural sinus *(arrowhead)*. There is also extracranial extension into the subperiosteal space *(arrow)* with a inflammatory changes in the skin soft tissues. (From Kaplan DM, Kraus M, Puterman M, et al. Otogenic lateral sinus thrombosis in children. *Inter J Pediatr Otorhinolaryngol.* 1999;49:177-183.)

will classify it as either epidural or intracranial. Epidural abscess can often be insidious in onset and will have symptoms and signs that are subtle when compared with a brain abscess. A brain abscess results from hematogenous spread of infection and is more likely to result from chronic otitis media, but it can occur with AOM. Brain abscesses most frequently occur in the temporal lobe or cerebellum and are diagnosed with contrast-enhanced CT or MRI.[10,67] MRI is superior in the diagnosis of brain abscesses, and CT gives valuable information on the bony structure of the mastoid.[64] Mastoidectomy is indicated, and collaboration with a member of the neurosurgical team is often necessary.

Otitic Hydrocephalus

Otitic hydrocephalus is a poorly understood complication described as the signs and symptoms of hydrocephalus with normal cerebrospinal fluid (CSF) opening pressure and lack of dilated ventricles. It is a diagnosis of exclusion, and it is likely made only by an investigator with a high degree of suspicion. Otitic hydrocephalus is possibly related to irritation of the sagittal sinus that interrupts absorption of CSF through the arachnoid villi. As with other causes of intracranial hypertension, presentation is often with neurologic symptoms of headache, vision changes, and nausea and vomiting. The use of antibiotics has largely made this disease and sequelae a rare phenomenon, but urgent management is necessary to preserve vision, often requiring surgery with mastoidectomy.[64,68]

Extracranial (Extratemporal)

Extracranial complications of AOM and mastoiditis can be further classified as extratemporal and intratemporal.

Subperiosteal Abscess

Subperiosteal abscess is the most common type of mastoid abscess.[69] It is an extension of the infection as it erodes the overlying mastoid bone.[70] Clinically, a subperiosteal abscess may manifest as postauricular tenderness and/or purulence with displacement of the pinna.[69] Patients will usually also show systemic signs of infection. This abscess is often seen as an extension of AOM in children but may also occur secondary to chronic otitis media. CT scan is recommended to determine the full extent of the abscess and to rule out other pathologic conditions (see Figure 13-6). Intravenous antibiotics are the mainstay of treatment for a subperiosteal abscess. Surgical intervention has lost popularity over the past decades, with intervention often limited to myringotomy without insertion of a ventilation tube.[71] Needle aspiration or incision and drainage may be performed in certain cases, with mastoidectomy reserved for refractory cases or those presenting with associated cholesteatoma or intracranial complications.[72]

Bezold Abscess

Extension of an AOM or mastoiditis through the mastoid tip may cause tracking of an abscess into the neck, deep to the sternocleidomastoid muscle. This is known as a Bezold abscess, named after the nineteenth-century otologist Friedrich Bezold.[70] Despite the well-described pathophysiology of this entity, it is rare in today's era. With the introduction of antibiotics and imaging and an improved health care system, the incidence of Bezold abscesses has declined over the past century.[73] Thus, workup of a Bezold abscess should include initiation of broad-spectrum antibiotic with adequate CSF penetration and imaging to determine its location and size. Management includes a complete mastoidectomy and a transcervical incision for incision and drainage of the abscess.[74]

Extracranial (Intratemporal)

Facial Paralysis

The facial nerve courses through the middle ear and temporal bone and is covered by the bony *fallopian canal*. When there is an AOM, edema and pressure is exerted on the nerve, sometimes resulting in weakness or paresis. A small area of dehiscence is often present, which may predispose to this complication of AOM. Facial paralysis is more likely to develop in children with congenital dehiscence. The lack or presence of associated complications, such as subperiosteal abscess, determines treatment choice, which may range from conservative medical management to surgical intervention.[57] While an adequately powered study investigating facial paresis/paralysis as a complication of AOM has yet to be completed, small-scale studies suggest that the deficit typically resolves after treatment.[75,76] Imaging is useful here to evaluate for cholesteatoma and/or any component of chronic middle ear disease that may require more extensive surgical intervention. It is important to delineate a facial paralysis secondary to an acute infection in a patient with a dehiscent fallopian canal versus a facial weakness in a patient with underlying chronic ear disease, since management defers between the two cases. Eye care should not be overlooked with facial nerve paralysis.

Acute Suppurative Labyrinthitis

Acute suppurative labyrinthitis is an inflammatory process involving bacterial invasion of the inner ear, which subsequently leads to necrosis of its structures.[77] Through a mechanism similar to that of other complications, there is often invasion of infection through a dehiscent area within the labyrinth. In a retrospective investigation of 285 patients, labyrinthitis was found to be the most common extracranial complication of AOM.[78] Acute suppurative labyrinthitis is often seen in patients who have an underlying congenital ear anomaly or have had otologic surgical intervention. Patients exhibit acute vestibular symptoms of vertigo, nausea, and vomiting, as well as permanent sensorineural hearing loss.[79] There is no indication for imaging, although many patients may have imaging if they are evaluated in the emergency department. With that said, imaging may help differentiate labyrinthitis caused by acute infection versus cholesteatoma eroding the labyrinth. Treating the associated middle ear infection is the only intervention typically necessary.[21] Although disconcerting to the patient, the vestibular system often undergoes central compensation as the infection resolves.

Petrous Apicitis

When AOM infection erodes into a well-pneumatized petrous apex, it may create a complex of symptoms that occur with or without mastoiditis symptoms. Clinically, extension of infection leading to petrous apicitis may manifest as Gradenigo syndrome, characterized by the triad of: (1) deep retro-orbital pain, (2) ipsilateral abducens palsy, and (3) purulent otorrhea. Petrous apicitis is associated with a high rate of mortality, so intervention is critical. Imaging modalities, including CT and MRI, play an important role in diagnosis. The former determines the bone structure, and the latter identifies concomitant cranial involvement. First-line management often includes a combination of middle ear ventilation and intravenous broad-spectrum antibiotics.

Acute Otitis Externa

Epidemiology

AOE affects roughly 1 in 123 persons in the United States per year.[80] It may occur in any age group, but tends to occur in children and teenagers, with a second peak of incidence in patients older than 65 years.[32] Factors predisposing to AOE depend on the age group. Children who have anatomic ear abnormalities, such as external canal stenosis, are at risk. Adult patients who wear hearing aids are at particular risk as well, due to repetitive mild ear canal trauma. Self-induced trauma with cotton swabs and exposure to swimming pools in the summer are also risk factors for otitis externa.[32,80]

Pathophysiology

The introduction of pathogens to the external auditory canal is often a result of local trauma or exposure to contaminated water. The anatomy and chemical environment of the external ear may also predispose to infection. Narrowed or stenotic ear canals prevent the natural self-migratory mechanism of otic debris, thus predisposing to infection. Hearing aid use in hearing-impaired individuals creates a similar situation. The normal pH of the external ear is slightly acidic from the production of cerumen and other sebaceous gland products of the cartilaginous external auditory canal. This acidity creates an inhospitable environment for bacteria. However, when the local environment is disrupted, the pH is altered, creating an environment conducive to bacterial growth.[11,32] With the growth of bacteria, local inflammation and edema occur, thus worsening infection and symptoms. EOM may continue to spread through the junction of the cartilaginous and bony canal via the fissures of Santorini. As infection reaches the bony canal medially, the periosteum lies immediately deep to the skin, leading to increasing pain. If the infection continues to spread through the periosteum, an osteomyelitis of the underlying temporal bone may occur, resulting in the dreaded complication of malignant otitis externa (MOE).

Microbiology

AOE is often a polymicrobial infection, with the most common pathogens involved being *P. auruginosa* (20 to 60% prevalence) and *S. aureus* (10 to 70% prevalence).[80] Over the past decades, there has been a decline in *P. aeruginosa* and an associated increase in *S. aureus*.[81] The reason for this change is unclear but is likely related to resistance patterns with frequent use of fluoroquinolones. In an AOE that does not resolve with otic antibiotic drops or in individuals with chronic AOE, secondary fungal infection should be considered.[32] In this situation, clinical symptoms will be similar. Pruritus may be more pronounced. In fungal infections, *Aspergillus* and *Candida* species are often cultured.[80]

Diagnosis

Acute infection of the EAC is defined as diffuse inflammation of the ear canal that is rapid in onset in the past 3 weeks with signs and symptoms of canal inflammation. The hallmark of AOE is tenderness of the tragus, pinna, or both, disproportionate to what is expected based on inspection.[80] Symptoms may also include pruritus, discharge, and fullness.[32] Uncomplicated AOE is a clinical diagnosis, and there is no need for imaging or additional workup unless predisposing factors lead to concern for malignant otitis externa.[11] History will often include reports of swimming or water exposure, water irrigations, or cotton swab use. On examination, visual inspection of the external anatomy of the ear will demonstrate edema, erythema, and discharge. Otoscopy is necessary to evaluate the TM and rule out chronic drainage from the middle ear with perforation of the TM. Palpation of the pinna and tragus will often elicit extreme discomfort for the patient, a helpful diagnostic sign. The canal may be cultured to confirm infection, but this is not essential in uncomplicated cases. The clinician should be vigilant not to overlook other causes of external canal inflammation that may cause overlapping symptoms, such as contact dermatitis, eczema, or more serious processes such as carcinoma or Ramsay Hunt syndrome caused by herpes simplex virus.[32,80] These other causes should be considered in AOE that is not responsive to topical therapy.

Treatment

Medical

There are three treatment modalities in uncomplicated AOE: (1) canal debridement, (2) topical otic preparations, and (3) pain control and analgesia (Table 13-1). Canal debridement facilitates normal migratory function of the EAC by removing obstruction. In cases in which patients are unable to tolerate debridement because of extreme pain,

TABLE 13-1	Topical Therapies in the Treatment of Acute Otitis Externa		
Component	Brand Name	Dose	Notes
Acetic acid 2%	Vosol/Acetasol	3-5 drops q 4-6 h	Irritation if tympanic membrane ruptured
Acetic acid 2%/hydrocortisone	Vosol HC/Acetasol HC	4-6 drops q 6-8 h	Irritation if tympanic membrane ruptured
Neomycin/Polymyxin B/ hydrocortisone	Otosporin/Cortisporin	4 drops q 6-8 h	Potential ototoxicity; maximum of 10-day course
Ciprofloxacin/hydrocortisone	Cipro HC	3 drops twice daily	7-day course adequate
Ciprofloxacin/dexamethasone	Ciprodex	4 drops twice daily	7-day course adequate
Ofloxacin	Floxin Otic	10 drops daily	7-day course adequate

a combination of acetaminophen, nonsteroidal antiinflammatory drugs, and opioids may be used. Although topical anesthesia, such as benzocaine otic solution, exists, this has not been approved by the U.S. Federal Drug Administration (FDA) in the treatment of AOE.[80] Pain management in AOE should not be overlooked.

Topical therapy is recommended as initial therapy for diffuse, uncomplicated AOE, with numerous studies supporting its clinical and bacteriologic success. Regarding topical preparations for the treatment of AOE, options are numerous, with little clinical evidence to support the use of one preparation over another.[80] These preparations include acidifying agents, antibiotics, and steroids. When using an antibiotic, *Pseudomonas* coverage is essential.

An acidic pH creates a hostile environment that prevents growth of microorganisms. For this reason, acetic acid solution is a valid first-line treatment option. This therapy creates an environment similar to the natural environment of the EAC and is most useful in patients who have mild symptoms of AOE, with minimal underlying pain. Studies differ regarding the superiority of topical antibiotics compared to acidifying agents, with some finding no significant difference.[80]

Topical antibiotics used in the treatment of AOE include aminoglycosides, polymyxin B, and quinolones. These are often found in combination with steroids, including hydrocortisone or dexamethasone. Neomycin is commonly formulated with polymyxin B and hydrocortisone. Of note, neomycin may induce permanent sensorineural hearing loss as a result of cochlear damage, so it should not be used in patients with a perforated TM ipsilateral to the site of infection.[32,80] Quinolone-containing otic drops that are FDA approved in the use of AOE include Floxin (ofloxacin otic solution, approved 1990), Ciprodex (ciprofloxacin and dexamethasone, approved 2003), and Otovel (ciprofloxacin and fluocinolone acetonide, approved 2016).[80,82,83] There is no known risk for ototoxicity with these products, making them useful in patients with TM perforations.

When comparing otic preparations, Ciprodex (ciprofloxacin-dexamethasone) has been shown to reduce pain and infection more quickly than neomycin/polymyxin/hydrocortisone.[84]

However, neomycin/polymyxin/hydrocortisone is significantly cheaper. Oral antibiotic coverage is not necessary in uncomplicated AOE, unless there is infectious extension outside the EAC or the patient has high-risk comorbidities, including diabetes mellitus or immunosuppression.[80] Multiple studies have found no statistically significant difference between topical and systemic antibiotics in the treatment of diffuse, uncomplicated AOE.[85,86]

Surgical

There is rarely an indication for surgical management in AOE. Surgical intervention is indicated in cases of malignant otitis externa, which may require surgical debridement in recalcitrant cases and cases with concomitant middle ear disease. With advancements in antipseudomonal antibiotic therapy, these situations are rare.[87]

Complications

Malignant Otitis Externa

Although there are few concerning complications of AOE, infection in patients with poorly controlled diabetes or who are immunocompromised raises concern for progression to malignant otitis externa (MOE), a life-threatening disease.[88] MOE occurs through extension of the AOE through the skin overlying the bony-cartilaginous junction, resulting in an osteomyelitis of the underlying temporal bone. It is hypothesized that the higher pH of the cerumen and poor leukocyte function in diabetic and immunocompromised patients predisposes them to MOE.[11] *P. aeruginosa* is the usual culprit, accounting for 50 to 90% of cases, with *S. aureus, Proteus mirabilis, Proteus* species, *Aspergillus fumigatus,* and *Klebsiella* species reported in some cases.[88,89] For nondiabetic patients with MOE, an increased suspicion for atypical organism involvement should exist.[81]

Clinically, the presentation of MOE may vary, with common symptoms including otalgia, otorrhea, aural fullness, and hearing loss.[88] Many of these symptoms also coexist in AOE, making diagnostic distinction difficult. Distinguishing characteristics of MOE include AOE refractory to treatment, as well as associated complications, such as osteomyelitis, cranial nerve palsies (most commonly of the facial nerve), meningitis, and intracranial abscesses.[90] On physical exam, there may be granulation tissue at the bony-cartilaginous junction

No single confirmatory diagnostic test exists for MOE. The clinician should have increased suspicion in a patient who has pain out of proportion to the findings on examination, especially in diabetic and immunocompromised patients. When MOE is on the differential, workup should include laboratory analysis, including inflammatory markers, such as white blood cell count, erythrocyte sedimentation rate (ESR), and C-reactive protein (CRP), which may all be elevated with MOE.[91] CT is often favored for diagnostic and prognostic prediction, with MRI useful in evaluation of soft tissue involvement (Figure 13-7). Bony changes may be detected on imaging as early as 3 to 5 days from disease onset.[88] Although several decades ago nuclear medicine studies, including technetium-99m (^{99m}Tc) and gallium-67 ([Ga]67) were preferred modalities in the workup of MOE, their use has fallen out of favor.[92,93] However, ^{99m}Tc may continue to be used for diagnosis because of its high sensitivity and [Ga]67 for its usefulness in deciding the end point of antibiotic therapy for MOE, which is typically 4 to 6 weeks after the initiation of treatment.[11,88] The use of positron emission tomography (PET) with 2-deoxy-2[fluorine-180] fluoro-D-glucose integrated with CT ([18F]FDG-PET/CT) in MOE is currently under investigation, with one study finding a sensitivity of 96% and a specificity of 91%, the highest reported accuracy for confirming or excluding MOE.[94]

Treatment of MOE may include a combination of medical and surgical interventions. For diabetic patients, strict glucose control is a necessity. Both topical and oral fluoroquinolones are commonly used, and their demonstrated efficacy has decreased the need for hospitalization in many situations.[95] In cases of fluoroquinolone resistance, third-generation cephalosporins with antipseudomonal activity may be considered.[88] Although the optimal length of antibiotic treatment in MOE remains controversial, a common time frame is 4 to 6 weeks.[88,96] For cases in which no clinical improvement is seen after 6 weeks of conventional treatment, the MOE is deemed refractory. In this situation, as well as cases of aggressive or advanced disease and facial nerve paralysis, surgical intervention including at least a mastoidectomy is indicated.[97] Clinicians should follow up with MOE patients for at least a year post-treatment, since MOE may reoccur as long as one year after treatment completion.[98] Monitoring may include a combination of physical examination, inflammatory marker monitoring, and nuclear imaging to assess for treatment response and disease resolution.[88,93,94]

Conclusions

Acute infections of the ear are a common presenting complaint. AOM occurs more often in young children, because of unfavorable anatomy of the eustachian tube. It is often medically managed and self-limited in many cases. However, it may result in severe complications and sequelae that require surgical intervention. Awareness of potential complications is a necessity, because AOM may rapidly progress if not recognized early, resulting in devastating neurologic complications. Mastoiditis is a complication that occurs as an extension of AOM. Management of mastoiditis is trending toward more conservative therapies with good results. Treatment options for AOM and mastoiditis will likely continue to evolve as antibiotic resistance increases and vaccines create a changing microbiologic environment.

AOE may be seen in a variety of age groups, with certain populations being predisposed to this infection. Diagnosis is made by clinical assessment, and the disease is often uncomplicated with excellent response to topical treatments. In diabetic or immunocompromised patients, there is concern that the infection will spread beyond the confines of the EAC, creating an osteomyelitis of the underlying temporal bone, known as MOE. Treatment of MOE typically involves antibiotics, with surgical intervention being rare. As with AOM, the profile of the organisms causing AOE continues to evolve.

In an era of improving antibiotics and preventive measures, such as vaccines, the profile of these acute infections will likely change. It will be the responsibility of the clinician to follow the evolution of these diseases to prevent their acute complications. Doing so will be a challenge, but a worthwhile undertaking. New solutions to old problems are the future of these infections.

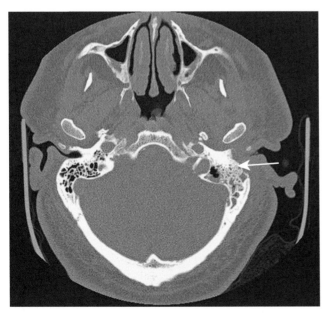

• **Figure 13-7** Malignant Otitis Externa. There is bony erosion of the posterior canal and extension of inflammation into the mastoid cortex *(arrow)*. (From Carfrae MJ, Kesser BW. Malignant otitis externa. *Otolaryngol Clin North Am.* 2008;41:537-549, viii-ix.)

References

1. Tahtinen PA, Laine MK, Huovinen P, Jalava J, Ruuskanen O, Ruohola A. A placebo-controlled trial of antimicrobial treatment for acute otitis media. *N Engl J Med*. 2011;364(2):116-126. Available at: http://doi.org/10.1056/NEJMoa1007174.

2. Hoberman A, Paradise JL, Rockette HE, et al. Treatment of acute otitis media in children under 2 years of age. *N Engl J Med*. 2011; 364(2):105-115. Available at: http://doi.org/10.1056/NEJMoa 0912254.

3. Hendley JO. Clinical practice: otitis media. *N Engl J Med*. 2002;347(15):1169-1174. Available at: http://doi.org/10.1056/ NEJMcp010944.

4. Celind J, Sodermark L, Hjalmarson O. Adherence to treatment guidelines for acute otitis media in children: the necessity of an effective strategy of guideline implementation. *Int J Pediatr Otorhinolaryngol*. 2014;78(7):1128-1132. Available at: http://doi.org/10.1016/j.ijporl.2014.04.029.

5. Coker TR, Chan LS, Newberry SJ, et al. Diagnosis, microbial epidemiology, and antibiotic treatment of acute otitis media in children: a systematic review. *JAMA*. 2010;304(19):2161-2169. Available at: http://doi.org/10.1001/jama.2010.1651.

6. Tong S, Amand C, Kieffer A, Kyaw MH. Trends in healthcare utilization and costs associated with pneumonia in the United States during 2008-2014. *BMC Health Serv Res*. 2018;18(1):715. Available at: http://doi.org/10.1186/s12913-018-3529-4.

7. Chesney J, Black A, Choo D. What is the best practice for acute mastoiditis in children? *Laryngoscope*. 2014;124(5):1057-1058. Available at: http://doi.org/10.1002/lary.24306.

8. Geva A, Oestreicher-Kedem Y, Fishman G, Landsberg R, DeRowe A. Conservative management of acute mastoiditis in children. *Int J Pediatr Otorhinolaryngol*. 2008;72(5):629-634. Available at: http://doi.org/10.1016/j.ijporl.2008.01.013.

9. Luntz M, Bartal K, Brodsky A, Shihada R. Acute mastoiditis: the role of imaging for identifying intracranial complications. *Laryngoscope*. 2012;122(12):2813-2817. Available at: http://doi.org/ 10.1002/lary.22193.

10. Minks DP, Porte M, Jenkins N. Acute mastoiditis: the role of radiology. *Clin Radiol*. 2013;68(4):397-405. Available at: http:// doi.org/10.1016/j.crad.2012.07.019.

11. Carfrae MJ, Kesser BW. Malignant otitis externa. *Otolaryngol Clin North Am*. 2008;41(3):537-549, viii-ix. Available at: http:// doi.org/10.1016/j.otc.2008.01.004.

12. Kaur R, Morris M, Pichichero ME. Epidemiology of acute otitis media in the postpneumococcal conjugate vaccine era. *Pediatrics*. 2017;140(3):e20170101. Available at: http://doi.org/10.1542/peds. 2017-0181.

13. Pichichero ME. Ten-year study of acute otitis media in Rochester, NY. *Pediatr Infect Dis J*. 2016;35(9):1027-1032. Available at: http://doi.org/10.1097/INF.0000000000001216.

14. Kyaw MH, Lynfield R, Schaffner W, et al. Effect of introduction of the pneumococcal conjugate vaccine on drug-resistant *Streptococcus pneumoniae*. *N Engl J Med*. 2006;354(14):1455-1463. Available at: http://doi.org/10.1056/NEJMoa051642.

15. Ben-Shimol S, Givon-Lavi N, Leibovitz E, Raiz S, Greenberg D, Dagan R. Impact of widespread introduction of pneumococcal conjugate vaccines on pneumococcal and nonpneumococcal otitis media. *Clin Infect Dis*. 2016;63(5):611-618. Available at: http://doi.org/10.1093/cid/ciw347.

16. Roland PS, Stroman DW. Microbiology of acute otitis externa. *Laryngoscope*. 2002;112(7 Pt 1):1166-1177. Available at: http:// doi.org/10.1097/00005537-200207000-00005.

17. Lieberthal AS, Carroll AE, Chonmaitree T, et al. The diagnosis and management of acute otitis media. *Pediatrics*. 2013;131(3): e964-e999. Available at: http://doi.org/10.1542/peds.2012-3488.

18. Marchisio P, Galli L, Bortone B, et al. Updated guidelines for the management of acute otitis media in children by the Italian Society of Pediatrics: treatment. *Pediatr Infect Dis J*. 2019;38(suppl 12S):S10-S21. Available at: http://doi.org/10.1097/INF.0000000000002452.

19. Goldman RD. Acute otitis media in children 6 months to 2 years of age. *Can Fam Physician*. 2022;68(8):589-590. Available at: http://doi.org/10.46747/cfp.6808589.

20. Rosenfeld RM, Tunkel DE, Schwartz SR, et al. Clinical practice guideline: tympanostomy tubes in children (update). *Otolaryngol Head Neck Surg*. 2022;166(suppl 1):S1-S55. Available at: http:// doi.org/10.1177/01945998211065662.

21. Cummings CW. *Cummings Otolaryngology: Head and Neck Surgery*. 5th ed. Philadelphia: Mosby/Elsevier; 2010.

22. Pan WR, le Roux CM, Levy SM, Briggs CA. Lymphatic drainage of the external ear. *Head Neck*. 2011;33(1):60-64. Available at: http://doi.org/10.1002/hed.21395.

23. Gaddey HL, Wright MT, Nelson TN. Otitis media: rapid evidence review. *Am Fam Physician*. 2019;100(6):350-356.

24. Gisselsson-Solen M, Henriksson G, Hermansson A, Melhus A. Risk factors for carriage of AOM pathogens during the first 3 years of life in children with early onset of acute otitis media. *Acta Otolaryngol*. 2014;134(7):684-690. Available at: http://doi. org/10.3109/00016489.2014.890291.

25. Pichichero ME. Otitis media. *Pediatr Clin North Am*. 2013;60(2): 391-407. Available at: https://doi.org/10.1016/j.pcl.2012.12.007.

26. McCormick DP, Jennings K, Ede LC, Alvarez-Fernandez P, Patel J, Chonmaitree T. Use of symptoms and risk factors to predict acute otitis media in infants. *Int J Pediatr Otorhinolaryngol*. 2016;81:55-59. Available at: http://doi.org/10.1016/j.ijporl.2015.12.002.

27. Paul CR, Moreno MA. Acute otitis media. *JAMA Pediatr*. 2020;174(3):308. Available at: http://doi.org/10.1001/jamapediatrics.2019.5664.

28. Prins-van Ginkel AC, Bruijning-Verhagen PC, Uiterwaal CS, van der Ent CK, Smit HA, de Hoog ML. Acute otitis media during infancy: parent-reported incidence and modifiable risk factors. *Pediatr Infect Dis J*. 2017;36(3):245-249. Available at: http://doi.org/10.1097/INF.0000000000001412.

29. Kobayashi M, Farrar JL, Gierke R, et al. Use of 15-valent pneumococcal conjugate vaccine and 20-valent pneumococcal conjugate vaccine among U.S. adults: updated recommendations of the Advisory Committee on Immunization Practices—United States, 2022. *MMWR Morb Mortal Wkly Rep*. 2022;71(4):109-117. Available at: http://doi.org/10.15585/mmwr.mm7104a1.

30. Marom T, Tan A, Wilkinson GS, Pierson KS, Freeman JL, Chonmaitree T. Trends in otitis media-related health care use in the United States, 2001-2011. *JAMA Pediatr*. 2014;168(1):68-75. Available at: http://doi.org/10.10.1001/jamapediatrics.2013.3924.

31. Pontefract B, Nevers M, Fleming-Dutra KE, Hersh A, Samore M, Madaras-Kelly K. Diagnosis and antibiotic management of otitis media and otitis externa in United States Veterans. *Open Forum Infect Dis*. 2019;6(11):ofz432. Available at: http://doi.org/10.1093/ofid/ofz432.

32. Lee H, Kim J, Nguyen V. Ear infections: otitis externa and otitis media. *Prim Care*. 2013;40(3):671-686. Available at: https://doi.org/10.1016/j.pop.2013.05.005.

33. Thomas NM, Brook I. Otitis media: an update on current pharmacotherapy and future perspectives. *Expert Opin Pharmacother*. 2014;15(8):1069-1083. Available at: https://doi.org/10.1517/14 656566.2014.903920.

34. Sone M, Kato T, Nakashima T. Current concepts of otitis media in adults as a reflux-related disease. *Otol Neurotol.* 2013;34(6):1013-1017. Available at: https://doi.org/10.1097/MAO.0b013e318299aa52.

35. Cohen R, Varon E, Doit C, et al. A 13-year survey of pneumococcal nasopharyngeal carriage in children with acute otitis media following PCV7 and PCV13 implementation. *Vaccine.* 2015;33(39):5118-5126. Available at: https://doi.org/10.1016/j.vaccine.2015.08.010.

36. Wald ER, DeMuri GP. Antibiotic recommendations for acute otitis media and acute bacterial sinusitis: conundrum no more. *Pediatr Infect Dis J.* 2018;37(12):1255-1257. Available at: https://doi.org/10.1097/INF.0000000000002009.

37. Klein A, Tamir SO, Sorek N, Hanun G, Yeshayahu Y, Marom T. Increase in *Haemophilus influenzae* detection in 13-valent pneumococcal conjugate vaccine immunized children with acute otitis media. *Pediatr Infect Dis J.* 2022;41(8):678-680. Available at: https://doi.org/10.1097/INF.0000000000003561.

38. Kaur R, Fuji N, Pichichero ME. Dynamic changes in otopathogens colonizing the nasopharynx and causing acute otitis media in children after 13-valent (PCV13) pneumococcal conjugate vaccination during 2015-2019. *Eur J Clin Microbiol Infect Dis.* 2022;41(1):37-44. Available at: https://doi.org/10.1007/s10096-021-04324-0.

39. Zevallos JP, Vrabec JT, Williamson RA, et al. Advanced pediatric mastoiditis with and without intracranial complications. *Laryngoscope.* 2009;119(8):1610-1615. Available at: https://doi.org/10.1002/lary.20259.

40. Tawfik KO, Ishman SL, Tabangin ME, Altaye M, Meinzen-Derr J, Choo DI. Pediatric acute mastoiditis in the era of pneumococcal vaccination. *Laryngoscope.* 2018;128(6):1480-1485. Available at: https://doi.org/10.1002/lary.26968.

41. Choi SS, Lander L. Pediatric acute mastoiditis in the post-pneumococcal conjugate vaccine era. *Laryngoscope.* 2011;121(5):1072-1080. Available at: https://doi.org/10.1002/lary.21727.

42. Cavel O, Tauman R, Simsolo E, et al. Changes in the epidemiology and clinical features of acute mastoiditis following the introduction of the pneumococcal conjugate vaccine. *Int J Pediatr Otorhinolaryngol.* 2018;104:54-57. Available at: https://doi.org/10.1016/j.ijporl.2017.10.025.

43. Harmes KM, Blackwood RA, Burrows HL, Cooke JM, Harrison RV, Passamani PP. Otitis media: diagnosis and treatment. *Am Fam Physician.* 2013;88(7):435-440.

44. Danishyar A, Ashurst JV. Acute otitis media. In: *StatPearls.* Treasure Island, FL: StatPearls; 2022.

45. Schilder AG, Chonmaitree T, Cripps AW, et al. Otitis media. *Nat Rev Dis Primers.* 2016;2(1):16063. Available at: https://doi.org/10.1038/nrdp.2016.63.

46. McCormick DP, Chonmaitree T, Pittman C, et al. Nonsevere acute otitis media: a clinical trial comparing outcomes of watchful waiting versus immediate antibiotic treatment. *Pediatrics.* 2005;115(6):1455-1465. Available at: https://doi.10.1542/peds.2004-1665.

47. Shah-Becker S, Carr MM. Current management and referral patterns of pediatricians for acute otitis media. *Int J Pediatr Otorhinolaryngol.* 2018;113:19-21. Available at: https://doi.org/10.1016/j.ijporl.2018.06.036.

48. Frost HM, Bizune D, Gerber JS, Hersh AL, Hicks LA, Tsay SV. Amoxicillin versus other antibiotic agents for the treatment of acute otitis media in children. *J Pediatr.* 2022;251:98-104.e5. Available at: https://doi.org/10.1016/j.jpeds.2022.07.053.

49. Perkins JA. Medical and surgical management of otitis media in children. *Otolaryngol Clin North Am.* 2002;35(4):811-825. Available at: https://doi.org/10.1016/s0030-6665(02)00051-8.

50. Wald ER. Management of recurrent acute otitis media. *N Engl J Med.* 2021;384(19):1859-1860. Available at: https://doi.org/10.1056/NEJMe2104952.

51. Rubin LG, Papsin B; Committee on Infectious D, Section on Otolaryngology-Head and Neck Surgery. Cochlear implants in children: surgical site infections and prevention and treatment of acute otitis media and meningitis. *Pediatrics.* 2010;126(2):381-391. Available at: https://doi.org/10.1542/peds.2010-1427.

52. Harley EH, Sdralis T, Berkowitz RG. Acute mastoiditis in children: a 12-year retrospective study. *Otolaryngol Head Neck Surg.* 1997;116(1):26-30. Available at: https://doi.org/10.1016/S0194-59989770347-4.

53. Daniel M, Gautam S, Scrivener TA, Meller C, Levin B, Curotta J. What effect has pneumococcal vaccination had on acute mastoiditis? *J Laryngol Otol.* 2013;127(suppl 1):S30-S34. Available at: https://doi.org/10.1017/S0022215112002654.

54. Balsamo C, Biagi C, Mancini M, Corsini I, Bergamaschi R, Lanari M. Acute mastoiditis in an Italian pediatric tertiary medical center: a 15-year retrospective study. *Ital J Pediatr.* 2018;44(1):71. Available at: https://doi.org/10.1186/s13052-018-0511-z.

55. King LM, Bartoces M, Hersh AL, Hicks LA, Fleming-Dutra KE. National incidence of pediatric mastoiditis in the United States, 2000-2012: creating a baseline for public health surveillance. *Pediatr Infect Dis J.* 2019;38(1):e14-e16. Available at: https://doi.org/10.1097/INF.0000000000002049.

56. Anthonsen K, Hostmark K, Hansen S, et al. Acute mastoiditis in children: a 10-year retrospective and validated multicenter study. *Pediatr Infect Dis J.* 2013;32(5):436-440. Available at: https://doi.org/10.1097/INF.0b013e31828abd13.

57. Loh R, Phua M, Shaw CL. Management of paediatric acute mastoiditis: systematic review. *J Laryngol Otol.* 2018;132(2):96-104. Available at: https://doi.org/10.1017/S0022215117001840.

58. Ghadersohi S, Young NM, Smith-Bronstein V, Hoff S, Billings KR. Management of acute complicated mastoiditis at an urban, tertiary care pediatric hospital. *Laryngoscope.* 2017;127(10):2321-2327. Available at: https://doi.org/10.1002/lary.26365.

59. Psarommatis IM, Voudouris C, Douros K, Giannakopoulos P, Bairamis T, Carabinos C. Algorithmic management of pediatric acute mastoiditis. *Int J Pediatr Otorhinolaryngol.* 2012;76(6):791-796. Available at: https://doi.org/10.1016/j.ijporl.2012.02.042.

60. Anne S, Schwartz S, Ishman SL, Cohen M, Hopkins B. Medical versus surgical treatment of pediatric acute mastoiditis: a systematic review. *Laryngoscope.* 2019;129(3):754-760. Available at: https://doi.org/10.1002/lary.27462.

61. Edwards S, Kumar S, Lee S, Pali BL, Marek RL, Dutta A. Epidemiology and variability in management of acute mastoiditis in children. *Am J Otolaryngol.* 2022;43(5):103520. Available at: https://doi.org/10.1016/j.amjoto.2022.103520.

62. Luntz M, Brodsky A, Nusem S, et al. Acute mastoiditis: the antibiotic era: a multicenter study. *Int J Pediatr Otorhinolaryngol.* 2001;57(1):1-9. Available at: https://doi.org/10.1016/s0165-5876(00)00425-0.

63. Zanetti D, Nassif N. Indications for surgery in acute mastoiditis and their complications in children. *Int J Pediatr Otorhinolaryngol.* 2006;70(7):1175-1182. Available at: https://doi.org/10.1016/j.ijporl.2005.12.002.

64. Smith JA, Danner CJ. Complications of chronic otitis media and cholesteatoma. *Otolaryngol Clin North Am.* 2006;39(6):1237-1255. Available at: https://doi.org/10.1016/j.otc.2006.09.001.

65. Brouwer MC, McIntyre P, Prasad K, van de Beek D. Corticosteroids for acute bacterial meningitis. *Cochrane Database Syst Rev.* 2015;(9):CD004405. Available at: https://doi.org/10.1002/14651858.CD004405.pub5.

66. Ulanovski D, Yacobovich J, Kornreich L, Shkalim V, Raveh E. Pediatric otogenic sigmoid sinus thrombosis: 12-year experience. *Int J Pediatr Otorhinolaryngol.* 2014;78(6):930-933. Available at: https://doi.org/10.1016/j.ijporl.2014.03.016.

67. Duarte MJ, Kozin ED, Barshak MB, et al. Otogenic brain abscesses: a systematic review. *Laryngoscope Investig Otolaryngol.* 2018;3(3):198-208. Available at: https://doi.org/10.1002/lio2.150.

68. Sadoghi M, Dabirmoghaddam P. Otitic hydrocephalus: case report and literature review. *Am J Otolaryngol.* 2007;28(3):187-190. Available at: https://doi.org/10.1016/j.amjoto.2006.07.007.

69. Cassano P, Ciprandi G, Passali D. Acute mastoiditis in children. *Acta Biomed.* 2020;91(suppl 1):54-59. Available at: https://doi.org/10.23750/abm.v91i1-S.9259.

70. Spiegel JH, Lustig LR, Lee KC, Murr AH, Schindler RA. Contemporary presentation and management of a spectrum of mastoid abscesses. *Laryngoscope.* 1998;108(6):822-828. Available at: https://doi.org/10.1097/00005537-199806000-00009.

71. Enoksson F, Groth A, Hultcrantz M, Stalfors J, Stenfeldt K, Hermansson A. Subperiosteal abscesses in acute mastoiditis in 115 Swedish children. *Int J Pediatr Otorhinolaryngol.* 2015;79(7):1115-1120. Available at: https://doi.org/10.1016/j.ijporl.2015.05.002.

72. Psarommatis I, Giannakopoulos P, Theodorou E, Voudouris C, Carabinos C, Tsakanikos M. Mastoid subperiosteal abscess in children: drainage or mastoidectomy? *J Laryngol Otol.* 2012;126(12):1204-1208. Available at: https://doi.org/10.1017/S0022215112002332.

73. Lin YH, Lin MY. Bezold abscess. *Ear Nose Throat J.* 2015;94(6):E45-E46. Available at: https://doi.org/10.1177/014556131509400621.

74. Valeggia S, Minerva M, Muraro E, et al. Epidemiologic, imaging, and clinical issues in Bezold's abscess: a systematic review. *Tomography.* 2022;8(2):920-932. Available at: https://doi.org/10.3390/tomography8020074.

75. Spratley J, Silveira H, Alvarez I, Pais-Clemente M. Acute mastoiditis in children: review of the current status. *Int J Pediatr Otorhinolaryngol.* 2000;56(1):33-40. Available at: https://doi.org/10.1016/s0165-5876(00)00406-7.

76. Palma S, Bovo R, Benatti A, et al. Mastoiditis in adults: a 19-year retrospective study. *Eur Arch Otorhinolaryngol.* 2014;271(5):925-931. Available at: https://doi.org/10.1007/s00405-013-2454-8.

77. Xiao Q, Zhang Y, Lv J, Yang J, Zhang Q. Case report: suppurative labyrinthitis induced by chronic suppurative otitis media. *Front Neurol.* 2022;13:892045. Available at: https://doi.10.3389/fneur.2022.892045.

78. Wu JF, Jin Z, Yang JM, Liu YH, Duan ML. Extracranial and intracranial complications of otitis media: 22-year clinical experience and analysis. *Acta Otolaryngol.* 2012;132(3):261-265. Available at: https://doi.org/10.3109/00016489.2011.643239.

79. Leskinen K, Jero J. Acute complications of otitis media in adults. *Clin Otolaryngol.* 2005;30(6):511-516. Available at: https://doi.org/10.1111/j.1749-4486.2005.01085.x.

80. Rosenfeld RM, Schwartz SR, Cannon CR, et al. Clinical practice guideline: acute otitis externa. *Otolaryngol Head Neck Surg.* 2014;150(suppl 1):S1-S24. Available at: https://doi.org/10.1177/0194599813517083.

81. Hobson CE, Moy JD, Byers KE, Raz Y, Hirsch BE, McCall AA. Malignant otitis externa: evolving pathogens and implications for diagnosis and treatment. *Otolaryngol Head Neck Surg.* 2014;151(1):112-116. Available at: https://doi.org/10.1177/0194599814528301.

82. Dohar JE, Garner ET, Nielsen RW, Biel MA, Seidlin M. Topical ofloxacin treatment of otorrhea in children with tympanostomy tubes. *Arch Otolaryngol Head Neck Surg.* 1999;125(5):537-545. Available at: https://doi.org/10.1001/archotol.125.5.537.

83. Graham DB, Tripp J. Ofloxacin. In: *StatPearls.* Treasure Island, FL: StatPearls; 2022.

84. Roland PS, Younis R, Wall GM. A comparison of ciprofloxacin/dexamethasone with neomycin/polymyxin/hydrocortisone for otitis externa pain. *Adv Ther.* 2007;24(3):671-675. Available at: https://doi.org/10.1007/BF02848792.

85. Pottumarthy S, Fritsche TR, Sader HS, Stilwell MG, Jones RN. Susceptibility patterns of *Streptococcus pneumoniae* isolates in North America (2002-2003): contemporary in vitro activities of amoxicillin/clavulanate and 15 other antimicrobial agents. *Int J Antimicrob Agents.* 2005;25(4):282-289. Available at: https://doi.org/10.1016/j.ijantimicag.2004.12.001.

86. Roland PS, Belcher BP, Bettis R, et al. A single topical agent is clinically equivalent to the combination of topical and oral antibiotic treatment for otitis externa. *Am J Otolaryngol.* 2008;29(4):255-261. Available at: https://doi.org/10.1016/j.amjoto.2007.09.002.

87. Rubin Grandis J, Branstetter BF IV, Yu VL. The changing face of malignant (necrotising) external otitis: clinical, radiological, and anatomic correlations. *Lancet Infect Dis.* 2004;4(1):34-39. Available at: https://doi.org/10.1016/s1473-3099(03)00858-2.

88. Trevino Gonzalez JL, Reyes Suarez LL, Hernandez de Leon JE. Malignant otitis externa: an updated review. *Am J Otolaryngol.* 2021;42(2):102894. Available at: https://doi.org/10.1016/j.amjoto.2020.102894.

89. Yang TH, Xirasagar S, Cheng YF, et al. Malignant otitis externa is associated with diabetes: a population-based case-control study. *Ann Otol Rhinol Laryngol.* 2020;129(6):585-590. Available at: https://doi.org/10.1177/0003489419901139.

90. Adegbiji WA, Aremu SK, Nwawolo CC, Alabi SB, Lasisi AO. Malignant otitis externa in developing country. *Clin Otorhinolaryngol.* 2017;1(1):003.

91. Honnurappa V, Ramdass S, Mahajan N, Vijayendra VK, Redleaf M. Effective inexpensive management of necrotizing otitis externa is possible in resource-poor settings. *Ann Otol Rhinol Laryngol.* 2019;128(9):848-854. Available at: https://doi.org/10.1177/0003489419846143.

92. Moss WJ, Finegersh A, Narayanan A, Chan JYK. Meta-analysis does not support routine traditional nuclear medicine studies for malignant otitis. *Laryngoscope.* 2020;130(7):1812-1816. Available at: https://doi.org/10.1002/lary.28411.

93. Sturm JJ, Stern Shavit S, Lalwani AK. What is the best test for diagnosis and monitoring treatment response in malignant otitis externa? *Laryngoscope.* 2020;130(11):2516-2517. Available at: https://doi.org/10.1002/lary.28609.

94. Stern Shavit S, Bernstine H, Sopov V, Nageris B, Hilly O. FDG-PET/CT for diagnosis and follow-up of necrotizing (malignant) external otitis. *Laryngoscope.* 2019;129(4):961-966. Available at: https://doi.org/10.1002/lary.27526.

95. Sylvester MJ, Sanghvi S, Patel VM, Eloy JA, Ying YM. Malignant otitis externa hospitalizations: analysis of patient characteristics. *Laryngoscope.* 2017;127(10):2328-2336. Available at: https://doi.org/10.1002/lary.26401.

96. Arsovic N, Radivojevic N, Jesic S, Babac S, Cvorovic L, Dudvarski Z. Malignant otitis externa: causes for various treatment responses. *J Int Adv Otol.* 2020;16(1):98-103. Available at: https://doi.org/10.5152/iao.2020.7709.

97. Singh J, Bhardwaj B. The role of surgical debridement in cases of refractory malignant otitis externa. *Indian J Otolaryngol Head Neck Surg.* 2018;70(4):549-554. Available at: https://doi.org/10.1007/s12070-018-1426-0.

98. Peled C, Parra A, El-Saied S, Kraus M, Kaplan DM. Surgery for necrotizing otitis externa-indications and surgical findings. *Eur Arch Otorhinolaryngol.* 2020;277(5):1327-1334. Available at: https://doi.org/10.1007/s00405-020-05842-x.

14

Nasal and Paranasal Sinus Infections

WALTER M. JONGBLOED, KYLE JOHNSON, AND KOUROSH PARHAM

Infection of the nasal cavity and paranasal sinuses is extremely common. In the United States alone, it affects an estimated 35 million adults each year and accounts for close to 16 million office visits annually.[1] When considering vital etiologies, the overall prevalence is much higher; most people have experienced this personally and potentially annually, because approximately 90% of patients with colds have an element of viral sinusitis.[2] The cost to the health system is significant. Roughly $11 billion is spent each year for direct management of acute and chronic sinusitis[1] in the diagnosis and management of sinusitis in adults each year, predominantly in the form of ambulatory and emergency department visits, but this also includes the nearly 500,000 surgical procedures performed each year. Annually, there is an estimated 73 million restricted activity days.[2] More than 1 in 5 antibiotic prescriptions is written in the United States for the treatment of sinusitis, making sinusitis the fifth most common diagnosis cited for antibiotic use, consequently contributing to the growing antibiotic resistance in the community and hospitals nationwide.[3] This chapter discusses the pathophysiology and management of nasal and paranasal sinus infections.

Nasal and Paranasal Sinus Anatomy and Physiology

The nose is a pyramidal structure anchored to the anterior center portion of the face (Figure 14-1). It consists of a bony skeleton superiorly and a cartilaginous framework inferiorly, covered by the facial skin envelope. The interior of the nose is lined by ciliated respiratory epithelium. The nasal cavity is divided in the midline by the nasal septum, which is constructed of a bony and cartilaginous midline structure and an overlying mucopericondrial layer. The lateral walls of the nasal cavity have bony outgrowths called the nasal conchae or turbinates (Figure 14-2). There are three or four turbinates on either side, the inferior, middle, and superior turbinates, with a fourth, known as the supreme turbinate, present in a minority of individuals. These are covered in respiratory epithelium and function to help regulate nasal resistance and airflow through the nasal cycle, a process by which swelling of the turbinates alternates from one side to the other through the engorgement of the turbinate mucosa similar to erectile tissue in the reproductive system. The increased surface area afforded by the turbinates also helps warm and humidify air as it enters the upper respiratory tract. Air travels medial to the anterior aspect of the inferior turbinate, lateral to the nasal septum, and inferomedial to the lateral nasal wall through an area of the highest resistance to airflow, otherwise known as the internal nasal valve. Small changes in this valve can have significant clinical implications: Swelling of one or more structures can lead to significant nasal obstruction. The cavity anterior to the inferior turbinate constitutes the nasal vestibule.

The paranasal sinuses consist of four paired normally air-containing spaces in the bones of the facial skeleton (Figure 14-3). The sinuses are named for the bones in which they are found and are the maxillary, ethmoid, frontal, and sphenoid sinuses. The function of the paranasal sinuses is uncertain. Proposed functions or benefits of these aerated sinuses in the face include resonance for speech production, decreased weight and mass of the head, and provision of an area to absorb force and thus protect the intracranial contents from trauma.[4] The cavities are lined by ciliated respiratory epithelium, which sweeps mucus produced in each cavity toward the sinus opening, or ostium. This mucociliary transport then proceeds along the lateral nasal walls and posteriorly into the nasopharynx and subsequently into the oropharynx, where it is swallowed. Nasal mucous production may exceed 1 to 2 quarts per day! Disruption in mucociliary transport can occur due to swelling or obstruction in the region of the sinus ostia with subsequent symptoms of fullness, pressure, and pain, many of the cardinal symptoms of sinusitis. The ethmoid and maxillary sinuses are the first to form, both of which are present at birth and continue to grow into adolescence. The frontal and sphenoid sinuses are the last to become aerated, and this process does not occur until adolescence. Thus, sinus disease in children is primarily encountered in the maxillary and ethmoid sinuses. Frontal and sphenoid sinus disease is isolated almost exclusively to adults.

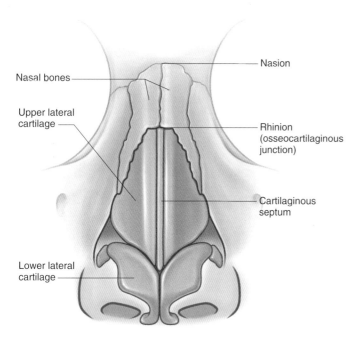

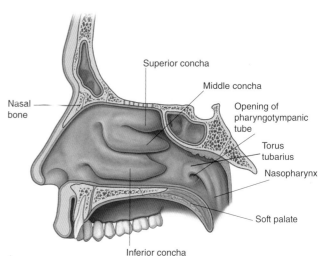

• **Figure 14-2** Right Lateral Nasal Wall Anatomy. (From Drake RL, Vogl AW, Mitchell AWM. *Grey's Anatomy for Students*. 3rd ed. Philadelphia: Churchill Livingstone; 2015.)

• **Figure 14-1** Bony and Cartilaginous Structure of the Nose. (From Aston SJ, Steinbrech DS, Walden JL. *Aesthetic Plastic Surgery*. Philadelphia: Saunders; 2009.)

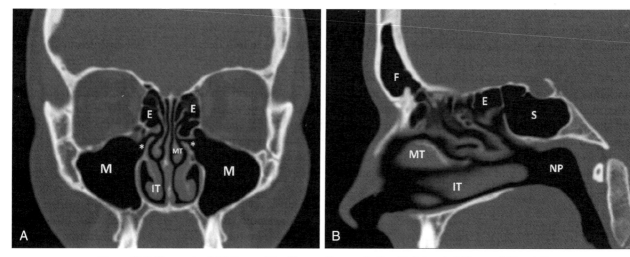

• **Figure 14-3** Noncontrast CT Scan of the Sinuses Demonstrating Well-Aerated Sinuses Without Air-Fluid Levels or Thickening of the Sinus Mucosa in a Patient Without Nasal Symptoms. **A,** Coronal cut. **B,** Sagittal cut. *, Maxillary sinus ostia; *E,* air cells of the ethmoid sinuses; *F,* frontal sinus; *IT,* inferior turbinate; *M,* maxillary sinuses; *MT,* middle turbinate; *NP,* nasopharynx. *S,* sphenoid sinus.

Etiology and Pathophysiology

Acute infection in the paranasal sinuses is most commonly due to viral infection. In a small subset of these, between 0.5 and 3%, bacterial infection may complicate the viral infection. The three most common pathogens in adults with initial episodes of acute bacterial rhinosinusitis (ABRS) are *Streptococcus pneumoniae, Haemophilus influenzae,* and *Moraxella catarrhalis,* each found in 20 to 43%, 22 to 25%, and 2 to 10% of aspirates, respectively.[5] *M. catarrhalis* is

found more frequently in children. *Staphylococcus aureus* and various anaerobes are also frequently isolated in cultures from sinus aspirates.

Chronic rhinosinusitis (CRS) has a more complicated pathophysiology, and represents a spectrum of disease, with the medical literature primarily distinguishing chronic rhinosinusitis with nasal polyposis (CRSwNP) from that without polypoid disease (CRSsNP). However, this too is proving to be somewhat of an oversimplification of the disease spectrum. Contributing factors to the development of

CRS may include multiple players, with infection itself not necessarily representing the main offender. When cultures are obtained in patients with CRS, the result is commonly polymicrobial consisting of both aerobic and anaerobic pathogens. However, polymicrobial isolates have also been discovered in nondiseased sinuses, calling in question the role of bacterial infection in the pathogenesis of CRS. Other possible contributing causes include excessive host response to *Alternaria* fungi, the production of exotoxins by staphylococcal superantigens, altered host immune response to normal flora or common pathogens such as defects in the eicosanoid pathway, discoordination of mucociliary transport, sinonasal mucosal inflammation, and the presence or development of biofilms.[6] Furthermore, other host diseases also contribute to the severity and frequency of exacerbations of CRS or recurrent acute rhinosinusitis (RARS) such as allergic rhinitis, diabetes, and immune suppression.[6]

Acute Rhinosinusitis

History and Physical

Patients with rhinosinusitis may complain of nasal obstruction, rhinorrhea, facial pain, fullness or pressure, fever, malaise, fatigue, halitosis, hyposmia, anosmia, maxillary dental pain, and/or ear fullness or pain. Characterizing the duration of symptoms is important for classifying the type of infection, with acute infections defined as lasting no longer than 4 weeks, chronic infections classified as lasting beyond 3 months, and subacute infections making up the difference in between. Physical examination findings may include fever, turbinate edema, nasal secretions, postnasal drip, or tenderness of the cheeks, forehead, or teeth. Other physical examination findings suggestive of a complicated infection with extrasinus involvement include orbital proptosis, periorbital edema and erythema, limitation of extraocular movements or other cranial neuropathies, and neck stiffness.

Of these possible history and examination findings, the cardinal symptoms of up to 4 weeks of purulent nasal drainage (anterior, posterior, or both) accompanied by nasal obstruction; facial pain, pressure, and fullness; or both has been proposed by the American Academy of Otolaryngology–Head and Neck Surgery (AAO-HNS) Clinical Practice Guideline on Adult Sinusitis in 2015 as the most sensitive and specific for the diagnosis of ABRS. Further, additional signs and symptoms include fever, cough, fatigue (malaise), reduced sense of smell (hyposmia), lack of sense of smell (anosmia), maxillary dental pain, and ear fullness or pressure.[7] Combinations of major and minor symptoms were used to define ARS in early consensus reports but have since been abandoned to focus on the three cardinal features.

Only about 0.5 to 2.0% of viral rhinosinusitis (VRS) episodes are complicated by bacterial infection.[8] Intriguingly, although viral illness more commonly manifests with clear rhinorrhea, the opacification of mucus does not occur because of the presence of bacteria in the mucus but rather as a result of the presence of neutrophils, which is not specific to bacterial infections and may be present in VRS as well. Therefore, the color of the rhinorrhea alone is not sufficient to differentiate bacterial from viral infection. On the other hand, a finding of purulent secretions in the nasal cavity or posterior oropharynx correlates higher than any other examination finding with positive bacterial cultures from sinus aspiration as well as predicting radiographic findings consistent with ABRS in research studies.[6] Historically, a system of major and minor criteria has been used to differentiate viral from bacterial acute sinus infections. However, more recent publications have focused on the previously three cardinal symptoms and signs of ABRS and have shown a high correlation between the presence of these three findings with culture results and radiographic imaging.[9] Of note, fever has been shown to have a sensitivity and specificity of only approximately 50% for the diagnosis of acute bacterial sinusitis versus viral infection, and therefore the presence or absence of fever alone is insufficient to rule in or rule out bacterial infection.[10,11]

Another important distinction in differentiating viral from acute bacterial infections is the progression of symptoms. Viral illnesses tend to improve and resolve within 7 to 10 days, whereas ABRS is characterized by a history of symptoms persisting beyond 10 days without improvement or a so-called "double worsening" of symptoms, when the patient's symptoms worsen within 10 days after an initial improvement in symptoms.[12] Although fever alone is not sufficient to differentiate between viral and bacterial infections, patients who present with more severe symptoms or signs and high fever ($\geq$39°C [102°F]) with purulent nasal discharge or facial pain in the first 3 to 4 days of their illness do tend to benefit from antibiotic therapy before the 10-day mark.[13] Therefore, assessing the time course and severity of the patient's symptoms is another important clue in differentiating viral from bacterial acute rhinosinusitis. Figure 14-4 summarizes a diagnostic/management algorithm for sinusitis.

Cultures

Direct sinus aspiration, primarily of the maxillary sinuses, is a method used as the gold standard for diagnosing ABRS, predominantly in the research of sinonasal diseases and much less in clinical practice. Cultures of fluid from the nasal cavity or nasopharynx correlates poorly with directly obtained sinus aspirates, and as such fails to reliably differentiate ABRS from VRS in clinical trials. Other studies have demonstrated better correlation of endoscopically obtained middle meatal cultures with direct aspirates, but this technique has yet to find an established role in the care of patients with uncomplicated ABRS, given that procedure is costly, time-consuming, potentially painful to the patient, and requires equipment not generally readily available in the offices of most primary care physicians.[14] However, in patients who fail treatment with first- and second-line empiric antibiotic therapy, culture-directed therapy should be the next step. In this situation, sinus puncture is still considered the gold standard with endoscopically guided cultures of the middle meatus considered as an alternative

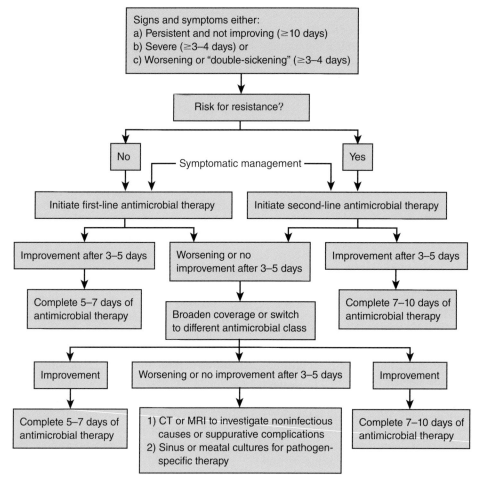

Signs and symptoms either:
a) Persistent and not improving (≥10 days)
b) Severe (≥3–4 days) or
c) Worsening or "double-sickening" (≥3–4 days)

Risk for resistance?

No   Symptomatic management   Yes

Initiate first-line antimicrobial therapy

Initiate second-line antimicrobial therapy

Improvement after 3–5 days

Worsening or no improvement after 3–5 days

Improvement after 3–5 days

Complete 5–7 days of antimicrobial therapy

Broaden coverage or switch to different antimicrobial class

Complete 7–10 days of antimicrobial therapy

Improvement

Worsening or no improvement after 3–5 days

Improvement

Complete 5–7 days of antimicrobial therapy

1) CT or MRI to investigate noninfectious causes or suppurative complications
2) Sinus or meatal cultures for pathogen-specific therapy

Complete 7–10 days of antimicrobial therapy

• **Figure 14-4** Decision Tree for the Management of Acute Bacterial Rhinosinusitis. (Adapted from the Infectious Disease Society of America Clinical Practice Guideline for Acute Bacterial Rhinosinusitis in Children and Adults, 2012.)

according to the Infectious Diseases Society of America (IDSA) guidelines.[13]

Imaging

Radiographic imaging is not recommended for the diagnosis of acute RS primarily because of the inability to distinguish viral from bacterial infection. However, in suspected ABRS with extrasinus complications suggested by severe headache, proptosis, cranial nerve palsies, or facial swelling, contrast-enhanced computed tomography (CT) or gadolinium-enhanced magnetic resonance imaging (MRI) is indicated to diagnose and characterize the extent of extrasinus involvement and to allow for appropriate treatment planning.[15] CT scan is preferred over MRI, given the utility of CT scan for surgical planning and intraoperative navigation.[6] CT scans are also generally much more readily available, do not generally require sedation for children, and can help to confirm the diagnosis more quickly, helping to expedite surgical treatment when necessary. MRI should not be overlooked as a complementary imaging modality, particularly when intracranial complications are suspected as discussed in the later section on complications.

Treatment

Medical Management

Antibiotics

Antibiotics have no role in the treatment of VRS, and for patients diagnosed with VRS, supportive therapy is indicated, as discussed later. Amoxicillin was long considered the first-line antibiotic of choice for ABRS given its low cost, safety, efficacy, and appropriately narrow microbiologic spectrum. However, the clinical practice guideline on ABRS published in 2012 by the IDSA recommends standard dosing of amoxicillin-clavulanate as first-line treatment instead of amoxicillin in both children and adults given the increased prevalence of β-lactam–resistant *H. influenzae* and *M. catarrhalis* in ABRS infections. Respiratory fluoroquinolones (levofloxacin and moxifloxacin) and doxycycline both have excellent activity against the usual pathogens causing uncomplicated ABRS and are therefore considered appropriate alternatives in the event of penicillin allergy. The third-generation oral cephalosporins cefixime or cefpodoxime may be used in conjunction with clindamycin for children with non–type I penicillin allergy or in geographic regions with high endemic rates of penicillin nonsusceptible *S. pneumoniae*. However, oral cephalosporins are no longer recommended for empiric monotherapy of ABRS.[13] Other alternatives that have been traditionally used in patients with penicillin allergy that are no longer recommended because of unacceptably high rates of resistance in *S. pneumoniae* and *M. catarrhalis* are trimethoprim-sulfamethoxazole (TMP-SMX) and macrolides (azithromycin and clarithromycin). The Sinus and Allergy Partnership Guidelines recommend using a fluoroquinolone or high-dose amoxicillin-clavulanate (4 g/250 mg per day or two extended-release tablets every 12 hours in adults and 90 mg/kg/day for children) for patients who have received antibiotics in the 4 to 6 weeks before the start of their current episode of sinusitis. The IDSA extended the recommendation for high-dose amoxicillin-clavulanate to include treating patients in geographic regions with high endemic rates (≥10%) of invasive penicillin nonsusceptible *S. pneumoniae,* those with severe infection (defined as systemic toxicity with high fever of 39°C (102°F) or higher, and threat of suppurative complications), age younger than 2 or older than 65 years, children who attend day care, recent hospitalization, or immunocompromised state.[13]

The AAO-HNS Clinical Practice Guideline on Adult Sinusitis in 2015 reports no difference in outcomes among different antibiotic agents, more specifically between amoxicillin or amoxicillin-clavulanate when compared with cephalosporins or macrolides.[16] Amoxicillin is often preferred by prescribers due to safety, efficacy, low cost, and narrow microbiologic spectrum. The decision to add clavulanate

for adults is for those at high risk of being infected by an amoxicillin-resistant organism. These risks include antibiotic use in past month, close contact with treated individuals, health care providers or a health care environment, failure of prior antibiotic therapy, breakthrough infection despite prophylaxis, close contact with a child in a day care facility, smoker or smoker in the family, and high prevalence of resistant bacteria in community.[17,18]

Duration of antibiotic therapy is not universally agreed upon, with the majority of clinical trials administering antibiotics for 10 days. Other trials have used shorter duration of therapy and show no significant difference in outcomes between 6 and 10 days of antibiotics versus 3 to 5 days of antibiotics (azithromycin, telithromycin, or cefuroxime) at up to 3 weeks after completion of treatment.[19] Importantly, shorter duration of therapy is correlated with lower incidence of adverse reactions such as diarrhea, nausea/vomiting, and vaginal discharge. In fact, some authors have advocated for a "watch and wait" approach for patients with nonsevere presentation (mild-moderate pain, fever <101°F), reserving antibiotics for patients whose symptoms are more severe at presentation or fail to improve or worsen within 7 days after diagnosis. This approach is strengthened by data showing up to 73% improvement in symptoms on placebo 7 to 12 days after initiation of therapy in patients with nonsevere ABRS.[20] For these reasons, the IDSA guidelines recommend a 5- to 7-day course of antibiotics for uncomplicated ABRS in adults (see Tables 14-1 and 14-2). However, evidence of efficacy of shorter courses of antibiotics is lacking in the pediatric population, so 7 to

TABLE 14-1   Antibacterial Regimens for Acute Bacterial Rhinosinusitis in Children

Indication	First-Line (Daily Dose)	Second-Line (Daily Dose)
Initial empiric therapy	Amoxicillin-clavulanate (45 mg/kg/day PO bid)	Amoxicillin-clavulanate (90 mg/kg/day PO bid)
β-Lactam allergy		
Type I hypersensitivity		Levofloxacin (10-20 mg/kg/day PO every 12-24 h)
Non–type I hypersensitivity		Clindamycin* (30-40 mg/kg/day PO tid) plus cefixime (8 mg/kg/day PO bid) or cefpodoxime (10 mg/kg/day PO bid)
Risk for antibiotic resistance or failed initial therapy		Amoxicillin-clavulanate (90 mg/kg/day PO bid)
		Clindamycin (30-40 mg/kg/day PO tid) plus cefixime (8 mg/kg/day PO bid) or cefpodoxime (10 mg/kg/day PO bid)
		Levofloxacin (10-20 mg/kg/day PO every 12-24 h)
Severe infection requiring hospitalization		Ampicillin/sulbactam (200-400 mg/kg/day IV every 6 h)
		Ceftriaxone (50 mg/kg/day IV every 12 h)
		Cefotaxime (100-200 mg/kg/day IV every 6 h)
		Levofloxacin (10-20 mg/kg/day IV every 12-24 h)

bid, Twice daily; *IV*, intravenously; *PO*, orally; *tid*, three times daily.
Adapted from the Infectious Disease Society of America Clinical Practice Guideline for Acute Bacterial Rhinosinusitis in Children and Adults, 2012.

TABLE 14-2	Antibacterial Regimens for Acute Bacterial Rhinosinusitis in Adults	
Indication	**First-Line (Daily Dose)**	**Second-Line (Daily Dose)**
Initial empiric therapy	Amoxicillin-clavulanate (500 mg/125 mg PO tid, or 875 mg/125 mg PO bid)	Amoxicillin-clavulanate (2000 mg/ 125 mg PO bid)
		Doxycycline (100 mg PO bid or 200 mg PO daily)
β-Lactam allergy		Doxycycline (100 mg PO bid or 200 mg PO daily)
		Levofloxacin (500 mg PO daily)
		Moxifloxacin (400 mg PO daily)
Risk for antibiotic resistance or failed initial therapy		Amoxicillin-clavulanate (2000 mg/125 mg PO bid)
		Levofloxacin (500 mg PO daily)
		Moxifloxacin (400 mg PO daily)
Severe infection requiring hospitalization		Ampicillin-sulbactam (1.5-3 g IV every 6 h)
		Levofloxacin (500 mg PO or IV daily)
		Moxifloxacin (400 mg PO or IV daily)
		Ceftriaxone (1-2 g IV q 12-24 h)
		Cefotaxime (2 g IV q 4-6 h)

bid, Twice daily; *IV,* intravenously; *PO,* orally; *tid,* three times daily.
Adapted from the Infectious Disease Society of America Clinical Practice Guideline for Acute Bacterial Rhinosinusitis in Children and Adults, 2012.

10 days remains the duration recommended by the IDSA for children with ABRS.[13] Literature to date shows no difference in clinical success for antibiotics given for 3 to 7 days versus 6 to 10 days.[21]

Using the same data and rationale, worsening of symptoms 48 to 72 hours after starting appropriate initial empiric antimicrobial therapy or failure to improve 3 to 5 days after initiation of antibiotic therapy should prompt the clinician to consider nonbacterial cause or infection with organisms resistant to the initially prescribed antibiotic. In the case in which the patient was initially treated with amoxicillin-clavulanate, the clinician should suspect β-lactamase–producing *H. influenzae* or *M. catarrhalis,* as well as β-lactam, macrolide, tetracycline, or TMP-SMX–resistant *S. pneumoniae,* because these organisms have been identified in aspirates in studies that have evaluated initial treatment failure for presumed ABRS.[22] Therefore, the IDSA guidelines recommend switching to a second-line antibiotic (see Figure 14-4) and treat for 7 to 10 days instead of the usual 5- to 7-day course.[13] Treatment failure, especially worsening of symptoms, should also prompt the clinician to evaluate for possible complications of sinusitis as evidenced by severe headaches, restricted extraocular muscle movement, orbital proptosis, mental status changes, vision changes, and/or periorbital edema, erythema or inflammation. This investigation may include further diagnostic studies as discussed previously.

A discussion on antibiotic stewardship is warranted as sinusitis is the fifth most common reason for antibiotic prescription. Especially in the urgent care setting, providers are pressured to see patients quickly. Further, an emphasis is placed on patient satisfaction, which is often tied to meeting patient's expectations. Patients with signs and symptoms of sinusitis usually expect antibiotics. Educational initiatives have shown significant reductions in antibiotic prescribing for ARS when provided with a simple education intervention and algorithmic tools.[23] The coronavirus disease 2019 (COVID-19) pandemic has created a need for virtual care to decrease exposure, and therefore many visits to urgent care and primary care offices have been replaced by either video visits, which allow for two-way communication between patient and provider, or E-visits, which are asynchronous visits that occur through a secure patient portal for minor acute illnesses, such as sinusitis. Interventions to encourage antibiotic stewardship in this setting also have been implemented, include a multifaceted stewardship bundle for E-visits, which has shown a direct improvement in guideline-concordant prescribing for sinusitis.[24] This shows that even in the setting of an ever-changing health care landscape with the added challenge of a global pandemic, there is opportunity for antibiotic stewardship.

Adjunctive Therapies

Symptomatic relief is indicated for the treatment of acute bacterial and VRS. Seeking relief from symptoms of ARS should begin with counseling on optimizing hydration (e.g., 6 to 8 glasses of water daily) and optimizing immune system function by promoting healthy lifestyle (including adequate sleep/nutrition and avoiding irritants such as tobacco smoke). Other treatments may include the use of topical or systemic decongestants to mitigate symptoms of nasal congestion and possibly prevent secondary bacterial infection, although these have not been shown to consistently prevent progression to ABRS. Oxymetazoline and neosynephrine are topical nasal decongestant sprays that both have the advantage of negligible systemic absorption, and also tend to be more effective in symptomatically improving nasal congestion than oral systemic decongestants. Topical decongestants, however, have not been shown to prevent development of ABRS, and the data in support of their use as an adjunct for symptomatic relief is not very strong.[20] An important consideration is the possible development of rhinitis medicamentosa, or rebound nasal congestion, after concluding use of topical decongestant sprays. Therefore, treating clinicians often limit their use to 3 to 5 days at a time. Furthermore, the sprays themselves may induce further inflammation in the sinus mucosa. Systemic decongestants, while avoiding the risk of rhinitis medicamentosa, should be avoided in patients with known hypertension because these may cause exacerbation of the same. Guidelines differ in their recommendations for using decongestants, with the AAO-HNS guidelines leaving decongestants as an option, although the more recently released IDSA guidelines recommend against their use entirely.

Systemic and topical steroids also have been used as adjunctive therapies to improve symptoms in patients with acute rhinosinusitis. Theoretically, the use of steroids could reduce the swelling of the nasal mucosa because of the allergic response in patients with allergic rhinitis. The medical literature, however, does not support the use of systemic steroids for the treatment of VRS, and the evidence is not very strong in support of topical steroid sprays in this setting either.[25] In the case of ABRS, there are no trials that have studied systemic glucocorticoids, but there are several that have evaluated the benefits of topical corticosteroid sprays in combination with antibiotics. Agents studied include mometasone, fluticasone, flunisolide and beclomethasone. One of the highest quality of these studies specifically demonstrated significantly improved mean symptom scores during days 2 to 15 in patients with nonsevere ABRS treated with topical mometasone fuorate nasal spray twice daily compared to patients treated with amoxicillin or placebo.[26] Patients with a strong history of allergic rhinitis are the most likely to benefit from the addition of intranasal topical steroid sprays.

Nasal saline irrigation is another adjunctive measure that may be beneficial for improved quality of life and decreased symptom severity for patients with acute rhinosinusitis. Two clinical trials showed modest improvement in mucociliary transport and symptoms in patients with acute rhinosinusitis treated with hypertonic (3 to 5%) saline irrigation.[27,28] Another randomized controlled trial, however,

found no difference in outcomes for hypertonic saline, normal saline, or observation for patients with the common cold and acute rhinosinusitis.[29] In the studies that show benefit, patients with frequent bouts of rhinosinusitis tended to have the greatest improvement, and therefore may be those whom the clinician should particularly recommend use nasal saline irrigations.

Antihistamines also have been considered for symptomatic treatment of acute rhinosinusitis symptoms because of a drying effect, but the data to support this practice are lacking. To date, no studies have been published specifically assessing this possible benefit in VRS. In ABRS, there are no studies that support the use of antihistamines in non-atopic patients, and these may, in fact, worsen symptoms by drying nasal mucosa and exacerbating nasal congestion. However, one RCT showed improvement in sneezing and nasal congestion for loratadine versus placebo in combination with antibiotics and oral steroids in allergic patients with ABRS.[30] Therefore, antihistamine therapy, particularly second-generation histamine$_1$-antagonists, given their decreased drowsiness and fewer anticholinergic side effects compared to first-generation drugs, may be considered for patients whose symptoms suggest a significant allergic component but are likely not helpful in patients without atopy.

Finally, pain management is an important consideration in these patients, because this is commonly a major factor that leads them to seek medical care. There are no data specifically evaluating different pain management approaches in acute rhinosinusitis, but acetaminophen and nonsteroidal antiinflammatory drugs (NSAIDs) alone are usually sufficient to control mild to moderate pain. The use of fixed-combination medications with opioids (e.g., acetaminophen or ibuprofen with codeine, oxycodone, or hydrocodone) is also appropriate in patients with moderate pain. Severe pain not responding to oral medications should prompt the clinician to investigate other possible causes for the patient's symptoms, including the possibility of development of extrasinus complications.

Chronic Rhinosinusitis and Recurrent Acute Rhinosinusitis

CRS and recurrent acute rhinosinusitis (RARS) generally require a different approach to treatment and thus will be considered separately from acute viral and bacterial rhinosinusitis. The impact of these disease processes is perhaps more dramatic on public health and well-being, with affected patients experiencing suffering from worsening mood, bodily pain, decreased energy levels, and poorer physical and social function in addition to their sinonasal complaints. Furthermore, costs related to treatment of CRS and recurrent ARS are high because of the need for multiple physician office visits, prescription and over-the-counter medications, and the need for surgical therapy (which is much less often indicated in the care of acute rhinosinusitis, except in the presence of extrasinus complications).

History and Physical

Symptoms of CRS are similar to those of patients with ARS, with nasal obstruction (81 to 95%); facial congestion, pressure, and/or fullness (70 to 85%); discolored rhinorrhea (51 to 83%); and hyposmia (61 to 69%) being the most common.[31] The persistence of two or more of these symptoms for 12 weeks or longer is highly sensitive for diagnosing CRS. But patients may additionally complain of headache, fever, cough, bad breath, fatigue, dental pain, and other nonspecific symptoms. The differential diagnosis for these symptoms is broad and includes allergic rhinitis, nonallergic rhinitis, vasomotor rhinitis, eosinophilic nonallergic rhinitis, nasal septal deformity, allergic fungal rhinosinusitis, invasive fungal rhinosinusitis and other nonrhinogenic causes of facial pain, such as the neurologic disorders vascular headache, migraine, trigeminal neuralgia, and other facial pain syndromes. Therefore, unlike in acute rhinosinusitis, the symptoms alone are insufficiently specific to diagnose CRS, and the diagnosis ultimately requires objective findings of sinonasal inflammation.[32,33] Such findings include purulent mucus or edema visualized in the middle meatus or ethmoid region, polyps in the nasal cavity or middle meatus, and/or radiographic imaging demonstrating inflammation of the paranasal sinuses.

The diagnosis of RARS is made when a patient experiences 4 or more episodes of ABRS in a year, without signs or symptoms of rhinosinusitis between episodes. Experts have debated in the literature whether to set the cutoff for RARS between 2 and 4 episodes per year. Studies evaluating the common cold document an average incidence of 1.4 to 2.3 episodes of cold per adult per year. Given that bacterial infection complicates a viral upper respiratory infection (URI) between 0.5% and 2.0% of the time,[8] the average adult is expected to suffer an ABRS infection less than once a year. Furthermore, because it is sometimes difficult to differentiate a viral illness from ABRS, setting a cutoff as low as 2 infections per year (the natural frequency of the common cold), could readily lead to overdiagnosis of RARS. For these reasons, both a multidisciplinary panel and the AAO-HNS have set the cutoff at 4 or more infections per year for the diagnosis of RARS. Additionally, each episode must meet the diagnostic criteria listed in the previous section regarding ABRS to fully make a diagnosis of RARS.[6] Therefore, the clinician is encouraged to confirm true bacterial infection to establish this diagnosis, which may be difficult, but can be aided through consultation with an otolaryngologist.

Another important consideration when managing CRS and RARS, is that these conditions are more likely to have other factors predisposing to more severe disease burden than isolated acute rhinosinusitis. These may include allergic rhinitis, cystic fibrosis, immunocompromised state, and ciliary dyskinesia, as well as anatomic variations. Allergic rhinitis may cause edema that can obstruct the paranasal sinus ostia, predisposing to RARS and CRS. Cystic fibrosis has a well-established association with CRS, and the immunodeficient states of IgA and IgG deficiencies have also been documented in patients with CRS and RARS.[34] Increased mucociliary transport time found in CRS may be due to ciliary dyskinesia, and studies have shown that surgical correction of anatomic obstruction of the paranasal sinuses improves objective measure of CRS.[35] For these reasons, the clinician should assess for these disease-modifying factors in patients with RARS and CRS.

Diagnostic Tests

Nasal Endoscopy

In contrast to ARS, nasal endoscopy as a diagnostic technique has a well-established role in the management of CRS to provide objective documentation of the presence of inflammation in the sinonasal cavity indicated by the presence of purulent mucus or edema in the middle meatus or ethmoid region, or polyps in the nasal cavity or middle meatus. Anterior rhinoscopy, consisting of the use of a light source and an instrument to dilate the nasal vestibule, only allows evaluation of the anterior one third of the nasal cavity, and given there is a presumed underlying cause in patients with RARS or CRS, this evaluation does not provide enough information to properly manage these conditions. The AAO-HNS 2015 guidelines strongly recommend confirming a clinical diagnosis of CRS with objective documentation of sinonasal inflammation, which may be accomplished using anterior rhinoscopy, nasal endoscopy, or CT. Nasal endoscopy is a technique using a rigid or flexible lighted endoscope to gain visualization that includes the posterior nasal cavity and nasopharynx and in many instances permits visualization of the sinus drainage pathways themselves, including the sphenoid ostium in the sphenoethmoidal recess and the uncinate process, semilunar hiatus, and ethmoidal bulla in the middle meatus that may be performed in the office under topical decongestant and anesthetic sprays. The information obtained during nasal endoscopy can be vital in planning surgical management for patients with pathologic conditions such as posterior nasal septal deviation, polyps in the nasal cavity, middle meatus, or sphenoethmoidal recess, neoplasms, soft tissue masses, foreign bodies, tissue necrosis, purulent discharge, and findings consistent with autoimmune or granulomatous disease. Furthermore, nasal endoscopy may permit directed cultures. Biopsy also may be performed, but complications such as damage to CNS structures, orbital contents, and potentially life-threatening hemorrhage make endoscopic nasal biopsy a procedure often performed under general anesthesia in the operating suite.[36] Other downsides to the use of nasal endoscopy for the confirmation of the diagnosis of CRS and RARS are the need for costly equipment, training in the use and care of the equipment, and the potential for minor complications, including bleeding and mild patient discomfort. For these reasons, referral to an otolaryngologist for nasal endoscopy is a useful adjunct in the diagnosis of CRS and RARS.

Imaging

CT scan without intravenous contrast of the paranasal sinuses is considered the gold standard imaging modality of choice for evaluating the paranasal sinuses (Figure 14-5). The medical literature provides strong support for the use of noncontrast CT to evaluate patients with CRS or RARS. Strengths of this technique include the ability to provide excellent anatomic detail for evaluating the patency of sinus ostia, presence of sinonasal polyposis, mucosal thickening, and anatomic variants. The superior anatomic detail afforded by CT scans also may be used to provide image guidance during endoscopic surgery. CT imaging may be used to exclude other more worrisome processes that might mimic CRS or RARS such as aggressive infections or neoplastic disease. Destruction of bony structures, extension of disease beyond the sinuses, and local invasion alert the clinician to a possible malignant process, and these should be evaluated further with MRI, whereas MRI is otherwise infrequently indicated in the evaluation paranasal sinus disease.[6]

There is some controversy in the medical literature regarding the use of CT scans versus nasal endoscopy for the evaluation and surveillance of patients with CRS and RARS. Benefits of nasal endoscopy over CT scan include avoidance of radiation, and a higher positive predictive value of nasal endoscopy over CT imaging.[37] On the other hand, a recently published cost-analysis estimated an average cost savings of $326 to $503 per patient for whom primary care clinicians confirmed the diagnosis of CRS with CT without contrast before treating or referring to an otolaryngologist for further evaluation and treatment.[38] Further research has concluded that once referred to the otolaryngology office, nasal endoscopy should be a first-line confirmatory test for CRS, reserving CT scanning for patients with a prolonged or complicated clinical course.[37]

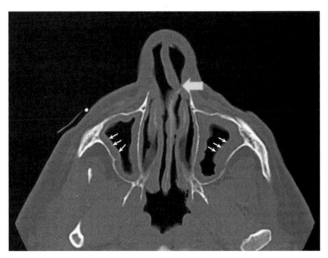

• **Figure 14-5** Axial CT scan without contrast demonstrating significant thickening of the maxillary sinus mucosa *(small arrows)* and a significant nasal septal deviation to the left *(large arrow)* in a patient with chronic sinusitis.

Allergy and Immune Function Testing

Patients with concomitant immune dysfunction or allergy often suffer more severe or unremitting bouts of RARS and flares of their CRS. Allergic rhinitis in particular has a very close association with CRS, with allergic rhinitis being more prevalent among patients with CRS than controls, and a higher prevalence of CRS among patients with allergic rhinitis than controls.[39] Furthermore, patients with allergic rhinitis and CRS tend to have more severe symptoms than their nonallergic counterparts.[40] Clinicians should therefore consider obtaining allergy skin testing in patients with CRS and RARS, and recommend management strategies such as allergen avoidance, immunotherapy, or both. The prevalence of AR is 40 to 84% in adults with CRS and 25 to 31% in young adults with sinusitis.[41] Unfortunately, however, despite a preponderance of data demonstrating a relationship between CRS and allergic rhinitis, there is a paucity of data showing improvement in RARS and CRS symptoms in allergic patients who practice allergen avoidance, undergo immunomodulating therapy, or both.[42]

Failure to respond to aggressive management of CRS and RARS should raise the suspicion of an immunodeficient state. Between 30 and 68% of patients with HIV suffer from CRS or RARS,[43] and one study found that 10% and 6% of patients refractory to medical and surgical therapy of their sinusitis were ultimately diagnosed with common variable immunodeficiency and immunoglobulin A (IgA) deficiency, respectively.[44] Hypogammaglobulinemia is another common primary immunodeficiency with a known association with RARS. Other clues as to the presence of a possible immune-deficient state include comorbid infections such as bronchitis, bronchiectasis, or recurrent otitis media. In this setting, the clinician should consider laboratory studies such as quantitative immunoglobulin measurements, preimmunization and postimmunization specific antibody responses to tetanus toxoid and pneumococcal vaccine, and tests such as delayed hypersensitivity skin tests and flow cytometric enumeration of T cells to measure T cell number and function.[6]

Nasal Polyposis

The AAO-HNS recommends that clinicians should confirm the presence of absence of nasal polyps in a patient with CRS. The presence of nasal polyps affects need for further diagnostic testing and treatment management. Roughly 4% of patients with CRS have polyposis.[45] Association among asthma, nasal polyps, and aspirin sensitivity is a recognized entity. AERD, otherwise known as aspirin triad or Samter's triad, is characterized by hypersensitivity to aspirin and other NSAIDs, asthma and CRSwNP.[46] Unilateral polyps should prompt investigation for other conditions such as carcinoma, inverting papilloma, and antrochoanal polyp, to name a few.

Treatment

Strategies to prevent recurrence or flare-ups are a mainstay of management in RARS and CRS. Good hand hygiene in the form of soap and water or the use of an alcohol-based hand rub can help reduce the risk of contracting a viral infection that may precede an episode of ABRS. Smoking cessation is also an important preventive measure to discuss with patients, because the prevalence of ABRS, RARS, and CRS has been shown to be higher in cigarette smokers.[47] Gastroesophageal reflux disease (GERD) also may be related to sinusitis, with some evidence suggesting that the use of PPI in patients with GERD may prevent CRS.[48]

Nasal Saline

The use of nasal saline in the management of CRS and RARS has a well-established track record. Potential benefits of using nasal saline include improved mucociliary function, decreased nasal mucosal edema, and mechanical rinsing of infection debris and allergens. There are also some data demonstrating a decreased reliance on other medications when nasal saline irrigations are employed.[49] Delivery methods include sprays, nebulization, nasal douching, and bulb syringe irrigation. Some studies report improved symptoms with hypertonic saline compared to isotonic saline, but the data are insufficient to establish superiority of hypertonic saline over isotonic preparations for nasal irrigation.[50] Side effects of nasal saline use includes nasal irritation, nosebleeds, nasal burning, tearing, headaches, and nasal drainage.[20]

Antibiotics

Antibiotic treatment of CRS is an important part of managing acute flare-ups of CRS and RARS. However, given the chronic nature of the disease, long-term antibiotic treatment is often indicated for CRS. Studies have particularly evaluated long-term treatment with macrolide antibiotics in patients with CRS without nasal polyposis (CRSsNP), citing a response rate between 60 and 80%.[42] This most frequently consists of a 12-week regimen beginning with 2 weeks of erythromycin 500 mg twice daily, followed by 250 mg twice daily for the remaining 10 weeks, but other macrolides (azithromycin, roxithromycin, clarithromycin) have also demonstrated similarly encouraging results. TMP-SMX also has been studied and demonstrates efficacy comparable to that of the macrolides.[51] Longer duration of treatment seems to show better outcomes, with one study showing improved outcomes on up to 1 year of antibiotic therapy.[52] Short-term antibiotic use is indicated in the management of exacerbations, and regimens studied in the literature include ciprofloxacin, amoxicillin/clavulanic acid, and cefuroxime for a duration of 9 to 14 days, each showing improvement in acute exacerbations and recidivism.[53] The data for use of antibiotics in patients with nasal polyps (CRSwNP) is less encouraging, showing only modest improvement in polyp size or statistically insignificant improvement in quality-of-life measures.[54] Topical preparations of antibiotics also have been studied, but data thus far lack significant benefit over nasal saline alone.[55]

Corticosteroids

Steroid therapy is a mainstay in the management of CRS. A preponderance of data support the use of topical intranasal steroids for treating patients with and without nasal polyps. No studies have demonstrated any superiority of one preparation over another, aside from negligible systemic absorption of the second-generation corticosteroids such as mometasone, fluticasone, and ciclesonide compared to up to 34 to 39% systemic absorption of first-generation steroids such as budesonide, betamethasone, beclamethasone, triamcinolone, and dexamethasone. Several options for delivery of topical steroid medications include nasal aerosols, turbuhalers, and sprays, with sprays being the least effective at delivering medication to the sinuses. Of note, penetration of medication to the sinuses is markedly improved after sinus surgery and may even be as low as 2 to 3% preoperatively regardless of the delivery method employed.[56] Side effects of nasal steroid sprays are generally minimal and include nasal irritation or dryness and epistaxis, as discussed earlier.

Oral corticosteroids may sometimes also be employed in the management of CRS. Data are sparse to support its use in patients without nasal polyps.[57] However, mounting data support the use of oral steroids to rapidly shrink polyps to allow for improved access of topical steroid therapy.[58] Typical courses studied in the medical literature start at 30 to 50 mg daily or tapered for a total of approximately 2 weeks.

Bioabsorbable Sinus Implants

Corticosteroid-eluting implants are placed into the sinus cavity to allow for consistent delivery of corticosteroids to the target organ. Many of the products are intended to be used in the immediate postoperative period. They have shown improved outcomes with reduced need for additional medical and surgical interventions in CRSsNP and CRSwNP.[59] Implants placed in the frontal outflow tract have also shown improved outcomes in the short term, and longer-lasting implants designed to elude corticosteroids over 90 days have also shown efficacy.[60]

Immunotherapy

The emergence of immunotherapy for treatment of CRS has developed considerably in the last 10 years. Dupilumab is a monoclonal anti–interleukin-4 (anti–IL-4) antibody that functions by preventing binding of IL-4 and IL-13, thereby blocking signaling for type 2 inflammation. It was approved for treatment of CRSwNP in 2019 after showing positive effects in phase 2 and phase 3 clinical trials.[61,62] It remains the only biologic medication approved by the U.S. Food and Drug Administration for the treatment of CRSwNP; others such as omalizumb, mepolizumab, and benralizumab are currently being investigated for this use.

Surgery

Surgery is often an important part of the long-term management of CRS and particularly serves as an effective means for allowing improved delivery of medications to the sinus cavities.[56] Sinus surgery has been shown to be safe and effective for improving symptoms scores and quality of life for patients with CRS with and without polyps.[63] The exact role of surgery is still somewhat debated in the literature as our understanding of the pathophysiologic contributors and our ability to address them improves. Many authors advocate for surgery as a last resort when maximal medical therapy has failed,[64] although a large amount of data exist illustrating that early surgery with maintenance medical therapy is as good as medical therapy alone, with the possible additional benefits of improvements in nasal obstruction.[65]

Odontogenic Sinusitis

Dental infection is another important cause of sinus infections that deserves consideration. This process is generally recalcitrant to initial medical and surgical treatments and is usually limited to a unilateral maxillary sinus. Up to half of patients will complain of a persistent rotten smell, but as few as one third will complain of maxillary dental pain.[66] Although physical examination of the dentition may elicit tenderness to palpation, this is unfortunately also surprisingly not sensitive for the identification of maxillary sinusitis. In fact, dental imaging in the form of a panoramic x-ray is also notoriously poor at picking up dental causes of sinusitis, and dental pathologic conditions are often initially overlooked on CT scans. Nevertheless, along with a high index of suspicion, CT may be nearly 100% sensitive for identifying odontogenic causes of sinusitis.[67] Dental implants, especially with maxillary sinus augmentation, bear the risk of implant-related odontogenic sinusitis.[68] Implant exposure of more than 4 mm, onset of peri-implantitis, and a bone graft disruption or extrusion are significantly more prevalent in those with odontogenic sinusitis.[69] This study also showed that molar implants show a significantly higher rate of complications than premolar implants. Infections are typically polymicrobial, and generally these consist of normal oropharyngeal flora. Endoscopically guided cultures may be useful but often fail to isolate anaerobic pathogens. Antibiotic therapy such as clindamycin or amoxicillin-clavulanate is usually recommended because of their excellent coverage of typical oral flora.[53]

Fungal Rhinosinusitis

Fungi are an important group of pathogens that may cause infections of the sinonasal tract. These infections may be invasive or noninvasive, with invasive infections almost exclusively limited to patients with compromised immune function. Fungal infections may be further classified as localized fungal colonization, fungal ball, allergic fungal rhinosinusitis (AFRS), acute invasive fungal rhinosinusitis (AIFRS), chronic invasive fungal rhinosinusitis (CIFRS), or granulomatous invasive fungal rhinosinusitis (GIFRS).[70]

Localized Fungal Colonization

Localized fungal colonization most commonly occurs in previously operated sinus cavities in areas that may suffer from poor mucociliary clearance. Fungal elements then grow in the mucus or mucous crusts within the nasal or paranasal sinus cavities. The condition is usually asymptomatic; although it may manifest with malodor, which is why it is most often diagnosed incidentally on nasal endoscopy.[71] Findings demonstrate a grossly visible collection of fungal hyphae that often appear as a clump of mold on the sinonasal mucosa. Treatment consists of simple debridement and subsequent sinus rinses to prevent reaccumulation of crusts and fungal elements.

Fungal Ball

A fungal ball consists of a noninvasive dense accumulation of fungal hyphae usually in a solitary maxillary sinus, although the process has been described to involve other and multiple sinuses much less commonly. Diagnostic criteria include (1) sinus opacification with or without heterogeneity on radiographic imaging, (2) mucopurulent cheesy or clay-like material within the sinus cavity, (3) a dense collection of fungal hyphae separate from the sinus mucosa, (4) nonspecific chronic inflammation of the mucosa, (5) no predominance of eosinophils or granuloma or allergic mucin, and (6) an absence of fungal invasion of the mucosa on histopathologic examination.[72] Several other terms have been used historically, including mycetoma, aspergilloma, and chronic noninvasive granuloma, but more recent publications have sought to standardize the term as fungus ball.[70] Patients are often asymptomatic, but some patients develop chronic mucopurulent rhinorrhea. Treatment is surgical, with removal of the fungal contents of the involved sinus, and no subsequent treatment is indicated, given the process is noninvasive by definition. Recurrence is infrequent, reported at about 1%, and complications are uncommon, but there are reports of the infection becoming invasive after substantial immunosuppression.

Allergic Fungal Rhinosinusitis

Some individuals may develop an IgE-mediated allergic reaction to fungal elements leading to mucosal inflammation. Sensitized individuals may experience generalized sinonasal inflammation combined with thick mucinous secretions that obstruct outflow pathways of the sinuses. The fungi continue to proliferate within the sinus cavity, leading to host responses to the organisms and associated locally destructive immune responses. This may proceed to cause sinus expansion and bone erosion. Often the presentation is mild, consistent with CRS with or without polyps, usually in patients who are young with significant atopy but immunocompetent. Occasionally, however, patients may present with more dramatic signs or symptoms, including acute visual loss, gross facial dysmorphia, or complete nasal obstruction.[73] The disease also has somewhat of a geographic disposition, affecting patients in warm, humid climates such as in India and the southern United States.

The diagnostic criteria for AFRS originally proposed by Bent and Kuhn are (1) type I hypersensitivity to fungi, (2) nasal polyps, (3) characteristic findings on CT scan, (4) presence of

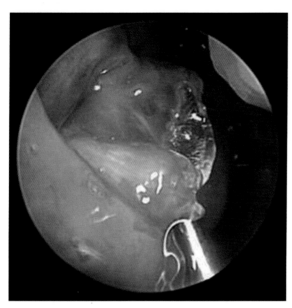

• **Figure 14-6** Allergic Mucin in a Pediatric Patient with Allergic Fungal Rhinosinusitis as Viewed with an Endonasal Endoscope. (From Thorp BD, McKinney KA, Rose AS, Ebert Jr CS. Allergic fungal sinusitis in children. *Otolaryngol Clin N Am.* 2012;45[3]:631-643, Fig. 2, with permission.)

fungi on direct microscopy or culture, and (5) allergic mucin (Figure 14-6) containing fungal elements without tissue invasion.[74] Previously operated patients may not demonstrate polyps, however, and because the proposal of these original criteria, other investigators have noted many patients lacking one or more of the criteria noted previously but whose disease process seems to behave similarly. These entities have been named eosinophilic fungal rhinosinusitis (EFRS) for those without type I hypersensitivity to fungi[75] and eosinophilic mucinous rhinosinusitis (EMRS) for those with neither hypersensitivity nor identifiable fungal hyphae.[76] The International Society for Human and Animal Mycology met in 2009 to establish a consensus regarding these terms and determined that they are poorly defined and require further investigation to refine the criteria to distinguish each entity from the others.[70] Considerable overlap exists among the three, however, specifically with regard to the presence of the thick eosinophilic mucin defined as the presence of eosinophil or eosinophil-degraded products in mucus. This usually appears thick and brown to black in color, with a consistency often compared to that of peanut butter.

Characteristic radiographic findings on CT scan include unilateral or asymmetric involvement of the sinuses, bone expansion and thickening of the bony walls of the sinuses, orbit and skull base, and heterogeneous density of the soft tissues usually without the metallic densities often noted in fungal balls. MRI will commonly demonstrate central hypointensity of the sinus cavity on T1 and an apparent signal void on T2, with peripheral enhancement on gadolinium-enhanced T1 sequences.[73]

Laboratory and immunologic studies are of special use for confirming the diagnosis of AFRS. Cultures of the eosinophilic mucin, usually obtained at the time of surgery, most commonly yield *Aspergillus* species, as well as *Alternaria, Bipolaris, Curvularia, Paecilomyces, Fusarium,* and *Scedosporium.*[71] Confirmation of type I hypersensitivity may be accomplished by either skin testing or in vitro tests such as mRAST or ImmunoCAP assays. These tests will often demonstrate sensitivities to multiple fungal allergens. Histopathologic evaluation of the mucin shows sheets of eosinophils, often with Charcot-Leyden crystals representative of eosinophilic breakdown products.[77] Special stains are often required to identify fungal hyphae on histopathologic examination.

Treatment is similar to that for non–fungal-related CRS. Patients are usually treated medically initially with nasal saline irrigations, topical steroids, and short courses of oral steroids and antibiotics. Many patients require surgery to help improve outflow from the sinuses and remove as much of the antigenic and inflammatory load as possible. This is to be followed by continued aggressive medical therapy as in nonfungal CRS. The role of desensitization therapy has yet to be confirmed by randomized controlled trials, but retrospective data suggest it may be beneficial for reducing symptom scores, improving endonasal signs of inflammation as observed on endoscopy, and decreasing the need for revision surgeries.[78] Studies to evaluate the role of antifungal therapies are lacking. There are, however, a handful of studies that demonstrate a benefit to using topical nasal fluconazole and high-dose oral itraconazole or voriconazole.[79] More research is required to establish the role of antifungal therapies in the care of patients with AFRS, however.

Acute Invasive Fungal Rhinosinusitis

Acute invasive fungal rhinosinusitis (AIFRS) is a locally aggressive disease occurring predominantly in immunocompromised patients. It is distinguished from chronic fungal infections by a duration of less than 4 weeks. The process may progress over a course of several hours and be life threatening to the patient. Patients with neutrophil dysfunction or neutropenia are especially susceptible as in the case of hematologic malignancies, aplastic anemia, uncontrolled diabetes mellitus, hemochromatosis, those undergoing antineoplastic chemotherapy, or after transplantation. However, the disease also has been reported to occur as a complication of HIV infection and in apparently immunocompetent hosts.[80] *Mucor* species are the classic pathogens at fault, but more recently *Aspergillus* species has been reported more frequently, with *Rhizopus* also among the most commonly isolated organisms.[71] Patients often have nonspecific symptoms, so a high index of suspicion is required to make the diagnosis early in any patient who is immunocompromised with fever and sinonasal symptoms.

Imaging studies generally demonstrate fairly nonspecific findings as well, such as varying degrees of soft-tissue opacification, particularly in the maxillary and ethmoid sinuses. Other findings more suggestive of AIFS, such as osseous erosion, facial soft-tissue thickening, and soft-tissue infiltration of periantral fat, unfortunately often do not manifest

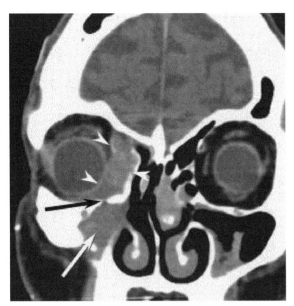

• **Figure 14-7** Coronal Reformats of a Contrast-Enhanced CT Scan in a Patient with Invasive Fungal Sinusitis. The infectious process *(white arrow)* has eroded from the maxillary sinus into the medial orbit *(arrowheads).* Dehiscence in the orbital floor where the infection has eroded through *(black arrow).* (From Branstetter IV BF, Weissman JL. Role of MR and CT in the paranasal sinuses. *Otolaryngol Clin N Am.* 2005;38[6]:1279-1299, Fig. 19, with permission.)

fungal elements invading blood vessels, vasculitis with thrombosis, hemorrhage, tissue necrosis, and acute neutrophilic infiltrates.[82] Tissue culture is necessary to identify the causative pathogen.

Treatment consists of seeking to reverse the underlying immunocompromised state, initiation of systemic antifungal therapy, and aggressive surgical debridement of all devitalized tissue. Aggressive treatment with repeated surgical debridement may be indicated in the setting of persistent disease (Figure 14-8). Amphotericin B, voriconazole, or isavuconazonium is often used, with therapy tailored to culture results.[83] Duration of antifungal therapy remains an area of uncertainty, but oral antifungal agents are often continued until immunosuppression improves. However, the persistence of immune suppression is often accompanied by dismal prognosis, with mortality rates as high as 50% reported in the literature.[84] Significant morbidity related to the aggressive surgical debridement required is also an important consideration, as orbital exenteration or resection of large portions of the palate or maxilla are often necessary to establish clear margins.

Chronic Invasive Fungal Rhinosinusitis

CIFRS has a more indolent course lasting longer than 12 weeks. It is much less frequent than the acute invasive variety and tends to infect patients with less overt immunosuppression such as diabetes mellitus, chronic corticosteroid use, and AIDS.[85] Any of the paranasal sinuses may be involved, but the ethmoid and sphenoid sinuses are most frequently affected and orbital involvement is not infrequent. Radiographic imaging will usually reveal a soft tissue density. A dense accumulation of hyphae with inflammatory reaction, occasional presence of vascular invasion, and

until late in the disease course (Figure 14–7).[81] MRI is useful for evaluating possible orbital or intracranial involvement. Biopsy is indicated to confirm the diagnosis. This is usually accomplished endoscopically, and attention is given to areas of necrosis or ischemia that often will not bleed when a biopsy is performed. Tissue samples are then sent for microscopic and histopathologic examination and culture. Microscopic examination of involved tissue is characterized by

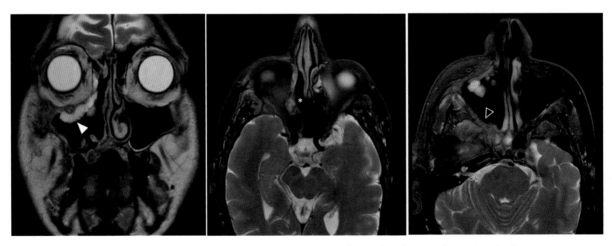

• **Figure 14-8** MRI of the Brain and Face with and Without Gadolinium Contrast Demonstrating Postoperative Changes of Right Medial Wall Maxillary Antrostomy, Right Middle and Inferior Turbinectomy, and Right Partial Ethmoidectomy. Soft tissue enhancement centered primarily within the right retromaxillary space surrounding devitalized bone fragment of the right maxillary alveolar process. There is absence of enhancement associated with the posterior wall of the right maxillary sinus *(open arrow)* that extends up toward the orbital apex *(asterisk),* which represents devitalized bone. Rim of enhancement surrounding the diseased V2 segment of the right trigeminal nerve *(solid arrow).* Findings suggestive of acute invasive fungal sinusitis.

involvement of local structures is characteristic on histo-pathologic examination.[70] *Aspergillus* is most commonly isolated in culture, with the Mucorales, *Penicillium* species, and *Candida* also reported. Treatment is similar to that for acute invasive FRS, consisting of surgical debridement of affected tissue and systemic antifungal therapy.[86] Fortunately the prognosis is significantly better than for AIFRS, but some patients may suffer from recurrence.

Granulomatous Invasive Fungal Rhinosinusitis

This disease entity is also characterized by a course lasting at least 12 weeks but affects immunocompetent patients. Presenting features consist of a slow-growing fibrous mass in the cheek, orbit, nose, and/or paranasal sinuses and often includes significant orbital proptosis. For unknown reasons, the disease is primarily diagnosed in Sudan, India, Pakistan, and Saudi Arabia, but *Aspergillus flavus* is the most commonly indicted pathogenic agent isolated in culture.[71] CT findings are often similar to those in CIFRS, but the histopathologic picture is distinguished by noncaseating granulomas and Langerhans giant cells, with vasculitis, vascular proliferation, and perivascular fibrosis sometimes seen as well.[70] Patients are treated by surgical removal of all involved tissue and structures. Recurrence has been reported to be as high as 80%, but some data suggest this may be improved with the use of postoperative systemic itraconazole.[87]

Complications of Sinusitis

Complications of sinusitis are fortunately rare in the era of antibiotics. Complications are often divided into orbital complications and intracranial complications, with orbital complications occurring more frequently than intracranial.[88] Orbital complications tend to manifest more frequently in the pediatric population, whereas complications occurring in adults may frequently be more severe than those occurring in children. Intracranial complications are more common in adolescents than younger children and tend to be due to ABRS, whereas older adult patients with intracranial complications often suffer from preceding CRS. For unclear reasons, extrasinus complications of sinusitis are more common in males than females. Given the close physical proximity of the paranasal sinuses to the orbits and skull base, it is easy to see why infections may spread from the sinuses to these neighboring structures. Direct spread, however, is more thought to be the exception rather than the rule, and spread is most often secondary to retrograde thrombophlebitis through the extensive valveless venous network among the sinuses, orbit, and skull base.[89] Ethmoid sinusitis is the most frequent offender in patients with orbital complications of their sinusitis,[90] whereas frontal sinusitis is the most commonly involved sinus in patients whose disease progresses to cause intracranial complications.[91] Orbital complications of ABRS as delineated in the Chandler classification include (1) preseptal cellulitis, (2) orbital cellulitis, (3) subperiosteal abscess, (4) orbital abscess, and (5) cavernous sinus thrombosis. This classification schema does not necessarily represent a natural progression from one stage to the next. Rather it is a useful framework for evaluating the degree of orbital involvement to aid in management decisions. Intracranial complications of sinusitis include meningitis, cerebritis, epidural abscess, subdural empyema, cerebral abscess, and Pott's puffy tumor. An important consideration, however, is that complicated cases of sinusitis are more frequently due to *Staphylococcus* and *Streptococcus* species, with methicillin-resistant *S. aureus*, *Streptococcus milleri,* and polymicrobial and anaerobic infections increasingly prevalent as well. Prognosis is generally still very good for patients with orbital complications of sinusitis, with modern rates of mortality and blindness near zero since the advent of antibiotics.[92] Intracranial complications, however, tend to have a poorer prognosis, with between 8 and 45% of patients suffering persistent neurologic deficits and the mortality rate often higher than 10%.[93]

Preseptal Cellulitis

Anatomically, the orbit is separated from its neighboring structures by a protective barrier in the form of the periorbita, which is simply the periosteum of the bones that constitute the orbital skeleton. Anteriorly, this protective sheath merges with the periosteum of the bones external to the orbit to form the orbital septum. Infection isolated to the soft tissues anterior to this septum is termed preseptal cellulitis and may also include preseptal abscess. Patients with preseptal cellulitis present with eyelid erythema, edema, and tenderness. Careful ophthalmologic examination is necessary to evaluate the patient's vision and extraocular movements, and consultation from an ophthalmologist is often warranted. Imaging is not generally indicated except to rule out orbital involvement, particularly when the patient exhibits additional worrisome signs or symptoms such as diplopia, decreased vision, limited extraocular muscle function, and/or orbital proptosis. CT with contrast and MRI will both demonstrate swelling of the eyelids as well as thickening and stranding of the periorbital soft tissues, with an absence of the same intraconally.[89] Treatment generally consists of broad-spectrum systemic and topical antibiotics to cover typical flora of the upper respiratory tract, with excellent prognosis expected.

Orbital Cellulitis

Patients with orbital cellulitis have inflammation and edema of the postseptal orbital contents. These patients will present with varying degrees of orbital proptosis and limitation of extraocular muscle function, depending on the extent of orbital inflammation. Imaging is indicated in these patients to determine the degree of infection and will appear as stranding of the orbital fat on CT with contrast and ill-defined T2 hyperintensity with concomitant postcontrast enhancement on T1-weighted images on MRI (Figure 14-9).[89] These inflammatory changes may be diffuse or localized to an area adjacent to the most severely affected sinus. Management of these patients includes frequent evaluation of extraocular

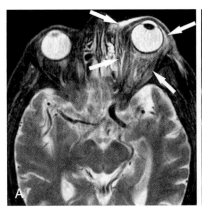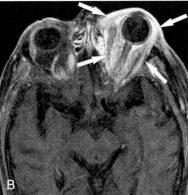

• **Figure 14-9** Orbital Cellulitis in a 55-Year-Old Man with Chronic Pansinusitis. **A,** Axial T2-weighted fat-suppressed sequence showing diffuse edema within the left orbital fat and extraocular muscles *(arrows).* **B,** Post-contrast axial T1-weighted images demonstrating infiltrative enhancement throughout the postseptal tissues *(arrows)* without discrete fluid collection. (From Hoxworth JM, Glastonbury CM. Orbital and intracranial complications of acute sinusitis. *Neuroimaging Clin N Am.* 2010;20[4]:511-526, Fig. 2, with permission.)

motion and vision in conjunction with intravenous antibiotics and treatment of the patient's sinus infection. Surgery is generally not indicated unless the examination findings deteriorate, suggesting failure of the infection to respond to therapy and worsening of the infection. Repeat imaging is often indicated in this situation to determine whether the infection has evolved to require surgical decompression of an orbital or an adjacent subperiosteal abscess as discussed in the following section.

Subperiosteal Abscess

The presentation of a subperiosteal abscess may be subtle and indistinguishable from a mild orbital cellulitis, or may include frank orbital proptosis, significantly impaired extraocular motion and loss of vision, depending on the size and degree of orbital compression from the abscess. These most commonly develop from spread across the lamina papyracea from ethmoid sinusitis, and less commonly via the orbital roof or floor from an adjacent frontal or maxillary sinusitis, respectively. The infectious process is limited by the resilient periorbita, which is stripped from the bone and displaced inward. CT imaging of the maxillofacial region should be performed with contrast. The appearance on imaging may range from a subtle rim-enhancing fluid collection to a large, lenticular-shaped lesion with significant orbital mass effect (Figure 14-10). Coronal and sagittal reformats of CT images are particularly useful to identify subtle collection, especially when arising from a frontal or maxillary sinus.[89] Treatment is as with orbital cellulitis, but more frequently includes surgery to open the sinus drainage pathways as well as decompression of large abscesses to alleviate mass effect on the orbital contents. Decreasing vision of 20/60 or worse and progression of symptoms despite adequate initial medical therapy are also important indications to proceed to surgery.[94] Intraoperative cultures of purulent drainage allow

for tailoring of antibiotic therapy and assist in choosing appropriate oral antibiotics when the patient is stable enough for discharge home. Close clinical evaluation is warranted postoperatively to identify recurrence early on, and repeat imaging may be necessary to evaluate for recurrence.

Orbital Abscess

Patients with orbital abscess present with proptosis, ophthalmoplegia, and visual impairment. Orbital apex syndrome may also manifest as the infectious process exhibiting mass effect on cranial nerves II, III, IV, and VI, as well as the ophthalmic branch of cranial nerve V, as they exit the skull base through the optic foramen and superior orbital fissure. CT imaging of the maxillofacial and orbital region should be performed with contrast. MRI is indicated to further evaluate for intracranial concerns (Figure 14-11). The radiologic appearance is that of a discrete rim-enhancing fluid collection within the orbital fat with extensive surrounding inflammation.[89] Treatment involves surgical drainage of the abscess with or without debridement of the involved sinuses, as well as medical management of the sinusitis with decongestants and intravenous antibiotics as described earlier.

Cavernous Sinus Thrombosis

Clinical presentation of cavernous sinus thrombosis typically includes fever, headache, periorbital swelling, diplopia, chemosis, and/or proptosis. Cranial nerve palsies also may be clinically apparent, most commonly involving the abducens nerve, but may also include palsies of third, fourth, and fifth cranial nerves. Acute-onset bilateral cranial nerve involvement in the setting of acute sinusitis is considered pathognomonic for cavernous sinus thrombosis. Findings on CT with contrast may be subtle, especially early in the clinical course, but may include heterogeneously decreased enhancement and thickening of the cavernous sinus, with

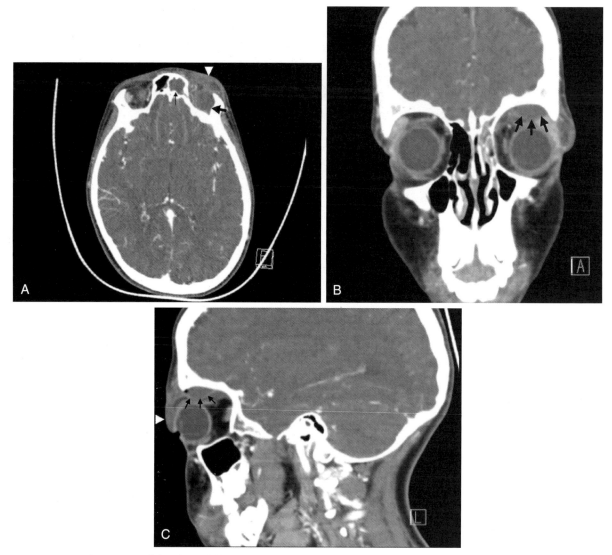

• **Figure 14-10** Subperiosteal Abscess in an 11-Year-Old Female with Acute Frontal and Ethmoid Sinusitis. **A,** Axial CT with contrast of the maxillofacial area demonstrating opacification of the left frontal sinus *(small arrow),* edema of the upper eyelid *(arrowhead),* and fluid collection within the orbit *(large arrow).* **B,** Coronal reformatted image showing rim-enhancing lenticular fluid collection in the superior aspect of the left orbit *(arrows)* as well as opacification of the ethmoid air cells on the left. **C,** Sagittal reformatted image again demonstrating the lenticular fluid collection with rim-enhancement *(arrows)* and edema of the upper eyelid *(arrowhead).* The remainder of the postseptal orbital fat is dark and free of stranding. Note that reviewing images from all three planes helps to distinguish the extent of the abscess and allows for identification of a fluid collection that may be missed when evaluating images only in the axial plane.

an area of nonopacification greater than 7 mm in greatest dimension suggestive of cavernous sinus thrombosis, especially when noted near the posterior aspect of the cavernous sinus.[95] This widening of the cavernous sinus may also lead to a convex contour of the lateral aspect of the sinus. Filling defects or dilation of the superior ophthalmic vein, inferior petrosal sinus, and sphenoparietal sinus are other findings that may help clue the radiologist in to a potential cavernous sinus thrombosis.[89] MR findings are similar to those of CT scan, with post-contrast T1-weighted imaging also showing increased dural enhancement along the lateral border of the cavernous sinus, and convexity in the same area

most readily apparent in the coronal plane (Figure 14-12). Treatment usually requires intravenous antibiotics, surgical management of the sinuses, decongestants, and saline rinses. Most patients do not require anticoagulation for the thrombosis. Worsening of the inflammation in the cavernous sinus may lead to narrowing and occlusion of the ipsilateral internal carotid artery, so frequent neurologic checks are an important part of management.

Pott's Puffy Tumor

Patients with frontal sinusitis may develop a subperiosteal abscess of the frontal bone, termed Pott's puffy tumor for

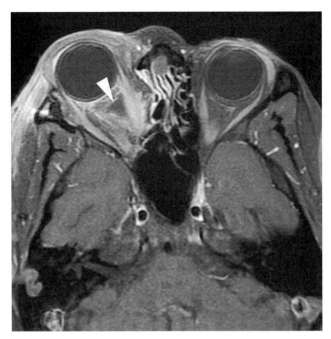

• **Figure 14-11** Orbital Abscess in a 34-Year-Old Woman 4 Days After Open Reduction and Internal Fixation of Traumatic Facial Fractures. Postcontrast axial T1-weighted image shows rim-enhancing fluid collection *(arrowhead)* and significant enhancement and thickening of the medial rectus muscle. (From Hoxworth JM, Glastonbury CM. Orbital and intracranial complications of acute sinusitis. *Neuroimaging Clin N Am.* 2010;20[4]:511-526, Fig. 5, with permission.)

Sir Percivall Pott, who first described such an abscess in the eighteenth century. Infection of the frontal sinus may also lead to thrombophlebitis through the valveless diploic veins that propagates either anteriorly to the subperiosteal space or posteriorly into the subdural or subarachnoid spaces with or without frank erosion of the anterior or posterior tables of the frontal sinus. Patients with Pott's puffy tumor will present with headache, fever, nasal congestion and drainage, and frontal swelling with tenderness of the swelling and frontal sinus.[96] They may also exhibit focal neurologic findings and depressed level of consciousness, which should alert the examiner to the potential presence of intracranial involvement as well. Radiographic imaging is indicated to confirm the diagnosis and evaluate for possible intracranial findings. CT with contrast will demonstrate rim-enhancing fluid collection in the subperiosteal space of the frontal bone (Figure 14-13). CT is also valuable for identifying bone destruction in the anterior and posterior tables of the frontal sinus. Frontal sinusitis may erode through the frontal table, resulting in cellulitis overlying the frontal sinus (Figure 14-14). CT is also helpful for evaluating for possible intracranial extra-axial fluid collections or parenchymal involvement. MRI, however, is more sensitive and specific for intracranial involvement and is also useful for identifying frontal osteomyelitis, which is evident as bone marrow edema and enhancement of the frontal bone.[89] Treatment involves empiric broad-spectrum intravenous antibiotic

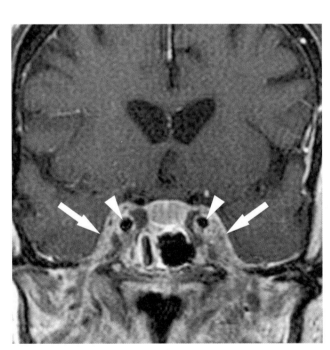

• **Figure 14-12** Cavernous Sinus Thrombosis in a 62-Year-Old Woman with History of Chronic Sinusitis. Postcontrast T1-weighted coronal image with fat saturation demonstrating convexity of the lateral aspect of the cavernous sinuses bilaterally *(arrows)*. Normal flow voids through the internal carotid arteries are noted as well *(arrowheads)*. (From Hoxworth JM, Glastonbury CM. Orbital and intracranial complications of acute sinusitis. *Neuroimaging Clin N Am.* 2010;20[4]:511-526, Fig. 6, with permission.)

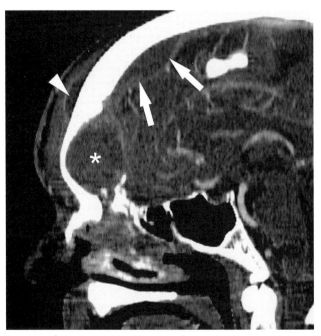

• **Figure 14-13** Pott's Puffy Tumor and Intracranial Epidural Abscess in a 46-Year-Old Man with Chronic Rhinosinusitis. Sagittal reformat of CT scan with contrast shows expansion of the frontal sinus with erosion of the interior table but sparing of the anterior table *(*)*. A rim-enhancing fluid collection overlying the frontal bone is consistent with frontal subperiosteal abscess, or Pott's puffy tumor *(arrowhead)*. There is also an epidural abscess intracranially *(arrows)*. (From Hoxworth JM, Glastonbury CM. Orbital and intracranial complications of acute sinusitis. *Neuroimaging Clin N Am.* 2010;20[4]:511-526, Fig. 8, with permission.)

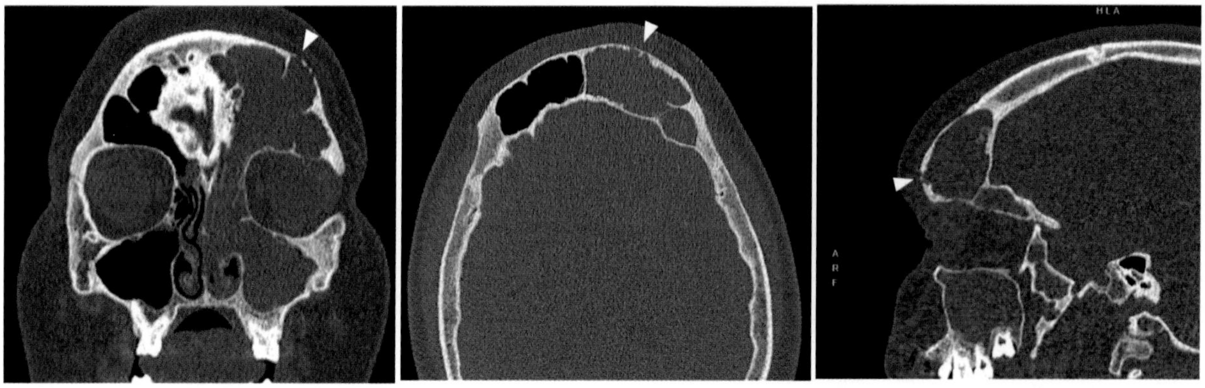

• **Figure 14-14** CT Scan of the Facial Bones Without Intravenous Contrast Demonstrating Opacification of the Left Maxillary Sinus and Ethmoid Air Cells with Opacification and Expansion of the Left Frontal Sinuses. There is irregular thinning to the anterior wall of the left frontal sinus and overlying soft tissue thickening concerning for osteomyelitis *(arrowheads)* with associated overlying soft tissue thickening concerning for cellulitis. Findings suggestive of frontal sinusitis with osteomyelitis and cellulitis without formation of the subperiosteal abscess.

therapy later tailored to surgically obtained culture results and surgical drainage of the abscess and affected sinus(es), with removal of infected bone.

Epidural Abscess and Subdural Empyema

Patients with epidural abscesses often have a surprisingly benign clinical presentation of headache and an absence of CNS symptoms. The abscess collects between the calvarium and dura (which is partially made up of the periosteum of the calvarium) and is limited by suture lines. Imaging demonstrates a lenticular-shaped low-density fluid collection on CT (Figure 14-15), with MRI findings demonstrating hyperintensity on T2 and variable signal intensity on T1, with rim enhancement on postcontrast T1 sequences.[89]

Subdural empyema has the distinction of being the most common intracranial complication of rhinosinusitis.[93] Patients may present with seizures, focal neurologic deficits, and coma if untreated within 24 to 48 hours of onset, because the infection can rapidly spread through the subdural space, leading to elevated intracranial pressures. Findings on non–contrast-enhanced CT may include a subtle low-density crescent-shaped collection that can cross suture lines, usually in the supratentorial compartment. MRI findings are similar to those described previously for epidural collection, making it difficult to distinguish the two when the collection is small and does not overlie a cranial suture (Figure 14-16).[89] Treatment of epidural and subdural infected fluid collections consists of intravenous antibiotics and surgical drainage of the sinuses and intracranial fluid collections.

Meningitis

Patients presenting with the classic signs of fever, headache, and meningismus are often readily diagnosed with meningitis, which is an infrequent isolated complication of ARS and more commonly accompanies subdural empyema. Imaging is generally unrevealing but may demonstrate meningeal enhancement or hydrocephalus on CT or MRI.[97] Lumbar puncture will aid to confirm the diagnosis, and treatment involves the usual medical management. Surgery is rarely indicated in these cases.

Cerebritis and Cerebral Abscess

Patients with cerebritis and cerebral abscess may present with fever, headache, and focal neurologic deficits, although this classic triad is more commonly seen in adults than children. New-onset seizure should also prompt the clinician to evaluate for intracranial infection, even in patients without sinusitis. However, rhinosinusitis is the most common process leading to cerebral abscess.[98] The patient's condition may rapidly deteriorate if the abscess ruptures into the ventricular system. Imaging with contrast-enhanced CT scan will demonstrate a rim-enhancing intraparenchymal lesion that is sometimes difficult to distinguish from a cystic tumor. MRI with contrast demonstrates hypointense T1 signal and hyperintense T2 signal in the abscess contents (Figure 14-17). Extensive diffusion restriction helps differentiate abscess from cystic tumor on MRI.[99] Treatment again requires intravenous broad-spectrum antibiotic coverage coupled with surgical drainage of the sinuses and intraparenchymal abscess.

Infections of the Soft Tissues of the Nose

Nasal Vestibulitis, Furunculitis, and Nasal Abscess

The soft tissues of the nose are susceptible to cellulitic infections just like the rest of the face. However, given the hair-bearing portion of the anterior portion of the soft tissues of the nose known as the vestibule, furunculitis is another type of soft tissue infection of the nose. This manifests as pain, tenderness to palpation, and often marked erythema, giving the tip of the nose a "Rudolph

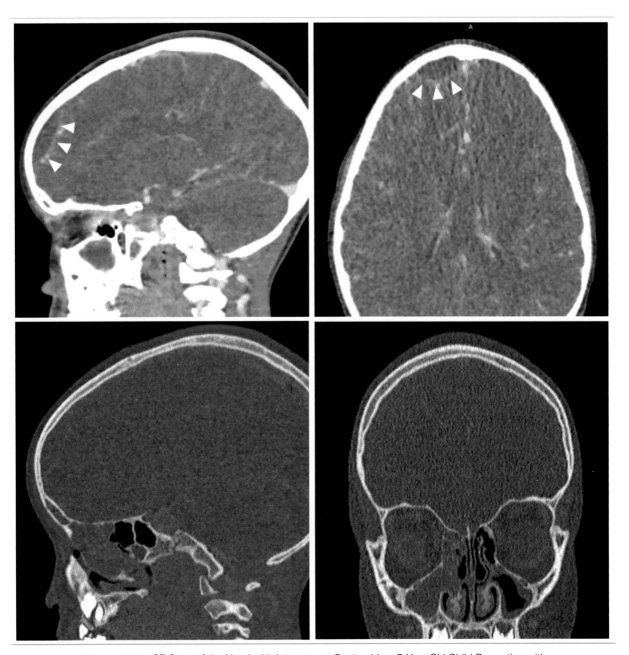

• **Figure 14-15** CT Scan of the Head with Intravenous Contrast in a 7-Year-Old Child Presenting with Eye Pain and Headache. Image demonstrates a 3.5- × 0.8- × 3.1-cm extra-axial collection in the right frontal region *(arrowheads)* extending slightly past the midline concerning for epidural abscess with mild mass effect on the underlying right frontal lobe. Complete opacification of the right maxillary sinus and bilateral anterior ethmoid air cells, right greater than left. Complete opacification of the bilateral frontal sinuses and mild indistinctness of the right cribriform plate are present. This patient ultimately required frontal craniotomy, endoscopic sinus surgery, and frontal trephination.

the red-nosed reindeer" appearance. When limited to the soft tissue lateral alar wall, the infection is termed vestibulitis. Occasionally the infection may progress to develop into an abscess. *S. aureus,* including methicillin-resistant strains, is the most common offending agent, with community-acquired MRSA (CA-MRSA) increasingly common.[100] CT with contrast may be helpful to determine whether a drainable fluid collection is present. Topical and oral antibiotics are otherwise the treatment of choice.

Clindamycin has been considered a useful antimicrobial, but resistance to this drug is increasing. TMP-SMX, tetracycline and rifampin are other options to which there has been reported less resistance in CA-MRSA infections.[100] Topical mupirocin is also considered first-line treatment for these infections. Prognosis is excellent when the infection is diagnosed and adequately treated early on. However, given the presence of valveless veins connecting the nose to the intracerebral dural venous sinuses, including

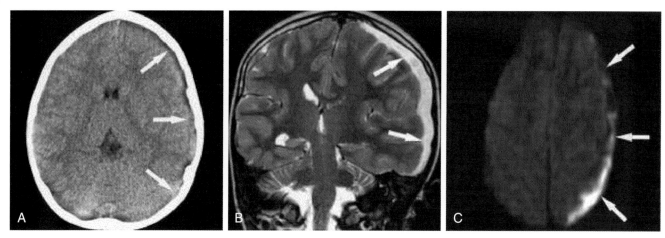

• **Figure 14-16** Subdural Empyema in a 5-Year-Old Boy Who Presented with Periorbital Swelling and Seizure. **A,** Noncontrast axial CT image showing diffuse cerebral swelling and slight left to right midline shift. A subtle, thin intermediate-to-low-density collection is identified on the left *(arrows)*. **B,** T2-weighted coronal image of the brain showing a left subdural convex fluid intensity collection *(arrows)*. **C,** Diffusion-weighted image showing restricted diffusion *(arrows)* helps distinguish the empyema from an effusion. (From Hoxworth JM, Glastonbury CM. Orbital and intracranial complications of acute sinusitis. *Neuroimaging Clin N Am*. 2010;20[4]:511-526, Fig. 10, with permission.)

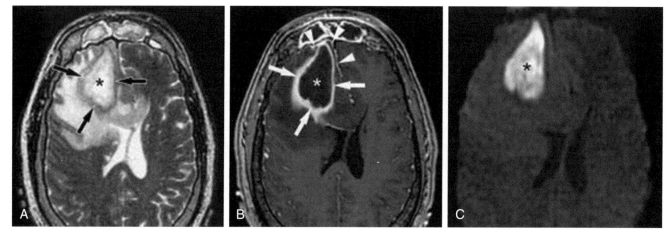

• **Figure 14-17** Cerebral Abscess in a 55-Year-Old Man Initially Thought to Have a High-Grade Frontal Glioma. **A,** T2-weighted sequence. **B,** Postcontrast T1 image. **C,** Diffusion-weighted sequence. The lesion is hyperintense on T2 and hypointense on T1 *(*)*, with surrounding rim that is isointense to slightly hyperintense to normal white matter on T2 and enhances on postcontrast T1 imaging *(arrows)*. Dural enhancement *(arrowheads)* and restricted diffusion, combined with sinus opacification, help differentiate this infectious abscess from a neoplasm. (From Hoxworth JM, Glastonbury CM. Orbital and intracranial complications of acute sinusitis. *Neuroimaging Clin N Am*. 2010;20[4]:511-526, Fig. 12, with permission.)

the cavernous sinus, patients should be cautioned against attempting to rupture or squeeze any abscesses collecting in this area, and appropriate medical and/or surgical therapy (i.e., incision and drainage when indicated) should be promptly initiated.

Nasal Septal Abscess

The nasal septum is made up of a midline cartilage and bony septum covered on either side by a mucoperiocondrial/mucoperiosteal membrane. Infection may develop deep in the mucopericondrial layer and most commonly develops in the setting of septal hematoma as a result of trauma or surgery on the nasal septum, with the rate of septal abscess after septoplasty estimated to range from 0.4% to 12.0%. Postoperative antibiotics used as routine prophylaxis have not been shown to reduce this rate.[101] Patients will complain of nasal obstruction and may also experience fever and facial pain. Treatment consists of prompt surgical drainage with or without packing and systemic antibiotic therapy usually targeted to treat *S. aureus,* a common pathogen in soft tissue infections of the nose.[102]

If left untreated, potential complications include septal perforation and loss of nasal dorsal support leading to saddle nose deformity, as well as progression to cavernous sinus thrombosis, meningitis, or cerebral abscess from thrombophlebitis progressing retrograde into the cranial vault.[103]

Rhinosporidiosis

Rhinosporidiosis is a benign disease caused by infection with the organism *Rhinosporidium seeberi* that may involve the nose, throat, ear, or genitalia in both males and females. It is endemic to India and Sri Lanka, but has been reported in Europe, Africa, and the Americas.[104] This infection causes a chronic and localized process of the mucous membranes, commonly resulting in a polypoid soft tissue mass of the affected area. Infection is thought to be acquired as the pathogen passes from its natural aquatic habitat and penetrates traumatized epithelium. The organism grows in the submucosa, developing into thick-walled sporangia ranging from 10 to 200 mm in diameter. These may be observed grossly as white dots with smaller dots within them. These smaller dots are often referred to as "daughter cells" or "sporangiospores." These white spots often give a strawberry-like appearance to the sessile or pendunculated friable, vascular polyp. Infection may be present for years as the lesion grows, before the patient develops symptoms of nasal obstruction, epistaxis, or grossly evident mass. Diagnosis is confirmed by tissue biopsy and characteristic appearance on standard hematoxylin and eosin or fungal stains. Imaging helps delineate the extent of the lesion. Wide local excision with electrocautery of the base is the only known method of cure because the organism is fastidious and efforts at isolating it in culture have failed, thus preventing attempts to test sensitivity to antimicrobial agents in vitro. However, empiric adjuvant therapy with the antilepromatous agent dapsone and antifungal agents griseofulvin, amphotericin B, trimethoprim-sulphadiazine, and sodium stibogluconate in conjunction with more limited surgery has been reported with varying degrees of success. Complications of the disease include recurrence or possible dissemination by autoinoculation of spores, hematogenous spread, lymphatic spread, or sexual contact.[105]

Tuberculosis

Tuberculosis is caused by the bacillus *Mycobacterium tuberculosis* and may involve the nose internally or externally. When internal, the primary targets are the cartilaginous nasal septum and anterior aspect of the inferior turbinates, with the nasal floor classically spared.[105] Patients with internal nasal manifestations of tuberculosis will present with pain, rhinorrhea, and nasal septal perforation. When manifestations are external, patients will present with lupus vulgaris, a chronic progressive form of cutaneous tuberculosis that manifests as a smooth-surfaced brownish-red, soft or friable plaque or patch with an overlying scale. This may occur as a result of hematogenous or lymphatic spread from other infected organs or from direct inoculation from another infected individual, with primary nasal tuberculosis being extremely rare. The infection often progresses from a soft, friable nodule to destroy the cartilage, leading to parrot-beak nasal deformity, ectropion, and atrophied lips. Diagnosis often requires biopsy, as swabs and nasal secretions are of low yield for isolating the bacillus. Treatment with four-drug regimen of rifampin, isoniazid, pyrazinamide, and ethambutol is usually curative, although more advanced lesions may leave scarring and deformity in their wake as described above.[106]

Leprosy

Nasal involvement with *Mycobacterium leprae* is an extremely common early finding in the development of the lepromatous form of the infection and may manifest with chronic nasal congestion, crusting, intermittent epistaxis, hyposmia, anosmia, and rhinorrhea.[105] The nasal discharge harbors large numbers of the bacilli and is believed to play an important role in the transmission of the disease. Leprous rhinitis on examination may appear consistent with other forms of CRS, including possible nasal crusting or septal perforation. More specific findings may include multiple nodules or plaques with yellowish thickening of the nasal mucosa that later develop into more generalized nodularity of the anterior aspect of the inferior turbinate and nasal septum. If left untreated, the disease often progresses to destroy the nasal septal cartilage, leading to septal perforation, saddle nose deformity, and atrophic rhinitis. Biopsy is diagnostic of the disease, and nasal swabs are useful for isolating and identifying the offending organism. Treatment consists of a 12-month multidrug regimen of rifampin, clofazimine, and dapsone.[107] Cure rates are excellent, but long-term sequelae of atrophic rhinitis and septal perforation with resultant saddle nose deformity may still result.

Syphilis

Involvement of the nose and nasal cavities is uncommon in syphilis, with patients most commonly experiencing chancres, inguinal lymphadenopathy, and secondary widespread mucocutaneous lesions. However, invasion of the nasal septum by the sexually transmitted agent *Treponema pallidum* has been described, leading to cartilaginous destruction and subsequent nasal septal perforation and saddle nose deformity.[105] Another possible presentation consisting of a smooth intranasal mass with cervical lymphadenopathy has been described in the literature as well.[108] Diagnosis is made with positive rapid plasma reagin (RPR) or Venereal Disease Research Laboratory (VDRL) tests and confirmed with positive fluorescent treponemal antibody-absorption (FTA-ABS), quantitative VDRL/RPR, microhemagglutination assay *T. pallidum* (MHA-TP), *T. pallidum* hemagglutination (TPHA), or *T. pallidum* particle agglutination (TPPA) tests.[108] First-line treatment is penicillin G monotherapy.

Leishmaniasis

Another organism with a predilection for nasal infection is the protozoan *Leishmania.* The disease is transmitted by the bite of sand flies and may manifest in one of several forms including visceral, cutaneous, and mucocutaneous, with multiple possible variations of each.[105] Mucocutaneous leishmaniasis (ML) is more common in the Americas and is more likely to involve the nose and nasal cavities, whereas visceral leishmaniasis is predominantly found in the Indian subcontinent and Sudan, and cutaneous leishmaniasis is particularly frequent in the Mediterranean countries. Nasal ML most commonly results in septal perforation and facial deformity from destruction of the underlying cartilages, with *Leishmania braziliensis* reported as the most common agent resulting in nasal septal perforation. Intranasal mass is another potential examination finding (Figure 14-18). Imaging can further characterize the mass (Figure 14-19). Biopsy and culture may be useful to identify the causative agent, but polymerase chain reaction has a sensitivity of 80 to 98%—double that of culture.[109] Owing to the specific nature of this test for identifying the pathogen, a high degree of suspicion is often required to make the diagnosis based on a history of potential exposure in an endemic area. The antiparasitic pentavalent antimonials are first-line agents against the disease. These include sodium stibogluconate and meglumine antimonate. Cure rates are excellent, but resulting deformity may not be avoidable unless the disease is diagnosed and treated early.

Rhinoscleroma

Inhalation of the organism *Klebsiella rhinoscleromatis,* a gram-negative bacterium endemic to the tropical and temperate zones of Africa, Asia, Eastern Europe, South America,

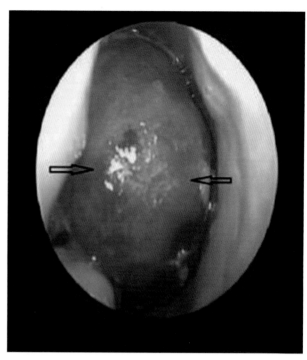

• **Figure 14-18** Endoscopic View of Fleshy, Hyperemic Mass *(Arrows)* Obstructing the Left Nasal Cavity in a Patient with Mucosal Leishmaniasis. (From Gul HC, Tosun F, Karakas A, et al. A case of mucosal leishmaniasis: mimicking intranasal tumor with perforation of septum. *J Microbiol Immunol Infect.* 2013;S1684-1182[13]:230-232, with permission.)

and Central America, can lead to the slowly progressive disease known as rhinoscleroma. Many modern authors prefer to refer to the disease simply as *scleroma* because although it primarily affects the nasal cavity in 95 to 100% of affected patients, it may also involve the nasopharynx (18 to 43%), oropharynx (13 to 35%), larynx (15 to 40%), trachea

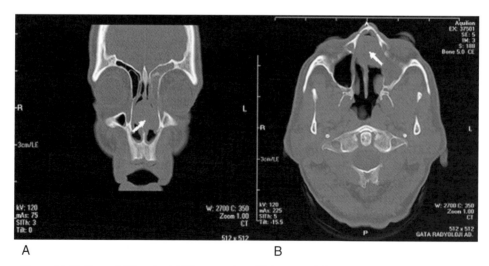

• **Figure 14-19** Coronal **(A)** and axial **(B)** noncontrast CT images of the patient with the nasal lesion in Figure 14-15, showing a soft tissue density mass obstructing the left nasal cavity and eroding through the septum to the right nasal cavity. (From Gul HC, Tosun F, Karakas A, et al. A case of mucosal leishmaniasis: mimicking intranasal tumor with perforation of septum. *J Microbiol Immunol Infect.* 2013;S1684-1182[13]:230-232, with permission.)

(12%), and bronchi (2 to 7%), as the disease process occurs at the transitional regions between two types of epithelium (e.g., squamous, ciliary, and respiratory).[110] For unclear reasons, males more commonly suffer from nasal and pharyngeal scleroma (male-to-female ratio, 2:1), whereas females are more commonly afflicted with the laryngotracheal variant (female-to-male ratio, 4:1). Both tend to manifest in the second to fourth decades of life. Patients may present initially in the first stage of the disease (rhinitic) with nasal congestion, crusting, and foul smell. As the disease progresses to the granulomatous stage, patients begin to suffer more marked nasal obstruction, deformity, epistaxis, anosmia, and/or numbness of the soft palate, as masses form of granulation tissue containing plasma cells, Russell bodies (elliptical bodies thought to represent degenerated plasma cells), and Mikulicz cells (large histiocytes with foamy cytoplasm containing the *K. rhinoscleromatis* bacilli). The final, sclerotic stage leads to scarring throughout the upper aerodigestive tract, with patients suffering nasal vestibular stenosis, hoarseness, and possibly stridor. MRI may reveal a high-intensity signal on T1-weighted images and aids to determine the extent of disease.[110] Tetracycline is the antibiotic of choice after diagnosis has been confirmed with tissue cultures from biopsy. Surgical management may be indicated to restore function when scarring has resulted in narrowing of the nasal and upper airways. Unfortunately, even with appropriate treatment the disease tends to exhibit a progressive, remitting-relapsing course.[105]

References

1. Blackwell DL, Lucas JW, Clarke TC. Summary health statistics for U.S. adults: national health interview survey, 2012. *Vital Health Stat*. 2012;10:1-171.
2. Battisti AS, Modi P, Pangia J. Sinusitis. [Updated 2022 Aug 8]. In: *StatPearls*. Treasure Island, FL: StatPearls Publishing; 2022.
3. Sinus and Allergy Health Partnership (SAHP). Antimicrobial treatment guidelines for acute bacterial rhinosinusitis. *Otolaryngol Head Neck Surg*. 2004;130(suppl 1):1-45.
4. van Cauwenberge P, Sys L, De Belder T, Watelet JB. Anatomy and physiology of the nose and the paranasal sinuses. *Immunol Allergy Clin North Am*. 2004;24(1):1-17.
5. Brook I. Microbiology and management of sinusitis. *J Otolaryngol*. 1996;25:249-256.
6. Rosenfeld RM, Piccirillo JF, Chandrasekhar SS, et al. Clinical practice guideline (update): adult sinusitis. *Otolaryngol Head Neck Surg*. 2015;152(suppl 2):S1–S39.
7. Lanza DC, Kennedy DW. Adult rhinosinusitis defined. *Otolaryngol Head Neck Surg*. 1997;117:S1-S7.
8. Gwaltney JM Jr. Acute community-acquired sinusitis. *Clin Infect Dis*. 1996;23:1209-1223.
9. Lindbaek M, Hjortdahl P, Johnsen UL. Use of symptoms, signs, and blood tests to diagnose acute sinus infections in primary care: comparison with computed tomography. *Fam Med*. 1996;28:183-188.
10. Axelsson A, Runze U. Comparison of subjective and radiological findings during the course of acute maxillary sinusitis. *Ann Oto Rhinol Laryngol*. 1983;92:75-77.
11. Williams J, Simel DL, Roberts L, et al. Clinical evaluation for sinusitis: making the diagnosis by history and physical examination. *Ann Intern Med*. 1992;117:705-710.
12. Meltzer EO, Hamilos DL, Hadley JA, et al. Rhinosinusitis: establishing definitions for clinical research and patient care. *Otolaryngol Head Neck Surg*. 2004;131(suppl 6):S1-S62.
13. Chow AW, Benninger MS, Brook I, et al. IDSA clinical practice guideline for acute bacterial rhinosinusitis in children and adults. *Clin Infect Dis*. 2012;54(8):e72-e112.
14. Benninger MS, Payne SC, Ferguson BJ, et al. Endoscopically directed middle meatal cultures versus maxillary sinus taps in acute bacterial maxillary rhinosinusitis: a meta-analysis. *Otolaryngol Head Neck Surg*. 2006;134:3-9.
15. Setzen G, Ferguson BJ, Han JK, et al. Clinical consensus statement: appropriate use of computed tomography for paranasal sinus disease. *Otolaryngol Head Neck Surg*. 2012;147:808-816.
16. Ahovuo-Saoranta A, Rautakorpi UM, Borisenko OV, et al. Antibiotics for acute maxillary sinusitis in adults. *Cochrane Database Syst Rev*. 2014;11:CD000243.
17. Jenkins SG, Farrell DJ, Patel M, et al. Trends in anti-bacterial resistance among *Streptococcus pneumoniae* isolated in the USA, 2000-2003: PROTEKT US years 1-3. *J Infect*. 2005;51:355-363.
18. Brook I, Foote PA, Hausfeld JN. Frequency of recovery of pathogens causing acute maxillary sinusitis in adults before and after introduction of vaccination of children with the 7-valent pneumococcal vaccine. *J Med Microbiol*. 2006;55:943-946.
19. Ah-see K. Sinusitis (acute). *Clin Evid*. 2006;15:1-11.
20. Rosenfeld RM, Singer M, Jones S. Systematic review of antimicrobials for patients with acute rhinosinusitis. *Otolaryngol Head Neck Surg*. 2007;137(suppl 3):S32-S45.
21. Falagas ME, Karageorgopoulos DE, Grammatikos AP, et al. Effectiveness and safety of short vs. long duration of antibiotic therapy for acute bacterial sinusitis: a meta-analysis of randomized trials. *Br J Clin Pharmacol*. 2009;67:161-171.
22. Nava JM, Bella F, Garau J, et al. Predictive factors for invasive disease due to penicillin-resistant *Streptococcus pneumoniae*: a population-based study. *Clin Infect Dis*. 1994;19:884-890.
23. Seybold ML, Tse HF. Antibiotic stewardship and sinusitis: a quality improvement project. *J Urgent Care Med*. 2020. https://www.jucm.com/antibiotic-stewardship-and-sinusitis-a-quality-improvement-project/. [Accessed 1 February 2023].
24. Wasylyshyn AI, Kaye KS, Chen J, et al. Improving antibiotic use for sinusitis and upper respiratory tract infections: a virtual-visit antibiotic stewardship initiative. *Infect Control Hosp Epidemiol*. 2022;43(12):1890-1893.
25. Malm L. Pharmacological background to decongesting and anti-inflammatory treatment of rhinitis and sinusitis. *Acta Otolaryngol*. 1994;515:53-55.
26. Meltzer EO, Charous BL, Busse WW, et al. Added relief in the treatment of acute recurrent sinusitis with adjunctive mometasone furoate nasal spray. The Nasonex Sinusitis Group. *J Allergy Clin Immunol*. 2000;106:630-637.
27. Inanli S, Öztürk O, Korkmaz M, et al. The effects of topical agents of fluticasone propionate, oxymetazoline, and 3% and 0.9% sodium chloride solutions on mucociliary clearance in the therapy of acute bacterial rhinosinusitis in vivo. *Laryngoscope*. 2002;112:320-325.
28. Rabago D, Zgierska A, Mundt M, et al. Efficacy of daily hypertonic saline nasal irrigation among patients with sinusitis: a randomized controlled trial. *J Fam Pract*. 2002;51:1049-1055.
29. Adam P, Stiffman M, Blake RL Jr. A clinical trial of hypertonic saline nasal spray in subjects with the common cold or rhinosinusitis. *Arch Fam Med*. 1998;7:39-43.

30. Haye R, Lingass E, Hoivik HO, et al. Azithromycin versus placebo in acute infectious rhinitis with clinical symptoms but without radiological signs of maxillary sinusitis. *Eur J Clin Microbiol Infect Dis.* 1998;17:309-312.

31. Bhattacharyya N. The economic burden and symptom manifestations of chronic rhinosinusitis. *Am J Rhinol.* 2003;17:27-32.

32. Arango P, Kountiakis SE. Significance of computed tomography pathology in chronic rhinosinusitis. *Laryngoscope.* 2001;111:1779-1782.

33. Stankiewicz JA, Chow JM. Nasal endoscopy and the definition and diagnosis of chronic rhinosinusitis. *Otolaryngol Head Neck Surg.* 2002;126:623-627.

34. Wang L, Freedman SD. Laboratory tests for the diagnosis of cystic fibrosis. *Am J Clin Pathol.* 2002;117(suppl):S109-S115.

35. Sipila J, Antila J, Suonpaa J. Pre- and postoperative evaluation of patients with nasal obstruction undergoing endoscopic sinus surgery. *Eur Arch Otorhinolaryngol.* 1996;253:237-239.

36. Orlandi RR. Biopsy and specimen collection in chronic rhinosinusitis. *Ann Otol Rhinol Laryngol.* 2004;113(suppl):24-26.

37. Wuister AM, Goto NA, Oostveen EJ, et al. Nasal endoscopy is recommended for diagnosing adults with chronic rhinosinusitis. *Otolaryngol Head Neck Surg.* 2014;150(3):359-364.

38. Leung RM, Chandra RK, Kern RC, Conley DB, Tan BK. Primary care and upfront computed tomography scanning in the diagnosis of chronic rhinosinusitis: a cost-based decision analysis. *Laryngoscope.* 2014;124(1):12-18.

39. Newman LJ, Platts-Mills TAE, Phillips CD, et al. Chronic sinusitis: relationship of computed tomographic findings to allergy, asthma, and eosinophilia. *JAMA.* 1994;271:363-368.

40. Krouse JH. Computed tomography stage, allergy testing, and quality of life in patients with sinusitis. *Otolaryngol Head Neck Surg.* 2000;123:389-392.

41. Savolainen S, Schlerter WW, Man WJ, et al. Allergy in patients with acute maxillary sinusitis. *Allergy.* 1989;44:1116-1122.

42. Fokkens WJ, Lund VJ, Mullol J, et al. European position paper on rhinosinusitis and nasal polyps 2012. *Rhinol Suppl.* 2012;23:3 pp. preceding table of contents, 1-298.

43. Zurlo JJ, Feuerstein IM, Lebovics R, et al. Sinusitis in HIV infection. *Am J Med.* 1992;93:157-162.

44. Chee L, Graham SM, Carothers DG, et al. Immune dysfunction in refractory sinusitis in a tertiary care setting. *Laryngoscope.* 2001;111:233-235.

45. Lange B, Holst R, Thilsing T, et al. Quality of life and associated factors in persons with chronic rhinosinusitis in the general population. *Clin Otolaryngol.* 2013;38(6):474-480.

46. Morales DR, Guthrie B, Lipworth BJ, Jackson C, Donnan PT, Santiago VH. NSAID-exacerbated respiratory disease: a meta-analysis evaluating prevalence, mean provocative dose of aspirin and increased asthma morbidity. *Allergy.* 2015;70(7):828-835.

47. Lieu JE, Feinstein AR. Confirmations and surprises in the association of tobacco use with sinusitis. *Arch Otolaryngol Head Neck Surg.* 2000;126:940-946.

48. Weaver EM. Association between gastroesophageal reflux and sinusitis, otitis media, and laryngeal malignancy: a systematic review of the evidence. *Am J Med.* 2003;115:81S-89S.

49. Papsin B, McTavish A. Saline nasal irrigation. *Can Fam Physician.* 2003;49:168-173.

50. Tomooka LT, Murphy C, Davidson TM. Clinical study and literature review of nasal irrigation. *Laryngoscope.* 2000;110:1189-1193.

51. Videler WJ, van Hee K, Reinartz SM, et al. Long-term low-dose antibiotics in recalcitrant chronic rhinosinusitis: a retrospective analysis. *Rhinology.* 2012;50(1):45-55.

52. Albert RK, Connett J, Bailey WC, et al. Azithromycin for prevention of exacerbations of COPD. *N Engl J Med.* 2011;365(8):689-698.

53. Mandal R, Patel N, Ferguson BJ. Role of antibiotics in sinusitis. *Curr Opin Infect Dis.* 2012;25(2):183-192.

54. Van Zele T, Gevaert P, Holtappels G, et al. Oral steroids and doxycycline: two different approaches to treat nasal polyps. *J Allergy Clin Immunol.* 2010;125(5):1069-1076.e4.

55. Desrosiers MY, Salas-Prato M. Treatment of chronic rhinosinusitis refractory to other treatments with topical antibiotic therapy delivered by means of a large-particle nebulizer: results of a controlled trial. *Otolaryngol Head Neck Surg.* 2001;125(3):265-269.

56. Grobler A, Weitzel EK, Buele A, et al. Pre- and postoperative sinus penetration of nasal irrigation. *Laryngoscope.* 2008;118(11):2078-2081.

57. Lal D, Hwang PH. Oral corticosteroid therapy in chronic rhinosinusitis without polyposis: a systematic review. *Int Forum Allergy Rhinol.* 2011;1(2):136-143.

58. Hissaria P, Smith W, Wormald PJ, et al. Short course of systemic corticosteroids in sinonasal polyposis: a double-blind, randomized, placebo-controlled trial with evaluation of outcome measures. *J Allergy Clin Immunol.* 2006;118(1):128-133.

59. Han JK, Marple BF, Smith TL, et al. Effect of steroid-releasing sinus implants on postoperative medical and surgical interventions: an efficacy meta-analysis. *Int Forum Allergy Rhinol.* 2012;2(4):271-279.

60. Kern RC, Stolovitzky JP, Silvers SL, et al. A phase 3 trial of mometasone furoate sinus implants for chronic sinusitis with recurrent nasal polyps. *Int Forum Allergy Rhinol.* 2018;8(4):471-481.

61. Bachert C, Mannent L, Naclerio RM, et al. Effect of subcutaneous dupilumab on nasal polyp burden in patients with chronic sinusitis and nasal polyposis: a randomized clinical trial. *JAMA.* 2016;315(5):469-479.

62. Bachert C, Han JK, Desrosiers M, et al. Efficacy and safety of dupilumab in patients with severe chronic rhinosinusitis with nasal polyps (LIBERTY NP SINUS-24 and LIBERTY NP SINUS-52: results from two multicentre, randomised, double-blind, placebo-controlled, parallel-group phase 3 trials. *Lancet.* 2019;394(10209):1638-1650.

63. Hopkins C, Browne JP, Slack R, et al. The national comparative audit of surgery for nasal polyposis and chronic rhinosinusitis. *Clin Otolaryngol.* 2006;31(5):390-398

64. Ragab SM, Lund VJ, Scadding G. Evaluation of the medical and surgical treatment of chronic rhinosinusitis: a prospective, randomised, controlled trial. *Laryngoscope.* 2004;114(5):923-930.

65. Georgalas C, Cornet M, Adriaensen G, et al. Evidence-based surgery for chronic rhinosinusitis with and without nasal polyps. *Curr Allergy Asthma Rep.* 2014;14(4):427.

66. Ferguson BJ, Narita M, Yu VL, et al. Prospective observational study of chronic rhinosinusitis: environmental triggers and antibiotic implications. *Clin Infect Dis.* 2012;54:62-68.

67. Longhini ABFB. Clinical aspects of odontogenic maxillary sinusitis: a case series. *Int Forum Allergy Rhinol.* 2011;1:409-415.

68. Anavi Y, Allon DM, Avishai G, Calderon S. Complications of maxillary sinus augmentations in a selective series of patients. *Oral Surg Oral Med Oral Pathol Oral Radiol Endod.* 2008;106:34-38.

69. Park MJ, Park HI, Ahn KM, et al. Features of odontogenic sinusitis associated with dental implants. *Laryngoscope.* 2023;133:237-243.

70. Chakrabarti A, Denning DW, Ferguson BJ, et al. Fungal rhinosinusitis: a categorization and definitional schema addressing current controversies. *Laryngoscope.* 2009;119(9):1809-1818.

71. Callejas CA, Douglas RG. Fungal rhinosinusitis: what every allergist should know. *Clin Exp Allergy.* 2013;43(8):835-849.

72. deShazo RD, O'Brien M, Chapin K, Soto-Aguilar M, Gardner L, Swain R. A new classification and diagnostic criteria for invasive fungal sinusitis. *Arch Otlaryngol Head Neck Surg.* 1997;123:1181-1188.

73. Manning SC, Merkel M, Kriesel K, Vuitch F, Marple B. Computed tomography and magnetic resonance diagnosis of allergic fungal sinusitis. *Laryngoscope.* 1997;107:170-176.

74. Bent JP, Kuhn FA. Diagnosis of allergic fungal sinusitis. *Otolaryngol Head Neck Surg.* 1994;111:580-588.

75. Ponikau JU, Sherris DA, Kern EB, et al. The diagnosis and incidence of allergic fungal sinusitis. *Mayo Clin Proc.* 1999;74:877-884.

76. Ferguson BJ. Eosinophilic mucin rhinosinusitis: a distinct clinicopathological entity. *Laryngoscope.* 2000;110:799-813.

77. Katzenstein AL, Sale SR, Greenberger PA. Allergic aspergillus sinusitis: a newly recognized form of sinusitis. *J Allergy Clin Immunol.* 1983;72:89-93.

78. Bassichis BA, Marple BF, Mabry RL, Newcomer MT, Schwade ND. Use of immunotherapy in previously treated patients with allergic fungal sinusitis. *Otolaryngol Head Neck Surg.* 2001;125:487-490.

79. Sacks PL, Harvey RJ, Rimme J, Gallagher RM, Sacks R. Topical and systemic antifungal therapy for the symptomatic treatment of chronic rhinosinusitis. *Cochrane Database Syst Rev.* 2011;8:CD008263.

80. Mignogna MD, Fortuna G, Leuci S, et al. Mucormycosis in immunocompetent patients: a case-series of patients with maxillary sinus involvement and a critical review of the literature. *Int J Infect Dis.* 2011;15:e533-e540.

81. DelGaudio JM, Swain RE Jr, Kingdom TT, Muller S, Hudgins PA. Computed tomographic findings in patients with invasive fungal sinusitis. *Arch Otolaryngol Head Neck Surg.* 2003;129:236-240.

82. deShazo RD, O'Brien M, Chapin K, et al. Criteria for the diagnosis of sinus mycetoma. *J Allergy Clin Immunol.* 1997;99:475-485.

83. Herbrecht R, Denning DW, Patterson TF, et al. Invasive fungal infections group of the European Organisation for Research and Treatment of Cancer and the Global Aspergillus Study Group. Voriconazole versus amphotericin B for primary therapy of invasive aspergillosis. *N Engl J Med.* 2002;347:408-415.

84. Valera FC, do Lago T, Tamashiro E, Yassuda CC, Silveira F, Anselmo-Lima WT. Prognosis of acute invasive fungal rhinosinusitis related to underlying disease. *Int J Infect Dis.* 2011;15:e841-e844.

85. Montone KT, Livolsi VA, Feldman MD, et al. Fungal rhinosinusitis: a retrospective microbiologic and pathologic review of 400 patients at a single university medical center. *Int J Otolaryngol.* 2012;2012:684835.

86. Li Y, Li Y, Li P, Zhang G. Diagnosis and endoscopic surgery of chronic invasive fungal rhinosinusitis. *Am J Rhinol Allergy.* 2009;23:622-625.

87. Gumaa SA, Mahgoub ES, Hay RJ. Post-operative responses of paranasal *Aspergillus* granuloma to itraconazole. *Trans R Soc Trop Med Hyg.* 1992;86:93-94.

88. Mortimore S, Wormald PJ. The Groote Schuur hospital classification of the orbital complications of sinusitis. *J Laryngol Otol.* 1997;111(8):719-723.

89. Hoxworth JM, Glastonbury CM. Orbital and intracranial complications of acute sinusitis. *Neuroimaging Clin N Am.* 2010;20(4):511-526.

90. Schramm VL, Myers EN, Kennerdell JS. Orbital complications of acute sinusitis: evaluation, management, and outcome. *Otolaryngology.* 1978;86(2):ORL221-ORL230.

91. Goldberg AN, Oroszlan G, Anderson TD. Complications of frontal sinusitis and their management. *Otolaryngol Clin North Am.* 2001;34(1):211-225.

92. Sultesz M, Csakanyi Z, Majoros T, et al. Acute bacterial rhinosinusitis and its complications in our pediatric otolaryngological department between 1997 and 2006. *Int J Pediatr Otorhinolaryngol.* 2009;73(11):1507-1512.

93. Bayonne E, Kania R, Tran P, et al. Intracranial complications of rhinosinusitis: a review, typical imaging data and algorithm of management. *Rhinology.* 2009;47(1):59-65.

94. Younis RT, Lazar RH, Bustillo A, et al. Orbital infection as a complication of sinusitis: are diagnostic and treatment trends changing? *Ear Nose Throat J.* 2002;81(11):771-775.

95. Schuknecht B, Simmen D, Yuksel C, et al. Tributary venosinus occlusion and septic cavernous sinus thrombosis: CT and MR findings. *AJNR Am J Neuroradiol.* 1998;19(4):617-626.

96. Bambakidis NC, Cohen AR. Intracranial complications of frontal sinusitis in children: Pott's puffy tumor revisited. *Pediatr Neurosurg.* 2001;35(2):82-89.

97. Herrmann BW, Chung JC, Eisenbeis JF, et al. Intracranial complications of pediatric frontal rhinosinusitis. *Am J Rhinol.* 2006;20(3):320-324.

98. Kocaeli H, Hakyemez B, Bekar A, et al. Unusual complications and presentations of intracranial abscess: experience of a single institution. *Surg Neurol.* 2008;69(4):383-391.

99. Bukte Y, Paksoy Y, Genc E, et al. Role of diffusion-weighted MR in differential diagnosis of intracranial cystic lesions. *Clin Radiol.* 2005;60(3):375-383.

100. Earley MA, Friedel ME, Govindaraj S, Tessema B, Eloy JA. Community-acquired methicillin-resistant *Staphylococcus aureus* in nasal vestibular abscess. *Int Forum Allergy Rhinol.* 2011;1(5):379-381.

101. Ketcham AS, Han JK. Complications and management of septoplasty. *Otolaryngol Clin North Am.* 2010;43(4):897-904.

102. Alshaikh N, Lo S. Nasal septal abscess in children: from diagnosis to management and prevention. *Int J Pediatr Otorhinolaryngol.* 2011;75(6):737-744.

103. Cochran CS, Landecker A. Prevention and management of rhinoplasty complications. *Plast Reconstr Surg.* 2008;122(2):60e-67e.

104. Das S, Kashyap B, Barua M, Gupta N, Saha R, Vaid L, Banka A. Nasal rhinosporidiosis in humans: new interpretations and a review of the literature of this enigmatic disease. *Med Mycol.* 2011;49(3):311-315.

105. Zargari O, Elpern DJ. Granulomatous diseases of the nose. *Int J Dermatol.* 2009;48(12):1275-1282; quiz 1282.

106. Alavi SM, Nashibi R. Nasal tuberculosis in a 56 year old woman. *Caspian J Intern Med.* 2014;5(1):49-51.

107. Suzuki J, Oshima T, Watanabe K, Suzuki H, Kobayashi T, Hashimoto S. Chronic rhinosinusitis in ex-lepromatous leprosy patients with atrophic rhinitis. *J Laryngol Otol.* 2013;127(3):265-270.

108. Pan X, Zhu X, Li QQ. Syphilis manifesting as a nasopharyngeal carcinoma with cervical lymphadenopathy: a case report. *Exp Ther Med.* 2012;3(6):1023-1025.

109. Gul HC, Tosun F, Karakas A, et al. A case of mucosal leishmaniasis: mimicking intranasal tumor with perforation of septum. *J Microbiol Immunol Infect.* 2016;49(4):604-607.

110. Abdel Razek AA. Imaging of scleroma in the head and neck. *Br J Radiol.* 2012;85(1020):1551-1555.

15

Salivary Gland Infections

THOMAS SCHLIEVE, ANTONIA KOLOKYTHAS, AND MICHAEL MILORO

Salivary Gland Infections

The majority of nonneoplastic disease of the major salivary glands involve acute or chronic infections of the parotid, submandibular, and, rarely, sublingual glands. Infections of these glands may be bacterial, viral, or mycobacterial in origin. Although any of the major and minor salivary glands may be affected, the parotid and submandibular glands are involved most frequently as acute bacterial parotitis (ABP) and acute bacterial submandibular sialadenitis (ABSS). The cause of sialadenitis may be related to a variety of factors, including decreased salivary flow (dehydration, malnutrition, obstruction, and medication side effect), trauma to the duct or ductal orifice (occupational, habitual, or dental), or obstruction to salivary flow (ductal trauma, mucous plug, sialolithiasis, or collagen vascular disease). The factors form the basis for the classification of infectious disorders of the salivary glands (Table 15-1).

A high index of suspicion is necessary to differentiate an infectious salivary gland process from other causes of salivary gland enlargement, including benign and malignant tumors. Infections of the submandibular gland usually are obstructive in origin, whereas those of the parotid gland result from nonobstructive causes. Sialodochitis, inflammation of the salivary gland ductal system, also may follow episodes of acute sialolithiasis. Acute and chronic sialadenitis are influenced by several factors, including patient age, past medical and surgical history, immune status, total body fluid balance, medications, and allergies. Other causative factors of salivary gland infection include congenital or acquired ductal abnormalities; the presence of foreign bodies affecting the gland, ducts, or both; concomitant dental therapy; systemic granulomatous diseases; human immunodeficiency virus (HIV); facial trauma; and recent hospitalization.

General Considerations

Routine patient evaluation includes a comprehensive medical history and physical examination. A chief complaint also should be elicited. Sialadenitis usually begins with pain because of swelling of the gland's innervated capsule. The timeline of symptoms should be determined to assess the chronicity of disease with a chronic process being that lasting longer than 1 month. The medical history may provide information regarding the assessment of the patient with salivary gland enlargement, because a variety of medical illnesses predispose patients to acute salivary gland infection (Table 15-2). Many cases of ABP occur in hospitalized patients who are debilitated with inadequate fluid intake and alteration of fluid balance with resultant dehydration. Patients who report postprandial submandibular edema and pain most likely have acute obstructive submandibular sialolithiasis. A previous history of salivary stone formation may aid in the diagnosis. Children with acute salivary gland edema and tenderness may have contracted mumps. Patients with acute gland edema should be questioned about contact with animals, specifically cats (see section on cat-scratch disease later in this chapter). Musicians who play wind instruments who report bilateral parotid swelling after a concert may have acute air insufflation of the parotid fascia in the classic "trumpet blowers syndrome." Patients who have undergone recent dental work, orthodontic bracket application, or with evidence of chronic cheek biting habit and salivary gland enlargement may have been infected by traumatic introduction of bacteria into the ductal system with resultant retrograde sialadenitis. Although uncommon, any odontogenic source should be eliminated by dental and radiographic examination and tooth vitality testing. Evidence of facial trauma with facial lacerations proximal to a line connecting the lateral canthus to the oral commissure and crossing a line from tragus to mid-philtrum may disrupt the Stensen duct and cause parotid region edema as a result of sialocele formation. The presence of a foreign body (e.g., dirt, glass, toothbrush bristles, food particles) may cause a physical obstruction to salivary flow. A patient history significant for collagen vascular disease or autoimmune disease may indicate the possibility of salivary gland obstruction as the cause of sialadenitis (e.g., a relationship between sarcoidosis and ranula formation in the sublingual glands). Finally, a thorough medical history may reveal a variety of medications that can lead to decreased salivary flow with stasis and retrograde sialadenitis (Table 15-3). Any constitutional signs and symptoms should be determined, including pain (prandial

TABLE 15-1	Classification of Salivary Gland Infections

Bacterial Infections

Acute bacterial parotitis
Chronic recurrent parotitis
Acute suppurative submandibular sialadenitis
Chronic recurrent submandibular sialadenitis
Chronic recurrent juvenile parotitis
Acute allergic sialadenitis (radiologic parotitis)
Actinomycosis
Cat-scratch disease

Viral Infections

Epidemic parotitis (mumps)
Benign lymphoepithelial lesion (HIV)
Cytomegalovirus
Coxsackie A virus
Influenza A virus
Echovirus

Fungal Infections

Mycobacterial Infections

Tuberculosis
Atypical mycobacteria

Parasitic Infections

Immunologically mediated infections
Systemic lupus erythematosus
Sjögren's syndrome
Necrotizing sialometaplasia
Sarcoidosis

TABLE 15-2	Risk Factors Associated With Salivary Gland Infections

Dehydration
Recent surgery and anesthesia
Chronic medical illnesses
Advanced age
Premature infants
Radiation therapy
Immunocompromised status
Long-term institutionalization
Renal failure
Hepatic failure
Congestive heart failure
Diabetes mellitus
Hypothyroidism
Malnutrition
Sialolithiasis
Oral infection
Oral neoplasm
Human immunodeficiency virus
Sjögren's syndrome
Depression
Psychiatric disorders
Anorexia nervosa/bulimia
Hyperuricemia
Hyperlipoproteinemia
Cystic fibrosis
Lead intoxication
Cushing's disease
Medications

TABLE 15-3	Medications Associated With Salivary Gland Infections

Antihistamines
Diuretics
Tricyclic antidepressants
Barbiturates
Phenothiazines
Antihypertensives
Anti-sialagogues
Anticholinergics
Chemotherapeutic agents

pain indicating an obstructive phenomenon) especially fever, malaise, diaphoresis, chills, and nausea.

After a thorough history has been obtained, the physical examination should begin with inspection to ascertain any asymmetries in the appearance and size of the glands bilaterally before palpation and possible introduction of iatrogenic edema. Any cardinal signs or symptoms of inflammation should be documented, including edema, erythema, tenderness, and warmth. In doing so, one can attempt to rule out the presence of a tumor of the gland. An infectious process will commonly manifest as a diffuse, tender, symptomatic swelling of the gland while a tumor is often a more discrete mass within the gland with or without symptoms. Evidence of facial trauma should be documented, including the presence of lacerations, ecchymosis, or abrasions (e.g., cat scratch or puncture). The examination should begin with an extraoral assessment followed by an intraoral examination. Palpation of the major salivary glands should begin with gentle bimanual examination of the glands, ducts, and ductal orifices. The clinician must observe carefully for spontaneous and evoked salivary flow while palpating the gland in a posterior to anterior direction ("milking" of the gland), expulsion of mucous plugs, small stones, or sludge, and the presence of purulence at the ductal orifice. In a nervous and anxious patient, it is important to recognize the sympathomimetic response to examination may result in decreased salivary flow. Finally, any potential odontogenic source of infection (secondary deep space involvement) for submandibular or posterior facial swelling must be ruled out.

The decision to perform instrumentation of the ductal orifice and probe the duct should not be made indiscriminately. The act of mechanical probing may be diagnostic and therapeutic if a calculus is present, a mucous plug is dislodged, or a ductal stricture is dilated. Conversely, this procedure may introduce bacteria that normally colonize the ductal orifice into the ductal system and allow retrograde contamination of the gland. Ductal probing is generally not indicated for epidemic mumps in children and is probably contraindicated in the setting of ABP. Finally, the head and neck examination should include palpation of the facial, preauricular, and cervical regions for any signs of associated lymphadenopathy.

Salivary gland radiography is guided by the history and physical examination findings and is useful in the diagnostic assessment of salivary gland enlargement. Plain film radiography may be useful for detection of salivary gland calculi in the glands and ductal system (Figures 15-1 and 15-2). The usefulness of this study is limited because only 80 to 85% of stones are radiopaque and therefore visible on plain film radiographs. A mandibular occlusal film can be used to detect calculi in the submandibular and sublingual glands and ducts. A "puffed cheek" view, in which the patient forcibly blows the cheeks laterally to distend the soft tissues over the lateral ramus and zygoma, may detect parotid gland and Stensen's duct calculi. Periapical and panoramic radiographs occasionally show calculi of the major salivary gland systems.

Computed tomography (CT) allows better distinction between salivary gland tissue and adjacent soft tissue than sialography, and although radiation exposure is increased, it is a less invasive procedure. CT scanning can distinguish

between intraglandular and extraglandular lesions. For example, the clinical appearance of a masticator space infection may mimic acute parotitis; however, a CT scan with soft tissue window attenuation differentiates the two entities. CT scanning may show posteriorly located submandibular hilar stones that were not visible on plain films. Because small calcification of the glands can be obscured in a contrast-enhanced CT, a noncontrast scan is often taken first to assist in visualization. The use of three-dimensional CT scanning has been applied to the salivary glands, with the ability to visualize ductal irregularities such as duct dilation and architectural alteration of the gland parenchyma in three dimensions (Figure 15-3).[1]

Ultrasonography is a straightforward, noninvasive imaging technique that may be useful in the evaluation of mass lesions of the parotid and submandibular glands. Ultrasonography can distinguish solid from cystic masses and localize an abscess cavity for potential drainage procedures. Parotid and submandibular gland cysts, stones, dilated ducts, and abscesses can be demonstrated. However, ultrasound images lack detailed image resolution and are operator dependent.

Magnetic resonance imaging (MRI) provides excellent soft tissue image resolution without radiation of the use of contrast media. The use of MRI in salivary gland infectious processes has been limited; however, recent use of MR sialography has gained popularity because of excellent resolution of salivary gland ductal anatomy. Several studies have documented the use of fast T2-weighted MRI to delineate ductal architecture and identify calculi.[2]

Over the past decade salivary endoscopy, or sialoendoscopy, has developed into a minimally invasive technique useful in the diagnosis and treatment of salivary gland disorders. Diagnostic and interventional procedures can be performed with a variety of sialoendoscopes. A semirigid endoscope

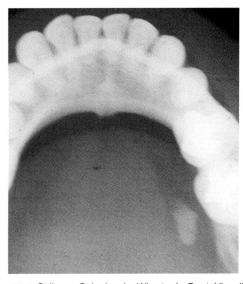

• **Figure 15-1** Salivary Calculus In Wharton's Duct Visualized on Mandibular Occlusal Radiograph.

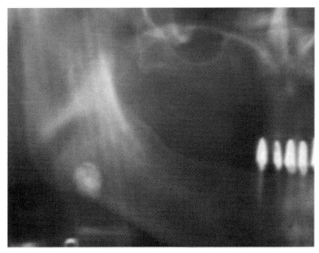

• **Figure 15-2** Salivary Calculus Within the Submandibular Salivary Gland Visualized on Panoramic Radiograph.

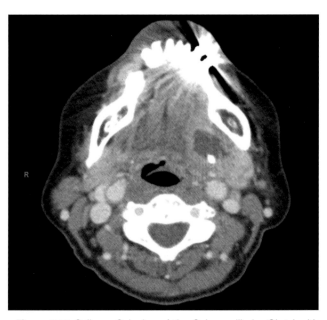

• **Figure 15-3** Salivary Calculus of the Submandibular Gland with Ductal Dilation.

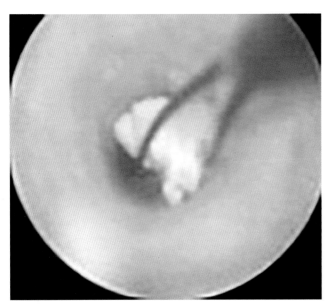

• **Figure 15-4** Sialoendoscopic View of Submandibular Sialolithiasis (Stone) Retrieval.

1 mm in diameter can be combined with exploration and surgical units, as well as devices with irrigation ports to allow for both ductal examination and treatment under direct visualization. Baskets, dilators, balloon catheters, and lasers can be used to crush, fragment, and retrieve stones; relieve ductal stenosis; wash out debris; remove mucous plugs; and place stents to maintain ductal integrity without major complications (Figure 15-4). Following sialoendoscopic intervention, a ductal stent should be placed to prevent stenosis from edema and allow any remaining debris to be washed out by saliva. The only contraindication to sialoendoscopy is acute parotitis. Relative contraindications include a ductal lumen that cannot be inflated adequately, stones larger than 1 cm, and intraparenchymal stones. The use of sialoendoscopy in the treatment of chronic recurrent parotitis as both a diagnostic and therapeutic technique is well-documented, and it has the potential to replace the need for sialography.[3-7]

Sialography was once considered the gold standard in diagnostic and salivary gland radiology; however, CT, MRI, and sialoendoscopy have now largely replaced it. Sialography is useful for the detection of radiolucent salivary calculi and mucous plugs or strictures. It provides excellent anatomic detail of the salivary gland parenchyma and ductal components while estimating the severity of ductal and parenchymal damage caused by obstructive, traumatic, inflammatory, and neoplastic diseases. Sialography is performed with water-soluble contrast media that contains between 28 and 38% iodine concentration. Because of the high iodine content of the contrast media, sialography is contraindicated in the setting of acute sialadenitis because contrast may extravasate outside the capsule of inflamed or damaged glands and ducts and cause severe pain and possibly soft tissue damage, with foreign body reaction and glandular necrosis. Other contraindications to sialography include iodine sensitivity and use before a planned thyroid scan study. In addition to

its diagnostic role in detection of calculi and possibly, mucous plugs, sialography may be therapeutic by dislodging small calculi or mucous plugs, thereby relieving the physical obstruction to salivary flow. Most contrast media are considered bacteriostatic (some contain a combination of contrast and antibiotics), but their bacteriostatic activity within the glands has not been proven. Sialography may be useful for determination of the degree of ductal and glandular destruction as a result of chronic and recurrent infectious or inflammatory processes. Sialadenitis, inflammation of the acinoparenchyma of the gland, results in saccular dilation caused by acinar atrophy; this is visible as "pruning" of the normal full arborization of the ductal system (Figure 15-5). The contrast does not penetrate into the peripheral ductules of the gland. Sialodochitis, inflammatory damage to the ductal system, classically displays a "sausage link" appearance on sialogram (Figure 15-6). The saccular enlargement of the ductal system

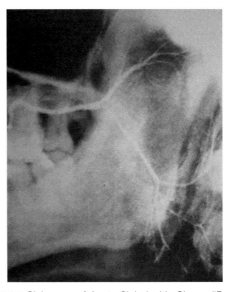

• **Figure 15-5** Sialogram of Acute Sialadenitis Shows "Pruning" of the Ductal System.

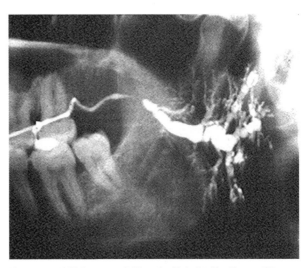

• **Figure 15-6** Sialogram of Chronic Sialadenitis Shows "Sausage Link" Appearance of Enlarged Ducts.

results from chronic inflammation, repetitive attempts to pump saliva out against a fixed obstruction, or both processes, with the resultant loss of ductal architecture and elasticity. Abscess cavities within the gland parenchyma may be seen as displacement and compression of normal glandular architecture peripherally around a radiolucent area. Finally, the retention of contrast media in the glandular system after the study (postevacuation phase) may indicate a decrease in the amount of residual salivary gland function. In the past, sialography has been combined with both CT and MRI to improve image resolution and details of the study; however, recent advancements in CT scanning such as multislice scanners and submillimeter-thick image capture have limited the need for these techniques.

Radioisotope scanning, or salivary scintigraphy, may be useful in the evaluation of salivary gland parenchyma. This study relies on the salivary glandular tissue's selective concentration of radioactive elements such as radioactive iodine; this selectivity is similar to that of thyroid tissue. In general, intraglandular lesions, such as benign mixed tumors, Warthin's tumor, and malignant salivary gland tumors, may be detected on intravenous injection of a radioactive isotope (technetium-99m [^{99m}Tc] pertechnetate). Salivary scintigraphy may show increased uptake of ^{99m}Tc in an acutely inflamed gland or decreased uptake in a gland with poor function as a result of chronic inflammation and scarring. The advantage of salivary scintigraphy is that all glands may be imaged simultaneously; however, the main problem with scintigraphy is poor detail resolution and therefore its use is limited.

Laboratory data may aid in the diagnosis of salivary gland infection. Peripheral leukocytosis may be expected in acute bacterial sialadenitis, and leukopenia and relative lymphocytosis may be present in cases of viral sialadenitis. In addition, serum amylase levels will be elevated in mumps infection with a peak during the first week of infection. In ABP, serum amylase levels will be normal. Sialochemistry, the evaluation of the electrolyte composition of saliva, measures sodium and potassium ion concentration changes with alterations in salivary flow rates. In general, noninflammatory disorders of the salivary glands result in elevations in potassium levels (normal potassium levels: parotid, 25 mEq/L; submandibular, 20 mEq/L), whereas inflammatory sialadenitis results in a decrease in potassium and an increase in sodium concentrations (normal sodium concentrations: parotid, 7 mEq/L; submandibular 5 mEq/L). Recurrent parotitis also may exhibit elevations in protein concentration (>400 mg/dL), and collagen sialadenitis (e.g., systemic lupus erythematosus) results in elevations of chloride concentrations greater than two to three times normal. Salivary flow also may be decreased in sialadenitis.

Bacteriology is of paramount importance in the diagnostic assessment of salivary gland infection. Routine acquisition of purulent material (i.e., aspiration or spontaneous or evoked drainage) is evaluated rapidly by Gram stain and aerobic, anaerobic, and fungal culture and antibiotic sensitivity testing. Acid-fast staining techniques may be used for

TABLE 15-4	Differential Diagnosis of Salivary Gland Enlargement
Salivary gland infection (see Table 15-1)	
Sialadenosis	
Hormonal	
Neurohormonal	
Malnutrition	
Mucoviscidosis (cystic fibrosis)	
Drug-induced	
Sialolithiasis	
Sialocele	
Ductal stricture	
Mucocele	
Ranula	
Megastenon	
Sialorrhea	
Xerostomia	
Trauma	
Odontogenic infection (secondary space involvement)	
Benign salivary gland tumors	
Malignant salivary gland tumors	
Lipoma	
Fibroma	
Mesenchymal tumors (hemangioma, neurofibroma)	
Lymph node hyperplasia	
Reactive lymphadenitis	
Infectious mononucleosis	
Lymphoepithelial cyst	
Dermoid cyst	
Epidermoid cyst	
Lymphoma	

suspected mycobacterial infections. The differential diagnosis of salivary gland enlargement includes many disorders that may cause clinical confusion (Table 15-4). In general, the presence of tumors and systemic diseases may be ruled out by the absence of cardinal signs of inflammation. Sialadenosis, or noninflammatory salivary gland enlargement, may result from a variety of systemic conditions. The presence of a benign tumor usually manifests as a slow growing, firm, painless mass, whereas a malignant tumor may enlarge more rapidly and include neurologic deficits (e.g., facial nerve weakness), pain, or fixation to the underlying tissues. The presence of postprandial gland edema and pain generally suggests obstructive sialadenitis. A proposed algorithm for assessment of salivary gland enlargement is outlined in Figure 15-7.

Bacterial Salivary Gland Infections

Acute Bacterial Parotitis

The history of ABP parallels the history of modern medicine. The first case of ABP was reported in *The Lancet* in 1829 and resulted in a gangrenous infection with facial paralysis. Treatment then consisted of leaches, emollient poultice, and surgical drainage.[8] ABP was distinguished from viral mumps by Brodie in 1834.[9] This entity has been referred to as suppurative parotitis, pyogenic parotitis, and

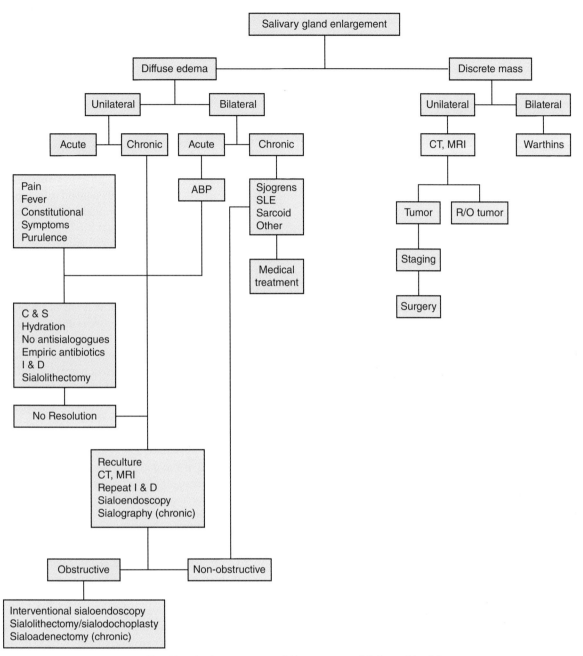

• **Figure 15-7** Algorithm for Assessment and Management of Salivary Gland Enlargement.

surgical mumps, because historically it has been attributed to postsurgical hypovolemia and dehydration. Before the modern surgical and antibiotic era of medicine, ABP was a common complication of abdominal surgery or intraabdominal trauma, with a mortality rate approaching 50%. Before the mid-twentieth century understanding of the physiology of fluid and electrolyte balance, postoperative dehydration was commonplace. The postoperative volume depletion was caused by inadequate volume replacement to compensate for sensible and insensible surgical losses in stasis and retrograde infection of the parotid gland through the Stensen duct. Salivary secretion is significantly decreased and may even cease when total body water decreases 8% or

more. In addition, being maintained nil per os, or NPO, results in decreased salivary stimulation and decreased detergent action of food, liquids and mastication. In July 1818, President Garfield suffered a gunshot wound to the abdomen in an assassination attempt. He underwent abdominal exploratory laparotomy surgery and developed peritonitis and dehydration. He died 10 weeks later as a result of sepsis, presumably as a result of suppurative parotitis.

Dehydration with resultant xerostomia has been associated with ABP in a report of seven cases caused by prolonged sun exposure in the Middle East in 1919.[10] By the late 1930s and during World War II, intravenous fluid resuscitation during and after surgery had become routine practice and the incidence of postsurgical ABP decreased dramatically. By 1955, with the routine use of perioperative prophylactic and therapeutic antibiotics, ABP was referred to by Robinson as "a vanishing disease,"[11] but by 1958, Petersdorf et al.[12] reported seven cases of penicillin-resistant staphylococcal parotitis and by the early 1960s, large series of cases of ABP were reported.[13,14] Currently, 0.03% of hospital admissions, of which 30 to 40% are postoperative patients, are due to ABP.[15]

In the past several decades, a dramatic change has occurred in the bacterial flora of the oral cavity. This change has largely been caused by the increased incidence of nosocomial and opportunistic infections in patients who are immunocompromised and those who are seriously ill in intensive care units whose mouths become colonized by microorganisms that were rarely found in the oral environment several decades ago. In addition, with the advent of antibiotics directed at some resident oral flora (e.g., streptococci), the voids became occupied by other bacterial species (e.g., gram-negative enteric organisms, *Escherichia coli, Klebsiella, Haemophilus influenzae*, diptheroids, *Neisseria* species), and iatrogenically induced, genetically altered organisms (i.e., penicillin-resistant staphylococci). Finally, with the improvement in culture techniques and laboratory analyses, the identification of anaerobic organisms (e.g., *Prevotella, Porphyromonas, Fusobacterium,* and *Peptostreptococcus*) in Stensen ductal discharge fluid and percutaneous needle aspiration material has increased. The most common bacteria isolated in cases of ABP using current techniques is *Staphylococcus aureus*. Also common, are the gram-negative bacilli (e.g., *Prevotella* and *Porphyromonas*), *Fusobacterium,* and *Peptostreptococcus*. Using aspiration culture techniques, approximately 1.7 isolates per specimen are obtained, with 47% producing β-lactamase; 100% of *S. aureus* and 50% of the *Prevotella* and *Porphyromonas* present in these aspirates were β-lactamase producing.[16,17]

ABP rarely occurs in children during the neonatal period. Usually, neonatal ABP begins during the first 2 weeks after birth and most often in premature infants. The transient bacteremia associated with birth is thought to play a role in development of neonatal ABP; but similar to adult ABP, the cause is thought to be dehydration in the majority of cases. The classic clinical presentation of parotid edema and erythema, with purulence expressible at Stensen duct, also may be observed but unlike adult ABP, neonatal ABP is more often bilateral. Although *S. aureus* is most commonly associated with neonatal ABP, *E. coli, Pseudomonas, Streptococcus pneumoniae*, and other organisms have been isolated. Systemic antibiotics and rehydration usually control the disease process, but in rare cases neonates may require surgical drainage.

In recent years, ABP has manifested in one of two forms: nosocomial and community-acquired variants. Most previous clinical and reported evidence, however anecdotal, suggests that the most common organism cultured from hospital-acquired cases of parotitis is *S. aureus*. In many cases, parotitis in patients who are debilitated and immunocompromised has been caused by gram-negative organisms, such as *Pseudomonas, Klebsiella, E. coli, Proteus, Eikenella,* and *H. influenzae*. Although rare, cases of fungal and mycobacterial parotitis have been reported.[16-23]

Several factors predispose the parotid gland to infectious processes. Retrograde infection of the parotid gland is postulated as the major cause of ABP. Dehydration, as a result of acute illness, surgery, trauma, or sepsis, may result in diminishing salivary flow, thereby eliminating the normal flushing action of saliva as it traverses through the Stensen duct. Another hypothesis is that parotid saliva has less intrinsic bacteriostatic activity than saliva produced by the other salivary glands. The serous parotid saliva contains less immunoglobulin-A (IgA), sialic acid (agglutinates bacteria), lysosomes, and glycoproteins that bind epithelial cells of the salivary duct and prevent bacterial adherence.[24] In healthy patients the content of parotid saliva includes high concentrations of fibronectin, which promote the adherence of *Streptococcus* spp. and *S. aureus* around the ductal orifice of Stensen duct.[24,25] Conversely, low levels of fibronectin promote the adherence of *Pseudomonas* and *E. coli*. This fact explains the clinical situation in which colonization as a result of dehydration leads to gram-positive parotitis versus the development of gram-negative parotid gland infections in patients who are debilitated or immunocompromised.[25,26]

Adherence of gram-negative rods to oropharyngeal cells is increased in critically ill patients.[27] Subsequent retrograde invasion of the Stensen duct and the parotid gland occurs with diminished salivary flow. The resultant ABP reflects the resident oral flora of the compromised host exposed to the opportunistic organisms of the hospital and intensive care unit.

Community-acquired ABP is much more common than hospital-acquired ABP. All the organisms associated with nosocomial ABO can cause community-acquired ABP, but most frequently it is associated with *S. aureus*. Although obstructive phenomenon such as sialoliths are uncommon in Stensen duct compared with Wharton duct, parotid duct obstruction may result from mucous plugs that form as a result of reduced salivary flow caused by dehydration or poor fluid balance. Salivary stasis may be the result of medications with antisialagogic side effects, such as diuretics, antihistamines, tricyclic antidepressants, antihypertensives (β-blocking agents), anticholinergics, and phenothiazines. These drugs may lead to increased salivary viscosity that causes stasis of flow and possible mucous plug formation. Hematogenous spread of infection to the parotid gland is unlikely in adults. Trauma to the Stensen duct may be responsible for 5 to 10% of cases of ABP. Ductal trauma, with subsequent periductal edema, may cause partial obstruction of salivary flow. Trauma may be the result of dental trauma, orthodontic appliances, cheek biting, toothbrush trauma, air insufflation during dental treatment, and "trumpet blowers syndrome." This entity should be differentiated from ABP, because it is merely a pneumoparotid with tissue emphysema and crepitus on physical examination and lacks the constitutional symptoms of ABP.[28] However, ABP may occur as the result of pneumoparotid if salivary stasis and bacterial infection are present. Finally, poor oral hygiene and immunocompromised states (e.g., diabetes mellitus, malnutrition, acute or chronic diarrhea) with resultant dehydration may be causative factors in ABP.

The diagnosis of ABP includes an assessment of history, physical examination, laboratory data, and radiographic studies when appropriate. A history of recent surgery or previous episodes of ABP may be significant. In postoperative patients the onset usually occurs after the third postsurgical day, commonly between the fifth and seventh day. The presence of an immunocompromised state or use of medications with antisialagogic effects should be ascertained. The onset of ABP is sudden and rapid with painful swelling and erythema of the preauricular region, classically at mealtime. Stretching of the parotid gland innervated capsule as a result of inflammation of the gland itself results in the sensation of pain. The physical findings of ABP usually are classic (Figure 15-8). The parotid gland is enlarged, possibly displacing the earlobe laterally, and tender to palpation. Both parotid glands can be affected (indicative of a systemic disorder), but if the infection is unilateral, the right gland seems to be infected more than the left. A predilection for males exists for ABP, and the mean age of presentation is 60 years.

The act of "milking" of the parotid gland with bimanual pressure to the Stensen duct intraorally and extraorally, in the posterior to anterior direction, may express purulent material if the duct is patent (Figure 15-9). Probing of the Stensen duct (with lacrimal probes) and catheter irrigation are generally contraindicated in ABP. Although ductal strictures may be dilated and small mucous plugs relieved, the risk of intro-

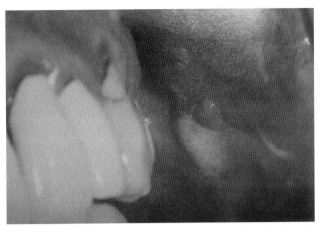

• **Figure 15-9** Intraoral View of Purulence Drainage from the Parotid Duct.

ducing purulent material into the proximal duct and gland should be considered. Constitutional symptoms, including fever, chills, and sweats, may occur if an established infection is present. Dehydration may be confirmed by the presence of xerostomia and poor skin turgor. Laboratory evaluation may reveal leukocytosis with a predominance of immature polymorphonuclear leukocytes and bandemia with true ABP. Further confirmation of dehydration is made by elevated hematocrit, increased blood urea nitrogen level, elevated urine specific gravity, decreased urinary flow rates, and possible contraction alkalosis on electrolyte examination.

Radiographic evaluation rarely demonstrates calculi in Stensen ducts; however, up to 20% of cases will demonstrate radiopaque stones while sialography is contraindicated in ABP (Figure 15-10). Ultrasonography may be useful for detection of stones when sialography is contraindicated or for the detection of fluid collections not appreciable on physical examination because of the multiple investments of fascia within the gland. CT scanning may help visualization of abscess formation (Figure 15-11) or tumors and can

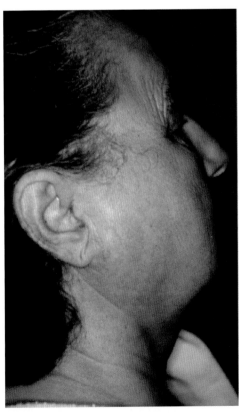

• **Figure 15-8** Clinical Example of Acute Bacterial Parotitis.

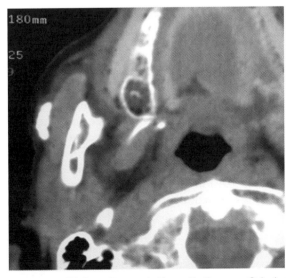

• **Figure 15-10** CT Scan Demonstrating a Radiopaque Calculus of the Parotid Duct.

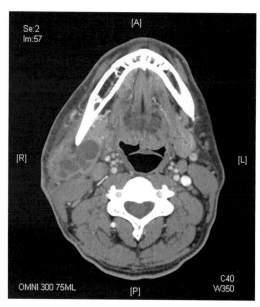

• **Figure 15-11** CT Scan Demonstrating Fluid Collection Within the Parotid Gland.

distinguish other secondary space infections (masticator, lateral pharyngeal, pterygomandibular spaces) from the glandular ABP. MRI may be more useful for delineating soft tissue pathologic conditions (tumors) and visualizing tissue planes. Bacteriologic studies are essential in the diagnosis of ABP. A Gram stain of purulent discharge may identify potential pathogens quickly and easily; however, culture and sensitivity studies should be performed as soon as possible. The culture studies confirm the Gram stain findings and identify specific organisms, whereas the sensitivity determines the most appropriate choice of antimicrobial agent. If the empiric antibiotic that is chosen pending culture and sensitivity results does not control the infection, antimicrobial therapy is guided by the culture and sensitivity findings. The best collection method for bacteriologic examinations is percutaneous needle aspiration with ultrasound guidance to precisely locate any fluid collections; however, percutaneous needle aspiration without ultrasound guidance is preferred to intraoral approaches. If no pus is obtained, injection of 0.5 mL of sterile saline and repeat aspiration of the same site may yield better material for culture. Alternatively, transductal aspiration using a small catheter introduced into the Stensen duct can be used; however, the possibility of oral contamination exists with this method. Unfortunately, in many circumstances, obtaining sufficient material for examination percutaneously is difficult and containing the sample for anaerobic analysis is problematic. If surgical drainage is required, direct needle aspiration through exposed parotid fascia may be performed with or without ultrasound guidance.[29]

The treatment of ABP consists of specific and nonspecific therapies. The historical description of nonspecific therapy included discontinuation of antisialagogic medications, increased fluid intake, heat packs, mouth rinses, sialogogues (such as sugar-free lemon drops or glycerin swabs), and analgesics as needed for pain. Radiation therapy, once considered a mainstay of therapy, no longer is warranted. The beneficial effects of radiation in cases of ABP in the early to mid-twentieth century were related to the simultaneous introduction and understanding of fluid and electrolyte balance. Rehydration remains a cornerstone of therapy for ABP, but caution must be exercised in patients who are elderly and debilitated who may not be able to appropriately redistribute the fluid load and may be at risk for acute cardiac overload and failure with resulting pulmonary edema. Fluid overload should be avoided by careful monitoring of urine output and specific gravity, electrolytes, and possible central venous pressure. Discontinuation of medications with antisialagogic side effects (or alteration of doses) should be undertaken after consultation with the prescribing physician and the determination of an appropriate alternative medication. These measures (rehydration and drug alteration) should act together to increase salivary flow while reducing salivary viscosity, resulting in the reestablishment of a physiologic salivary flushing action. In addition, improvement in oral hygiene with the use of chlorhexidine rinses may decrease the oral bacterial load and the potential for continued retrograde colonization of the gland. Specific therapy of ABP involves the removal of ductal obstructions such as mucous plugs (gentle ductal probing, irrigation, and possibly endoscopy) or sialoliths (endoscopic or open ductal surgery). These invasive procedures should be attempted only after the institution of empiric antimicrobial therapy.

Prompt species-specific antimicrobial therapy is the keystone of ABP treatment. Empiric therapy may be based on Gram stain results; alternatively, another antibiotic may be chosen based on the knowledge of contemporary flora of ABP discussed previously, including β-lactamase–producing organisms. In the past, community-acquired ABP and cases of suspected *Staphylococcus* involvement in nosocomial ABP, a semisynthetic antistaphylococcal penicillin (methicillin, oxacillin, or dicloxacillin) or a first-generation cephalosporin (cephalexin) was considered a reasonable choice for empiric therapy. If methicillin-resistant *Staphylococcus aureus* (MRSA) is identified, vancomycin or linezolid are the drugs of choice. Current antimicrobial trends indicate that β-lactamase–inhibiting drugs such as amoxicillin with clavulanic acid (Augmentin) for outpatient oral administration in the less severe case of ABP and ampicillin with sulbactam (Unasyn) for inpatient administration may be reasonable first-line choices for empiric therapy. Clindamycin also may be used in patients with severe penicillin allergy, but erythromycin should be avoided because of high bacterial resistance. As alternatives, other macrolide antibiotics such as azithromycin or clarithromycin may be used in the outpatient setting of community-acquired ABP, because they have an appropriate bacterial spectrum for ABP and a dosage frequency that improves compliance. Combination antibiotic therapy may be necessary in consultation with the hospital infectious disease service in cases of hospital-acquired ABP, in community-acquired ABP in the immunocompromised host, in nursing home patients because of the high incidence of MRSA, if generalized sepsis develops, or if nonroutine organisms are identified (e.g., *Pseudomonas*). Antibiotic therapy should be continued until at least 1 week after resolution of signs and symptoms of ABP. If ABP is recalcitrant to therapy or recurs, repeated culture of the abscess and obtaining a CT scan or ultrasound to rule out possible parenchymal abscess formation should be considered (Figure 15-12).

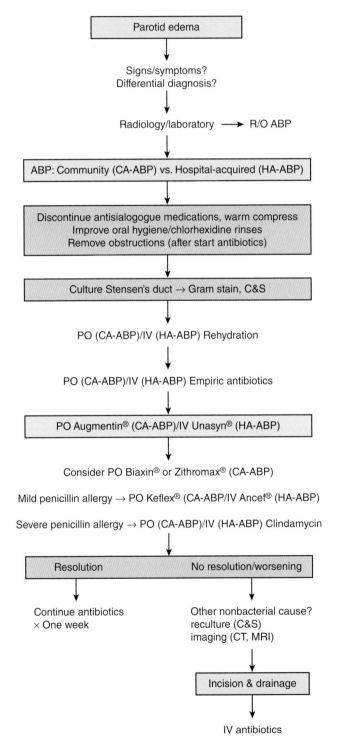

• **Figure 15-12** Algorithm for Management of Acute Bacterial Parotitis.

Despite rehydration and antibiotic therapy, progressive infection may lead to local extension into adjacent fascial spaces; osteomyelitis of the mandible, including temporomandibular joint; facial paralysis; internal jugular vein thrombosis; necrotizing fasciitis; generalized hematogenous sepsis; airway obstruction (with involvement of the lateral pharyngeal-retropharyngeal spaces); multiple organ dysfunction syndrome; and death. Therefore, if nonspecific and specific therapy fail to produce clinical improvement within 72 to 96 hours, if pain and edema increase, if temperature and white blood cell count increase, or if complications occur, surgical intervention may be necessary and lifesaving. Surgical drainage of ABP is performed much less frequently than in the past when antibiotic therapy was unavailable. However, as resistant strains of bacteria continue to develop because of overuse of antibiotics, incision and drainage may become more necessary, and surgeons should be familiar with these techniques.

The parotid gland is surrounded by a dense fibrous soft tissue capsule with multiple investments of fascia within the gland that makes fluctuance on physical examination uncommon and spontaneous drainage an unlikely phenomenon. Surgical exposure is necessary to ensure drainage of all potential loculations that may have developed under the dense parotid fascia. The presence of loculations may be confirmed with CT scanning or preoperative and/or intraoperative ultrasound. If the parotitis is severe enough to warrant surgical intervention, needle aspiration with or without drainage catheter placement under ultrasound guidance can be successful in select cases (Figure 15-13, A and B). These patients are relatively healthy individuals with unilocular abscess formation. It is difficult to drain a multiloculated abscess with needle drainage because of the difficulty in perforating and draining each loculation effectively.[29-31]

Incision and drainage of the parotid gland is usually performed with the patient under general anesthesia, but monitored anesthesia care with local anesthesia may be used if the patient's condition precludes the use of a general anesthetic. Drainage usually is accomplished through a retromandibular incision (a modified superficial parotidectomy incision) through skin and subcutaneous tissue, which exposes the underlying parotid fascia. Multiple penetrations are made through the parotid fascia with blunt dissection (with a closed Kelly clamp) to prevent injury to major vascular hazards and branches of the facial nerve. A useful technique is intraoperative ultrasound-guided drainage. This allows the surgeon to identify abscess cavities within the gland, minimize unnecessary dissection, identify vascular structures, and ensure all fluid has been drained.[29] Attention should be directed to any accessory parotid gland tissue that may contain abscess cavities and lie at or above the level of the zygomatic arch. This salivary gland tissue may require extension of the incision more cranially to gain access for adequate drainage. Although grossly purulent flow may not be obtained, serous drainage through the perforation in the parotid fascia may be sufficient to obtain "decompression" of the gland, which may result in immediate improvement

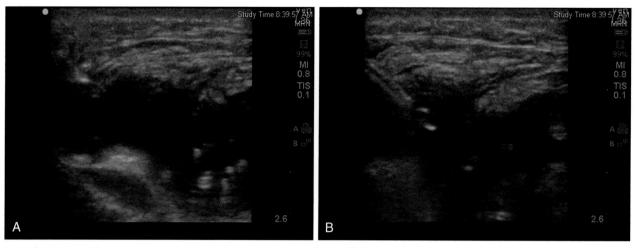

• **Figure 15-13　A,** Ultrasound demonstrating parotid gland fluid collection. **B,** Ultrasound-guided percutaneous drain placement.

in edema, pain, fever, and white blood cell count. The wound can be left open and packed with saline gauze changes 2 or 3 times daily. Occasionally, rubber drains are placed into the abscess cavities to allow for continued drainage and removed as drainage subsides. This method usually results in minimal scarring or cosmetic deformity, and the formation of a sialocele or persistent salivary fistulae are uncommon complications of surgery.

Acute Bacterial Submandibular Sialadenitis

ABSS is most commonly associated with physical obstruction of the Wharton duct. Sialolithiasis usually occurs in the submandibular gland and ductal system (80% of cases) for several reasons. The submandibular gland lies inferior to its ductal system, so that in the erect *Homo sapiens,* flow must occur against the forces of gravity. The length of the Wharton duct contributes to increased transit time of saliva in the ductal system, which may result in the formation of microcalculi and resultant coalescence causing mechanical obstruction to flow and eventual ABSS.[32] Two acute bends are present in the Wharton duct: one occurs as the gland courses posterior to the mylohyoid muscle, and the second occurs just proximal to the exit of the duct superiorly into the anterior floor of the mouth. A sphincteric mechanism at the orifice of the Wharton duct acts as a physical narrowing at this portion of the duct. The alkaline submandibular gland saliva contains a higher concentration of calcium salts (carbonates, phosphates, and oxalates) than the other major salivary glands. All these factors may contribute to salivary stasis, crystallization of precipitated calcium salts with calculus formation, obstruction to salivary flow, and infection. This disease process occurs twice as often in males, with a peak age of occurrence between 30 and 50 years. Interestingly, the left submandibular gland is more commonly affected than the right, and bilateral involvement in the absence of another systemic disorder is rare. Multiple occurrences of sialolith formation in the same glad is common:

two calculi are present in 20% of involved cases, and more than two calculi occur in approximately 5% of cases. With the advent of sialoendoscopy, the incidence of multiple stones has increased. This is partially due to the high incidence of radiolucent stones in both the parotid and submandibular ducts, as well as the ability to directly visualize stones, thus ensuring that no stone is left behind, something that occurred in up to 18% of traditional sialolithotomy procedures. Sialolithiasis may occur uncommonly in the parotid gland, sublingual glands, and minor salivary glands. Chronic stone formation may lead to ductal ulceration and strictures that may cause obstruction as a result of ductal stenosis.

The classic features of ABSS are pain and swelling in the submandibular region that occurs at mealtime (Figure 15-14); that is, flow is stimulated against a fixed obstruction. Patients may report a history of previous similar episodes. Associated cervical lymphadenopathy may be present. ABSS is a community-acquired disease that less frequently is associated with dehydration and hospitalization than ABP. Purulence may be

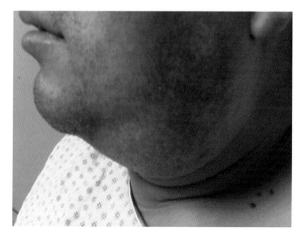

• **Figure 15-14** Acute bacterial submandibular sialadenitis of the left submandibular gland.

expressible from the orifice of the Wharton duct, but in many cases flow in completely obstructed. Any purulent material may be sent for Gram stain and culture and sensitivity studies, but any material collected intraorally is contaminated with resident oral flora. Therefore, the majority of cultures from Wharton duct demonstrate a mixed bacterial flora containing gram-positive cocci with *S. aureus* and *Peptostreptococcus* species most commonly isolated. In 56% of isolates, bacteria producing β-lactamase were present.[17] As a result, empiric antimicrobial therapy consists of choices similar to those for ABP depending on the severity of presentation. Choices include extended-spectrum penicillin with β-lactamase inhibition, a first-generation cephalosporin, clindamycin, or azithromycin. The diagnosis of ABSS as a result of sialolithiasis may be confirmed with mandibular occlusal radiograph (see Figure 15-1); however, only 80% of calculi are radiopaque, possibly less than 80% based on newer data available from sialoendoscopy demonstrating a 32% rate of occult radiolucent calculi in the submandibular gland. CT scanning may be useful in localization of a posterior stone in the proximal duct or at the hilum of the gland.

The treatment of ABSS consists of antibiotic therapy, maintenance of fluid intake, avoidance of antisialogogues, and removal of a sialolith, if present. Anterior calculi in the distal third of the duct may be removed in the office with the patient under local anesthesia. The procedure involves dilation of the ductal orifice with lacrimal probes, massage of the gland, milking of the duct from proximal to distal in an attempt to expel the stone. A suture ligature should be placed proximal to the suspected stone to prevent displacing the stone further proximally toward the gland hilum. If this method is unsuccessful, a sialolithotomy, or opening into the ductal system through the oral mucosa, is performed. Again, an attempt is made to gently deliver the stone though the surgically created opening. A sialodochoplasty, or ductal revision surgery, is also performed. This procedure involves suturing the edges of the duct to the oral mucosa in the area of the sialolithotomy. This approach provides several advantageous changes to the ductal anatomy in an attempt to prevent reoccurrence of the sialolithiasis. The sialodochoplasty effectively shortens the overall length of the Wharton duct and eliminates the narrow punctum and acute curvature at the orifice of the duct, so that flow can occur unimpeded though the new non-sphincteric opening. After a sialodochoplasty procedure, a stent may be inserted in the opening with a plastic catheter to ensure fistualization of the tract into the oral cavity. Patients are encouraged to use salivary stimulants such as lemon drops, glycerin swabs, and citrus fruits to encourage salivary flow postoperatively. An alternative to sialolithotomy and sialodochoplasty, sialoendoscopy, is a minimally invasive technique that can be used in the outpatient setting to examine the duct for abnormalities or polyps, remove stones and foreign material, dilate strictures, and irrigate the duct to remove any mucous plugs. It has a high success rate and should be considered a useful adjunct in the diagnosis and treatment of salivary gland disease.[4,5,7] In cases of posterior stones located in the middle or proximal

third of the Wharton duct (and in cases of recurrent ABSS), access through an intraoral approach may be technically difficult, and, in general, the submandibular gland and stone are removed through an extraoral approach with the patient under general anesthesia in the operating room. Although submandibular sialoadenectomy has several risks (extraoral scar; hypoglossal, marginal mandibular branch of facial and lingual nerve paresthesia; and facial and deep lingual artery vascular hazards), it results in far less morbidity than a parotidectomy.

Chronic Recurrent Bacterial Parotitis

Chronic recurrent bacterial parotitis (CRBP) is defined as repeat episodes of ABP that are separated by intervening periods of remission. This disorder usually is caused by an episode of ABP, but it may be idiopathic or result from Sjögren's syndrome, congenital ductal malformations, strictures, trauma (e.g., from orthodontic appliances), foreign bodies within the Stensen duct (including toothbrush bristles, popcorn kernels, grass, straw, and fish bones), or as an aftereffect of viral parotitis. Classically, two forms of CRBP have been described: an adult form and a juvenile form. The adult form has been more closely associated with infection from *S. aureus*, whereas *Streptococcus viridans* is the major pathogenic bacteria in the juvenile form, which usually occurs in children between the ages of 3 and 6 years. The juvenile form has a slight male predilection, is associated with unilateral parotid enlargement, and may resolve spontaneously at puberty with functional recovery of the parotid gland. If the condition persists beyond puberty, it is more common in females. CT scanning or MRI is useful to distinguish chronic infection from parotid tumors in children. Although gram-positive cocci have been implicated most frequently in this disease process, other species, including opportunistic organisms in the immunocompromised host have been identified in CRBP. Infection of the parotid gland may be subclinical at various times during the disease course, and therefore the gland may show evidence of latent infection during periods of clinical remission. CRBP may result in parenchymal destruction and loss of glandular function.

CRBP is characterized by unilateral or bilateral edema of the parotid gland that may last for days, weeks, or months with periods of exacerbation and remission. Constitutional symptoms may occur, and the white blood cell count and erythrocyte sedimentation rate may be elevated during times of exacerbation. Sialographic findings may include evidence of sialectasis with dilation of the ductal system and pooling of contrast media with the gland and ductal system, perhaps with cystic cavity formation.[33] Salivary scintigraphy with ^{99m}Tc pertechnetate may be used to assess the functional integrity of the gland and monitor for spontaneous functional recovery.

Treatment of CRBP is as controversial as the cause. One theory for its cause is based on bacterial infection, and therefore treatment includes species-specific systemic antibiotic therapy, guided by culture and sensitivity results when available. Any identified foreign bodies should be removed from the ductal system. Systemic antibiotics may be needed on an intermittent basis in the juvenile form of the disease until the patient reaches puberty. Similar to treatment of ABP, analgesics may be necessary, and avoidance of dehydration and the discontinuance of antisialagogic medications are recommended. Intraductal instillation of antibiotics may be useful during periods of remission; such treatment is begun between 1 and 2 weeks after resolution of an acute episode.[34] The procedure involves cannulation of the Stensen duct with a no. 50 polyethylene tube. Local anesthesia with 2% lidocaine may be used to anesthetize the periductal tissues. The irrigant solution may contain tetracycline or erythromycin. Generally, in adults approximately 3 to 4 mL of 15 mg/mL solution is used; in children 1.5 to 2.5 mL of 10 mg/mL solution is instilled into the ductal system. The solution is allowed to remain in the ductal system for between 5 and 10 minutes. This procedure may be repeated on a daily basis for 3 to 5 days.

A second theory for the cause of CRBP is based on inflammation resulting from ductal abnormalities, strictures, radiolucent stones, or mucous plugging. It has been noted in the literature that ductal irrigation with antibiotic solution when compared in randomized fashion to irrigation with normal saline has equivalent results in resolution of symptoms due to CRBP.[35] This would suggest that it is the irrigation and not the antibiotic that is producing the desired outcome. In addition, treatment with steroids to decrease inflammation combined with duct irrigation, sialography, or sialoendoscopy to remove precipitated material from the duct will improve patient symptoms without the need for antibiotics. The increasing use of sialoendoscopy has demonstrated that in these patients, up to 63% will have stones undetected by standard techniques of radiography, sialography, or ultrasonography. In addition, stricture and stenosis of the duct can be relieved with dilation and stenting techniques thereby making sialoendoscopy an ideal treatment approach for patients with CRBP.[5-7,35-38]

Historically, treatment was aimed at parotid gland destruction and atrophy using parotid duct ligation, glossopharyngeal nerve sacrifice, or low-dose radiation therapy to the gland. Current practice advocates parotidectomy with facial nerve preservation only in cases recalcitrant to other forms of nonsurgical therapy.

Chronic Recurrent Submandibular Sialadenitis

Chronic recurrent submandibular sialadenitis (CRSS) is associated with recurrent sialolithiasis and usually follows acute episodes of ABSS. CRSS occurs more commonly than CRBP. Sialography may be helpful in confirming the diagnosis by demonstrating evidence of sialadenitis and sialectasis, with decreased gland emptying rates indicative of poor gland function. Treatment of chronic recurrent submandibular sialadenitis consists of empiric antibiotic therapy, sialogogues, fluid replacement, and sialolithotomy, if indicated. Ultimately, for recurrent episodes or if the submandibular

gland is nonfunctional, sialoadenectomy is indicated. Interestingly, long-standing CRSS may produce a firm, tumor-like mass in the submandibular triangle, known as the Kuttner tumor.[39]

Actinomycosis

On rare occasions, *Actinomyces* (*A. israelii, A. naeslundii, A. propionicus, A. viscosus, A. odontolyticus, A. meyeri,* and *A. eriksonii*) may invade the salivary glands and cause infection. Involvement of the salivary glands, the parotid gland most frequently, may occur in up to 10% of cases of cervicofacial actinomycosis. This organism is a member of the resident oral flora and may lead to acute or chronic infection that may be difficult to distinguish from other forms of sialadenitis. Bacterial invasion of the salivary gland parenchyma may be odontogenic in organs or arise from inflammation of the tonsils. Diagnosis is based on Gram stain and biopsy culture, and sensitivity testing. *Actinomyces* are gram-positive, microaerophilic, non–acid-fast bacteria that grow slowly in culture and may demonstrate the classic "sulfur granules," which are aggregates of filamentous forms of the organisms. Culture material obtained from fistulous tracts may be contaminated and demonstrate a mixed bacterial flora. Sialography may show localized acinar destructive sialadenitis within the gland parenchyma. Treatment is the same as for cervicofacial actinomycosis, including incision and drainage if indicated, and long-term (4 to 6 months), high-dose penicillin therapy (other antibiotics have been used, including erythromycin and tetracycline). The avoidance of dehydration also is important in preventing the progression to chronic, irreversible sialadenitis.

Cat-Scratch Disease

First described in 1931, its etiology was not elucidated until 1983 when small gram-negative pleomorphic bacilli were detected with silver impregnation stains. Although the originally described organism, *Afipia felis* was later determined not to be the etiologic agent, further testing led to the discovery of the major etiologic agent, *Bartonella henselae.* Cat-scratch disease (CSD) is the most common cause of chronic lymphadenopathy among children and adolescents (80% of patients are under 21 years), often presenting with tender regional lymphadenopathy arising 2 weeks after the development of a distal inoculation site. This site, usually on the hands, arms, or chest is usually noted 3 to 10 days after the initial injury, with 65% of patients having a clinically visible inoculation site. Approximately 33 to 50% of patients will have fever, 33% have malaise/fatigue, most do not appear ill, and cervical lymphadenopathy ranging from 1 to 10 cm in size with overlying erythema is usually present.

Although CSD begins in the preauricular and cervical lymph node chains, it can subsequently involve the salivary glands, mostly the parotid, by contiguous spread.

Traditionally, the diagnosis of CSD was made based on four criteria: contact with a cat and a primary inoculation site, positive CSD skin test result (Rose-Hangar intradermal), negative for other causes of lymphadenopathy, and characteristic histologic features present on biopsy (silver impregnation stains positive for *Bartonella* organisms). More recently, the Rose-Hangar skin test (which was derived from human pus) has been replaced by an enzyme-linked immunoassay, as well as polymerase chain reaction (PCR) techniques because of concerns over transmission of other diseases and frequent false negative results early in the disease course. Tissue biopsy by a direct approach or fine-needle aspiration of involved nodes can be used for silver stains and PCR when necessary. Histologically, CSD demonstrates a highly characteristic pattern of stellate microabscesses surrounded by a rim of granulomatous inflammation. CSD is usually self-limiting with resolution of symptoms within 2 to 6 months, although analgesics and antipyretics are appropriate. Antibiotic administration is controversial with only a clear benefit in immunocompromised individuals. The most frequently used antibiotics are erythromycin, doxycycline, and rifampin, although gentamicin, trimethoprim-sulfamethoxazole, and quinolone use has been described. Fine-needle aspiration of necrotic debris and suppuration is preferred over open incision and drainage procedures to decrease the chance of fistula formation.[40,41]

Acute Allergic Sialadenitis/Radiologic Parotitis

On rare occasion, immunologic disorders may lead to involvement of the major salivary glands. This may occur after therapeutic radiation to distant organs, with an allergic response to circulating metabolites. Although food allergies are rare, allergies to heavy metals and medications occur more commonly (these include iodine, chloromycetin, terramycin, and thiouracil). This history generally is that of acute salivary gland enlargement, most commonly the parotid gland, and dyspnea after a contrast study such as an intravenous pyelogram. The course of this disease is usually self-limited.

Viral Salivary Gland Infections

Viral Sialadenitis/Epidemic Parotitis/Mumps

Viral mumps is an acute, nonsuppurative communicable infectious disease, primarily of the parotid gland tissue, that often occurs in epidemics during spring and winter months. Although the disease is usually considered a childhood disease occurring between 6 and 8 years of age, with an equal sex predilection, it can occur in any age group, including adults who may have avoided childhood illness. The disease usually is caused by a paramyxovirus, a ribonucleic acid virus related to the influenza and parainfluenza groups. A variety of other nonparamyxoviruses may cause parotid swelling similar to mumps, including coxsackie A and B viruses, Ebstein-Barr virus, influenza, and parainfluenza (type1 and 3) viruses, enteric cytopathic human orphanvirus (ECHO) virus, lymphocytic choriomeningitis virus,

and HIV. If initial testing for paramyxovirus is negative, serologic testing for these viruses should be considered.[42-44]

The virus is transmitted by infected saliva and urine. The viral incubation period between exposure and the development of signs and symptoms is 15 to 18 days. The disease includes a prodromal period that lasts 24 to 48 hours and includes fever, chills, headache, and preauricular tenderness. Infection is characterized by rapid, painful, nonerythematous unilateral or bilateral swelling of the parotid glands that may be severe enough to displace the earlobe. Purulent discharge from the Stensen duct is rare. Because influenza and other viruses may infect the parotid gland, viral serum titers for mumps virus should help to confirm the suspected diagnosis. Testing for IgG and IgM mumps virus antibodies can confirm infection or provide evidence of prior infection/immunization. Further testing by virus isolation in culture or detection of viral nucleic acid by PCR in throat, saliva, or urine specimens can be used. Laboratory evaluation generally is nonspecific, but may show leukopenia with a relative lymphocytosis. Serum amylase levels also may be elevated, irrespective of an associated pancreatitis, and peak during the first week of infection. This is in contrast to ABP, which does not cause an elevation of serum amylase levels.[42]

Attempts to eradicate the disease have resulted in routine administration of measles-mumps-rubella (MMR) vaccine in children at 12 months of age. The disease usually resolves spontaneously within 5 to 10 days; therefore, symptomatic treatment of pain and fever and the avoidance of dehydration are essential. Persistent or recurrent swelling may suggest the development of chronic bacterial sialadenitis of childhood.

Several untoward complications of viral mumps may result from generalized viremia. Mumps pancreatitis may manifest with abdominal pain and tenderness and elevated serum amylase levels. Diabetes mellitus is an uncommon complication of mumps pancreatitis. Orchitis, with testicular enlargement and tenderness, occurs in approximately 20% of adult men affected with mumps parotitis. Half of these individuals develop testicular atrophy, which, if bilateral, may lead to sterility. Priapism is an uncommon complication of mumps orchitis. Meningoencephalitis is an uncommon sequela of viral mumps, which may manifest as neck stiffness, lethargy, and headache. This disease generally is mild and self-limited but may lead to severe encephalitis. Other less common complications of viral mumps include mumps thyroiditis, mumps myocarditis, mumps nephritis, and mumps hepatitis.[42]

HIV-Associated Salivary Gland Infection

The head and neck manifestations of HIV occur in approximately 5 to 10% of HIV-positive patients. These clinical findings have been well described and include xerostomia; associated parotid intraglandular, and possibly cervical, lymphadenopathy; and painless parotid gland enlargement with or without cyst formation. Fine-needle aspiration samples positive for the presence of amylase in the cystic fluid can help to confirm the diagnosis. Immuno-fluorescence shows that this sicca-like syndrome is characterized by a diffuse lymphocytic infiltrate throughout the involved parotid gland acinar tissue, but without anti-Ro and anti-La autoantibodies, which are present in Sjögren's syndrome. The development of benign lymphoepithelial lesions (BLLs) in the parotid glands affected by the HIV virus may occur. The BLL-diffuse lymphocytic infiltration later may progress to acinar atrophy, ductal proliferation, and production of epimyoepithelial islands. The CD8 lymphocytic infiltration of the parotid parenchyma also may lead to lymphoepithelial cyst formation. In fact, in up to 5% of BLL lesions, malignant lymphomas may develop, most commonly non-Hodgkin's lymphoma, and up to 1% of all BLLs may progress to carcinoma. Therefore, BLL must be included in the differential diagnosis of parotid gland enlargement. The diagnosis may be aided with CT scanning, FNA, and MRI. Treatment of cystic lesions consists of observation, serial drainage, or sclerotherapy.[45,46]

Cytomegalovirus

Salivary gland inclusion disease may be caused by cytomegalovirus, a subgroup of herpes virus that produces latent disease. Most infections produce no symptoms except in the immunocompromised host (especially the terminal stages of HIV disease). Transmission may occur from blood or organ transplantation, and the salivary glands are frequently involved in this disease process. A mononucleosis-like syndrome occurs in the triad of fever, pharyngitis, and lymphadenopathy, but results of heterophile antibody testing for infectious mononucleosis are negative. No specific treatment is indicated, and cytomegalovirus is resistant to antiviral agents such as acyclovir, requiring treatment with IV ganciclovir or valganciclovir in the immunocompromised patient.

Mycobacterial Salivary Gland Infections

Tuberculosis

Primary involvement of the salivary glands with *Mycobacterium tuberculosis* is uncommon. Tuberculosis may manifest in two different forms: an infiltrative, disseminated form or a circumscribed, nodular form. The disseminated form is spread hematogenously, whereas the circumscribed form spreads through the lymphatics. The parotid gland and the preauricular lymph nodes usually are affected unilaterally, either in an acute of chronic form. Secondary involvement of the salivary glands with *M. tuberculosis,* associated with active pulmonary tuberculosis, most commonly affects the submandibular gland and cervical lymph node chain, resulting in a draining lesion known as scrofula (tuberculous cervical lymphadenitis) (Figure 15-15). Diagnosis is made with chest radiography, a positive blood Quantiferon TB Gold or positive findings from a purified protein derivative intradermal skin test, and identification of acid-fast bacilli in sputum. Treatment is similar to that for pulmonary

tuberculosis with long-term, multidrug therapy. Consultation with an infectious disease specialist should be made because these patients must be reported to the local health board and Centers for Disease Control and Prevention.

Atypical Mycobacterial Infections

Atypical mycobacteria may also affect the salivary gland, including both the submandibular and parotid glands. These infections are most common in the pediatric age groups and immunocompromised patients *(Mycobacterium avium).* Skin testing may aid in the diagnosis, and surgical excision is rarely indicated as an adjunct to antibacterial treatments.

Parasitic Salivary Gland Infections

Filariasis

Helminthic infestations with filariasis worms have been reported in salivary glands. Eight known filarial nematodes use humans as a definitive host. Filariasis is endemic in Africa and Central America. Definitive diagnosis is made by biopsy of the affected salivary gland nodule. Laboratory evaluation reveals eosinophilia. Treatment includes the use of antiparasitic drugs such as ivermectin, diethylcarbamazine, or albendazole, and excision of the salivary gland nodule.

Immunological Salivary Gland Disorders

Collagen Sialadenitis (Systemic Lupus Erythematosus)

The entire spectrum of collagen-vascular diseases may affect the salivary glands, including scleroderma, dermatomyositis, and polymyositis, but system lupus erythematosus is most common. This disease must be distinguished from Sjögren's syndrome. Collagen sialadenitis occurs most frequently in women in the fourth and fifth decades of life. The disorder may affect any of the major salivary glands and usually manifests as a slowly enlarging gland. The diagnosis is made by identification of the underlying systemic disorder, and sialochemistry studies may reveal sodium and chloride ion levels that are elevated two or three times normal values. Treatment involves addressing the causative systemic disease process.

Sarcoidosis

Sarcoidosis is a chronic, granulomatous disease characterized by noncaseating granulomas that may affect the salivary glands in up to 6% of cases. Heerfordt's syndrome, or uveoparotid fever, occurs in 10% of cases and consists of a triad of parotid enlargement, uveitis, and seventh cranial nerve palsy. The cause is unknown, and the disease is most common in the third and fourth decades of life and more common in black patients than white patients. The initial symptoms consist of prodromal constitutional symptoms of

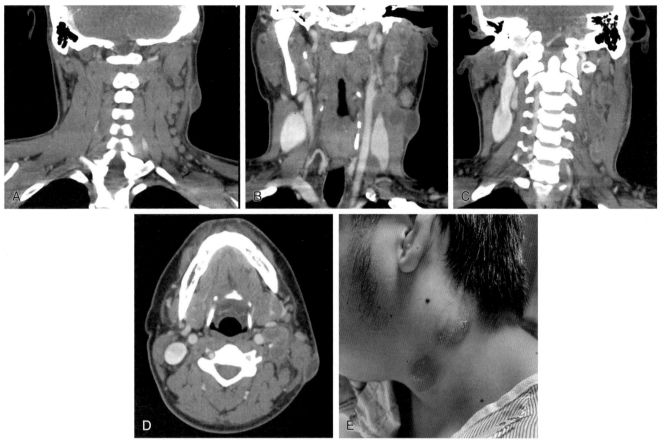

• **Figure 15-15 A,** Coronal CT scan demonstrating extensive left neck lymphadenopathy with superficial draining lesions (scrofula). **B,** Coronal CT showing internal jugular vein compression. **C,** Coronal CT and **(D)** axial CT showing carotid space involvement with *Mycobacterium bovis* infection. **E,** Clinical appearance of scrofula skin lesions.

fever, malaise, weakness, nausea, and night sweats that may last from weeks to months. Typical chest radiographic features include symmetric bilateral perihilar lymphadenopathy. Parotid enlargement usually is painless, firm, and bilateral, and the submandibular glands may be affected. The diagnosis can be confirmed with histopathologic evidence of lack of caseation and acid-fast bacilli to distinguish the disease from tuberculosis. Laboratory evaluation may reveal hypercalcemia, elevation of serum alkaline phosphatase, and serum angiotensin-converting enzyme concentration. The Kveim test involves intradermal injection of human sarcoid tissue antigen, but results are positive in only 75% of cases. Therapy consists of early administration of corticosteroids or methotrexate, particularly if uveitis (which can lead to glaucoma) and facial paralysis are present.

Granulomatosis With Polyangiitis

The initial presentation of granulomatosis with polyangiitis (Wegener's granulomatosis) can be extremely variable; however, because of the significant morbidity and mortality of this disease when left untreated, prompt diagnosis and treatment is essential. When parotid involvement is present, a unilateral, painful parotid gland mass may be noted.

Questioning for other findings associated with Wegener's granulomatosis such as rhinitis, strawberry gingivitis, hearing loss, and scleritis should be completed. Serologic testing for cytoplasmic antineutrophil cytoplasmic antibody (C-ANCA) and histopathologic examination of biopsy specimens confirm the diagnosis. Because Wegener's granulomatosis is a systemic inflammatory necrotizing vasculopathy, multiple organs can be affected with rapidly progressive glomerulonephritis and pulmonary hemorrhage the most serious complications. Treatment consists of immunosuppression with high-dose steroids, cyclophosphamide, and methotrexate. Before the development of diagnostic testing and effective treatments, the average survival was only 5 months with a 2-year mortality over 90%.[47]

References

1. Kawamata A, Ariji Y, Langlais RP. Three dimensional computer tomography imaging in children. *Dent Clin North Am*. 2000;44:395.
2. Yousem DM, Kraut MA, Chalian AA. Major salivary gland imaging. *Radiology*. 2000;216:19.
3. Marchal F, Becker M, Dulguerov P, et al. Interventional sialoendoscopy. *Laryngoscope*. 2000;110:318.

4. Nahlieli O, Baruchin AM. Endoscopic technique for the diagnosis and treatment of obstructive salivary gland disease. *J Oral Maxillofac Surg.* 1999;57:1394.

5. Ardekian L, Klein HH, Araydy S, Marchal F. The use of sialendoscopy for the treatment of multiple salivary gland stones. *J Oral Maxillofac Surg.* 2014;72(1):89-95.

6. Baurmash HD. Chronic recurrent parotitis: a closer look at its origin, diagnosis, and management. *J Oral Maxillofac Surg.* 2004;62(8):1010-1018.

7. Nahlieli O, Baruchin AM. Long-term experience with endoscopic diagnosis and treatment of salivary gland inflammatory diseases. *Laryngoscope.* 2000;110(6):988-993.

8. Hotel Dieu. Parotitis terminating in gangrene. *Lancet.* 1829; 2:540.

9. Brodie BC. Inflammation of the parotid gland and salivary fistulae. *Lancet.* 1834;1:450.

10. Cope VZ. Acute necrotic parotitis. *Br J Surg.* 1919;7:130.

11. Robinson JR. Surgical parotitis, a vanishing disease. *Surgery.* 1955;38(4):703-707.

12. Petersdorf RG, Forsyth BR, Bernanke D. Staphylococcal parotitis. *N Engl J Med.* 1958;259(26):1250-1254.

13. Krippaehne WW, Hunt TK, Dunphy JE. Acute suppurative parotitis: a study of 161 cases. *Ann Surg.* 1962;156:251-257.

14. Spratt JS. The etiology and therapy of acute pyonic parotitis. *Surg Gynecol Obstet.* 1961;112:391.

15. Rice D. Nonneoplastic diseases of the salivary glands. In: Bailey BJ, ed. *Head and Neck Surgery: Otolaryngology.* Philadelphia: Wolters Kluwer Health/Lippincott Williams & Wilkins; 2014.

16. Brook I. Aerobic and anaerobic microbiology of suppurative sialadenitis. *J Med Microbiol.* 2002;51(6):526-529.

17. Brook I. Anaerobic bacteria in upper respiratory tract and head and neck infections: microbiology and treatment. *Anaerobe.* 2012;18(2):214-220.

18. Brook I, Frazier EH, Thompson DH. Aerobic and anaerobic microbiology of acute suppurative parotitis. *Laryngoscope.* 1991;101(2):170-172.

19. Brook I, Finegold SM. Acute suppurative parotitis caused by anaerobic bacteria: report of two cases. *Pediatrics.* 1978;62(6): 1019-1020.

20. Marioni G, Rinaldi R, de Filippis C, Gaio E, Staffieri A. Candidal abscess of the parotid gland associated with facial nerve paralysis. *Acta Otolaryngol.* 2003;123(5):661-663.

21. Masters RG, Cormier R, Saginur R. Nosocomial gram-negative parotitis. *Can J Surg.* 1986;29(1):41-42.

22. Pruett TL, Simmons RL. Nosocomial gram-negative bacillary parotitis. *JAMA.* 1984;251(2):252-253.

23. Raad II, Sabbagh MF, Caranasos GJ. Acute bacterial sialadenitis: a study of 29 cases and review. *Rev Infect Dis.* 1990;12(4):591-601.

24. Carlson E, Ord R. Infections of the salivary glands. In: Carlson E, Ord R, eds. *Textbook and Color Atlas of Salivary Gland Pathology.* Ames, IA: Wiley-Blackwell; 2021.

25. Aly RL, Levit S. Adherence of *Staphylococcus aureus* to squamous epithelium: role of fibronectin and teichoic acid. *Rev Infect Dis.* 1987;9(suppl 4):S341-S350.

26. Simpson WA, Courtney HS, Beachey EH. *Fibronectin: A Modulator of the Oropharyngeal Bacterial Flora.* Microbiology 1982. Washington, DC: American Society for Microbiology; 1982:344.

27. Johanson WG, Pierce AK, Sanford JP. Changing pharyngeal bacterial flora of hospitalized patients: emergence of gram-negative bacilli. *N Engl J Med.* 1969;281(21):1137-1140.

28. Mandel L. Wind parotitis. *N Engl J Med.* 1973;289(20):1094-1095.

29. Graham SM, Hoffman HT, McCulloch TM, Funk GF. Intraoperative ultrasound-guided drainage of parotid abscess. *J Laryngol Otol.* 1998;112(11):1098-1100.

30. Yeow KM, Liao CT, Hao SP. US-guided needle aspiration and catheter drainage as an alternative to open surgical drainage for uniloculated neck abscesses. *J Vasc Interv Radiol.* 2001;12(5):589-594.

31. Yeow KM, Hao SP, Liao CT. US-guided percutaneous catheter drainage of parotid abscesses. *J Vasc Interv Radiol.* 2000;11(4):473-476.

32. Epivatianos A, Harrison JD, Dimitriou T. Ultrastructural and histochemical observations on microcalculi in chronic submandibular sialadenitis. *J Oral Pathol.* 1987;16(10):514-517.

33. Patey DH. Inflammation of the salivary glands with particular reference to chronic and recurrent parotitis. *Ann R Coll Surg Engl.* 1965;36:26-44.

34. Quinn JH, Graham R. Recurrent suppurative parotitis treated by intraductal antibiotics. *J Oral Surg.* 1973;31(1):36-39.

35. Antoniades D, Harrison JD, Papanayotou P, et al. Treatment of chronic sialadenitis by intraductal penicillin or saline. *J Oral Maxillofac Surg.* 2004;62:431.

36. Nahlieli O, Schacham R, Yoffe B, et al. Diagnosis and treatment of strictures and kinks in salivary gland ducts. *J Oral Maxillofac Surg.* 2001;57:484.

37. Plonowska KA, Ochoa E, Ryan WR, Chang JL. Sialendoscopy in chronic obstructive sialadenitis without sialolithiasis: a prospective cohort study. *Otolaryngol Head Neck Surg.* 2021;164(3):595-601.

38. Delagnes EA, Aubin-Pouliot A, Zheng M, Chang JL, Ryan WR. Sialadenitis without sialolithiasis: prospective outcomes after sialendoscopy-assisted salivary duct surgery. *Laryngoscope.* 2017;127(5): 1073-1079.

39. Yoshihara T, Kanda T, Yaku Y, Kaneko T. Chronic sialadenitis of the submandibular gland (so-called Küttner tumor). *Auris Nasus Larynx.* 1983;10(2):117-123.

40. English CK, Wear DJ, Margileth AM, Lissner CR, Walsh GP. Cat-scratch disease: isolation and culture of the bacterial agent. *JAMA.* 1988;259(9):1347-1352.

41. Lamps LW, Scott MA. Cat-scratch disease: historic, clinical, and pathologic perspectives. *Am J Clin Pathol.* 2004;121(suppl):S71-S80.

42. McQuone SJ. Acute viral and bacterial infections of the salivary glands. *Otolaryngol Clin North Am.* 1999;32(5):793-811.

43. Brill SJ, Gilfillan RF. Acute parotitis associated with influenza type A: a report of twelve cases. *N Engl J Med.* 1977;296(24): 1391-1392.

44. Buckley JM, Poche P, McIntosh K. Parotitis and parainfluenza 3 virus. *Am J Dis Child.* 1972;124(5):789.

45. Berg EE, Moore C. Office-based sclerotherapy for benign parotid lymphoepithelial cysts in the HIV-positive patient. *Laryngoscope.* 2009;119(5):868-870.

46. Frantz MC, Frank H, vonWeyhern C, et al. Unspecific parotitis can be the first indication of a developing Wegener's granulomatosis. *Eur Arch Otorhinolaryngol.* 2008;265(1):131-134.

47. Saha AK, Rachapalli S, Steer S, et al. Bilateral parotid gland involvement in Wegener's granulomatosis. *Ann Rheum Dis.* 2009; 68(7):1233-1234.

16

Odontogenic Infections of the Fascial Spaces

GABRIEL M. HAYEK, ELIE M. FERNEINI, AND MORTON GOLDBERG

Dental care largely consists of the treatment of dental infection or the restoration and replacement of dentition lost to bacterial infection. The prevention and treatment of orofacial infection involves every aspect of dental care: caries, pulpal disease, gingivoperiodontal conditions, pathology, trauma, and reconstructive and implant surgery. The surgeon routinely faces the realities of the potentially pathogenic flora of an odontogenic infection when surgical procedures are performed in or around the oral cavity. This chapter focuses on the cause, clinical manifestations, anatomic considerations, and treatment of odontogenic infections.

Dental infection has plagued humankind for as long as the species has existed. Little imagination is required to picture a primitive man suffering pain and swelling of the face because of fractured teeth, dental caries, or periodontal disease. Indeed, infection of dental origin is one of the most common diseases of humans and in underdeveloped countries is a frequent cause of death. The remains of Native Americans, unearthed in the American Midwest, and the remains of people who lived in early Egypt have revealed the bony crypts of dental abscesses and sinus tracts and the ravages of osteomyelitis of the jaws.

Treatment of localized infection was probably the first primitive surgical procedure performed, and it most likely involved the opening of bulging abscesses with sharp stones or pointed sticks. Today, the principle remains the same; fortunately, the techniques have improved. Not until the early twentieth century, however, was a causal relationship established between dental infection and the severe life-threatening neck swelling that Ludwig described nearly 70 years earlier.[1] Although therapy has progressed, the scalpel, extraction forceps, and the endodontic reamer remain the keystones of therapy for odontogenic infections, along with the judicious use of antibiotics.

Despite great advances in dental care in Western society, including fluoridation of water, early interception of caries, and periodontal prophylaxis, infection remains a major problem in dental practice. Although penicillin was considered the long-awaited panacea for dental infection, the bacteriologic spectrum of the oral flora and the understanding of its complexities have undergone rapid evolution since penicillin was introduced.

Before the antibiotic era, most serious odontogenic infections were known to be streptococcal, but the problem of bacterial resistance to antibiotics soon became obvious in the oral cavity, as elsewhere. The serious epidemic of penicillin-resistant staphylococcal infections of the 1950s and 1960s was finally resolved by the development of semisynthetic antibiotics, which are not metabolized by the penicillinase enzyme of the staphylococci. The widespread use of these drugs has resulted in the current plague of human infection from enteric (gram-negative) and opportunistic organisms, including vancomycin-resistant enterococci and methicillin-resistant staphylococci. Mutation and selective genetic pressure have resulted in bacterial species that exhibit resistance to multiple antibiotics, a situation complicated by deoxyribonucleic acid (DNA) exchange between species.

Nature abhors a vacuum, even a biologic one. The empty ecologic niche created by the decline of certain pathogenic bacterial species is soon filled by other organisms. The human oral cavity is a biologic system that supports life for as many as 400 species of microorganisms. Bacterial infection of dental origin is a constantly changing, but measurable, reflection of the modern evolution of the oral flora.[2-4]

During the past five decades, dangerous and life-threatening dental infections have been reported and are related to a variety of bacterial species, some opportunistic, others nosocomial, and a few anaerobic. These include *Escherichia coli* and *Pseudomonas, Proteus, Serratia, Acinetobacter (Mima), Klebsiella, Eikenella, Bacteroides (Prevotella),* and *Corynebacterium* and other less common organisms. For example, *Pseudomonas,* once thought to be a rare transient in the oral cavity, currently is found in the saliva of 5 to 10% of healthy persons. Similar changes have been observed in the pharyngeal flora that is probably related to an antibiotic-induced reduction of normal flora, acquisition of new flora during hospitalization, and use of immunosuppressive drugs. Aerobic gram-negative rods inhabit the pharynxes of 5% of normal nonhospitalized persons, but colonize the pharynxes of more than 60% of institutionalized older and hospitalized patients with serious illnesses, those who have undergone surgical procedures, and critical care health workers. Nevertheless, aerobic and anaerobic streptococci, *Bacteroides, Fusobacterium,* and *Eikenella,* and mixed aerobic-anaerobic flora are the organisms most commonly identified in odontogenic infections in otherwise healthy patients.[5] Quantitative estimations of the number of microorganisms in saliva and plaque range as high as 10^{11}/mL. In the depths of a periodontal pocket, the number of anaerobes per gram of curetted material may reach 1.8 times 10^{11}/mL, approximately the same concentration of anaerobes in human feces. Considering this plethora of microorganisms that grow luxuriantly in this wet, warm, dark, and debris-strewn cavity, the effectiveness of the systemic and oral host defense mechanisms in preventing serious infection from commonplace minor trauma, such as cheek biting or the shedding of deciduous teeth, is remarkable.

Recent investigational data gathered from molecular genetic methods, including gene sequencing from bacterial identification, suggests that there may be as many as 400 species of bacteria in the microflora of the human oropharynx.

Pathways of Dental Infection

The cause of, diagnosis of, and therapy for bacterial infection limited to the dental pulp or periodontal tissue are described elsewhere in the book.

The narrow pulpal foramen at the root apex, although of insufficient diameter to permit adequate drainage of infected pulp, does serve as a reservoir of bacteria and permits the egress of bacteria into periodontal tissue and bone. This access explains the occasional problem when antibiotics alone are used to treat draining fistulas from abscessed teeth. Once the drainage ceases, the bacteria harbored in the pulp chamber subsequently repopulate the periapical tissues from the untreated pulp, thus reinitiating the infection. Serious dental infection spreading beyond the socket is more commonly the result of pulpal infection than of periodontal infection. Once infection extends past the apex of the tooth, the pathophysiologic course of a given infectious process can vary, depending on the number and virulence of the organism, host resistance, and anatomy of the involved area (Figure 16-1).

If the infection remains localized at the root apex, a chronic periapical infection may develop. Frequently, sufficient destruction of bone develops to create a well-corticated radiolucency observable on dental radiographs. This process represents a focal bone infection, but "garden variety" radiolucencies associated with carious teeth should not be confused with true osteomyelitis.

Once infection extends beyond the root apex, it can proceed into deeper medullary spaces and evolve into widespread osteomyelitis. More commonly, this process forms fistulous tracts through the alveolar bone and enters into the surrounding soft tissue. This phenomenon often is associated with sudden soft tissue swelling and a reduction in

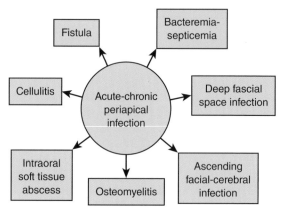

• **Figure 16-1** Pathways of Dental Infection.

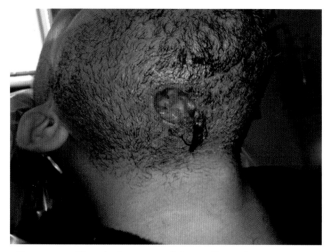

• **Figure 16-2** Chronic Cutaneous Submandibular Fistula of Dental Origin.

intrabony pressure, resulting in a lessening of pain. The fistula may penetrate the mucosa or skin and thus serve as a natural drain for the abscess (Figure 16-2). The puckered, ulcerated, and chronically indurated appearance of such dentocutaneous fistulae frequently leads the unwary or inexperienced examiner to diagnoses ranging from chancre to cancer. Unnecessary, time-consuming, and costly diagnostic procedures, including biopsy, can be avoided if dental radiographs and careful examinations are performed. Dental infection should be first on the list of possible diagnoses when facial swelling or a fistula is the initial sign.

Once beyond the confines of the dentoalveolar bone, infection can localize as an abscess or spread through soft tissue as cellulitis, or both. In common clinical usage, these terms are often confused or used interchangeably. An *abscess* is a thick-walled cavity containing pus, whereas *cellulitis* is a diffuse, erythematous submucosal or subcutaneous infection. Staphylococci are frequently associated with abscess formation. These microorganisms produce coagulase, an enzyme that can cause fibrin deposition in citrated or oxalated blood. Streptococci are associated more often with cellulitis because they produce enzymes such as streptokinase (fibrinolysin), hyaluronidase, and streptodornase. These enzymes break down fibrin and connective tissue ground substance and lyse cellular debris, thus facilitating the rapid spread of bacterial invaders. These organisms are not restricted to one type of reaction. Oral infections frequently are composed of mixed flora, or the bacteria can behave in any untraditional fashion. Thick-walled abscesses, with little or no blood supply to their lumen, respond slowly or poorly to antibiotic therapy, whereas cellulitis usually responds well without surgical drainage.

Erysipelas is a specific form of cellulitis (lymphangitis) caused by β-hemolytic streptococci. A discrete entry injury usually occurs on the face, violating this barrier to bacteria. Marked interstitial edema of the subcutaneous tissues occurs, but relatively little evidence of necrosis is present. Characteristically, the tissues have a sharply demarcated, brawny, edematous swelling that is intensely red because of vasodilation. The lesion often is associated with profound toxemia.

Treatment of Odontogenic Infections

Treatment of odontogenic infections can involve medical, surgical, or dental therapy or combinations thereof. Any infection of dental origin requires definitive treatment of the affected tooth if the source of the infection is to be eliminated. Once the tooth has been identified, endodontic elimination of the infected pulp, deep periodontal scaling, or extraction must be performed. The method of tooth treatment is a question of judgment, determined by factors such as the extent of the infection, the patient's general health status, the degree of trismus present, and the biomechanical necessity of retaining the tooth. The last factor must not sway the surgeon's judgment to the detriment of the patient's well-being. The clinician must avoid "tunnel vision" when diagnosing dental disease because it can have serious consequences if a major infection is present. Extraction of the involved tooth is the most rapid method of establishing drainage, while simultaneously removing the nidus of microorganisms within the pulp chamber and canals. Alternatively, endodontic therapy can be used to eliminate the source of infection.

Reliable evidence indicates that extractions of lower molar teeth in the presence of infection increases the incidence of alveolar osteitis. Therefore, antibiotic therapy should be used when a tooth is to be extracted during the acute stage of diffuse or deep infections, especially those involving the mandibular third molars.

Incision and Drainage

Incision and drainage rids the body of toxic purulent material and decompresses the tissues, allowing better perfusion of blood containing antibiotics and defensive elements and increases oxygenation of the infected area.

The abscess should be drained surgically at the same time that dental therapy is performed. Incision and drainage are the oldest and usually the simplest surgical procedures. Rapid, sharp incision through the oral mucosa adjacent to the alveolar bone usually is sufficient to produce "laudable pus"—an eighteenth-century phrase that is both descriptive and exclamatory. The surgeon who could produce instant relief and probably cure by the evacuation of pus from an abscess was also praiseworthy and, therefore, was more renowned than less skillful colleagues who incised prematurely or in the wrong place.

A thorough knowledge of facial and neck anatomy is necessary to properly drain a deep abscess, but an abscess confined to the dentoalveolar region presents no anatomic mysteries to the surgeon. Only the thin, bulging mucosa separates the scalpel from the infection. Ideally, abscesses should be drained when fluctuant before spontaneous rupture and drainage. Incision and drainage are best performed at the earliest sign of this ripening of the abscess, although surgical drainage also can be effective early, before the development of classic fluctuance.

The following principles should be used when possible with incision and drainage:

1. Incise in healthy skin and mucosa when possible. An incision placed at the site of maximum fluctuance where the tissues are necrotic or beginning to perforate can result in a puckered, unaesthetic scar.
2. Place the incision in an aesthetically acceptable area, such as under the shadow of the jaw or in a natural skinfold or crease.
3. When possible, place the incision in a dependent position to encourage drainage by gravity.
4. Dissect bluntly, with a closed surgical clamp or finger, through deeper tissues and explore all portions of the abscess cavity thoroughly so that compartmentalized areas of pus are disrupted and excavated. Extend the dissection to the roots of the teeth responsible for the infection.
5. Place a drain and stabilize it with sutures.
6. Consider the use of through-and-through drains in bilateral, submandibular space infections.
7. Do not leave drains in place for an overly extended period; remove them when drainage becomes minimal. The presence of the drain itself can produce some exudate and can be a portal for secondary bacterial invaders.[6]
8. Clean wound margins daily under sterile conditions to remove clots and debris. Note that there is no evidence that formally irrigating drains improves outcomes.[6]

Another approach to drainage of well-localized abscesses is the use of a computed tomographic (CT)-guided catheter. It is introduced percutaneously and guided into deep neck abscesses. CT-guided catheterization allows precise location of the lesion without extensive dissection and subsequent scarring. In select patients, it can be performed in a radiology suite. Specimens for Gram staining and culture are readily obtained, and the catheter can be left in place to serve as a drain.

The use of heat to "draw" an abscess to the surface has been discussed and debated extensively. The physiology of heat application to infection appears rational because the resulting dilation of small vessels intensifies host defenses through increased vascular flow and diffusion. However, the hope of converting an extraoral abscess into an intraoral one by the use of warm mouth rinses is not well-based; no scientific evidence exists that any application of heat will produce the desired effect.

Fenestration of the alveolar bone with a high-speed dental drill, although uncommon, occasionally can be used to relieve pain. Fenestration is best accomplished through the soft tissue drainage wound at the level of the tooth root apex. Medical therapy for localized dentoalveolar abscesses consists mainly of supportive care: hydration, a soft diet, analgesics, and good oral hygiene.

Antibiotic Therapy

The use of antibiotics in the treatment of a well-localized and easily drained dentoalveolar abscess is probably unnecessary because surgical drainage and dental therapy resolve the infection in most patients. Abscesses and cellulitis in patients who are immunocompromised and in those with systemic signs and symptoms, such as trismus or elevated temperature, usually indicate the need for antibiotics. Poorly localized, extensive abscesses and those associated with diffuse cellulitis require antibiotic therapy.

In patients with diminished host defenses, such as those with poorly controlled diabetes, patients who are immunosuppressed or immunoincompetent, those receiving renal dialysis, or seriously ill or hospitalized patients, supplemental antibiotics are required for a dentoalveolar infection because of the fear of sudden, overwhelming sepsis spreading from even a small focus. Fatal dental infection may be observed in immunosuppressed patients.[7-11]

Ideally, the choice of antibiotic for the therapy of odontogenic infection depends on the definitive laboratory results of culture and sensitivity testing. Because most dentoalveolar infections occur in otherwise healthy outpatients seen in offices and clinics, cultures are not routinely performed and usually are not needed. A pragmatically rational approach to empiric antibiotic selection is acceptable, both ethically and legally, if the choice is based on scientific data and contemporary experience with the microbiology of the flora of oral infection.

It is also important to note that a longer duration of antibiotics does not equate with better care.[12] A total course of 3 to 5 days often results in the same clinical outcome as courses of 7, 10, or even 14 days. Every day of antibiotics increases the risk for *Clostridioides difficile* infection and antibiotic resistance, and antibiotic courses longer than 5 days should be the exception, not the rule. There is growing evidence that antibiotics prescribed for pain and swelling should be discontinued 24 hours after the symptoms resolve. Antibiotics should not be prescribed if the only symptom is pain.

The constantly evolving flora of oral infection has been well documented. Numerous studies have revealed that the majority of infections in the immunocompetent patient consist of mixed aerobic and anaerobic flora. Most contain some anaerobes. The most frequently and consistently isolated organisms are aerobic streptococci (α-, β-, and γ-), anaerobic streptococci (*Peptostreptococcus*), *Bacteroides (Porphyromonas, Prevotella)*, *Fusobacterium,* and *Eikenella*. Less frequently, *Bacteroides fragilis,* the gram-negative anaerobic rod that normally inhabits the bowel and pelvis, is found. Skin organisms, such as *Staphylococcus aureus* and *Staphylococcus epidermidis,* currently are reported less frequently than in previous decades of the antibiotic era but have a high incidence in nonodontogenic facial infections in children. Aerobic *Corynebacterium* and anaerobic *Propionibacterium*, both gram-positive rods, are encountered occasionally.

Penicillin has been the antibiotic of empiric choice for dental infections for nearly five decades, with a proven record of efficacy. However, the microorganism population of any ecosystem can and does evolve in response to environmental selection or through mutatory influences, whether on the floor of a tropical rainforest or in the gingival sulcus of *Homo sapiens.* The population of some oral microspecies has demonstrated a profound and measurable change in susceptibility to penicillin, and β-lactamase–producing organisms such as *Bacteroides* now are frequently noted to be insensitive to penicillin, with some published series reporting 40% resistance. Even streptococci, which historically have been exquisitely sensitive to penicillin, are occasionally reported as penicillin-resistant. Several strains of clindamycin-resistant *Bacteroides* also have been observed.[13-15]

Facial surgeons should read and interpret these data with a critical eye. If some 40% of *Bacteroides* are reported to be resistant, 60% must be sensitive—a ratio that still has therapeutic validity in a mixed aerobic-anaerobic infection treated with penicillin or amoxicillin.

The humoral and cellular host defense mechanisms, if normal, are far more essential to the demise of invading organisms than the antibiotic disk applied in the laboratory. In addition, obtaining material (pus) for culture usually implies that surgical drainage (or aspiration) has been performed, a procedure that ranks equal in importance to the presence of normal defenses in the successful therapeutic outcome of dentoalveolar infection.

Most of these infections are a mixed flora of aerobes and anaerobes; therefore, the bacterial synergism that enhances the growth of these different types of organisms can be disrupted with penicillin. Whether the aerobic streptococci produce essential nutrients for the anaerobes, provide enzymes, clear metabolites, or reduce the oxygen tension in the tissue, their destruction by penicillin secondarily diminishes the growth and reproduction of the anaerobes.

Therefore, penicillin or amoxicillin remains the empiric antibiotic of choice in the treatment of most dentoalveolar infections in the noncompromised host. In fact, there is now evidence that penicillin is such an appropriate antibiotic of choice and that penicillin allergy alone is associated with increased risk of surgical site infection.[16] As stated succinctly and scientifically by Moenning, "It would seem presumptuous to state that penicillin is currently not effective against most odontogenic infections and premature to consider substituting another antibiotic as the drug of first choice for mild to moderate odontogenic infections (in non-compromised hosts), especially when cost and lack of toxicity are also considered."[17] That statement remains as valid in 2023 as it was in 1989. For more severe or recalcitrant infections seen in an outpatient environment, culture and antibiotic sensitivity studies may be necessary. Metronidazole is an effective supplement to penicillin and enhances the destruction of anaerobes.

Oral clindamycin has long been considered an excellent choice for both aerobic and anaerobic destruction. If a β-lactam antibiotic (e.g., penicillins, cephalosporins) has been used for 2 to 3 days without any resolution of odontogenic infection, the use of another β-lactam or β-lactamase–stable antibiotic (e.g., clindamycin) should be considered.[18] There has been some pushback on this largely related to evidence of increasing resistance to clindamycin. One study found a serious increase in clindamycin resistance (30%) to viridans streptococci and *Staphylococcus* species.[19] Furthermore, the 2021 American Heart Association/American Dental Association (AHA/ADA) and 2017 American Dental Association/American Academy of Orthopaedic Surgeons (ADA/AAOS) guidelines have removed clindamycin as recommendation for dental prophylaxis or therapeutic use because of black box warnings for *C. difficile*.[12,20,21] Azithromycin, doxycycline, and cephalexin have been inserted into the guidelines instead.

The paradox of antibiotic therapy often leads to clinical situations in which the solution to problem *A* creates problem *B*. Recent observations show that the use of antianaerobic antibiotics (clindamycin, metronidazole, amoxicillin-clavulanate) can create high-density colonization of the stools by vancomycin-resistant enterococci in patients who are already colonized by these organisms (i.e., patients in intensive care units), thus enhancing the infection's morbidity and mortality and placing other patients and intensive care unit personnel at greater risk of colonization.[22]

Erythromycin is poorly absorbed and less effective in odontogenic infection than penicillin or clindamycin, but other macrolides (azithromycin) are tolerated better than erythromycin, resulting in higher compliance rates.[23] Amoxicillin-clavulanic acid (Augmentin), a potent inhibitor of β-lactamases, is efficacious, but its cost and usefulness in severe infections should inhibit its use in routine odontogenic infections. First- and second-generation cephalosporins are also useful in odontogenic infections. Tetracycline is not recommended for severe anaerobic infection therapy, but its analogs, minocycline and doxycycline, can be useful in low-grade dentoalveolar infections.

For patients who are sufficiently ill to require hospitalization for an odontogenic infection and for compromised hosts (including patients with insulin-dependent diabetes, those with chronic alcoholism, intravenous drug abusers, recently hospitalized patients, and those receiving prophylactic antibiotics in the previous 4 weeks), ampicillin-sulbactam (Unasyn) can be used parenterally, as well as first- or second-generation cephalosporins. Amoxicillin-clavulanate (Augmentin) is an excellent oral drug for outpatient discharge.

Quinolones have limited activity against anaerobes, and it is difficult to justify their use for odontogenic infections.

Fourth-generation quinolones, although useful against anaerobes, have created serious hepatic toxicity in some patients. For the recalcitrant infection that does not respond rapidly to penicillin therapy and in the compromised host, aerobic and anaerobic culture and sensitivity studies are necessary to determine whether antibiotics other than penicillin are indicated.

The use and abuse of antibiotic therapy and the indications for therapy are discussed at length in Chapter 8. Antibiotics are indicated in combination with surgery both therapeutically and prophylactically in the following situations:
1. Acute cellulitis of dental origin
2. Acute pericoronitis with elevated temperature and trismus
3. Deep fascial space infections
4. Extensive, deep, or old (>6 hours) orofacial lacerations
5. Dental infection or oral-maxillofacial surgery in the compromised host
6. Prophylaxis for dental surgery for some patients with valvular cardiac disease or a prosthetic valve and also for some class II and all class III and IV operative wounds

The 2021 Surgical Society Infection Guidelines have significantly addended their recommendations for the use of antibiotics in craniomaxillofacial fractures:[24]
1. Nonoperative facial fractures should not be prescribed antibiotics (Level 2C)
2. Operative, nonmandibular facial fractures should not receive preoperative antibiotics more than 1 hour from incision time (Level 2C).
3. Operative mandibular fractures should not receive preoperative antibiotics more than 1 hour from incision time (Level 2C).
4. Operative, nonmandibular fractures should not receive postoperative antibiotics more than 24 hours after surgery (Level 1B).
5. Operative, mandibular fractures should not receive postoperative antibiotics more than 24 hours after surgery (Level 1B).
6. All operative facial trauma should receive perioperative prophylactic antibiotics within 1 hour of incision.

Whether treatment is medical (antibiotics), surgical (incision and drainage, extraction, or endodontics), or both, another important decision is whether hospitalization for the therapy is warranted or ambulatory (office) care is sufficient. Recent studies have revealed that odontogenic pain or infection may account for as much as 2% of adult and pediatric emergency department (ED) visits. Extrapolating, this may represent hundreds of thousands of ED visits annually, at the cost of considerable time and money for overburdened health care facilities.

One university hospital has reported averaging 40 hospital admissions annually for severe odontogenic infections. Other studies reveal that, when admitted, 14% of patients remain intubated for an average of 2.3 days, with an average stay in the intensive care unit lasting 3 days. Length of stay correlates with an increased number of involved fascial spaces. In patients with a length of stay greater than 5 days, 55% were related to preoperative or postoperative extraction infections of third molars. More than 70% of patients hospitalized for odontogenic deep space infections are uninsured, whereas 22% are covered by Medicare. Reported hospital billings ranged from $18,000 to $28,000, with one case as high as $611,000.[25]

The decision regarding whether to treat odontogenic infections in an ambulatory (office, clinic, ED) or inpatient environment is multifactorial and depends on well-recognized criteria, although educated and experienced surgical judgment remains a flexible influence. The criteria for admission with one or more deep space infections include:

1. Airway obstruction or an impending threat to airway patency based on clinical examination, including dyspnea, dysphagia, tongue displacement, uvular deviation, and severe trismus (CT scan confirmation of a narrowed airway is obligatory for planning therapy, including anesthesia. Inability to swallow oral antibiotics may tilt the judgmental balance toward admission.)
2. Severe dehydration or electrolyte imbalance
3. Comorbid medical issues (i.e., loss of glycemic control)
4. Core temperature greater than 101°F
5. Elevated white cell count
6. Necrotizing fasciitis
7. Descending mediastinitis or ascending orbital-cerebral infection
8. Altered or obtruded state of consciousness
9. Social or psychiatric issues (e.g., homelessness, psychosis) or the potential for noncompliance with outpatient therapy

See Appendix I for an illustrative case report.

Anatomic Considerations in Dentoalveolar Infections

Localization of a dentoalveolar abscess is related to the anatomic position of the dental root from which it originated, especially in relation to muscle attachments, particularly the buccinator and mylohyoid muscles (Figure 16-3). Although a diffuse infection can cause some diagnostic consternation, the appearance of an acute dental abscess or fistula distant from its site of origin is rare. Familiarity with dental root anatomy is helpful in the occasional case in which an abscess develops in a less common position. Infection usually follows the path of least resistance; the data presented in Table 16-1 represent clinical experience and anatomic realities. For example, any acute swelling or fistulous formation of the posterior hard palate should prompt an investigation of the palatal roots of the adjacent maxillary molar.

Infection of mandibular incisors and canines usually appears as a bulging erythematous mass deep in the labial sulcus. These infections are obvious to the surgeon and are accessible to drainage by a scalpel. Ideally, the incision should be carried to the bone, but deep sharp dissection at the lower canine-premolar region should be avoided because of the presence of the sensory (mental) nerve to the lip. If the infection spreads from bone deep to the origin of the mentalis muscle, the submental space becomes involved. A lingual site for infection of the mandibular anterior teeth is less common and is usually caused by periodontal sepsis rather than periapical sepsis. A routine gingival incision usually is adequate for drainage on the lingual surface, unless the sublingual space is involved.

The mandibular premolars generally demonstrate buccal infection. Incision into the buccal vestibule is indicated, but again discretion must be used because of the presence of the

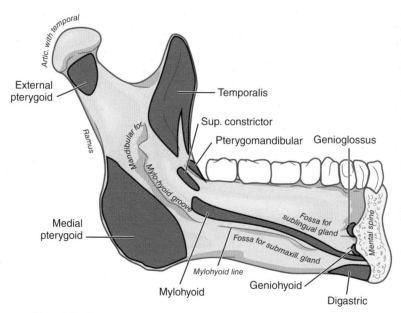

• **Figure 16-3** Lingual Surface of the Mandible Showing the Relationship of the Mylohyoid Muscle Attachment to the Apices of the Teeth. This is an important factor in determining whether a sublingual or a submandibular abscess will form.

TABLE 16-1	Localization of Dental Abscesses	
Teeth	**Common Abscess Site**	**Less Common Site**
Mandibular incisors	Labial	Lingual
Mandibular canines	Labial	Lingual
Mandibular premolars	Buccal	Lingual
Mandibular molars	Buccal	Lingual
Maxillary incisors	Labial	Palatal
Maxillary canines	Labial	Palatal
Maxillary first premolars	Labial (buccal roots) Palatal (palatal roots)	— —
Maxillary second premolars	Buccal	Palatal
Maxillary molars	Buccal (buccal roots) Palatal (palatal roots)	— —

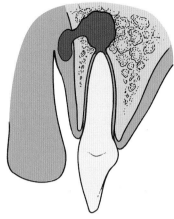

• **Figure 16-5** Schematic Illustration of Maxillary Incisor Periapical Infection with Labial Surface Dentoalveolar Abscess Formation. (From Hupp JR, Ellis E, Tucker MR. *Contemporary Oral and Maxillofacial Surgery*. 6th ed. St Louis: Mosby; 2014.)

mental nerve and its foramen. If the infection extends inferior to the buccinator muscles laterally or inferior to the mylohyoid muscle lingually, deep infections of the buccal space and submandibular space can occur.

Infection of mandibular third molars frequently is periodontal (pericoronitis), but can be related to the root apices if caries has invaded the pulp of an erupted or partially erupted tooth. The pathways of infection from mandibular third molars may involve the buccal vestibule, buccal fascial space, masticator space, and pharyngeal space.

The manifestation of infections of the upper teeth also depends on the anatomic location of their root apices (Figures 16-4 and 16-5). Maxillary incisor and canine roots lie closer to the thin labial plate of bone than to the thicker palatal bone, and infections therefore usually are observed as

bulging submucosal (vestibular) abscesses or fistulae in the labial sulcus. The muscles of the upper lip, arising from the alveolar bone, are thin and have little influence on the spread of infection. Generalized cellulitis of the upper lip or midface can occur, but penetration of infection into the floor of the nose is rare. Drainage is accomplished easily by a sharp incision into the labial sulcus. When palatal migration of infection does occur from an anterior tooth, it may vary in appearance from minimal swelling to massive bulging of the anterior palate (Figure 16-6). Incision of the palatal mucosa provides adequate drainage. The palatal vessels can be avoided by making the incision parallel to the vessels.

A maxillary premolar and molar infection may extend buccally or palatally because multiple roots are usually present. Infection from maxillary premolars usually extends into the connective tissue of the buccal vestibule and can spread superiorly, causing cellulitis to the level of the eyelids. This situation is best resolved by incising high in the buccal vestibule, which usually is the area of dependent fluctuance. The attachment of the buccinator muscle usually is well

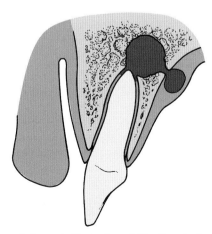

• **Figure 16-4** Schematic Illustration of Maxillary Incisor Periapical Infection with Palatal Surface Dentoalveolar Abscess Formation. (From Hupp JR, Ellis E, Tucker MR. *Contemporary Oral and Maxillofacial Surgery*. 6th ed. St Louis: Mosby; 2014.)

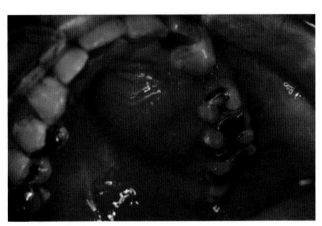

• **Figure 16-6** Palatal Dentoalveolar Abscess Originating from a Premolar (Root) Infection. (From Topazian RG, Goldberg MH, Hupp JR. *Oral and Maxillofacial Infection*. 4th ed. Philadelphia: Saunders; 2002.)

above the root apex of maxillary premolars, but penetration into the buccal space can occur.

A maxillary molar infection may exit from the alveolar bone buccally, palatally, or posteriorly. The buccal vestibule is the most common site for the appearance of abscesses, but invasion of the buccal space occurs commonly. Molar infection of the palatal region is surprisingly uncommon, considering the length of most molar palatal roots. Superior spread of pus into the maxillary sinus also is uncommon. Posterior spread of infection can involve the masticator and pharyngeal spaces, and superior extension into the infratemporal space also can occur.

In all odontogenic infections, examination usually reveals the presence of deep caries, periodontal inflammation, or impacted or fractured teeth as the cause. Bone fractures or gingival trauma should not be overlooked in the search for the causative factors of abscesses or cellulitis. Careful examination of the oral cavity, radiographs, and a high index of suspicion for all restored teeth help localize the origin of the infection. An easily overlooked cause of facial infection is the eruption of the maxillary third molar in an extreme buccal or posterior position, thereby causing erosion of the buccal mucosa, cellulitis, deep space infection, and severe trismus. Because of the difficulties of performing an adequate examination of the posterior oral cavity in such circumstances and the inadequacies of radiographs, frequently only the suspicious, experienced, and persistent examiner is successful in discovering the cause of the infection.

Fascial Space Infection

When a dental infection spreads deeply into soft tissue rather than exiting superficially through oral or cutaneous routes, fascial spaces can be affected (Box 16-1). Following the path of least resistance through connective tissue and along fascial planes, the infection can spread distantly from its dental source, causing considerable morbidity and occasionally death. A thorough knowledge of the anatomy of the face and neck is necessary to predict the pathways of spread of these infections accurately and to drain these deep spaces adequately.

The spread of infection through deep fascial spaces is determined by the presence and patterns of loose connective tissue. Fasciae develop in planes of connective tissue subjected to muscular movement and contraction. Surrounding or separating muscles, the fasciae and fascial planes offer an anatomically defined highway for infection to spread from superficial to deep parts of the face and neck. A description of deep fascial spaces essentially is an anatomic discussion of the various fasciae that surround or separate the anatomic boundaries of a given space. The concept of fascial "spaces" is based on the anatomist's knowledge that all spaces exist only potentially until fasciae are separated by pus, blood, drains, or a surgeon's finger.

Infections of fascial spaces are discussed here primarily in terms of their odontogenic origins. Teeth are the most common cause of these infections, and therapy is incomplete without definitive dental treatment. However, deep fascial space infections of the neck also can occur as a result of pharyngeal and tonsillar infections, trauma, reconstructive surgery, cancer surgery, and sialadenitis of major salivary glands.

Each fascial space infection described in this chapter is a clinical entity; case reports appearing in Appendix I illustrate the unique characteristic of each situation. In the treatment of infections of fascial spaces, including surgical treatment, the principles discussed earlier always should be considered. The following points also are germane:

1. Diffusion of antibiotics into close fascial spaces is limited because of poor vascularity. Penetration of antibiotics through thick-walled abscesses is minimal. "Average" doses may be inadequate.
2. Therapy of fascial space infections depends on adequate, open, and dependent drainage.
3. Large surgical incisions may be necessary to obtain adequate exposure of deep compartments.
4. Fascial spaces are contiguous, and infection spreads readily from one space to another. Multiple incisions may be necessary because frequently more than one space is involved in the infection.
5. Primary and secondary spaces must be drained.
6. The anatomy of the face or neck may be severely distorted by the swelling of the infectious process.
7. Repeated surgical drainage may be necessary.
8. The fascial spaces most commonly involved in odontogenic infections are the submandibular and buccal spaces. Less common are the parapharyngeal spaces and the temporal compartment of the masticator space.

Although observation and palpation can elicit the presence of superficial dentoalveolar and fascial space infections (i.e., buccal, canine, submental spaces), the presence of deep infections always must be a suspicion. The presence of

---

•BOX 16-1   Fascial Spaces of Clinical Significance

Face
- Buccal
- Canine
- Masticator
  - Masseteric compartment
  - Pterygoid compartment
  - Zygomaticotemporal compartment

Suprahyoid
- Sublingual
- Submandibular
  - Submaxillary
  - Submental
- Lateral pharyngeal
- Peritonsillar

Infrahyoid
- Anterovisceral (pretracheal)

Space of total neck
- Retropharyngeal
- Danger space
- Space of carotid sheath

dysphagia, dyspnea, prolonged white blood cell and temperature elevation, and unresolved trismus suggests the need for repeat imaging (CT, MRI) of deep spaces, because the presence of, or even surgical drainage of, a superficial infection may obscure a concomitant or secondary deep space involvement.

Canine Space

Canine space infections, although not rare, are less common than one might expect. Infections of the maxillary canine teeth usually appear as labial sulcus swelling and less commonly as palatal swelling (Figure 16-7). However, the levator muscle of the upper lip overlies the apex of the canine root. The origin of the muscle is high in the canine fossa of the maxillary wall, whereas its insertion is the angle of the mouth, intermingling with the fibers of the orbicularis oris and zygomatic muscles.

If the canine infection perforates the lateral cortex of the maxillary bone superior to the origin of the muscle, the potential canine space is affected. Whether this represents a true fascial space or simply a muscular compartment is debatable, but an abscess of this space requires surgical intervention. Canine space infections can cause marked cellulitis of the eyelids. Drainage is accomplished best through an intraoral approach, high in the maxillary labial vestibule by sharp and blunt dissection. This approach is an extension of that used for fenestration or apicoectomy of the canine root apex. Percutaneous drainage may be performed lateral to the nose, but this procedure does not afford dependent drainage and results in a visible scar.

See Appendix I for an illustrative case.

Cavernous Sinus Thrombosis

Although ascending infection (venous sinus thrombosis) is not a fascial space infection, it can be of odontogenic origin. Cavernous sinus infection, ascending from the maxillary teeth, upper lip, nose, or orbit through the valveless anterior and posterior facial veins, carries an extremely high mortality rate. Any patient with initial signs of proptosis, fever, obtunded state of consciousness, ophthalmoplegia, or paresis of the oculomotor, trochlear, and abducens nerves, especially after maxillary infections and exodontia, should have an emergency neurosurgical consultation (see Chapter 11).[26]

Buccal Space

Mandibular and maxillary premolar and molar teeth tend to drain in a lateral and buccal direction. The relation of the root apices to the origins of the buccinator muscle (the outer surfaces of the alveolar process of the maxilla and mandible) determines whether infection exits intraorally in the buccal vestibule or extends deeply into the buccal space. Molar infections exiting superiorly to the maxillary origin of the muscle or inferiorly to the mandibular origin of the muscle enter the buccal space.

The buccal space contains the buccal fat pad, the Stensen (parotid) duct, and the facial (external maxillary) artery. Infection of this space is diagnosed easily because of marked cheek swelling associated with a diseased molar or premolar tooth. When fluctuance occurs, strong consideration should be given to percutaneous drainage. Attempts to direct fluctuance intraorally by warm rinses are futile, and intraoral drainage through the mucosa, submucosa, and buccinator muscle may be difficult.

Cutaneous drainage should be performed inferior to the point of fluctuance with blunt dissection into the depth and extreme boundaries of the space. The purulent contents can expand the space to a surprising volume (Figures 16-8 and 16-9). The branches of the facial nerve should be avoided. The usual incision and drainage site is quite inferior to the Stensen duct. Aspiration of this space is performed easily.

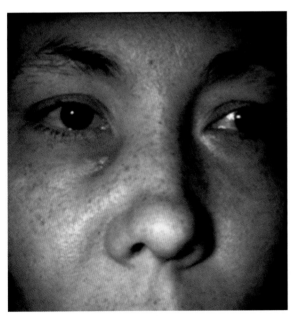

• **Figure 16-7** Chronic Fistula High in the Canine Space from a Periapical Infection of the Maxillary Canine Tooth. (From Topazian RG, Goldberg MH, Hupp JR. *Oral and Maxillofacial Infection*. 4th ed. Philadelphia: Saunders; 2002.)

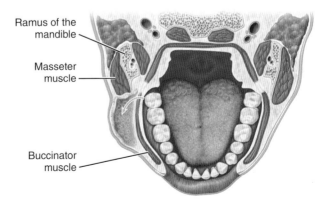

Ramus of the mandible

Masseter muscle

Buccinator muscle

• **Figure 16-8** Buccal Space Abscess Anatomy. (From Hargreaves KM, Cohen S. *Cohen's Pathways of the Pulp.* 10th ed. St Louis: Mosby; 2011.)

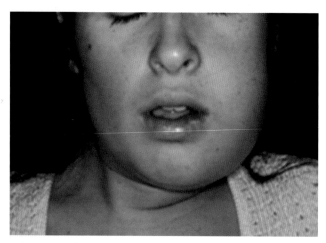

• **Figure 16-9** Buccal Space Infection. Notice the massive swelling and erythema.

Of special interest, and far from uncommon, is nonodontogenic buccal space infection or buccal cellulitis caused by *Haemophilus influenzae*. This infection, usually seen in infants or children younger than 3 years, is characterized by high fever for at least 24 hours before the appearance of clinical signs. The rapid onset of dark red swelling can be easily confused with an odontogenic infection or erysipelas. Otitis media frequently is also present or has occurred recently. Now commonly resistant to ampicillin, *H. influenzae* infection may respond well to amoxicillin-clavulanate (Augmentin) or a cephalosporin such as cefaclor. This process can occur in older children (Figure 16-10).

Recurrent buccal space abscesses can occur as a complication of Crohn's disease. This segmental transmural intestinal disease, whose clinical course includes intermittent abdomi-

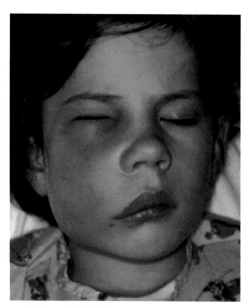

• **Figure 16-10** Buccal Cellulitis Caused by *Haemophilus Influenzae After Recent Otitis Media.* (From Topazian RG, Goldberg MH, Hupp JR. *Oral and Maxillofacial Infection.* 4th ed. Philadelphia: Saunders; 2002.)

nal pain, fever, weight loss, and diarrhea, is characterized by inflammatory granulomas, which can occur throughout the entire length of the gastrointestinal tract, from the mouth to the anus. Granulomatous lesions and ulcerations of the buccal mucosa can progress to true buccal space abscesses. A high recurrence rate of the granulomas or new abscess formation is possible despite antibiotic, corticosteroid, or surgical therapy.

See Appendix I for an illustrative case.

Masticator Spaces

The masticator spaces *(masseteric, pterygoid,* and *temporal)* are well differentiated, but communicate with each other and with the buccal, submandibular, and parapharyngeal spaces. Infection may be confined to any one of these compartments or may spread rather readily to any or all the other compartments.

Of the muscles of mastication, only the outer surface of the masseter and the inner surface of the medial (internal) pterygoid are covered by true fascia. Sicher[27] states that the temporal fascia is actually the suspensory bracing of the zygomatic arch rather than a muscle sheath. Although little space exists between the fibers of the masseter and temporalis muscles, considerable space is present between the temporalis muscle and the pterygoid muscles. The fatty connective tissue in this space extends anteriorly to the border of the buccinator muscle at the pterygomandibular raphe.

The masticator space as a unit is bound by fascia. It contains the muscles of mastication, the internal maxillary artery, and the mandibular nerve. If subdivided, the boundaries of the masseteric compartment are the masseter muscle laterally and the mandibular ascending ramus medially, whereas the pterygomandibular compartment is bounded medially by the pterygoid muscles and laterally by the mandible. Both compartments communicate freely with the superficial and deep temporal pouches superiorly, the buccal space anteriorly, and the lateral pharyngeal spaces posteriorly. Extension of infection into parotid and submandibular spaces can also occur.

Infection of the masticator space occurs most frequently from molar teeth, and infections of the third molars (wisdom teeth) are implicated most commonly as the cause. Pericoronitis of the gingival flap of third molars or caries-induced dental abscesses usually can be found in cases of masticator space infection. Infections of this space also have been reported as a result of contaminated mandibular block anesthetic injections, or infection may spread to this space from nearby contiguous spaces. Infection of the masticator space also can result from direct trauma to or through the muscles of mastication or surgery in the area (e.g., after temporal cranial flaps are made for neurosurgery or after orthognathic surgery).

Infratemporal space infections also can occur as a result of temporomandibular joint surgery or arthroscopy. The postulated mechanism is contamination from the external auditory canal flora (streptococci, staphylococci, *Haemophilus, Proteus,* and *Pseudomonas* organisms).

Clinically the hallmark of masticator space infection is trismus, the sine qua non of masticator space infection. If trismus is not present, these spaces are uninvolved with the infectious process. An exception would be an infection in a patient who is immunosuppressed, who might not exhibit the classic signs of inflammation or the unique signs of deep space infection.

Swelling may not be a prominent sign of a masticator space infection, especially in the masseteric compartment. In this area, the infectious process exists deep to large muscle masses that obscure or prevent much observable swelling. This process distinctly contrasts with infections of the buccal space, in which swelling is the cardinal sign of infection.

Surgical access to the various compartments of the masticator space is complicated by the containment of the infectious process by the muscle masses. Although drainage of the entire masticator space from the intraoral space is possible and occasionally practical, access from an extraoral incision is easier technically and more prudent. Some suggest an approach to all compartments through an incision along the pterygomandibular raphe. This incision is technically possible in a cadaver, but is less feasible in an infected patient with trismus and makes dependent drainage difficult. The masseteric and pterygoid compartments can be entered by superficial sharp and deep blunt dissection at the external angle of the mandible, avoiding the mandibular branch of the facial nerve. This approach allows dependent drainage of both spaces at the insertion of the muscle sling on the inferior border at the mandibular angle. Adequate local anesthesia can be accomplished at the mandibular angle (Figures 16-11 and 16-12).

The temporal spaces, although accessible through Sicher's intraoral incision, also can be drained percutaneously through an incision slightly superior to the zygomatic arch. The incision should be made parallel to the zygomatic arch and therefore parallel to the zygomatic branch of the facial nerve rather than perpendicular to it.

See Appendix I for an illustrative case.

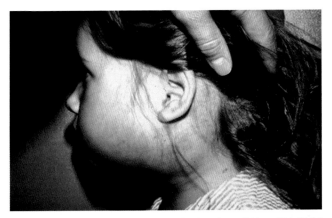

• **Figure 16-11** Masticator Space Infection in a 5-Year-Old Child Caused by an Infection from a Deciduous Mandibular Molar. (From Topazian RG, Goldberg MH, Hupp JR. *Oral and Maxillofacial Infection.* 4th ed. Philadelphia: Saunders; 2002.)

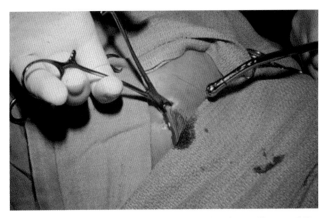

• **Figure 16-12** Incision and Drainage of a Masticator Space of the Child in Figure 16-11. Purulent flow occurred after blunt penetration of the masseteric compartment. (From Topazian RG, Goldberg MH, Hupp JR. *Oral and Maxillofacial Infection.* 4th ed. Philadelphia: Saunders; 2002.)

Submandibular and Sublingual Spaces

The submandibular (submaxillary) and sublingual spaces, although distinct anatomically, should be considered as a surgical unit because of their proximity and frequent dual involvement in odontogenic infection. Some confusion in nomenclature exists because some anatomists describe these spaces as compartments of the "submandibular space."

The mylohyoid muscle, which forms the floor of the oral cavity, is the key to the diagnosis and surgical management of these space infections. Separating the sublingual space above from the submandibular space below is the mylohyoid muscle, which attaches to the lingual surface of the mandible in an obliquely downward line from posterior to anterior. Thus, the root apices of the premolar and first molar teeth usually are superior to this attachment. As a result, lingual perforations of infections from these teeth penetrate the more superior (sublingual) compartment (see Figure 16-3). Only loose connective tissue rather than true fascia separates one side of the floor of the mouth from the other, an anatomic situation that permits infection to spread bilaterally with ease.

Anteriorly, the sublingual space communicates with the submental space. In this area, the sublingual space can be invaded by infection from incisor teeth, especially from periodontal infection. Posteriorly, the sublingual space communicates with the lateral pharyngeal spaces, in the neighborhood of the posterior edge of the mylohyoid muscle and the lesser wings of the hyoid bone.

Infection of the sublingual space appears clinically as brawny, erythematous, tender swelling of the floor of the mouth, beginning close to the mandible and spreading toward the midline or beyond. Some elevation of the tongue may be noted in late cases (Figure 16-13). Infection must be differentiated from the cellulitis that might accompany an impacted sialolith in the Wharton duct.

Surgical drainage of the sublingual space should be performed intraorally by an incision through the mucosa

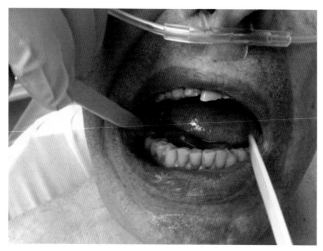

• **Figure 16-13** Clinical Appearance of a Sublingual Space Infection with Elevation of the Tongue by Indurated Sublingual Tissue.

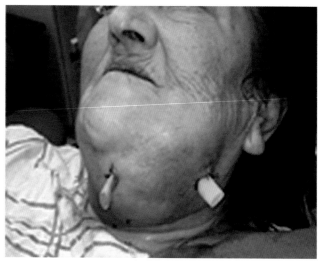

• **Figure 16-15** Clinical Appearance of a Submandibular Infection.

parallel to the Wharton duct bilaterally. If the submandibular space is to be drained, both spaces can be reached through a submandibular approach.

The submandibular space is separated from the overlying sublingual space by the fibers of the mylohyoid muscle. Odontogenic infections of this space are commonly caused by the second and third molar teeth (and, rarely, the first molar), because their root apices lie inferior to the mylohyoid line of muscle attachment. The space is bounded laterally by the submandibular skin, superficial fascia, platysma muscle, superficial layer of deep cervical fascia, and the lower border of the mandible. The contents of the submandibular space include the submandibular salivary gland and its lymph nodes, the facial (external maxillary) artery, the proximal portion of the Wharton duct, and the lingual and hypoglossal nerves as they course deep to the submandibular gland on the inferior surface of the mylohyoid muscle (Figures 16-14 and 16-15).

Diagnosis of submandibular space infection is made by finding the typical swelling of the space, either brawny or soft, and correlating it with the presence of a diseased mandibular molar. Infection can be related to sepsis in an

adjoining space, such as the sublingual, the submental, or the masticator space. Conversely, infection can spread from the submandibular space into any contiguous space, including the pharyngeal spaces. The infectious process commonly spreads across the midline into the contralateral submandibular space. If the spread is bilateral and involves all submandibular and sublingual spaces and the submental space, the result is the well-known Ludwig's angina.

Differential diagnoses should include acute sialadenitis, sublingual trauma or foreign body, and submandibular lymphadenitis; these can produce a secondary overlying cellulitis that further confuses the diagnosis.

Therapy for submandibular space odontogenic infection includes surgical drainage, antibiotics, and definitive care of the primary dental infection. An incision is performed through the skin below and parallel to the mandible. Blunt dissection is carried to the depths of the space and its anterior and posterior margins. Deep abscess loculations should be entered with a small closed clamp, probing in all directions while attempting to avoid damage to the submandibular gland, the facial artery, and the lingual nerve. The contralateral space should not be entered unless it is involved in the infection; if necessary, however, drains can be placed into both sides, as in the treatment of Ludwig's angina.

See Appendix I for an illustrative case.

Submental Space

A potential fascial space exists in the chin and occasionally becomes infected, either directly from a mandibular incisor or indirectly from the submandibular space. The submental space is located below the chin and is bound above by the skin and the chin (mentalis) muscles, laterally by the anterior bellies of the digastric muscles, deeply by the mylohyoid muscle, and superiorly by the deep cervical fascia, the platysma muscle, the superficial fascia, and the skin. Submental infection can spread easily to either or both submandibular spaces.

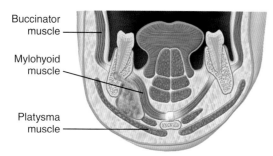

Buccinator muscle

Mylohyoid muscle

Platysma muscle

• **Figure 16-14** Schematic Drawing of a Submandibular Space Infection Originating from a Mandibular Molar Tooth. Surgical drainage is accomplished through skin and platysma muscle. (From Hargreaves KM, Cohen S. *Cohen's Pathways of the Pulp*. 10th ed. St Louis: Mosby; 2011.)

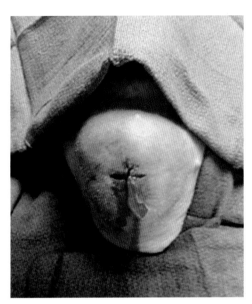

• **Figure 16-16** Submental space infection after an incision and drainage.

If infection from the incisors exits labially through the mandibular bone, inferior to the muscle attachments, the submental space becomes involved. The chin appears grossly swollen and is firm and erythematous (Figure 16-16). Percutaneous surgical drainage is the most effective approach. A horizontal incision in the most inferior portion of the chin, in a natural skin crease, provides dependent drainage and the most cosmetically acceptable scar. The space can be drained orally through the mentalis muscle through the labial vestibule, but dependent drainage cannot be established from this approach.

See Appendix I for an illustrative case.

Infections Associated With Impacted Third Molar Teeth

Lower third molars are a frequent cause of infection, even in otherwise healthy patients. In Western society, in which contemporary dental care and the widespread use of fluoridated drinking water have resulted in a remarkable decrease in dental caries and prevention of early loss of first and second molar teeth, a high rate of impacted third molars has resulted. Impaction is often associated with pericoronal infection (Figure 16-17). Bacteriologically the profuse colonization under the moist, poorly oxygenated pericoronal flap consists of the usual mixed aerobic-anaerobic flora, but can result in tissue destruction and pain to a level similar to that of acute necrotizing ulcerative gingivitis.[28] The use of antibiotics is recommended for third molar pericoronitis if body temperature is elevated or if trismus or adenopathy is present. Initially, gentle mechanical irrigation and debridement can be useful, as are incision and drainage, with extraction of the maxillary third molar (or cuspal reduction) if it is in occlusion with the edematous mandibular flap. Lower extraction usually is delayed until the trismus has resolved sufficiently to permit surgical access.

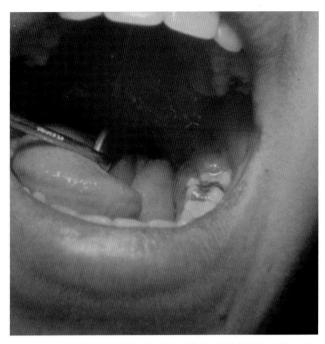

• **Figure 16-17** Pericoronitis of a Mandibular Third Molar. Note the swelling extending to the lingual surface of the mandible.

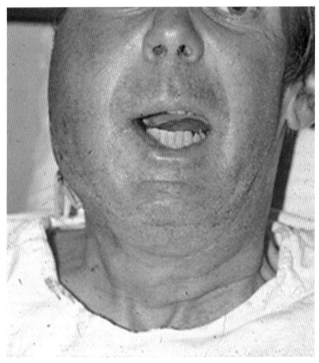

• **Figure 16-18** Pan-Space Infection from a Third Molar, Including Buccal, Parotid, Masticator, Submandibular, and Sublingual Spaces. (From Topazian RG, Goldberg MH, Hupp JR. *Oral and Maxillofacial Infection.* 4th ed. Philadelphia; Saunders: 2002.)

Pericoronitis occasionally spreads rapidly because of the anatomic location of the mandibular third molar at the crossroads of the masticator, submandibular, and buccal fascial spaces with adjacent anatomic access to contiguous parapharyngeal, parotid, submandibular, and other spaces (Figure 16-18).[29] Unfortunately, the same potentially serious sequelae exist as postextraction complications, which is an important issue in the risk-to-benefit ratio and medicolegal areas of surgery.

The role of prophylactic antibiotics in third molar surgery is controversial. If pericoronitis is present at the time of surgery or has been present recently, antibiotic therapy is indicated. However, removal of the truly asymptomatic and completely impacted third molar fits the category of clean-contaminated rather than contaminated surgery, and data exist to support the efficacy of nonuse of prophylactic antibiotics. If the mandibular marrow space has been widely exposed, especially during a lengthy extraction, "prophylactic" postoperative antibiotics would seem prudent. However, for true prophylaxis, the antibiotic ideally should be administered preoperatively.[30] The use of antibiotics after third molar extraction has not altered the infection rate. Advocates and dissenters continue the ongoing clinical debate.

Penicillin (or amoxicillin) remains the antibiotic of choice, administered as 2 g of amoxicillin orally (PO) 1 hour before the procedure, with no further doses given. Alternatively, 2 g of penicillin G can be given intravenously (IV) as a single dose. In patients who are allergic to penicillin, azithromycin, 500 mg PO or IV as a single dose, is suggested.

The overall third molar postoperative infection rate ranges from 4.2 to 6.3% with or without antibiotics, but most studies are subject to challenge because they fail to differentiate which patients have a history of pericoronitis and whether the extraction sites are profusely irrigated.[31]

Ludwig's Angina

Ludwig's angina is a firm, acute, toxic cellulitis of the submandibular and sublingual spaces bilaterally and of the submental space. As early as 1796, extraction of abscessed teeth was considered contraindicated because "it might give rise to extensive inflammation and angina, in a dangerous degree." Three Fs became evident even before the first written description of the disease: it was to be *feared*, it rarely became *fluctuant,* and it often was *fatal*. A sensation of choking and suffocation (angina) often was combined with the name of the author (Ludwig) who fully described it in 1836.[1]

The original description of the disease has not been improved since the observations of Wilhelm Friedrich von Ludwig were published while he was court physician to the King of Wurttemberg and president of that kingdom's medical association. His descriptive phrases ring true today, despite considerable improvements in therapy and mortality:

"Amidst the symptoms which herald the approach—an erysepalous angina, temperature swings . . . discomfort upon swallowing, there develops on one or both sides of the neck a firm connective tissue with which it comes in contact . . . it extends uniformly about the periphery of the neck . . . to a marked degree. It advances in similar fashion to involve the tissues which cover the small muscles between the larynx and the floor of the mouth . . . the tongue rests upon a red, indurated mass which feels like a hard ring adjacent to the inner surface of the jaw bone. It becomes difficult and painful to open the mouth . . . speech is impaired and hoarse . . . this is because the tongue is pressed backward and upwards, there is pressure upon the larynx . . . as the disease progresses . . . externally certain areas become, at times, softer . . . at other times more prominent and apparently fluctuant. Fever increases with morning exacerbations . . . swallowing continues to be difficult and the patient opens the mouth only with effort; dyspnea appears usually in paroxysms . . . and on the tenth to twelfth day of the disease, death occurs, with the patient in a comatose state with evidence of respiratory paralysis . . . there are nuances in the typical picture of the disease . . . particularly the onset and severity of the local lesion. . . . Among the cases in which autopsy was permitted . . . there were found abscess cavities whose walls were made up of gangrenous partly decomposed masses of muscle . . . the periosteum of the inner surface of the jaw was loosened from the bone and was discolored."

Ludwig refrained from suggesting a "scientifically valid" hypothesis of the cause of the disease, but stated that "it differentiates itself from other neck inflammations with symptomatic or idiopathic swelling of the salivary glands."[32] As therapy, he recommended local and general bloodletting, softening poultices, and external and internal use of mercurials, vesicants, cathartics, and diuretics. He described the case of Fraulein N.N., who suffered both the disease and the therapy, including leeches, bran poultices, tartar emetic, dry heat, a gargle of althea and honey, almond oil, ipecac, and finally, "a piece of silver nitrate the size of a six Krenzer coin over the middle of the swelling . . . which had created a splendid necrosis." Because of or despite the therapy (chemical incision and drainage), N.N. survived, and "three weeks after the onset, when the last traces of the induration could still be felt, the patient felt well and strong."

Almost 60 years passed before the causative relationship between dental disease and Ludwig's angina was established. Carious rotten teeth were ubiquitous in Ludwig's era, whereas his eponymous angina was comparatively uncommon; hence, he never recognized the association. Considering that the germ theory of disease had yet to be postulated, antibiotics were undiscovered, anesthesia did not exist, and contemporary surgeons were reluctant to incise without the certainty of finding "laudable pus," N.N. was indeed fortunate to have survived. Curiously, Ludwig did not survive a throat inflammation, and he died in 1865 at the age of 75.

Today, Ludwig's angina is a disease primarily of dental origin. Dental infection has been reported as the causative factor in 90% of cases in some series, either as primary dental infection or as a postextraction phenomenon. As was stated in 1943, "The dentist who is unfortunate enough to have performed extraction on a patient who subsequently develops Ludwig's angina is more likely to have been incidental to the train of events than to have been the responsible agent."[33]

Other causative factors include submandibular gland sialadenitis, compound mandibular fracture, oral soft tissue lacerations, puncture wounds of the oral floor, and secondary infections of oral malignancies. Ludwig's angina infection has been reported in a newborn. The term *pseudo-Ludwig's angina* has been applied to these cases of nondental origin; they also are referred to as *pseudo-Ludwig's phenomena*.

Fortunately, the incidence of Ludwig's angina remains low in this modern era of preventive dental care and antibiotic therapy. In the preantibiotic era, a mortality rate greater than 50% was reported, but this was reduced to approximately 5% with the use of penicillin. Most early cases probably are aborted by the use of antibiotics before the rapid, deep spread of infection occurs. Representing less than 1% of all admissions to oral-maxillofacial services, Ludwig's angina is observed most frequently in the contemporary compromised host. If the disease is untreated, the mortality rate is close to 100%. A true Ludwig's angina is an obligatory hospital admission.

Bilateral infection of the sublingual and submandibular spaces, as well as the submental space, with brawny edema, an elevated tongue, airway obstruction, and a paucity of pus are the clinical hallmarks of Ludwig's angina. Sepsis can spread rapidly to involve the masticator and pharyngeal spaces.

A veritable host of organisms have been implicated as the causative agents of this disease. Because Ludwig's angina is commonly of dental origin, streptococci or mixed oral flora are the most commonly reported organisms from cultures of whatever exudate can be obtained after surgical drainage. Contemporary reports of Ludwig's angina have demonstrated the presence of staphylococci, gram-negative enteric organisms such as *E. coli* and *Pseudomonas*, and anaerobes, including *Bacteroides* and *Peptostreptococcus* species. The isolation of these organisms may indicate the changing oral flora of the antibiotic era or reflect more sophisticated modern culture techniques. *Prevotella melaninogenica*, *Prevotella oralis*, and *Prevotella corrodens* also have been isolated from patients with Ludwig's angina or other odontogenic infections. Experimental data from studies of cutaneous infections similar to the ulcer of Meleney suggest that a synergistic or obligatory synergistic relationship may exist among anaerobes such as *Prevotella (P. melaninogenica)*, anaerobic streptococci, and fusospirochetes, all common organisms. Mixtures of oral organisms that did not include *Prevotella* could not create transmissible subcutaneous infections in experimental animals, whereas infection was produced by the addition of that organism. Whatever the role of anaerobes, primary or synergistic, a search for them should not be omitted when culturing specimens from Ludwig's angina or other serious odontogenic infections (see Geisler et al.[34] and Chow et al.[35]).

Treatment of Ludwig's angina includes early diagnosis of the incipient cases, maintenance of a patent airway, intense and prolonged antibiotic therapy, extraction of the affected teeth, hydration, and early surgical drainage (with life in the balance, a quick extraction is more rational than time-consuming tooth salvage). Empiric antibiotic therapy (intravenous) for Ludwig's angina should be intense; choices include penicillin plus metronidazole or imipenem used as single agents. Although black box warnings exist, there are growing numbers of surgeons who think moxifloxacin is an excellent choice in penicillin-allergic patients for severe odontogenic infections. It is a broad-spectrum, fourth-generation synthetic fluoroquinolone effective against *Eikenella, Bacteroides, Prevotella,* and most other strains of bacteria that produce β-lactamase.[14,36] It has been reported to have the highest rates of bacterial susceptibility, including penicillin; however, it remains quite expensive and must be used with caution in children. A combination of levofloxacin and metronidazole can achieve similar results, albeit with similar concerns and neither levofloxacin/metronidazole nor moxifloxacin should be considered first-line therapy.

The establishment and maintenance of an adequate airway are the sine qua non of therapy. Death is more likely to occur early from airway obstruction than from sepsis. Tracheostomy has been almost routine during most of the twentieth century, but it may prove difficult to perform in the late stage of the disease because of massive neck edema and tissue distortion. Attempts at blind endotracheal intubation can be time-consuming, unsuccessful, and fraught with danger, especially if attempted by an inexperienced anesthesiologist, because of the swollen elevated tongue and glottic edema. The danger of rupturing a bulging lateral pharyngeal or retropharyngeal abscess exists if the infection involves these fascial spaces. Cervical soft tissue plain radiographs and CT scanning should be done before attempted tracheostomy, if time permits. Fiberoptic laryngoscopy is useful in the airway management of Ludwig's angina but requires an anesthesiologist skilled in its use, and the patient must be cooperative and premedicated. Tracheal intubation with the patient under deep inhalation anesthesia may be successful, usually obviating the need for tracheostomy. The use of sedative and opioid agents, which can cause more rapid respiratory deterioration, is not recommended (see Chapter 31).

Although some authorities advocate high doses of antibiotics without surgery until fluctuance develops, in most surgeons' experience, fully developed Ludwig's angina requires prompt and deep surgical incision because fluctuance is uncommon and late. Ludwig's angina is a diffuse cellulitis of deep fascia. Seventy percent of cases still require surgical intervention and drainage. The submandibular and sublingual spaces and secondarily involved spaces must be explored bilaterally. The masticator spaces must be drained if trismus is present. The prudent and experienced surgeon recognizes the wisdom of the maxim "a chance to cut is a chance to cure" when confronted with Ludwig's angina.

A horizontal incision midway between the chin and the hyoid bone was the classic approach to the surgical drainage of Ludwig's angina, but this "cut-throat" incision has proved unnecessary and unaesthetic. Bilateral incision into the submandibular spaces with blunt dissection to the midline suffices if bilateral drains meeting in the midline are placed. This maneuver, combined with drainage of the sublingual spaces, relieves the intense pressure of edematous tissue on

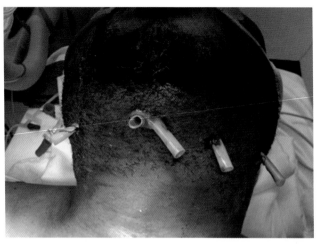

• **Figure 16-19** Surgical Therapy for Ludwig's Angina. The procedure involves incisions and placement of drains bilaterally into the submandibular spaces, meeting in the midline and draining the submental space.

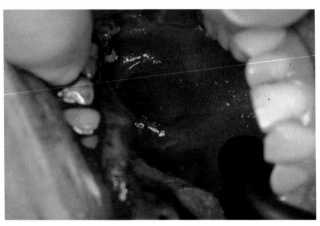

• **Figure 16-20** Lateral Pharyngeal Space Abscess Occurring Late After a Third Molar Extraction. Note the bulging of the lateral pharyngeal wall, soft palate, and tonsillar area with displacement of the uvula. (From Topazian RG, Goldberg MH, Hupp JR. *Oral and Maxillofacial Infection*. 4th ed. Philadelphia: Saunders; 2002.)

the airway and provides specimens for Gram staining and culture (Figure 16-19).

The platysma muscle and suprahyoid fasciae are incised by this approach, and the fascia of the submandibular gland is also entered. The mylohyoid muscle should be divided and the sublingual spaces entered. A closed clamp should be inserted through the median raphe of the mylohyoid muscle and advanced to the hyoid bone at the base of the tongue. Generally, little pus is obtained because the infection often represents cellulitis of the fascial spaces rather than true abscess formation. In some cases, especially late or fully developed ones, purulent flow is produced.

Needle aspiration of deep fascial space infections has been attempted, sometimes obviating open drainage procedures. However, Ludwig's angina, basically a rapidly spreading, deep cellulitis without localization of pus or formation of fluctuance is not amenable to this technique, even if the needle is CT guided.

Sequelae after adequate drainage and antibiotic therapy are uncommon. However, inadequate drainage or premature closure of the surgical wounds can lead to reinfection. Late spread to other fascial spaces or generalized sepsis can occur and are ever-present dangers. Failure to extract the offending tooth could cause reinfection. Secondary revision of scarring may be necessary for cosmetic reasons or to repair stenosis of the Wharton duct.

The mortality rate for Ludwig's angina has decreased since the advent of prompt surgical intervention, airway maintenance techniques, and antibiotic therapy. However, three fatal cases are discussed in Appendix I to illustrate the potential or actual lethality of this disease.

Lateral Pharyngeal Space Infection

The lateral pharyngeal space (pharyngomaxillary space) is a lateral neck space shaped like an inverted cone, with its base at the skull and its apex at the hyoid bone. Its medial wall is contiguous with the carotid sheath, and it lies deep to the pharyngeal constrictor muscle. It is divided, for surgical and anatomic purposes, into anterior and posterior compartments.

Infections of the lateral pharyngeal space can result from pharyngitis, tonsillitis, parotitis, otitis, mastoiditis, and dental infection, especially if the masticator spaces are primarily infected. Herpetic gingivostomatitis involving pericoronal tissue also has been reported as a cause of the lateral pharyngeal abscess. If the anterior compartment becomes infected, the patient exhibits pain, fever, chills, medial bulging of the lateral pharyngeal wall with deviation of the palatal uvula from the midline, dysphagia, swelling below the angle of the mandible, and usually trismus (Figure 16-20). Infection of the posterior compartment is noted for the absence of trismus and visible swelling, but respiratory obstruction, septic thrombosis of the internal jugular vein, and carotid artery hemorrhage can occur in patients at a late stage of infection. CT and MRI may prove useful in diagnosing lateral pharyngeal infections and may reveal confluence with other deep space infections and septic erosion of the wall of the great vessels.

Therapy consists of antibiotics, surgical drainage, and tracheostomy if indicated. The surgical approach may be oral, by incision of the lateral pharyngeal wall, or external, by exposure of the carotid sheath near the lateral tip of the hyoid bone after retraction of the sternocleidomastoid muscle. Blunt dissection along the posterior border of the digastric muscle leads to the lateral pharyngeal space. In the combined intraoral and extraoral approach, a mucosal incision is made lateral to the pterygomandibular raphe, and a large curved clamp is passed medial to the medial pterygoid muscle in a posterior-inferior direction. The tip of the clamp is delivered through the skin by a cutaneous incision between the angle of the mandible and the sternocleidomastoid muscle. A submandibular incision is also usually sufficient for drainage of a standard lateral pharyngeal abscess, particularly in cases simultaneously involving the submandibular space.

See Appendix I for an illustrative case.

Retropharyngeal Space

The esophagus and trachea are enclosed by the middle layer of the deep cervical fascia. A thick strand of connective tissue extends laterally from the esophagus to the carotid sheath, thus creating an anterior neck compartment known as the *pretracheal* (previsceral) space and a posterior or *retropharyngeal* (retrovisceral) space. The posterior space lies behind the esophagus and pharynx and extends inferiorly to the upper mediastinum and superiorly to the base of the skull.

Clinically, retropharyngeal space infections can result most commonly from nasal and pharyngeal infections in children (tonsillitis), dental infection diffusing through contiguous spaces, esophageal trauma or foreign bodies, and tuberculosis. Infection can also reach this space through the lymphatics to involve the retropharyngeal lymph nodes. Dysphagia, dyspnea, nuchal rigidity, esophageal regurgitation, and fever characterize infections of the retropharyngeal space. If the pharynx can be visualized, a bulging of the posterior wall may be observed and is usually more prominent unilaterally because of the adherence of the median raphe of the prevertebral fascia. Lateral soft tissue radiographs of the neck are extremely useful and may reveal considerable widening of the retropharyngeal space, well beyond the 3- to 6-mm width in normal adults at the second vertebra (or >14 mm in children; Figure 16-21). In adults, the ratio of the space width to the vertebra is 6 mm at C2 and 20 mm

at C6. The presence of gas in the prevertebral soft tissues and the loss of the normal lordotic curvature of the cervical spine also may be observed on plain radiographs and CT scans. CT scans reveal the presence of the infection in the retropharyngeal space and its inferior extent.

Although some reports indicate that 10 to 40% of retropharyngeal infections resolve with only medical management, these cases reflect early diagnosis and antibiotic therapy. Infection of the retropharyngeal space usually requires prompt surgical drainage and allows little time for delay, debate, or decision by committee. Because many anesthesiologists are reluctant to risk aspiration or airway obstruction by pus pouring from the ruptured space during passage of an endotracheal tube, tracheostomy may be indicated. However, drainage has been performed transorally with the patient under local anesthesia in the extreme Trendelenburg position and with constant suctioning. In the transoral technique, an incision is made through the midline of the posterior pharyngeal mucosa, and the abscess is opened by blunt dissection.

An external approach generally provides more dependent drainage. An incision is made along the anterior border of the sternocleidomastoid muscle and parallel to it, inferior to the hyoid bone. This muscle and the carotid sheath are retracted laterally, and blunt finger dissection is carried deeply, avoiding the hypoglossal nerve, to the level of the hypopharynx. Blunt finger dissection deep to the inferior constrictor muscles opens the retropharyngeal space abscess. Deep drains are placed and maintained until all clinical and laboratory signs of infection are no longer apparent. Needle aspiration with CT scan guidance has avoided open surgical drainage in a few cases. The overall mortality rate for retropharyngeal infections of all causes is approximately 10%.

See Appendix I for an illustrative case.

Mediastinitis

Extension of infection from deep neck spaces into the mediastinum is heralded by chest pain and severe dyspnea, unremitting fever, and radiographic demonstration of mediastinal widening. Rarely, mediastinitis can be caused by an odontogenic infection that spreads directly along the great vessels in the perivascular space of the carotid sheath (Figure 16-22). Intravenous drug abusers who inject into the major blood vessels of the neck are at risk for deep neck infections, including the carotid space, and may have septic thrombosis of the jugular veins.

The spread of an odontogenic infection to the mediastinum also is noteworthy because it is preceded by infection of other fascial spaces that may have been drained adequately. Therefore, mediastinitis may be a late complication and should be suspected in patients with exacerbation of fever associated with substernal pain. Progressive septicemia, mediastinal abscesses, pleural effusion, empyema, compression of mediastinal veins with decreased venous return to the heart, and pericarditis can occur, with death as the final outcome.

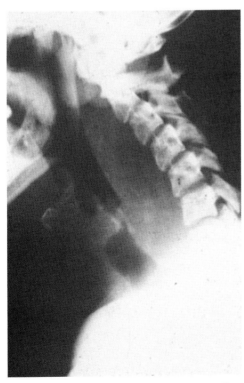

• **Figure 16-21** Retropharyngeal Space Abscess After Extraction of a Mandibular Third Molar. Note the massive soft tissue swelling with tracheal displacement. (From Topazian RG, Goldberg MH, Hupp JR. *Oral and Maxillofacial Infection.* 4th ed. Philadelphia: Saunders; 2002. Courtesy John F. DuPont, Jr.)

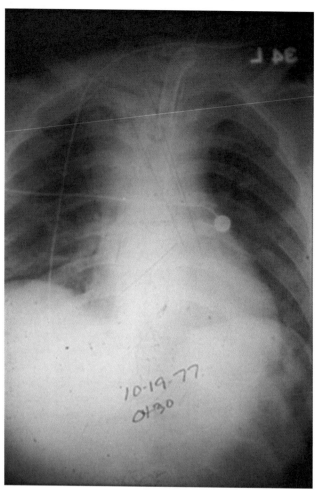

• **Figure 16-22** Mediastinitis Caused by a Retropharyngeal Space Infection. (From Topazian RG, Goldberg MH, Hupp JR. *Oral and Maxillofacial Infection*. 4th ed. Philadelphia: Saunders; 2002.)

Necrotizing mediastinitis of dental origin may be related to the synergistic effect of aerobic and anaerobic bacteria invading susceptible tissue far from their normal oral environment.[37-40] Passively commensal in the mouth, the bacteria can become synergistically aggressive and invasive elsewhere.

Treatment of suppurative mediastinitis consists of extensive, long-term antibiotic therapy and surgical drainage of the mediastinum. Specimens for culture should be obtained regularly during long-term therapy.

See Appendix I for an illustrative case.

Summary

The incidence and severity of odontogenic infections have diminished since the advent of antibiotic therapy. However, significant morbidity and mortality of these infections continue. Dentists and physicians constantly must be alert to the potential seriousness of these infections, which should never be dismissed as simple dental abscesses. Odontogenic infection therapy is based on the severity and anatomic location of the infection, the patient's general health status,

his or her response to therapy, and the assumed or laboratory-determined pathogenic microflora of the infection. Small superficial odontogenic infections differ greatly from deep space infections despite their common origins.

Deep space infections must be recognized promptly and treated as an emergency. Underlying medical problems must be controlled, a patent airway established, contemporary diagnostic imaging performed, and deep drainage performed. Repeated diagnostic and therapeutic measures may be necessary until the endpoint (absence of clinical, radiographic, and laboratory signs of infection) has been reached.

References

1. Ludwig WF. Medicinishe correspondenz. *Blatt de Wurtembergischen Arztlichen Vercins.* 1836;6:26.
2. Seppänen L, Rautemaa R, Lindqvist C, Lauhio A. Changing clinical features of odontogenic maxillofacial infections. *Clin Oral Investig.* 2010;14(4):459-465.
3. Storoe W, Haug RH, Lillich TT. The changing face of odontogenic infections. *J Oral Maxillofac Surg.* 2001;59(7):739-748.
4. Yuvaraj V, Mohan A, Pasupathy S. Microflora in maxillofacial infections   a changing scenario? *J Oral Maxillofac Surg.* 2012;70:119-125.
5. Al-Qamachi LH, Aga H, McMahon J, et al. Microbiology of odontogenic infections in deep neck spaces: a retrospective study. *Br J Oral Maxillofac Surg.* 2010;48:37-39.
6. Bouloux GF, Wallace J, Xue W. Irrigating drains for severe odontogenic infections do not improve outcome. *J Oral Maxillofac Surg.* 2013;71:42-46.
7. Carey JW, Dodson TB. Hospital course of HIV-positive patients with odontogenic infections. *Oral Surg Oral Med Oral Pathol Oral Radiol Endod.* 2001;91(1):23-27.
8. Chen MK, Wen YS, Chang CC, et al. Deep neck infections in diabetic patients. *Am J Otolaryngol.* 2000;21:169.
9. Huang TT, Tseng FY, Liu TC, et al. Deep neck infection in diabetic patients: comparison of clinical picture and outcomes with nondiabetic patients. *Otolaryngol Head Neck Surg.* 2005;132(6):943-947.
10. Rao DD, Desai A, Kulkarni RD, et al. Comparison of maxillofacial space infection in diabetic and nondiabetic patients. *Oral Surg Oral Med Oral Pathol Oral Radiol Endod.* 2010;110:e7.
11. Zheng L, Yang C, Zhang W, et al. Is there association between severe multispace infections of the oral maxillofacial region and diabetes mellitus? *J Oral Maxillofac Surg.* 2012;70:1565-1572.
12. Pappa H, Jones DC. Mediastinitis from odontogenic infection: a case report. *Br Dent J.* 2005;198(9):547-548.
13. Kuriyama T, Nakagawa K, Karasawa T, et al. Past administration of beta-lactam antibiotics and increase in the incidence of beta-lactamase-producing bacteria in patients with odontogenic infections. *Oral Surg Oral Med Oral Pathol Oral Radiol Endod.* 2000;89(2):186-192.
14. Kuriyama T, Karasawa T, Nakagawa K, et al. Bacteriology and antimicrobial susceptibility of gram-positive cocci isolated from pus specimens of orofacial odontogenic infections. *Oral Microbiol Immunol.* 2002;17(2):132-135.
15. Kuriyama T, Karasawa T, Nakagawa K, et al. Bacteriologic features and antimicrobial susceptibility in isolates from orofacial odontogenic infections. *Oral Surg Oral Med Oral Pathol Oral Radiol Endod.* 2000;90(5):600-608.

16. Kim MK, Chuang SK, August M. Antibiotic resistance in severe orofacial infections. *J Oral Maxillofac Surg.* 2017;75(5):962-968.

17. Moenning JE, Nelson CL, Kohler RB. The microbiology and chemotherapy of odontogenic infections. *J Oral Maxillofac Surg.* 1989;47(9):976-985.

18. Brook I, Lewis MAO, Sandor GKB, et al. Clindamycin in dentistry: more than just effective prophylaxis for endocarditis? *Oral Surg Oral Med Oral Pathol Oral Radiol Endod.* 2005;100(5):550-558.

19. Lockart PB, Tampa MP, Aminoshariae A, et al. Evidence-based clinical practice guidelines on antibiotic use for the management of plural- and periapical-related dental pain and intraoral swelling: a report from the American Dental Association. *J Am Dent Assoc.* 2019;150(11):906-921.

20. Roistacher DM, Heller JA, Ferraro NF, August M. Is penicillin allergy a risk factor for surgical site infection after oral and maxillofacial surgery? *J Oral Maxillofac Surg.* 2022;80(1):93-100.

21. Wilson WR, Gewitz M, Lockart PB, et al. Prevention of viridans group streptococcal infective endocarditis: a scientific statement from the American Heart Association. *Circulation.* 2021;143(20):963-978.

22. Donskey CJ, Chowdhry TK, Hecker MT, et al. Effect of antibiotic therapy on the density of vancomycin-resistant enterococci in the stool of colonized patients. *N Engl J Med.* 2000;343(26):1925-1932.

23. Al-Belasyand FA, Hairam AR. The efficacy of azithromycin in the treatment of acute infraorbital space. *J Oral Maxillofac Surg.* 2003;61(3):310-316.

24. Quinn RH, Murray JN, Pezold R, Sevarino KS. The American Academy of Orthopaedic Surgeons appropriate use criteria management of patients with orthopaedic implant undergoing dental procedures. *J Bone Joint Surg Am.* 2017;99(2):161-163.

25. Ahmad N, Abubaker AO, Laskin D, et al. The financial burden of hospitalization associated with odontogenic infections. *J Oral Maxillofac Surg.* 2013;71(4):656-658.

26. Desa V, Green R. Cavernous sinus thrombosis: current therapy. *J Oral Maxillofac Surg.* 2012;70(9):2085-2091.

27. Sicher H. *Oral Anatomy.* St Louis: Mosby. St. Louis: Mosby; 1965. 4th ed.

28. Peltroche-Llacsahuanga H, Reichhart E, Schmitt W, et al. Investigation of infectious organisms causing pericoronitis of the mandibular third molar. *J Oral Maxillofac Surg.* 2000;58(6):611-616.

29. Oshima A, Ariji Y, Goto M, et al. Anatomical considerations for the spread of odontogenic infection originating from the pericoronitis of impacted mandibular third molar: computed tomographic analyses. *Oral Surg Oral Med Oral Pathol Oral Radiol Endod.* 2004;98(5):589-597.

30. Halpern LR, Dodson TB. Does prophylactic administration of systemic antibiotics prevent postoperative inflammatory complications after third molar surgery? *J Oral Maxillofac Surg.* 2007;65(2):177-185.

31. Ren YF, Malmstrom HS. Effectiveness of antibiotic prophylaxis in third molar surgery: a meta-analysis of randomized controlled clinical trials. *J Oral Maxillofac Surg.* 2007;65(10):1909-1921.

32. Burke J. Angina Ludovici: a translation, together with a biography of Wilhelm Frederick von Ludwig. *Bull Hist Med.* 1939;7:1115-1126.

33. Williams AC, Guralnick WC. The diagnosis and treatment of Ludwig's angina. *N Engl J Med.* 1943;228:443.

34. Geisler PJ, Wheat P, Williams RA, et al. Isolation of anaerobes in Ludwig's angina. *J Oral Surg.* 1979;37(1):60-63.

35. Chow AW, Roser SM, Brady FA. Orofacial odontogenic infections. *Ann Intern Med.* 1978;88(3):392-402.

36. Forrester JD, Wolff CJ, Choi J, Colling KP, Huston JM. Surgical infection society guidelines for antibiotic use in patients with traumatic facial fractures. *Surg Infect.* 2011;22(3):274-282.

37. Colmenero Ruiz C, Labajo AD, Yanez Vilas I, et al. Thoracic complications of deeply situated serious neck infections. *J Craniomaxillofac Surg.* 1993;21:76-81.

38. Zeitoun IM, Dhanarajani PJ. Cervical cellulitis and mediastinitis caused by odontogenic infections: report of two cases and review of the literature. *J Oral Maxillofac Surg.* 1995;53(2):203-208.

39. Cai XY, Zhang WJ, Zhang ZY, et al. Cervical infection with descending mediastinitis: a review of six cases. *Int J Oral Maxillofac Surg.* 2006;35(11):1021-1025.

40. Warnke PH, Becker S, Springer IN, et al. Penicillin compared with other advanced broad spectrum antibiotics regarding antibacterial activity against oral pathogens isolated from odontogenic abscesses. *J Craniomaxillofac Surg.* 2008;36(8):462-467.

17

Infections of the Periodontium

JOSEPH V. CALIFANO, JAMES A. KATANCIK, AND PHILIP M. PRESHAW

Infections of the Periodontium

Periodontal diseases are prevalent throughout the world, affecting adults, adolescents, and children. Because of the significance of these diseases in the population, early diagnosis and treatment are extremely important. Periodontal diseases are multifactorial and can have both acute and chronic impacts on patients. Chronic and acute infections of the periodontium are discussed.

Overview of Periodontal Anatomy

The periodontium is a complex structure composed of the gingiva, periodontal ligament (PDL), cementum, and alveolar bone (Figure 17-1). The primary functions of the periodontium are to allow the tooth to be attached to the bone and to provide a barrier for the underlying structures from the oral microflora.

The gingival epithelium is composed of stratified squamous epithelium, which is primarily orthokeratinized or parakeratinized. The gingiva covers the supracrestal root surface and the alveolar bone, and consists of epithelial and connective tissue components. The gingival (oral) epithelium becomes the sulcular epithelium and junctional epithelium as it lines the gingival sulcus near the tooth surface (enamel or cementum) and ultimately attaches to it with hemidesmosomes. The gingival sulcus is a shallow crevice that is bound apically by the coronal aspect of the junctional epithelium, laterally by the sulcular epithelium, and medially by tooth surface, and it superiorly exits into the oral cavity. The junctional epithelium is supported by the supracrestal connective tissue fibers of the gingiva.

These structures create an initial barrier between the subgingival biofilm (bacterial plaque) and the subepithelial components of the periodontium. Apically, the PDL (connective tissue attachment) connects the root cementum to the alveolar bone, functionally supporting the tooth within the mandible or maxilla. The portions of the PDL fibers that are embedded in cementum and alveolar bone are called Sharpey's fibers.[1] In addition to providing tooth support, the unique design of the periodontium allows for the distribution of the forces of mastication.

Microbiology of the Periodontium

Dental biofilm (plaque) is the primary cause of the periodontal diseases, gingivitis and periodontitis. It is a tooth and dental restoration adherent soft mass composed primarily of microorganisms and their extracellular matrix. The biofilm has a biologically diverse, heterogeneous, organized structure that changes over time.[2] When there is a significant accumulation of dental biofilm, inflammation of the gingiva occurs, leading to gingivitis that, if untreated, may progress to periodontitis.[3,4] The mechanical removal of biofilm reverses the inflammatory process in the gingival tissues.[5,6]

When an adult prophylaxis (tooth cleaning) for a periodontally healthy patient is followed by a period of plaque accumulation of 21 days (i.e., an experimental gingivitis study), biofilm growth is established on the tooth surface by successive colonization of bacterial species in a specific, predictable manner.[6] Early colonizers are predominately gram-positive cocci and rods. Many of these organisms are facultative anaerobes. Examples are *Streptococcus sanguis* and *Actinomyces naeslundii*. These species have the ability to attach to salivary proteins that adsorb to the tooth surface. Once these early colonizers attach to the teeth, other species in turn become part of the biofilm by attaching to species that preceded them in biofilm accumulation. This succession of species accumulation occurs on the basis of the ability of each species to attach to the species that preceded it, thereby increasing the complexity of the biofilm. In addition, as plaque accumulates, environmental factors such as oxygen tension and substrate availability vary.[7] This is due in part to gingival inflammation and ulceration of the sulcular epithelium. As plaque accumulation continues, gram-negative cocci, filaments, rods (e.g., *Prevotella intermedia, Fusobacterium nucleatum, Campylobacter rectus, Porphyromonas gingivalis, Tannerella forsythia*), and finally spirochetes (e.g., *Treponema denticola*) become part of the biofilm. These latter bacteria include obligate anaerobes and motile bacteria.

The bacterial species that compose the naturally occurring tooth-associated biofilm are highly variable when

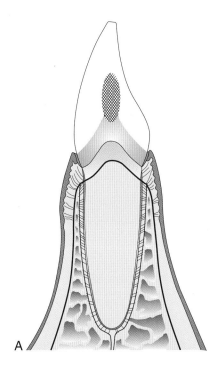

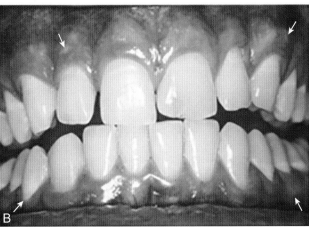

• **Figure 17-1** Healthy Periodontium. **A,** Cross-sectional illustration of healthy gingiva. **B,** Healthy gingiva. (**A,** From Wolf HF, Rateitschak EM, Rateitschak KH, Hassel TM, et al. Color Atlas of Dental Medicine Periodontology. 3rd ed. Stuttgart/New York: Theime; 2005. **B,** From Newman MG, Takei HH, Klokkevold PR, et al. *Newman and Carranza's Clinical Periodontology.* 13th ed. St Louis: Elsevier; 2019.)

comparing different subjects.[8] It is dependent on the level of oral hygiene and the genetic make-up of the host. There has been extensive research characterizing the species residing in the dental plaque biofilm in healthy individuals, patients with varying degrees of gingivitis, and periodontitis. Methods to identify bacterial species include culturing and characterizing each species by metabolic means,[9] immunofluorescence, DNA probes,[10,11] and polymerase chain reaction (PCR) of 16s rRNA.[12,13] Culturing techniques have identified in excess of 500 species associated with gingivitis and periodontitis; however, this count is limited to the organisms that can be cultivated in the laboratory.[8] Through PCR it has been estimated that more than 700 species may exist in the biofilm associated with teeth.[12,13]

Many of the species identified by PCR have not been described and studied, because they are uncultivable and therefore little is known about them. There is considerable debate regarding which of these species might be considered pathogenic in the cause of periodontitis. Although investigators have historically considered that certain bacterial species are largely responsible for periodontal destruction found in periodontitis, the modern consensus is that that bacteria are necessary, but not sufficient to cause periodontitis. There may be direct effects of periodontitis-associated bacteria on the periodontium; however, it is considered, as will be discussed later, that periodontitis is primarily the result of immunopathologic process.[14,15] In all individuals, plaque accumulation will result in gingivitis. Some patients will only have gingivitis. Others, in whom there is a persistent and dysregulated immune-inflammatory response, have destruction of their own tissues. It is likely that many bacterial species, especially those more associated with disease (e.g., gram-negative obligate anaerobes, motile bacteria, spirochetes), are more likely to elicit dysregulated immune responses that result in tissue destruction in some individuals.

When excellent oral hygiene is observed, bacterial biofilm accumulation is at a low level and is largely removed each day through brushing and flossing. In this case, tooth-associated bacterial biofilm is composed mostly of the initial colonizers described previously. This level of hygiene is, however, uncommon in humans. Most humans have a plaque biofilm that is well established. The biofilm is, in many individuals, only significantly disrupted during professional care (i.e., periodic adult prophylaxis or periodontal debridement based on the patient's need). Consequently, gingivitis at varying levels of severity is almost universal among humans, and a substantial proportion of these individuals also have periodontitis in which a portion of the periodontal tissues supporting the teeth (i.e., connective tissue and alveolar bone) has been lost.[16]

Chronic Infections of the Periodontium

Chronic periodontal infections are common and include dental biofilm-induced gingivitis and several forms of periodontitis. Dental biofilm-induced gingival inflammation or gingivitis is almost universal in humans. A large proportion of humans have periodontitis in addition to gingivitis. These diseases are usually asymptomatic and are often only detected by a dental professional during a routine examination. Gingivitis is completely reversible with professional debridement of the teeth and improved oral hygiene measures. In contrast, periodontitis results in permanent destruction of connective tissue and bone that support the teeth, and it can result ultimately in tooth loss if left untreated. The tissue destruction usually occurs slowly over a long period of time, although there can be short periods of more rapid destruction. As periodontitis is usually asymptomatic, regular routine periodontal examination is important to allow for early detection and treatment to avoid permanent loss of periodontal tissues.

Dental Biofilm–Induced Gingivitis

In health, histologically, the subepithelial connective tissue in the gingiva contains dense connective tissue fiber bundles called gingival fibers. Some of these fibers insert by Sharpey's fibers into the coronal aspect of the tooth root just apical to the cementoenamel junction (CEJ). This establishes the connective tissue attachment of the gingiva to the tooth. The junctional epithelium attaches to the tooth just coronal to the gingival fibers by hemidesmosomes. The epithelial attachment is to tooth enamel just coronal to the CEJ (see Figure 17-1). There is a normal level of vascular supply to these tissues and minimal numbers of immune cells (i.e., neutrophils, macrophages, lymphocytes, plasma cells). Clinically healthy gingiva is pink, can have physiologic pigmentation, has a firm consistency, and has normal tissue contours. A periodontal examination with a periodontal probe to measure the position of the gingival and epithelial attachment finds that the probe stops within the gingival sulcus on enamel at the junctional epithelium at or coronal to the CEJ. In some instances, the probe may penetrate into the junctional epithelium (see Figure 17-3, later). The sulcular epithelium lining the gingival sulcus is intact, and there is no bleeding on probing.

As described earlier, biofilm accumulation results in gingival inflammation or gingivitis at varying levels of severity dependent on the amount of biofilm and the host immunoinflammatory response. All humans with biofilm accumulation will have gingivitis, but the magnitude of the gingival inflammation for a given amount of biofilm varies between individuals based on genetic, systemic (e.g., diabetes, varying gonadotrophic hormone levels in puberty), and environmental (e.g., smoking, poorly contoured dental restorations, dental calculus) influences. Histologically, the gingival inflammation results in a decrease in the density of the gingival connective tissue fibers as a result of collagen breakdown. There is an increase in vascularity of the gingival tissues. In addition, there is vasodilation and an increase in vascular permeability. This results in edema and erythema within the gingival tissues, creating the clinical appearance of gingivitis. The sulcular epithelium becomes ulcerated and rete pegs that normally extend only modestly into the subepithelial connective tissue are elongated as epithelial basal cells proliferate into collagen-depleted zones of the connective tissue. The subepithelial connective tissue is infiltrated with immune cells that include neutrophils, macrophages, lymphocytes, and plasma cells. The plasma cell is the most numerous of these cells. Clinically, the gingiva is red to magenta, has an edematous consistency, and has gingival enlargement with changes in the gingival contour (Figure 17-2). A periodontal examination with a periodontal probe to measure the position of the epithelial and gingival connective tissue attachment finds that the probe often penetrates the junctional epithelium and perhaps the gingival connective tissue (Figure 17-3), because of the ulceration of the epithelium, decrease in connective tissue density, and edema found in gingivitis. The connective tissue attachment

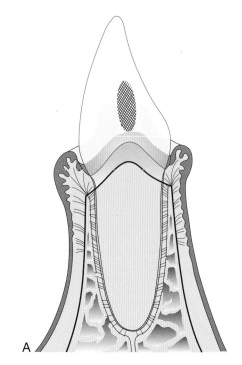

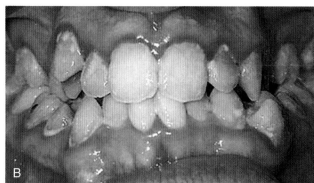

• **Figure 17-2** Gingivitis. **A,** Cross-sectional illustration of gingivitis. **B,** Gingivitis. (Used with permission from Color Atlas of Dental Medicine: Periodontology. 3rd edition, 9783136750032. Herbert F. Wolf, Edith M. & Klaus H. Rateitschak, Thomas M. Hassell.)

is, however, still at the level of the CEJ, and there is no connective tissue attachment loss. The sulcular epithelium lining the gingival sulcus is ulcerated, and there may be bleeding on probing.

Periodontitis

In the presence of biofilm-induced gingivitis, some individuals have periodontitis that results in detachment of gingival connective fibers apical to the CEJ, alveolar bone loss, and detachment of PDL fibers that connect the tooth root to the alveolar bone. The extent of this destruction can involve only a few or all teeth and can be slight, moderate, or severe depending on the amount of attachment loss. It is clear that some humans are susceptible to destructive periodontitis whereas others are resistant. There are likely genetic and environmental components to susceptibility.[14,15,17]

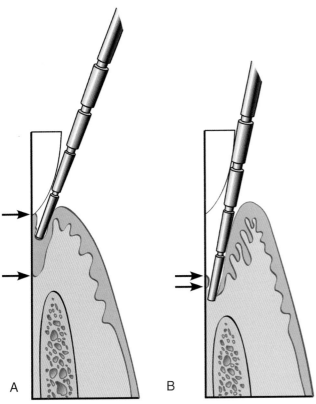

• **Figure 17-3** Periodontal Probing in Health, Gingivitis, and Periodontitis. **A,** Probing in healthy or gingivitis site. **B,** Probing periodontitis site. (From Newman MG, Takei HH, Klokkevold PR, et al. *Newman and Carranza's Clinical Periodontology.* 13th ed. St Louis: Elsevier; 2019.)

The genetic component likely may be related to an inherited tendency to dysregulation of the host response to the bacterial plaque residing in the gingival crevice.[14,15,17] Clinically the appearance of the gingiva will be the same as in gingivitis. The gingival margin may be in the same position as seen with gingivitis, or there may be gingival recession or interproximal blunting of papilla (Figure 17-4). A periodontal examination with a periodontal probe to measure the position of the gingival and epithelial attachment finds that the probe terminates at a point apical to the CEJ, as there has been detachment of gingival and PDL fibers and alveolar bone loss (see Figure 17-3). There may be radiographic evidence of alveolar bone loss (see Figure 17-4).

Periodontitis includes three types of disease: periodontitis, necrotizing periodontal diseases, and systemic diseases associated with loss of periodontal supporting tissue.[18]

Periodontitis can occur at any age after eruption of the permanent dentition, but it typically has an onset in early adulthood or older. Although it can have periods of more rapid attachment loss and periods of stability, the rate of destruction of periodontal attachment and alveolar bone is relatively slow. There is evidence of substantial heritability of periodontitis that is estimated to be as large as 50% in younger patients and up to 25% in older patients.[19]

In some cases, periodontitis can exhibit a rapid rate of attachment loss (grade C periodontitis). A subset of these patients with rapid attachment loss have periodontitis with a circumpubertal onset that results in severe periodontal destruction during adolescence and early adulthood.

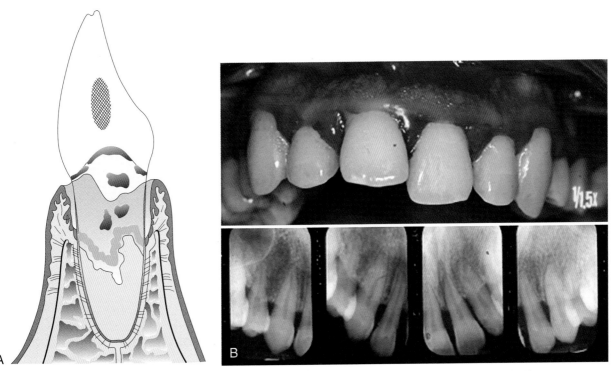

• **Figure 17-4** Periodontitis. **A,** Cross-sectional illustration of periodontitis. **B,** Periodontitis. (Used with permission from Color Atlas of Dental Medicine: Periodontology. 3rd edition, 9783136750032. Herbert F. Wolf, Edith M. & Klaus H. Rateitschak, Thomas M. Hassell.)

Periodontitis with this circumpubertal onset is often familial, and the pattern of expression in families with this disease is consistent with an autosomal dominant gene of major effect.[20] Periodontal destruction can follow a generalized pattern or can present with a first molar/incisor pattern of destruction. Both patterns can occur among siblings in the same family. It has been suggested by some investigators that periodontitis with this circumpubertal onset and rapid rate of destruction has a unique bacterial cause dominated by a specific JP2 clone of *Aggregatibacter actinomycetemcomitans*.[21,22] Others have not found a statistical difference in the bacterial species found in the dental biofilm associated with gingivitis, periodontitis, and periodontitis with circumpubertal onset.[9]

Periodontitis due to systemic diseases associated with loss of periodontal supporting tissue is a group of rare diseases associated with mendelian conditions in which the gene mutation or defect is known. Examples include Papillon-Lefèvre syndrome, leukocyte adhesion deficiency, cyclic neutropenia, and Ehlers-Danlos syndrome.[18,23] The genetic defects affect phagocyte function, immune regulation, or connective tissue metabolism. These patients typically have severe periodontitis that begins with the primary dentition and progresses rapidly.[24] Unlike other forms of periodontitis in which nonoral diseases do not occur concomitant with periodontitis, these patients often exhibit difficulty in managing bacterial infections at other anatomic locations. Treatment is typically unsuccessful in maintaining the natural dentition for these individuals.

Etiology of Periodontal Diseases

The pathogenesis of periodontal disease is multifactorial and complex. The host response to periodontitis-associated organisms is largely successful in confining the bacteria of the tooth-associated biofilm to the gingival sulcus or periodontitis lesion. In contrast to acute bacterial infections in which the infection is resolved as the immune response clears the pathogen from host tissues, dental biofilm persists on the tooth surface despite innate and adaptive immunity. This persistence results in persistent chronic inflammation in the periodontal tissues that in some patients is dysregulated and exaggerated, resulting in destruction of the connective tissue attachment and alveolar bone supporting the teeth (i.e., periodontitis), and in others only results in gingival inflammation without attachment loss (i.e., gingivitis). It appears that the tooth-associated dental biofilm is necessary but not sufficient to cause periodontitis in all individuals.[14,17]

As discussed in Chapter 1, several immune mechanisms act as part of innate immunity in response to the presence of bacteria and other microorganisms in tissues of the body. Pathogen-associated molecular patterns (PAMPs) that include many molecules unique to pathogens are recognized by pattern recognition receptors (PRRs). Examples of PRRs include Toll-like receptors (TLRs), nucleotide-binding oligomerization domain (NOD)-like receptors (NLRs),

retinoic acid-inducible gene 1 (RIG-1)-like receptors (RLRs), and the FMLP receptor. They are found on many cell types and include macrophages, neutrophils, fibroblasts, epithelial cells, endothelial cells, and dendritic cells, all of which are found in the periodontium. As the receptors on these cells are engaged by PAMPs, signal transduction from these receptors results in gene expression of proinflammatory cytokines. These cytokines include tumor necrosis factor α (TNF-α), type I interferons, interleukin (IL)-1, IL-6, IL-8, and IL-12. These cytokines activate phagocytes, recruit phagocytes to sites of infection, increase the resistance of cells to viral infection, activate natural killer cells, and support the development of adaptive immunity for the pathogen. In addition, complement proteins are activated as described in Chapter 1. Complement proteins elaborated in this process such as C3a, C3b, and C5a also serve as chemoattractants, opsonins, and promote vasodilation and an increase in vascular permeability. Lipid mediators (i.e., arachidonic acid metabolites) such as prostaglandins and leukotrienes are also released by macrophages and are proinflammatory.

As the biofilm bacteria are not cleared by innate immunity and persist in the periodontal lesion, adaptive immune responses occur that are specific for bacteria in the dental biofilm. Adaptive immune responses are highly regulated, in part to prevent autoimmunity but also to help resolve a robust immune response once the pathogen is cleared. This is largely at the level of the T helper cell subsets as described in Chapter 1. The T helper cell subsets work in concert with one another to orchestrate an immune response that is tailored to the specific infection (e.g., bacterial, viral, extracellular, intracellular). To regulate the response to an infection, a particular T helper cell subset may dominate the response. In periodontitis, for example, a response might be dominated by the T_h17 T helper cell subset and may promote inflammation, continued excessive recruitment of phagocytic cells to the periodontal tissues, and osteoclast activity through production of IL-17, IL-21, IL-26, TNF-α, and RANKL.[14,25,26]

Although not completely understood, emerging evidence suggests that the immunoregulatory process in periodontitis patients may be different from that of patients with only gingivitis and represents dysregulation of the immune response that results in destruction of periodontal connective tissue attachment and alveolar bone.[14,25-27] It is likely immune dysregulation in periodontitis is to some extent genetically controlled and therefore results from inherited risk for disease.[14,25-27] Some investigators have theorized that dysregulation of immunity is also partly due to dysbiosis of the periodontal microflora and the result of particular keystone pathogenic organisms.[28]

Treatment Approaches for Gingivitis and Periodontitis

Details of appropriate care for patients with gingivitis and periodontitis have been reviewed in detail in an American

Academy of Periodontology position paper,[24] and in recent publications including the European Federation of Periodontology S3 clinical practice guidelines.[29,30] A brief discussion of this topic follows.

The treatment of gingivitis and periodontitis begins with disrupting and removing dental biofilm and calculus, which is dental biofilm that has become calcified and therefore more difficult to remove. This is accomplished with professional debridement of the tooth surfaces (i.e., periodontal debridement) and oral hygiene instruction to help improve effectiveness of the patient's home care through improved toothbrushing and interproximal tooth cleaning with floss and/or interdental brushes. For patients with gingivitis, this is typically all the treatment that is needed. Some patients with stage I periodontitis (periodontitis severity that has minimal attachment/bone loss) also may need only this relatively limited care. If so, the patient is placed in an oral health maintenance program for which professional dental visits are completed at an interval appropriate for the individual patient's needs.

Treatment of more severe periodontitis may require additional therapy to achieve periodontal health.[29,30] Locally administered sustained-release antibiotics as an adjunct to subgingival instrumentation in patients with periodontitis may be considered in some cases. Because concerns about impacts of systemic antibiotics on both individual patients and public health, the routine use of systemic antibiotics as an adjunct to subgingival debridement in patients with periodontitis is not recommended. However, the adjunctive use of systemic antibiotics may be considered for specific patient categories (e.g., generalized periodontitis stage III grade C in young adults, likely as part of treatment by a specialist).[29] For many patients with a diagnosis of periodontitis, surgical therapy with flap access to the tooth root surfaces is needed to allow effective debridement. Osseous resection may be completed during the surgery, allowing for greater pocket reduction to facilitate future supportive periodontal therapy (maintenance care). In some cases, pocket reduction can instead be achieved by regenerative surgical procedures that use techniques, devices, materials, and biologics that serve to promote healing that may regenerate periodontal tissues lost to the disease process.[24,29,30]

Regardless of the type of active therapy used to achieve periodontal health, the long-term outcome of care largely depends on compliance with the supportive periodontal care program planned for the patient.

Acute Infections of the Periodontium

Acute periodontal infections are clinical conditions of rapid onset that involve the periodontium or associated structures and may be characterized by pain or discomfort. They may or may not be related to the underlying chronic conditions of gingivitis or periodontitis. They may be localized or generalized, with possible systemic manifestations. Although less common than chronic periodontal infections, such as gingivitis and periodontitis, acute periodontal infections are commonly encountered in oral health care practice and are much more likely to result in patients seeking urgent care than are chronic conditions. Acute infections must be treated promptly because they can be rapidly destructive to the periodontal attachment and supporting bone and treatment must be focused on the microbial cause, most commonly bacterial or viral. Once the acute infection is resolved, it is important for the clinician to address any underlying chronic disease that may be present.

Abscesses of the Periodontium

A periodontal abscess is defined as an acute lesion characterized by localized accumulation of pus within the gingival wall of the periodontal pocket/sulcus. Periodontal abscesses cause rapid tissue destruction and may be associated with systemic dissemination. They are classified according to cause and are most frequently associated with preexisting periodontitis, and can be a common finding in patients with stage III/IV periodontitis (i.e., severe disease).[31,32] The classification includes whether a periodontal abscess is occurring in a periodontitis patient (more common, as an acute exacerbation of periodontitis), or in a nonperiodontitis patient (e.g., as a result of impaction, harmful habits, gingival overgrowth, or alteration of the root surface).[32] Periodontal abscesses occurring as an acute exacerbation of periodontitis are localized within the tissues adjacent to the periodontal pocket and may involve the periodontal ligament and adjacent alveolar bone. An abscessed area can manifest the following signs and symptoms: swelling, suppuration, or visible redness of the soft tissue, extrusion or loosening, and tenderness to even slight percussion of the tooth involved.

Periodontal Abscess in a Patient Without Periodontitis

A periodontal abscess in a nonperiodontitis patient typically manifests as a localized, painful, rapidly expanding lesion involving the marginal gingiva or interdental papilla, in a previously disease-free area (Figure 17-5). The most

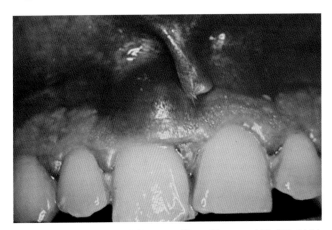

• **Figure 17-5** Periodontal Abscess. (From Newman MG, Takei HH, Klokkevold PR, et al. *Newman and Carranza's Clinical Periodontology.* 13th ed. St Louis: Elsevier; 2019.)

common etiologic factor associated with this type of periodontal abscess is impaction of a foreign body, such as a popcorn hull, toothbrush bristle, or shell fragments from shellfish.[33] Initially, the abscess appears as a red swelling with a smooth, shiny surface. Within 24 to 48 hours, the lesion is usually fluctuant and pointed, with a surface orifice from which a purulent exudate may be expressed. If permitted to progress, the lesion generally ruptures spontaneously. Symptoms can include pulpal hypersensitivity.[33] Diagnosis of this type of periodontal abscess is derived by the clinical examination of the affected site, patient report of symptoms, and a thorough history of the present illness. Treatment of the abscess includes removal of the foreign body by local debridement, drainage through the gingival sulcus, and in some cases incision and drainage of the abscess. Resolution of the abscess often occurs within 24 to 48 hours of effective treatment.[34,35]

Periodontal Abscess in a Patient With Periodontitis

The periodontal abscess in a patient with preexisting periodontitis is a localized purulent infection within the tissues adjacent to the periodontal pocket that can lead to the rapid destruction of the periodontal ligament and alveolar bone (see Figure 17-5). Clinical features can include the following signs and symptoms: a smooth, shiny swelling of the gingiva; pain, with the area of swelling tender to touch; a purulent exudate; and an increase in probing depth. The involved tooth may be sensitive to percussion and may be mobile.

Etiologic factors that can result in periodontal abscess formation include dental biofilm, soft tissue occlusion of the periodontal pocket orifice after incomplete debridement, teeth with advanced furcation involvement, anatomic tooth factors such as root grooves, endodontically involved teeth, and diabetes. Although a periodontal abscess is more common in patients with preexisting periodontal disease, they can also occur in a site that does not have a history of periodontitis. Patients with periodontitis may be unaware of the disease but will often see the dentist when they have an acute exacerbation associated with an abscess and pain. Teeth with advanced furcation involvement, teeth with anatomic variations, and teeth with a previous history of a periodontal abscess may be at higher risk.[32]

Diagnosis of a periodontal abscess can be challenging, because the clinical presentation can be similar to teeth with pulpal disease, teeth with pulpal and periodontal disease, and teeth with vertical root fracture. Determination of the diagnosis should include careful examination of the affected site to include probing, determination of attachment loss, palpation, percussion, assessment of the pulpal status, determination of mobility, and proper radiographic evaluation.

The goal of therapy for a periodontal abscess is elimination of the acute signs and symptoms as soon as possible. Treatment considerations include establishing drainage by debriding the pocket and disrupting and removing dental biofilm, calculus, and any impacted foreign objects and possibly incising the abscess. Other treatments can include irrigation of the pocket with an antimicrobial, limited occlusal adjustment, administration of antimicrobials, and management of patient comfort. A surgical procedure for access for debridement may be considered. If the involved tooth has advanced attachment and bone loss and is deemed hopeless, then extraction of the tooth would be indicated. A comprehensive periodontal evaluation should follow resolution of the acute condition given the likelihood of underlying periodontitis.

The use of systemic antibiotics may be indicated when there are signs of systemic involvement and if complete drainage cannot be established. The duration and type of antibiotic that is selected can vary because periodontal abscesses have a mixed bacterial etiology; however, an antibiotic from the penicillin family is empirically the drug of choice, whereas tetracyclines and metronidazole have also been advocated.[36]

Pericoronal Abscess (Pericoronitis)

Although not now classified as a type of periodontal abscess,[18] the pericoronal abscess (pericoronitis) may still be considered as an acute periodontal condition, though in a different category from periodontal abscesses. The pericoronal abscess is a localized purulent infection within the soft tissues surrounding the crown of a partially erupted tooth (Figure 17-6). This abscess is most commonly associated with a partially erupted mandibular third molar in which case the operculum, a flap of soft tissue covering a portion of the crown of the tooth, becomes infected. The gingival tissue surrounding the partially erupted mandibular third molar is often red, swollen, and painful to palpation or manipulation. In addition, the patient may exhibit suppuration, trismus, fever, malaise, or lymphadenopathy.[37] Pain can be compounded when the opposing maxillary third molar occludes on the operculum, causing trauma to the

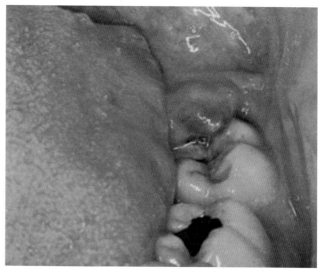

• **Figure 17-6** Pericoronal Abscess. (From Newman MG, Takei HH, Klokkevold PR, et al. *Newman and Carranza's clinical periodontology.* 13th ed. St Louis: Elsevier; 2019.)

already inflamed tissue. The bacteria associated with this type of abscess are primarily anaerobic, and spirochetes are often present. The infection is commonly found in younger patients, corresponding with the timing of eruption of the third molars. Evaluation of the pericoronal abscess should include determination of attachment loss, palpation, percussion, and the presence of suppuration; assessment of the pulpal status of adjacent teeth; determination of mobility; and a radiographic evaluation. The characteristic localization of the abscess to the mandibular third molar and on occasion the mandibular second molar, aids in determining a diagnosis. Treatment of a pericoronal abscess may include the use of analgesics, antibiotic therapy, irrigation or gentle debridement, and extraction of the opposing third molar if it is impinging on the operculum covering the mandibular third molar. Once the acute phase of the infection has been controlled, the definitive treatment is often extraction of the involved third molar, if normal eruption is deemed unlikely. This determination requires a careful analysis of arch space limitations and angulation of the involved third molar. Recurrence of the infection is common if the underlying cause is not resolved. Alternative treatment may include soft tissue exposure of the partially erupted tooth, if position and arch space are considered adequate; however, underlying tooth position can lead to recurrence of soft tissue hypertrophy and reinfection.

Necrotizing Periodontal Diseases

Necrotizing periodontal diseases are unique in their clinical presentation and course. Data suggest that the cause and pathogenesis of necrotizing periodontal diseases also may be distinctive from other periodontal diseases. Necrotizing gingivitis (NG) is a type of necrotizing periodontal disease in which the necrosis is limited to the gingival tissues and necrotizing periodontitis (NP) includes clinical attachment loss and involvement of the alveolar bone. The diseases are classified according to presentation in chronically, severely compromised patients (adults with HIV/AIDS with CD4 counts <200 cells/mm³ and detectable viral load, or other severe immunosuppression, or children with severe malnourishment, extreme living conditions or severe infections), or in temporarily and/or moderately compromised patients (gingivitis or periodontitis patients with uncontrolled factors such as stress, smoking, nutrition, habits, or previous necrotizing periodontal diseases).[31,32]

Necrotizing Gingivitis

NG has an acute clinical presentation with the distinctive characteristics of rapid onset of gingival pain; interdental gingival necrosis, commonly referred to as "punched-out" papillae, and bleeding. The ulcerated and necrotic papillary and marginal gingiva may be covered by a yellowish-white or grayish slough, or pseudomembrane. Pain, often intense and of sudden onset, is a critical diagnostic finding because it is rare with dental biofilm–induced gingivitis and periodontitis. The onset of NG has been associated with preexisting gingivitis, tissue trauma, increased psychological stress, immunosuppression, tobacco smoking, and malnutrition. Acute psychological stress in particular appears to be a predisposing factor and can contribute to poor eating habits, increased smoking, and poor oral hygiene. Other signs and symptoms in more severe cases can include fetid breath odor, fever, lymphadenopathy, and general malaise. Loss of attachment and bone are rare in NG, but may be associated with multiple episodes over time or NG may be superimposed upon existing periodontitis.

NG is an infectious disease most associated with a fusiform-spirochete bacterial flora. Four zones have been described within the gingival lesion:[38]
1. Superficial bacterial zone: large mass of bacteria of varying morphotypes
2. Neutrophil-rich zone: leukocytes, particularly neutrophils and many spirochetes between the cells
3. Necrotic zone: disintegrating cells and many spirochetes and fusiform bacteria
4. Spirochetal infiltration zone: tissue elements well preserved but with infiltrating spirochetes and cocci and rods in adjacent nonnecrotic connective tissue regions

Microbiologic studies have demonstrated the presence of an anaerobic microflora consisting of *Treponema* and *Selenomonas* species, *F. nucleatum*, *P. intermedia*, and *P. gingivalis*. NG is not considered to be communicable.

Immunosuppression can lead to a depression of neutrophil function, including chemotaxis, phagocytic activity, and bactericidal abilities. In addition, altered lymphocyte function and lack of protective antibodies also have been reported in NG.[39,40]

Treatment is conservative, including gentle tooth debridement, antimicrobial rinses, and possibly systemic antibiotics. Underlying causes, such as stress and malnutrition also must be addressed. The signs and symptoms of NG typically resolve quickly after treatment, often within a week of adequate therapy, and soft tissue defects will typically regenerate with proper home and professional care.

Necrotizing Periodontitis

NP is characterized by severe and rapidly progressive disease that has a distinctive erythema of the free gingiva, attached gingiva, and alveolar mucosa; extensive soft tissue necrosis; and severe loss of periodontal attachment, but deep pocket formation is not always evident (Figures 17-7 and 17-8).[32] In severe cases in severely immunocompromised and/or malnourished patients, bone sequestrum and extraoral signs may also occur. The prevalence and demographics of NP in a systemically healthy population is unclear. NP may have social and clinical demographics and microbiologic and immunologic characteristics that are distinct from NG and that predispose subjects to a more progressively destructive disease.

The evidence suggests that immunosuppression plays a clear role in the risk for NP. In an HIV-infected population with NP, patients were more than twentyfold more likely to have CD4⁺ counts less than 200 cells/mm³. However, most

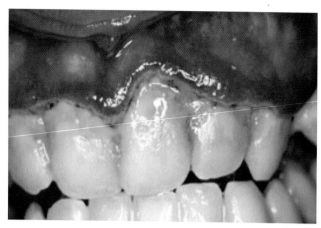

• **Figure 17-7** Necrotizing Gingivitis. (From Newman MG, Takei HH, Klokkevold PR, et al. *Newman and Carranza's Clinical Periodontology.* 13th ed. St Louis: Elsevier; 2019.)

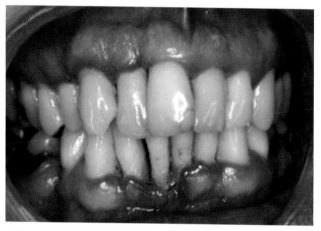

• **Figure 17-8** Necrotizing Periodontitis. (From Newman MG, Takei HH, Klokkevold PR, et al. *Newman and Carranza's Clinical Periodontology.* 13th ed. St Louis: Elsevier; 2019.)

HIV-infected individuals with CD4$^+$ cell counts below 200 cells/mm^3 do not have NP, suggesting other factors are involved in the cause and pathogenesis of NP.[41] The data suggest that an immunocompromised state may alter the rate of disease progression, but the initial clinical presentation of disease may be a function of its microbial cause.

Endodontic-Periodontal Lesions

Endodontic-periodontal lesions are clinical conditions involving both the pulp and periodontal tissues and may occur in acute (i.e., abscess) or chronic form.[32] The acute form is more likely to occur after a recent traumatic or iatrogenic event such as a perforation during dental treatment or a root fracture. In a patient with periodontitis, an endodontic-periodontal lesion more usually manifests with slow progression and lack of acute symptoms. Endodontic-periodontal lesions are classified according to the presence of root damage (e.g., root fracture, perforation, root resorption) or the absence of root damage in either periodontitis or nonperiodontitis patients.[31,32]

The periodontium communicates with pulp tissues through many channels and pathways in addition to the apical foramina, especially in the bifurcation and trifurcation regions of molars. These channels may be involved in extending pulpal infections to the periodontium and vice versa. Apical granulomas from necrotic pulps are extensive and can extend along the lateral aspects of roots, leading to extensive resorption of the alveolar crest.[42] Communication between the periodontium and pulp also can lead to periodontally derived endodontic lesions via lingual grooves, root and tooth fractures, cemental agenesis or hypoplasia, root anomalies, intermediate bifurcation ridges, and trauma-induced root resorption.[43] In most instances, lateral canals are found to be associated with the production of the periodontal lesions that result in the destruction of interradicular bone and bone in bifurcations.

Periodontal damage of pulpal origin has the potential to occur in the early stages of pulpal disease. An apical endodontic lesion may also extend and drain along the periodontium. This can result in a clinically detectable tract (e.g., a narrow pocket) into the furcation or any aspect of the tooth. The direct extension of periodontal inflammation through the apical foramen or lateral canals to the pulp, including subsequent pulpal necrosis, has been demonstrated; however, normal pulps are often observed in teeth with advanced periodontitis.[44] The initial effect of periodontal inflammation on the pulp may be degenerative.

The microbiota of an acute dentoalveolar abscess is usually polymicrobial similar to periodontal disease. *Fusobacterium, Prevotella, Porphyromonas, Peptostreptococcus, Cambylobacter, Tannerella,* and *Streptococcus* are the predominant genera that have been isolated. Spirochetes also reside in infected root canals.[45] Acute manifestations of root canal infections can result in rapid and extensive destruction of the attachment apparatus. Dental abscesses can form at any level of the periodontium, from the cervical region of the tooth to the apex, and may drain anywhere along this path, through the periodontal pocket or through the gingival tissue. This can manifest as increased probing depth, suppuration, increased tooth mobility, and loss of periodontal attachment.

A vertical root fracture can also appear as an endodontic-periodontal lesion. Root fractures occur frequently in previously endodontically treated teeth. Pain with mastication is often the primary complaint, and thermal sensitivity, gingival swelling, and a periodontal abscess or sinus tract are also common. Narrow or localized deep periodontal pockets are usually detected in the area of the fracture.

The endodontic-periodontal lesion may appear as a growing periapical area with secondary formation of a deep periodontal pocket. Determination of pulp vitality and periodontal probing characteristics are essential to establish a diagnosis and treatment plan. Deep periodontal probing depths with a vital pulp test would suggest a lesion of periodontal origin, but partial necrosis of the pulp in a multirooted tooth can confuse the diagnostic picture. Isolated deep and narrow periodontal probing depths with severe

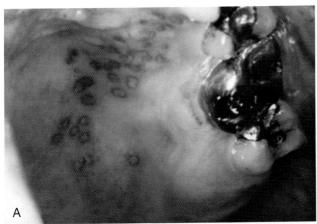

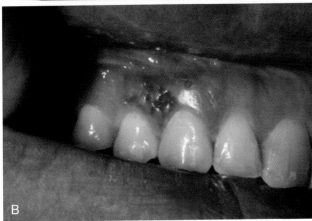

• **Figure 17-9** Herpetic Gingivostomatitis. (From Newman MG, Takei HH, Klokkevold PR, et al. *Newman and Carranza's Clinical Periodontology.* 13th ed. St Louis: Elsevier; 2019.)

localized bone loss are often associated with pulpal pathologic conditions, whereas circumferential deep probing is more characteristic of periodontitis.

Primary Herpetic Gingivostomatitis

Primary herpetic gingivostomatitis is an infection of the oral cavity caused by the herpes simplex virus (HSV) type 1 (Figure 17-9). In the primary infection, the virus ascends through sensory and autonomic nerves, where it persists as latent HSV in neuronal ganglia. Secondary manifestations result from various stimuli such as sunlight, trauma, fever, and stress. Secondary herpetic stomatitis can occur on the palate, gingiva, or oral mucosa.

Primary herpetic gingivostomatitis appears as a diffuse, erythematous, shiny involvement of the gingival and adjacent oral mucosa, with varying degrees of edema and gingival bleeding. Initial viral presentation appears as spherical clustered vesicles on the gingival, labial, and buccal mucosa; soft palate; pharynx; sublingual mucosa; or tongue. Approximately 24 hours later, the vesicles rupture and form painful, small ulcers with a red, elevated halo-like margin and a depressed, yellowish or grayish white central portion. Pain from the ruptured vesicles, cervical adenitis, body temperature as high as 40°C (~105°F), and generalized

malaise are common. The course of the disease is 7 to 10 days.

Early diagnosis is important, and treatment with antiviral medications can alter the course of the disease by reducing symptoms and potentially reducing recurrences. Primary herpetic gingivostomatitis is contagious. Acute herpetic gingivostomatitis usually occurs in infants and children, with most adults having developed immunity to HSV after a subclinical infection during childhood. Recurrent herpetic gingivostomatitis occurs and may be associated with immunosuppression. Secondary herpetic infection of the skin does occur, such as herpes labialis.

Gingival Diseases of Specific Bacterial Origin

Gingival diseases of specific bacterial origin include sexually transmitted diseases, such as gonorrhea *(Neisseria gonorrhoeae)* and syphilis *(Treponema pallidum).* Oral lesions may be secondary to systemic infection or occur through direct infection. Streptococcal gingivitis or gingivostomatitis can manifest as an acute condition with fever, malaise, and pain associated with acutely inflamed, diffuse, red, and swollen gingiva with increased bleeding and occasional gingival abscess formation. These gingival infections are usually preceded by tonsillitis and have been associated with group A β-hemolytic streptococcal infections.

Gingival Diseases of Fungal Origin

Gingival diseases of fungal origin occur more frequently in patients who are immunocompromised or who have had the normal flora disturbed by the long-term use of antibiotics. The most common oral fungal infection is candidiasis, caused by infection with *Candida albicans.* A generalized candidal infection can manifest as white patches on the gingiva, tongue or oral mucous membrane that can be removed with gauze, leaving a red, bleeding surface (Figure 17-10). In individuals infected with HIV, candidal infection can manifest as erythema of the attached gingiva that has been referred to as *linear gingival erythema* or *HIV-associated gingivitis.*

Peri-implant Health and Disease

Dental implants support dental prostheses that replace teeth that are congenitally missing or have been lost due to extensive dental caries, periodontal attachment loss, or trauma. By definition then they do not contain a periodontium but are discussed here because they can have disease that has similarities to the periodontal diseases. These devices are typically root form fixtures that are made of titanium, though more recently some have been made of ceramic materials. They usually have threads similar to a screw and also have a rough surface to increase their surface area. The dental implant also has an abutment attached that

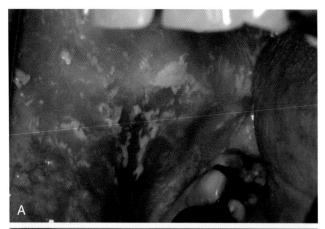

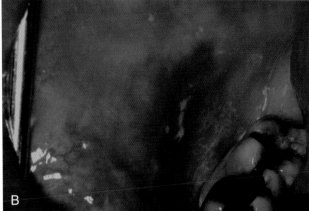

• **Figure 17-10** Candidiasis. (From Neville BW, Damm DD, Allen CM. *Oral and Maxillofacial Pathology.* 4th ed. St Louis: Saunders; 2016.)

extends out of the bone and gingiva, allowing a crown or other dental prosthesis to be attached. After surgical placement and optimal healing, these devices are osseointegrated into the alveolar bone. Osseointegration of a dental implant is defined as bone to implant contact at the light microscopic level. Gingival soft tissue surrounds the abutment connected to the dental implant and attaches to the abutment by hemidesmosomes of the gingival epithelium.[46] An important difference between the peri-implant tissues and periodontium is that although peri-implant tissues include bone and a gingival epithelial hemidesmosomal attachment, there is an absence of cementum, and connective tissue attachment of the gingival connective tissue and periodontal ligament. Therefore, there are no Sharpey's fibers that connect the implant to bone and gingival connective tissue in the same way as there are for teeth (Figure 17-11).[46]

The peri-implant–associated microflora in both health and disease is similar to that found in periodontal health, gingivitis, and periodontitis.[47,48] The 2018 classification of periodontal and peri-implant disease and conditions recognize peri-implant health, peri-implant mucositis, and peri-implantitis.[18] Dental implants exhibiting health have alveolar bone closely approximated to the dental implant surface with bone covering the entire dental implant rough surface from the apex to the platform (i.e., the full length of the implant or no more than 1.5 mm apical to the implant platform) and have an absence of signs of gingival inflammation similar to what is found in gingivitis around teeth (i.e., no

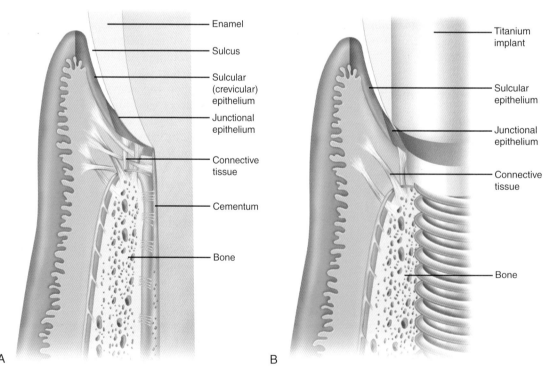

• **Figure 17-11** Comparison of the Periodontal and Peri-implant Tissues. **A,** Cross-sectional illustration of the periodontal tissues **B,** Peri-implant tissues. (From Newman MG, Takei HH, Klokkevold PR, et al. *Newman and Carranza's Clinical Periodontology.* 13th ed. St Louis: Elsevier; 2019.)

gingival enlargement, edema, erythema [red or magenta color], bleeding and/or suppuration on probing). With peri-implant mucositis there are signs of gingival inflammation with no change in the level of alveolar bone. This is analogous to gingivitis around teeth. Histologically, with peri-implant mucositis, the appearance is similar to that observed with gingivitis around teeth. Peri-implantitis exhibits gingival inflammation but also has destruction of alveolar bone.[18,46]

The cause of peri-implant diseases in many cases can be attributed to accumulation of bacterial biofilm. In addition, in the case of peri-implantitis, a dysregulated immune response resulting in bone destruction similar to that found with periodontitis may play a role. Although not fully established with evidence, it is likely that in many cases peri-implantitis has a genetic component to risk for disease as has been found for periodontitis.[17,19,20,49] Indeed, patients who have lost teeth as a result of periodontitis are at a greater risk for peri-implantitis if they have teeth replaced with dental implants, a fact that must always clearly be explained to patients who are seeking implants to replace teeth lost to periodontitis.[38,50,51] In addition, dental implants can have disease that results in peri-implant bone loss during the healing phase shortly after surgical placement. Peri-implantitis and potential failure and loss of the implant may also occur as a result of trauma during the implant surgery. Peri-implantitis in some cases also has been associated with design features of the implant-supported prosthesis that result in excessive, nonaxial, or otherwise unfavorable occlusal forces.[51]

Treatment of Peri-implant disease

Treatment of peri-implant mucositis is similar to gingivitis, given that it is reversible by professional cleaning to remove associated bacterial biofilm and improve the daily oral hygiene efforts of the patient. Debridement of the dental implant abutment and attached prosthesis to disrupt and remove biofilm and calculus must be ideally done with instruments that will not scratch the titanium abutment surface, typically titanium or plastic instruments and/or a glycine air polishing device.

Peri-implantitis presents a significant challenge to the clinician. Treatment often involves removal of the abutment and prosthesis supported by the implant. The dental implant may then need to be surgically exposed by reflection of the gingival soft tissue, and the bony defect adjacent to the implant curetted to remove any granulation associated with the implant. The exposed implant surface is then debrided of biofilm and calculus. The surface may be further treated with antimicrobial agents, and the bony defect may then be grafted with particulate bone allograft. Additional materials might include biologics (e.g., bone morphogenetic protein-2, enamel matrix derivative) and/or a barrier membrane to enhance bone regeneration.[52] Once there is bone loss and accumulation of peri-implant microflora, treatment efforts in resolving the implant-associated inflammation,

progressive bone loss, and regenerating lost bone are often of limited success, and although results from published trials are encouraging, further research is indicated to establish predictable and evidence-based protocols for treatment of peri-implantitis.

References

1. Fiorellini JP, Kim DM, Chang Y. Anatomy of the periodontium. In: Newman MG, Takei HH, Klokkevold PR, et al., eds. *Newman and Carranza's Clinical Periodontology*. 13th ed. St. Louis: Elsevier; 2019:19-48.
2. Jakubovics NS, Goodman SD, Mashburn-Warren L, Stafford GP, Cieplik F. The dental plaque biofilm matrix. *Periodontology 2000*. 2021;86:32-56.
3. Anerud A, Boysen H, Dunford RG, et al. The natural history of periodontal disease: the correlation of selected microbiological parameters with disease severity in Sri Lankan tea workers. *J Clin Periodontol*. 1995;22:678-974.
4. Loe H. Human research model for the production and prevention of gingivitis. *J Dent Res*. 1971;50:256-264.
5. Lindhe J, Axelsson P. Effect of controlled and hygiene procedures on caries and periodontal disease in adults. *J Clin Periodontol*. 1978;5:133-151.
6. Loe H, Theilade E, Jensen SB. Experimental gingivitis in man. *J Periodontol*. 1965;36:177-187.
7. Marsh PD. Dental plaque as a biofilm and a microbial community: implications for health and disease. *BMC Oral Health*. 2006;6(suppl 1):S14.
8. Kumar PS. Microbial dysbiosis: the root cause of periodontal disease. *J Periodontol*. 2021;92:1079-1087.
9. Moore LVH, Moore WEC. The bacteria of periodontal diseases. *Periodontol 2000*. 1994;5:66-77.
10. Haffajee AD, Cugini MA, Smith C, et al. Microbial complexes in subgingival plaque. *J Clin Periodontol*. 1998;25:134-144.
11. Colombo AP, Boches SK, Cotton SL, et al. Comparisons of subgingival microbial profiles of refractory periodontitis, severe periodontitis, and periodontal health using the human oral microbe identification microarray. *J Periodontol*. 2009;80:1421-1432.
12. Choi BK, Paster BJ, Dewhirst FE. Diversity of cultivable and uncultivable oral spirochetes from a patient with severe destructive periodontitis. *Infect Immun*. 1994;62:1889-1895.
13. Aas JA, Paster BJ, Stokes LN, et al. Defining the normal bacterial flora of the oral cavity. *J Clin Microbiol*. 2005;43:5721-5732.
14. Preshaw PM. Periodontal disease pathogenesis. In: Newman MG, Takei HH, Klokkevold PR, et al., eds. *Newman and Carranza's Clinical Periodontology*. 13th ed. St. Louis: Elsevier; 2019:89-111.
15. Hajishengallis G, Chavakis T, Lambris JD. Current understanding of periodontal disease pathogenesis and targets for host-modulation therapy. *Periodontol 2000*. 2020;84:14-34.
16. Kassebaum NJ, Bernabé E, Dahiya M, Bhandari B, Murray CJL, Marcenes W. Global burden of severe periodontitis in 1990-2010: a systematic review and metaregression. *J Dent Res*. 2014;93(11):1045-1053.
17. Loos BG, Van Dyke TE. The role of inflammation and genetics in periodontal disease. *Periodontol 2000*. 2020;83:26-39.
18. Caton J, Armitage G, Berglundh T, et al. A new classification scheme for periodontal and peri-implant diseases and conditions: introduction and key changes from the 1999 classification. *J Periodontol*. 2018;89(suppl 1):S1-S8.

19. Michalowicz BS, Diehl SR, Gunsolley JC, et al. Evidence of a substantial genetic basis for risk of adult periodontitis. *J Periodontol.* 2000;71:1699-1707.

20. Marazita ML, Burmeister JA, Gunsolley JC, et al. Evidence for autosomal dominant inheritance and race-specific heterogeneity in early-onset periodontitis. *J Periodontol.* 1994;65:623-630.

21. Zambon JJ. *Actinobacillus actinomycetemcomitans* in human periodontal disease. *J Clin Periodontol.* 1985;12:1-20.

22. Haubek D, Johansson A. Pathogenicity of the highly leukotoxic JP2 clone of *Aggregatibacter actinomycetemcomitans* and its geographic dissemination and role in aggressive periodontitis. *J Oral Microbiol.* 2014:6:23980-24002.

23. Hart TC, Atkinson JC. Mendelian forms of periodontitis. *Periodontol 2000.* 2007;45:95-112.

24. Rosen PS. Treatment of plaque-induced gingivitis, chronic periodontitis, and other clinical conditions. *J Periodontol.* 2001;72:1790-1800.

25. Gaffen SL, Hajishengallis G. A new inflammatory cytokine on the block: rethinking periodontal disease and the Th1/Th2 paradigm in the context of Th17 cells and IL17. *J Dent Res.* 2008;87:817-830.

26. Preshaw PM, Taylor JJ. How has research into cytokine interactions and their role in driving immune responses impacted our understanding of periodontitis? *J Clin Periodontol.* 2011;38(suppl 11):60-84.

27. Meyle J, Chapple I. Molecular aspects of the pathogenesis of periodontitis. *Periodontol 2000.* 2015;69(1):7-17.

28. Lamont RJ, Hajishengallis G. Polymicrobial synergy and dysbiosis in inflammatory disease. *Trends Mol Med.* 2015;21(3):172-183.

29. Sanz M, Herrera D, Kebschull M, et al. On behalf of the EFP Workshop participants and methodological consultants: treatment of stage I–III periodontitis—The EFP S3 level clinical practice guideline. *J Clin Periodontol.* 2020;47:4-60.

30. Herrera D, Sanz M, Kebschull M, et al; EFP Workshop participants and methodological consultants. Treatment of stage IV periodontitis: the EFP S3 level clinical practice guideline. *J Clin Periodontol.* 2022;49(suppl 24):4-71.

31. Papapanou PN, Sanz M, Buduneli N, et al. Periodontitis: consensus report of Workgroup 2 of the 2017 World Workshop on the Classification of Periodontal and Peri-Implant Diseases and Conditions. *J Clin Periodontol.* 2018;45(suppl 20):S162-S170.

32. Herrera D, Retamal-Valdes B, Alonso B, Feres M. Acute periodontal lesions (periodontal abscesses and necrotizing periodontal diseases) and endo-periodontal lesions. *J Clin Periodontol.* 2018;45(suppl 20):S78-S94.

33. Melnick PR, Takei HH. Treatment of periodontal abscess. In: Newman MG, Takei HH, Klokkevold PR, et al., eds. *Newman and Carranza's Clinical Periodontology.* 13th ed. St. Louis: Elsevier; 2019:493-497.

34. Van House RL, Gillette WB. Ill effects of improper hygiene procedure. *J Am Dent Assoc.* 1980;101:476-480.

35. Hilgeman JL, Snyder JD, Ahl DR. Periodontal emergencies. *Dent Clin North Am.* 1986;30:459-472.

36. Roldan S, Gonzalez I, Sanz M, et al. The periodontal abscess. Part I: clinical and microbiological findings. *J Clin Periodontol.* 2000;27:387-394.

37. Phillips C, Proffit WR, Koroluk LD, et al. Effect of quality of life measures on the decision to remove third molars in subjects with mild pericoronitis symptoms. *J Oral Maxillofac Surg.* 2014;72:1235-1243.

38. Schwarz F, Derks J, Monje A, Wang H. Peri-implantitis. *J Periodontol.* 2018;89(suppl 1):S267-S290.

39. Maltha JC, Mikx FHM, Kuijpers FJ. Necrotizing ulcerative gingivitis in beagle dogs. Part III. Distribution of spirochetes in interdental gingival tissue. *J Periodont Res.* 1985;20:522-531.

40. Cogen RB, Stevens Jr AW, Cohen-Cole S, et al. Leukocyte function in the etiology of acute necrotizing ulcerative gingivitis. *J Periodontol.* 1983;54:402-407.

41. Riley C, London JP, Burmeister JA. Periodontal health in 200 HIV-positive patients. *J Oral Pathol Med.* 1992;21:124-127.

42. Bender IB, Seltzer S. The effect of periodontal disease on the pulp. *Oral Surg Oral Med Oral Pathol.* 1972;33:458-474.

43. Dongari A, Lambrianidis T. Periodontally derived pulpal lesions. *Endod Dent Traumatol.* 1988;4:49-54.

44. Langeland K, Rodrigues H, Dowden W. Periodontal disease, bacteria and pulpal histopathology. *Oral Surg Oral Med Oral Pathol.* 1974;37:257-270.

45. Sakko M, Tjaderhane L, Rautemaa-Richardson R. Microbiology of root canal infections. *Prim Dent J.* 2016;5:84-89.

46. Ivanovski S, Lee R. Comparison of peri-implant and periodontal marginal soft tissues in health and disease. *Periodontol 2000.* 2017;76:116-130.

47. Lafaurie G, Sabogal M, Castillo D, et al. Microbiome and microbial profiles of peri-implantitis: a systematic review. *J Periodontol.* 2017;88:1066-1089.

48. Melo F, Milanesi F, Angst P, Oppermann R. A systematic review of the microbiota composition in various peri-implant conditions: data from 16s rRNA gene sequencing. *Arch Oral Biol.* 2020;117:1-12.

49. Fourmousis I, Vlachos M. Genetic risk factors for the development of peri-implantitis. *Implant Dent.* 2019;28:103-114.

50. Belibasakis G. Microbiological and immune-pathological aspects of peri-implant diseases. *Arch Oral Biol.* 2016;59:66-72.

51. Hammerle C, Tarnow D. The etiology of hard- and soft-tissue deficiencies at dental implants: a narrative review. *J Periodontol.* 2018;89(suppl 1):S291-S303.

52. Figuero E, Graziani F, Sanz I, Herrera D, Sanz M. Management of peri-implant mucositis and peri-implantitis. *Periodontol 2000.* 2014;66:255-273.

18

Osteomyelitis of the Jaws

MICHAEL T. GOUPIL AND MOHAMMAD BANKI

Osteomyelitis of the jaws (OMJ), a bone infection of the marrow space, is an ancient disease that has been noted in animals millions of years ago. It was discussed by Hippocrates (460 to 370 BC) as a disease in humans.[1] Osteomyelitis is fortunately a relatively rare condition in Western societies. This is primarily due to the advent of antibiotics and increased access to improved dental health care.[2] However, in those areas of the world where health care, especially dental care, is limited or nonexistent, osteomyelitis continues to be a significant problem. Dental caries continues to be the leading infectious disease in the world and is a major contributor to the cause of osteomyelitis. This chapter will review OMJs, focusing on the etiology, recognition, and management of this serious and significant condition. Noninfectious osteonecrosis, such as osteoradionecrosis and medication-related osteonecrosis, are briefly touched upon because of similar radiographic appearance.

Noninfectious Osteonecrosis

In making the diagnosis of OMJ, several other disease processes may mimic the presenting signs and symptoms of osteomyelitis, especially osteonecrotic radiographic changes. These include primary or metastatic cancer, osteoradionecrosis (ORN), and medication-related osteonecrosis of the jaws (MRONJ).[3]

ORN and medication-induced osteonecrosis can usually be ruled out based on a thorough medical history. ORN is characterized by a history of head and neck radiation exceeding 50 gray, xerostomia, increased dental caries, and lack of facial hair growth. The area of osteonecrosis needs to be within the radiation port. Medication-related osteonecrosis is characterized by the use of medications known to influence bone physiology. The most common are bisphosphonates and other medications used to treat osteoporosis and steroids.

The angle of the jaw is a frequent site for metastatic cancer disease such as breast and prostate. Biopsy of the affected osteonecrotic bone is required to help identify causative organisms of OMJ. These same biopsies should be used to rule-out the possibility of a neoplastic process.

Infection-Induced Osteomyelitis

Osteomyelitis is an inflammatory process of the medullary portion of the bone and is more frequently seen in the mandible. A bacterial source is introduced into the bone frequently from a dental infection, traumatic event, or surgical intervention. Because of the availability of antibiotics, the incidence of osteomyelitis has decreased.[4-6] However, there appears to be an increase in OMJ in Western countries related to the recent COVID pandemic.[2]

The literature contains a variety of osteomyelitis classifications in part related to the uniqueness of anatomic regions. The focus of this chapter is on OMJs. The most simplistic classification system divides the disease into two major categories: acute and chronic. The division between acute and chronic OMJ has been established as 4+ weeks. Acute osteomyelitis is characterized with an onset of fever, malaise, facial cellulitis, trismus, and leukocytosis. Usually, chronic OMJ is preceded by the acute phase and is characterized by swelling, deep pain, purulence, intraoral and/or extraoral fistulae, and overlying soft tissue wounds. Because of the purulence and fistulae this form of the disease is also referred to as suppurative osteomyelitis. A primary form of chronic OMJ also has been described in which there is no preceding acute phase.[7]

The key to successful treatment of OMJ is early detection, which translates to early suspicion more so with a patient with a positive history of COVID infection. Identification of the causative bacterial or fungal organisms can be difficult but is imperative to direct appropriate antibiotic management. Surgical intervention is almost always required, especially in the chronic form of the disease.[8]

Acute Osteomyelitis

Acute osteomyelitis requires a bacterial inoculation of the bone. The bacterial inoculation is usually from an odontogenic source secondary to pulpal or periodontal involvement of a diseased tooth. The bacterial inoculation also may be from a traumatic event such as a bone fracture or extraction of a tooth. With an increasing number of dental implants being placed, it follows that a failing implant will increase the incidence of OMJ.

The bacterial inoculation precipitates an inflammatory process in the medullary portion of the bone. Edema, which is part of the inflammatory process, results in venous stasis as the rigid cancellous portion of the bone does not allow for expansion. This is particularly true of the mandible, where the primary vascular supply is located within the bone. This vascular stasis diminishes nutrient supply to the bone and the final result is osteonecrosis. This vascular stasis interferes with recruitment of leukocytes to the area and results in further compromise to the body's ability to mount an immune response. This lack of blood flow also causes a decrease in available oxygen and thus encourages anerobic bacterial growth and colonization.[7]

Dental caries is still considered the most prevalent infection worldwide and one would expect to see significant numbers of cases of OMJ. The advent of antibiotics and the increased access to dental health care has fortunately led to a decrease in osteomyelitis. Another factor that needs to be considered in the resulting outcome of localized dental infection verses acute osteomyelitis is the presence of morbidity cofactor. One of the following may be instrumental or required for the development of OMJ[4]:

1. A systemic disease process, such as diabetes mellitus, cancer, or ethyl alcohol abuse, that leads to an impaired immune system.
2. A disease that compromises microcirculation or microcirculation-like sickle cell disease or an underlying collagen vascular disease.
3. An osteopathy such as osteopetrosis.

The increase of osteomyelitis in patients with COVID-19 has been attributed to immune system dysfunction and tissue hypoxia secondary to decreased blood flow vascular coagulopathy and increased perivascular tissue edema from an increased vascular permeability.[2]

The clinical presentation of OMJ consists of deep intense pain, high intermittent fever, paresthesia or anesthesia of the lower lip (when located in the mandible), increased white blood cell count, elevated erythrocyte sedimentation rate (ESR), and usually an identifiable source. The paresthesia/anesthesia of the lower lip is secondary to the edema and increased pressure on the inferior alveolar neurovascular bundle within a confined space. The early detection and diagnosis of OMJ is based on a high degree of suspicion.[5,9]

In the early state of acute osteomyelitis, plain film radiographs are usually nondiagnostic, but an orthopanographic radiograph is still recommended as the first imaging modality. A period of 4 to 7 days, and even longer, is required before sufficient calcium is lost from the bone to be detectable as an irregular radiolucency on plain radiographic films. This radiolucency is usually adjacent to the odontogenic cause, frequently a tooth extraction site, or jaw fracture line, including the hardware that might have been used to treat the fracture.[4,7]

Magnetic resonance imaging (MRI) has a high degree of sensitivity for detecting intramedullary inflammation. It should be considered to be the single most effective imaging modality for early diagnosis of acute osteomyelitis and should be used early when the suspicion for OMJ is high. MRI is not the best imaging method for surgical treatment planning because it can overestimate the amount of intramedullary infection as opposed to widespread edema.[4,7,10]

High-resolution computed tomography (CT), including cone-beam CT (CBCT), can also depict bony changes before they are evident on plain film radiographs. Fine-cut CT can define small sequestra, the margins of the infectious process, and cortical erosions. CT is essential when surgery is part of the treatment plan.[4]

Isotope scanning (scintigraphy) historically was considered the imaging technique for the diagnosis of acute osteomyelitis. However, because of its lack of specificity, scintigraphy has been replaced by more reliable imaging techniques. It still should be considered when multiple focal sites are suspected.

Because OMJ is an infection, identification of the causative organism is still the gold standard. Identification of the specific causative organism is difficult because of the contamination of the culture specimen by normal oral flora, especially when an intraoral technique is used. Surgical intervention is usually required to obtain a reasonably contaminant-free specimen. Multiple bone samples (three to five) should be obtained free of salivary contamination. In spite of obtaining noncontaminated samples, there is a 28 to 50% chance that no causative organisms will be identified. Hence the need for multiple samples and prolonged culture time (up to 14 days) to isolate slow-growing or dormant organisms.[11-13] The most frequent encountered organisms are viridians streptococci and oral anaerobes such as *Peptostreptococcus, Fusobacterium,* and *Prevotella* species. *Actinomyces* species and *Eikenella corrodens* may be contaminants in the original specimens but take on increased importance if antibiotic therapy is subtherapeutic. If dental implants are part of the infectious process, *Staphylococcus aureus* and coagulase-negative staphylococci need to be considered. The close collaboration with the microbiologic laboratory is necessary to ensure that specimens are handled appropriately and are incubated for a sufficient time and that special techniques are used when necessary.[5,6,14]

The treatment of acute osteomyelitis is contingent upon early suspicion and recognition. Osteomyelitis, though an infection, needs to be considered a surgical disease. Treatment should be aimed at obtaining contaminant-free specimens for microbiologic assessment. At the same time, specimens should be taken for histologic examination. Histologic examination may identify *Actinomyces* species or tuberculosis when culturing is ineffective. The same specimens can be used to rule out a neoplastic process. Empiric use of a penicillin-type antibiotic should be considered. True penicillin allergy should be established. There is a high failure rate for patients who are penicillin allergic. This may be attributed to multiple rounds of clindamycin that produced increased resistance in polymicrobial staphylococcal infections.[15]

Surgical intervention based on CT planning has two other goals in addition to obtaining contaminant-free microbiologic specimens. Removal of the necrotic bone reduces the bioburden and allows the bone immune response to be more effective. As one of the initiating factors of osteomyelitis is a compromised blood supply, surgical intervention should be designed to decompress the medullary portion of the bone and to increase the blood flow to the area. Sequestrectomy, saucerization, and decortication have all been described in the literature to accomplish this goal.[5]

Removal of the precipitating cause of the infection is the basis of all infection treatment. If the initial source of the infection is odontogenic, this must be addressed. Extraction of the offending tooth is usually the treatment of choice. If the infection is related to fracture fixation hardware or a dental implant, removal of this foreign material needs to be considered.

The patient's immune status needs to be assessed. Undiagnosed diseases such as human immunodeficiency virus (HIV) or diabetes (and now COVID-19) need to be considered. Systemic health should be optimized through nutrition assessment and identification of substance abuse issues, including tobacco and alcohol. Consider early consultation with an infectious disease specialist or other internal medicine physician.

Secondary Chronic Osteomyelitis

Chronic OMJs have been arbitrarily defined as a bone marrow infection of at least bone six weeks in duration. It is normally preceded by the acute phase. Secondary chronic osteomyelitis of the jaw (SCOMJ) is characterized by dead bone that is colonized by organisms that can no longer be treated by antibiotics alone.[7]

SCOMJ manifests with facial swelling, pain, possibly intraoral fistulae with purulent drainage, nonhealing exposed bone, and overlying soft tissue wounds with draining fistulae. The pain characterization may have changes along with changes in paresthesia/anesthesia. The focused medical history reveals the condition has been present for at least 1 month with signs and symptoms consistent with acute OMJ. The acute phase may have been treated unsuccessfully with antibiotics. Initial treatment may have been unsuccessful for a variety of reasons, including the causative bacteria was not identified or may now have mutated, the antibiotic choice was inappropriate or an insufficient dose and/or duration, and a lack of identification of cofactors that alter the body to mount an effective immune response.[5]

Because of the reclassification of the infection process from acute to chronic has been arbitrarily defined as 1 month, there is an overlay and overlap of signs, symptoms, and other diagnostic criteria. Biopsies and radiographic image interpretation take on the important role of ruling out a neoplastic process. Further biopsy under sterile conditions is necessary to obtain contaminant-free specimens for microbiologic culturing and histologic examination for organisms, including fungi, that are difficult to culture, such as *Mycobacterium* and *Actinomyces*.

Surgery now becomes the primary treatment of SCOMJ with antibiotics taking on the role as adjunctive therapy.[16] Plain films, including panoramic radiographs, continue to have a role in patient evaluation. They may indicate a bony fracture that was the initiating event of the OMJ or a fracture resulting from the osteonecrotic process. Fine-cut CT scans are essential for the surgical treatment planning. CT is also useful for postsurgical follow-up and planning of any required reconstruction procedures (Figure 18-1).

Clinical Case of Osteomyelitis of the Jaws

A 65-year-old man was referred to the oral and maxillofacial surgery service by his general dentist for the extraction of a symptomatic right mandibular third molar. The tooth had communication with the oral cavity and had a history of prior episodes of pericoronitis that had been successfully treated with enteral antibiotics. The patient was otherwise in good general health and his list of medications only contained supplemental vitamins. He denied tobacco or alcohol use. The patient underwent an uncomplicated surgical extraction of the third molar and was placed on a 7-day

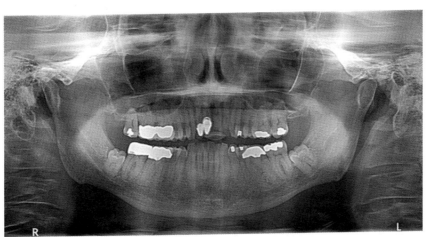

• **Figure 18-1** Preoperative Panoramic Radiograph of Impacted Mandibular third Molar Teeth.

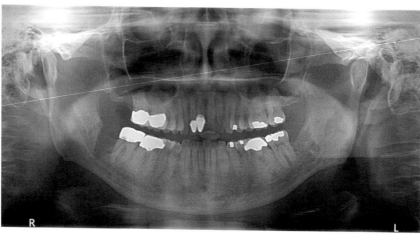

• **Figure 18-2** Panoramic Radiograph. Postoperative week 1: image revealing no fractures in the right mandibular angle region.

course of amoxicillin. His postoperative course was remarkable for pain and trismus mostly because of muscle spasm (Figure 18-2).

Panoramic radiographs obtained at postoperative week 1 and repeated at postoperative week 4 revealed the mandible to be intact and devoid of any obvious signs of osseous pathologic condition (Figure 18-3).

At the eighth postoperative week, the patient returned to clinic with a complaint of sudden return of right mandibular pain and malocclusion of 3 days duration. The patient denied any history of trauma and was afebrile. Examination of the mandible was difficult because of trismus and the presence of focal intense pain. Additionally, a small quantity of a purulent exudate was noted at the site of the previous extraction. A sample of the drainage was obtained and submitted to the laboratory for culture and sensitivity studies (Figure 18-4).

A radiograph revealed a nondisplaced fracture involving the right mandibular angle region. Radiolucencies consistent with osteolysis and ragged osseous borders and presence of a sequestrum were noted. The patient was asked to return to the clinic the following morning, and under intravenous sedation the wound was explored and a sample obtained for repeat culture. Additionally, the fracture site was debrided and curettage was performed of granulation tissue. Sequestrectomy and saucerization were performed, and specimens were also submitted for biopsy to rule out other noninfective pathology conditions. The patient was then placed into maxilla-mandibular fixation (Figure 18-5).

Two days after debridement, the patient reported increased malaise and a decision was made to have the patient admitted for further workup. The patient had a low-grade fever with a slight leukocytosis (13,000 mm^{-3} consisting of 78% polymorphonuclear leukocytes and 16% bandemia). CT scan was interpreted by the radiologist as being most consistent with a diagnosis of osteomyelitis of the mandible due to the soft and hard tissue changes present. An infectious disease consult was obtained to assist with the management of the patient. The patient was treated presumptively for osteomyelitis pending the results of the biopsy and the culture and sensitivity studies. He was empirically placed on intravenous broad-spectrum antibacterial coverage.

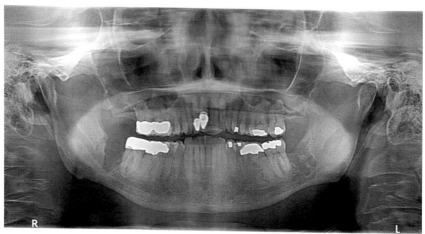

• **Figure 18-3** Panoramic Radiograph. Postoperative week 4: image revealing no gross evidence of osseous pathologic condition.

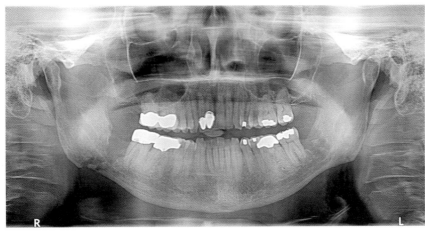

• **Figure 18-4** Panoramic Radiograph Obtained on Postoperative Week 8 Demonstrating a Pathologic Fracture of the Right Mandibular Angle and Presence of Sequesterae.

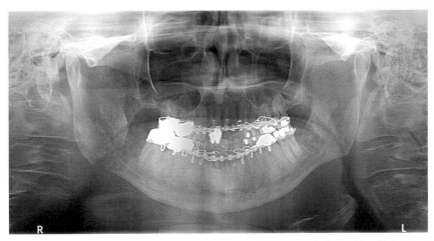

• **Figure 18-5** Panoramic Radiograph: Application of Erich Archbars and Maxillo-Mandibular Fixation.

Vancomycin and ampicillin-sulbactam (Unasyn) were recommended by the infectious disease consultant and implemented. Rigid fixation was also applied to the fracture site on post-admission day 4. Bone biopsy result returned consistent with osteomyelitis, and the culture revealed mixed oral flora. The patient was placed on a 4-week course of intravenous penicillin followed by a 3-month regimen of amoxicillin-clavulanate (Augmentin). The patient tolerated the antibiotic course and had a full recovery from the infection. The pathologic fracture of the mandible fully healed without any sequelae. He has been symptom-free for 12 months since the initial presentation.

Treatment of Secondary Osteomyelitis

Surgery

Surgery is the primary treatment modality for SCOMJ. The removal of dead, infected bone decreases the bioburden which the patient's immune system needs to deal. Every attempt needs to be made to obtain multiple contamination-free bony specimens that can be used for microbiologic

analysis. Similar specimens are needed for histologic evaluation to rule out a neoplastic process and to identify bacterial and fungal organisms that are difficult to culture. Lack of blood flow to the area is one of the etiologic factors in the development of OMJ. This lack of blood flow inhibits the body's ability to deliver nourishment and antibiotics to the affected bony site, inhibits the patient's immune system to react, and sets up an environment conducive for anaerobic bacterial growth. Surgical procedures should be designed to increase blood flow to the affected area. Additionally, consideration must be given to the stabilization of the bone remaining after surgery to prevent the potential of further complicating fractures. Fractures present at the time of the initial surgery should be treated appropriately.

Several surgical procedures are available, and they may be used singularly or in combination. Saucerization is the "unroofing" of bone in the affected site to expose the medullary cavity through debridement. This also decompresses the area and improves circulation. For saucerization procedures the exposed bone is packed open to allow for exfoliation of recognized sequestrum. Sequestrectomy is the removal of obvious nonviable bone. Decortication is the removal of chronically infected bone cortex with exposure of the medullary cavity. After thorough and aggressive debridement, primary closure is obtained as opposed to a saucerization procedure. For more aggressive disease, a resection procedure should be considered to remove all infected and nonviable bone. Bone stabilization must be obtained as part of the reconstructive plan. Bone grafting and dental implant placement are part of the reconstructive plan.[5-7] Conservative surgical procedures appear to have a lower success rate.[17]

Antibiotics

Antibiotic therapy is part of the SCOMJ treatment plan, but it must be considered as adjunctive therapy and not the primary modality. Antibiotic choice becomes a challenge for a variety of reasons. Previous antibiotic therapy may have been inadequate as to antibiotic choice, dosage level, duration of treatment, and/or lack of patient compliance. Current organisms may have developed antibiotic resistance. The primary causative organisms have been addressed, and now the causative organism is an opportunistic species or a previous contaminant. With soft tissue breakdown and bone exposure, other organisms may contaminate the site be it of an oral and/or skin origin. The development of a biofilm, abscess formation, and presence of dead bone have a dramatic negative effect on the ability of antibiotic penetration.[13]

To select the proper antibiotic, extra care needs to be taken to obtain contamination-free specimens. Multiple specimens should be obtained under sterile conditions. They should be obtained deep within the bone during the surgical phase of treatment. Ideally the patient should not have received any antibiotics for at least 14 days before obtaining the specimens.[12] There should be close coordination between the surgeon and the laboratory for proper culture and sensitivity testing. Particular attention is necessary in the identification of anaerobes because long culturing times are required. Histopathologic examination may be helpful in organism identification.[8] The presence of the same organism in more than one specimen increases the probability that the causative organism has been identified. It is not unusual to have negative culture results in spite of the best technique.[13]

Other laboratory tests are required to monitor the effectiveness of the treatment plan. Antibiotic blood levels should be monitored to determine that dose levels are sufficient to penetrate the biofilm and to ensure patient compliance. Although blood cell count and ESRs are useful, they are not the most sensitive tests to assess outcome. C-reactive protein may be a more reliable test for assessing treatment efficacy.[16]

The optimal duration of antibiotic is still undefined; however, there appears to be consensus that at least 6 weeks of therapy is required. Frequently therapy is started with intravenous antibiotics and then followed by longer-term oral antibiotics. There is evidence that oral antibiotics only is very successful and much more cost effective.[15] The length of treatment should be guided by the clinical signs and symptoms, C-reactive protein levels, and CT.[7-9,14,18]

Altered Immune Response

Altered immune response always must be considered in SCOMJ. Treatment of the source of an odontogenic infection usually results in its resolution, increasingly so with the addition of an appropriate antibiotic. When these infections do not resolve with appropriate treatment (assuming patient compliance), alterations in the body's immune system should be considered. A thorough patient medical and social history may reveal substance abuse and/or poor nutrition. Laboratory assessment may reveal undiagnosed diabetes, HIV, or COVID infection. When possible the patient's immune response system should be optimized.

Hyperbaric Oxygen

Hyperbaric oxygen (HBO) therapy might be considered as a treatment adjunct, especially when the treatment of the initial acute phase appears to have been appropriate. One of the precursors of osteomyelitis is decreased vascular flow that then results in localized hypoxia, which not only can lead to tissue death but also is excellent for anerobic bacteria to thrive. The addition of HBO has the potential to increase oxygen availability in the affected site. This increased oxygen improves cellular metabolism of the hypoxic tissue and produces a poor environment for anaerobic bacterial proliferation. HBO has the ability to enhance angiogenesis.[19-22]

Primary Chronic Osteomyelitis

Chronic osteomyelitis can manifest de novo without evidence of a preceding episode of acute osteomyelitis. Patients may be asymptomatic with the condition noted on a routine oral radiographic assessment. Focal sclerosing osteomyelitis (condensing osteitis) appears as sclerotic bone adjacent to the apex of a tooth.

Chronic recurrent osteomyelitis of children is usually multifocal. This is seen in the preteen and teen years. Assessment by radionuclide scintigraphy is indicated. This is an inflammatory process in which no infection source is readily identified. Hematogenous spread should be considered.

Diffuse sclerosing osteomyelitis is primarily seen in the mandible of women. It is an infectious process involving the bone and appears radiographically with a characteristic sclerotic pattern. The infection is most likely caused by *Actinomyces* species and *Eikenella corrodens*. The condition can be painful, and bone may be exposed to the oral cavity with a secondary infection from normal oral flora. Treatment is aimed at symptomatic relief. Therapy consists of localized surgical debridement and antibiotics.[14,18,23]

Conclusion

Although osteomyelitis has been recognized as a significant bone infection over the centuries, little in the literature has changed concerning its diagnosis and treatment. Even with antibiotics, for the most part OMJ is considered a surgical disease. Multiple bone biopsy samples taken under sterile conditions may improve the identification of a causative organism. Successful treatment outcomes appear to rely more on the surgical intervention than the antibiotic choice. The COVID-19 pandemic, with its unknown long-term consequences may result in an increase of OMJ worldwide. Early suspicion, early detection, and early surgical intervention are required.

References

1. Schmitt S. Osteomyelitis. *Infect Dis Clin North Am*. 2017;31: 325-338.
2. Pavic AK, Zučić V. Osteomyelitis of the jaws in Covid-19 patients: a rare condition with a high risk for severe complications. *Front Surg*. 2022;9:867088. Available at: https://doi.org/10.3389/fsurg.2022.867088.
3. Assouline-Dayan Y, Chang C, Greenspan A, Shornfeld Y, Gershwin ME. Pathogenesis and natural history of osteonecrosis. *Semin Arthritis Rheum*. 2001;32(2):94-124.
4. Schuknecht B, Valavanis A. Osteomyelitis of the mandible. *Neuroimaging Clin N Am*. 2003;13:605-618.
5. Topazian RG. Osteomyelitis of the jaws. In: Topazian RG, Goldberg MH, Hupp JR, eds. *Oral and Maxillofacial Infections*. 4th ed. Philadelphia: Saunders; 2002.
6. Wallace-Hudson J. Osteomyelitis. In: Fonseca RJ, ed. *Oral and Maxillofacial Surgery: Surgical Pathology*. Vol 5. Philadelphia: Saunders; 2000.
7. Baltensperger MM, Eyrich GH. *Textbook on Osteomyelitis of the Jaws*. Leipzig: Springer-Verlag; 2009.
8. Lew DP, Waldvogel FA. Osteomyelitis. *Lancet*. 2004;364: 369-379.
9. Hudson JW. Osteomyelitis of the jaws: a 50-year perspective. *J Oral Maxillofac Surg*. 1993;52:1294-1301.
10. Qaisi M, Montague L. Bone margin analysis for osteonecrosis and osteomyelitis of the jaw. *Oral Maxillofac Surg Clin North Am*. 2017;29:301-313.
11. Bertrand K, Lamy B, De Boutray M, et al. Osteomyelitis of the jaw: time to rethink the bone sampling strategy? *Eur J Clin Infect Dis*. 2018;37:1071-1080.
12. Lucidarme Q, Lebrun D, Vernet-Garnier V, et al. Chronic osteomyelitis of the jaws: pivotal role of microbiological investigation and multidisciplinary management—a case report. *Antibiotics*. 2022;11(5):568. Available at: https://doi.org/10.3390/antibiotics11050568.
13. Urish KL, Cassat JE. *Staphylococcus aureus* osteomyelitis. *Infect Immunol*. 2020;88(7):1-10.
14. Chiu CT, Chiang WE, Chuang CY, Chang SW. Resolution of oral bisphosphonate and steroid-related osteonecrosis of the jaws: a serial case analysis. *J Oral Maxillofac Surg*. 2010;68:1055-1063.
15. Lim R, Mills C, Burke AB, et al. Are oral antibiotics an effective alternative to intravenous antibiotics in the treatment of osteomyelitis of the jaw? *J Oral Maxillofac Surg*. 2021;79:1882-1890.
16. Hogan A, Hepport VC, Suda AJ. Osteomyelitis. *Arch Orthop Trauma Surg*. 2023;133:1183-1196.
17. Baur DA, Altay MA, Flores-Hidalgo A, Ort Y, Queresby FA. Chronic osteomyelitis of the mandible: diagnosis and management—an institution's exposure over years. *J Oral Maxillofac Surg*. 2015;73:655-665.
18. Lazzarini L, Lipsky BA, Mader JT. Antibiotic treatment of osteomyelitis: what have we learned from 30 years of clinical trials. *Int J Infect Dis*. 2005;9:127-138.
19. Uçkay I, Jugun K, Gamulin A, Wagener J, Hoffmeyer P, Lew D. Chronic osteomyelitis. *Curr Infect Dis Rep*. 2012;14:566-575.
20. Gaetti-Jardim Jr E, Landucci LF, de Oliveira KL, et al. Microbiota associated with infections of the jaws. *Int J Dent*. 2012;2012:369751. doi: 10.1155/2012/369751. Epub 2012 Jul 8. PMID: 22829824; PMCID: PMC3399405
21. Hudson JW. Osteomyelitis of the jaws: a 50-year perspective. *J Oral Maxillofac Surg*. 1993;52:1294-1301.
22. Wallace-Hudson J. Osteomyelitis. In: Fonseca RJ, ed. *Oral and Maxillofacial Surgery: Surgical Pathology*. Vol 5. Philadelphia: Saunders; 2000.
23. Bevin CR, Inwards CY, Keller EE. Surgical management of primary chronic osteomyelitis: a long-term retrospective analysis. *J Oral Maxillofac Surg*. 2008;66:2073-2085.

19

Oropharyngeal and Tonsillar Infections

DANIEL P. RUSSO, JAMES G. NAPLES, AND KOUROSH PARHAM

Infections of the oropharynx and tonsils are common infections that account for a significant amount of health care costs. Acute pharyngitis occurs in both children and adults and is one of the most frequent reasons for a physician visit, with an estimated 15 million outpatient visits per year.[1] It is often considered a disease of the pediatric population, with some estimates that it accounts for 7.3 million pediatric visits each year and 37% of all children presenting to an outpatient clinic.[2,3] Children are commonly 5 to 12 years old, and the incidence is estimated to be 12.8 per 100,000 patient years. It is also a relatively common complaint in the adult population, with an incidence of 4.7 per 100,000 patient years.[4]

A variety of infectious agents are responsible for acute oropharyngeal infections, and differentiating among the pathogens is a challenge to even the most experienced physician. The constellation of symptoms is often concerning to the affected patient, but the disease is often self-limited. Viral causes of pharyngitis are more common than bacterial.[5-7] Bacterial causes can have unwanted systemic and locally advanced sequelae if not treated appropriately. In an era of increasing antibiotic resistance, the workup of pharyngitis should be thorough and the treatment options should be carefully considered. A more complete thought process on the part of the physician will ultimately lead to improved diagnostic ability and a more judicious use of antibiotics.

Complications do occur with pharyngitis. They are uncommon overall, but can be life threatening. Suppurative complications resulting from rapid spread of infection to deeper spaces of the neck can result in airway compromise if not recognized in a timely manner. There are also systemic, nonsuppurative complications for bacterial and viral pharyngitis that need to be considered when evaluating acute oropharyngeal infections. Fortunately, improving antibiotic therapies and recognition of worsening symptoms has decreased complications of pharyngitis.[8]

The economic impact of pharyngitis is significant. Because it accounts for such a large percentage of patient visits to a physician, it has a large economic burden. Most of the economic burden comes from time lost at work for parents of children with strep throat, and this has been estimated to be 224 to 539 million dollars per year in the United States.[9,10]

It is clear that acute infections of the oropharynx and tonsils play a significant role in pathologic conditions of the head and neck. The discussion of oropharyngeal infections is broad and has become a much broader topic with the introduction of human papillomavirus (HPV) as a causative agent in oropharyngeal cancer. This chapter focuses on acute oropharyngeal infections. Appropriate workup and diagnostic measures will be reviewed, along with medical and surgical therapies. Finally, the chapter discusses specific complications and how they can be avoided and managed.

Anatomy

The anatomy of the pharynx can be cumbersome because of the great number of structures in a crowded anatomic space. There are three distinct regions of the pharynx: the nasopharynx, the oropharynx, and the hypopharynx. The oropharynx starts at the anterior tonsillar pillars bilaterally, which consist of the palatoglossus muscles. It includes the tonsils, thus making tonsillar infections a specific subsite of the oropharynx. Superiorly it extends from the soft palate to the posterior pharyngwall, where it is separated from the nasopharynx. Inferiorly, its boundary is the hyoid bone to the posterior pharyngeal wall, where it lies above the hypopharynx (Figure 19-1). The major subsites of the oropharynx include soft palate/uvula, tongue base, tonsils, and lateral/posterior pharyngeal wall.[11]

The blood supply of the oropharynx comes mostly from the ascending pharyngeal branch of the external carotid. The sensory innervation is via the glossopharyngeal plexus and includes cranial nerves IX and X.[5] A majority of the lymphatic drainage is unilaterally to levels II, II, and IV in the neck, which explains why infections may manifest with anterior cervical adenopathy.

Causes (See Table 19-1)

Viral

Viruses are the most common cause of oropharyngeal and tonsillar infections.[1,4-6,12,13] These infections occur as a constellation of symptoms related to the common cold or upper respiratory tract illness, but some warrant particular

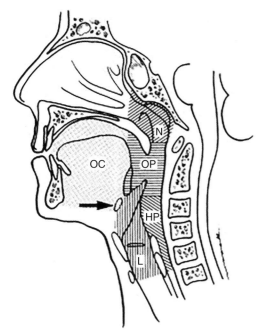

• **Figure 19-1** Anatomy Demonstrating the Boundaries of the Oropharynx in Relation to Other Upper Aerodigestive Anatomy. *HP,* Hypopharynx; *L,* larynx; *N,* nasopharynx; *OC,* oral cavity; *OP,* oropharynx. (Borrowed from Anderson JC, Homan JA. Radiographic correlation with neck anatomy. *Oral Maxillofac Surg Clin N Am.* 2006;20[3]:311-319.)

TABLE 19-1	Infectious Causes of Acute Pharyngitis	
Bacteria	**Viral**	**Atypical Bacteria**
Group A β-hemolytic Streptococcus	Adenovirus	*Mycoplasma pneumonia*
Group C Streptococcus	Herpes simplex virus 1 and 2	*Chlamydiophila pneumoniae*
Neisseria gonorrhoeae	Coxsackievirus	*Chlamydiophila psittaci*
Corynebacterium diphtheriae	Rhinovirus	
Fusobacterium necrophorum	Coronavirus	
Francisella tularensis	Influenza A and B	
Yersinia pestis	Parainfluenza	
Treponema pallidum	Respiratory syncytial virus	
Mixed anaerobes	Epstein-Barr virus	
	Cytomegalovirus	
	Human immunodeficiency virus	

Data adapted from Weber R. Pharyngitis. *Prim Care Clin Office Pract.* 2014;41(1):91-98.

attention and different treatments. The viruses most often responsible are respiratory viruses: rhinovirus, adenovirus, coronavirus, parainfluenza, influenza, and respiratory syncytial virus (RSV). These are the organisms that cause some variation of the common cold. They are usually self-limited and of little clinical significance because they do not require intervention on the part of the physician. The viral causes of oropharyngeal infections that have more clinically significant implications are Epstein-Barr virus (EBV), human immunodeficiency virus (HIV), cytomegalovirus (CMV), and herpes simplex virus (HSV). Most recently, the pandemic-inducing novel coronavirus-19 (2019-nCoV) has also demonstrated episodes of acute pharyngitis, in children predominantly.[14]

EBV (mononucleosis) is a herpesvirus. The virus infects B cells, which serves as a reservoir for the virus. These infected B cells circulate throughout a person's lifetime. The body's T cells respond by attacking the infected B cells, and in the acute setting it often causes an infection that can have severe complications involving a variety of organ systems. It often presents in the second decade of life with nonspecific symptoms of fatigue and cervical adenopathy in addition to pharyngotonsillitis. Data suggest that up to 95% of adults worldwide are infected with EBV.[15] In some cases the complications can become life threatening with upper airway obstruction or splenic rupture.[12,14]

HIV is the causative agent of acquired immunodeficiency syndrome (AIDS) and can manifest in the acute setting with an acute retroviral syndrome.[12,13] Symptoms include fever, pharyngitis, rash, headache, and adenopathy.[16] These symptoms can manifest within a few days after incubation of the virus, but occur more often 3 to 5 weeks after acquisition of the infection.[12] They occur as a result of the immune system's response to a large viral load. Cytokine release and inflammatory mediators manifest initially as nonspecific symptoms. It can mimic EBV and mononucleosis with its symptoms of sore throat and pharyngitis in addition to malaise and fatigue.

Herpes simplex virus-1 (HSV-1) is another viral cause of acute oropharyngeal infection. HSV-1 is an infection that manifests with oral lesions, pharyngitis with a prodrome, and adenopathy. This infection is termed *herpetic gingivostomatits* and can be quite severe and cause pain and dehydration. It is often seen in children with a painful swollen vesicle on an erythematous base, but asymptomatic seroconversion may occur in many people.[17] The vesicles of this virus often help differentiate it from other causes of pharyngitis or tonsillitis.

CMV is an infection that often manifests itself in immunocompromised patients; however, it can occur in patients with a competent immune system. In fact it has been reported that the seroprevalence of CMV is 60 to 100% worldwide. Most patients with a competent immune system have a benign course, but in severe cases, it can mimic a mononucleosis type of infection with pharyngitis.[18]

The 2019-nCoV is a novel enveloped virus responsible for COVID-19 and one of the largest pandemics in modern history. The condition resulted in significant morbidity and mortality, specifically in those with preexisting health conditions. Although the significant effects of this illness lie in its impact on the respiratory tract overall, sore throat and pharyngitis is a common finding, estimated to be the presenting symptoms in 28 to as high as 48% of cases.[14]

Bacterial

Several bacteria cause pharyngitis and tonsillitis, but the overwhelming majority of cases are due to group A *Streptococcus* (GAS). The traditional method for detecting bacterial colonization and infection of tonsil and adenoid tissue has been culture and polymerase chain reaction. However, recent advancement in molecular studies focused on DNA extraction has resulted in a more accurate and holistic picture of these surfaces' microbiomes. Results of such studies have demonstrated that adenotonsillar tissue is colonized by a diverse milieu of potentially pathogenic bacteria, even in healthy children. In fact, specimens of tissue collected from patients undergoing adenotonsillectomy has demonstrated collections of bacteria and purulent foci in the absence of

acute infection (Figure 19-2).[19,20] In children this organism is estimated to be responsible for 15 to 36% of cases of sore throat,[9,21] whereas in adults it is reported to account for 5 to 15% of cases of pharyngitis. Overall, GAS accounts for approximately 15 to 30% of pharyngitis in all cases of pharyngitis, regardless of age.[12]

This pathogen occurs among children aged 5 to 15 years old[10] and is frequently seen in the winter and early spring months. Unlike viral causes, it manifests without any prodrome, cough, or nasal congestion. One of the reasons that GAS is of such great clinical concern is that it can cause nonsuppurative complications of rheumatic fever and poststreptococcal glomerulonephritis. In fact, prevention of rheumatic fever is one of the most compelling reasons to treat GAS pharyngitis. Fortunately, these complications are rare, especially in developed countries.[11,12,22]

Streptococcal species such as group C and G β-hemolytic *Streptococcus* are also thought to be responsible for about 5% of pharyngitis and oropharyngeal infections,[4,6] but the clinical presentation is often milder. These also have been reported to cause nonsuppurative complications such as rheumatic fever.[7] Other bacteria species that should be considered in

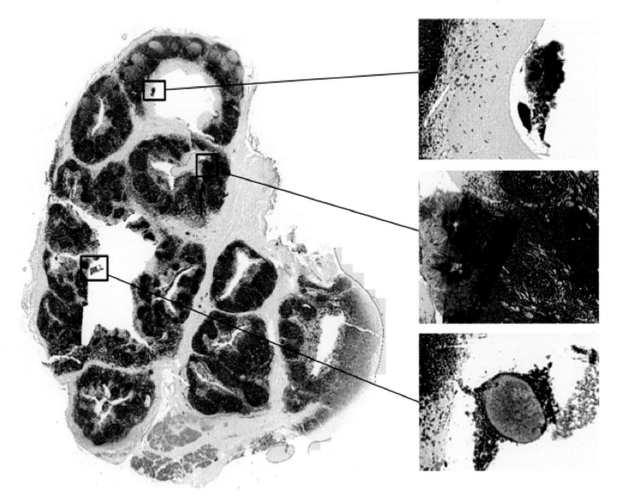

• **Figure 19-2** Coronal Section of a Palatine Tonsil from a Child with Recurrent Tonsillitis. CD-3 cells stained brown. CD-20 cells stained black. Bacteria stained in blue within the tonsillar parenchyma and crypts. (Borrowed from Johnson JJ, Douglas R. Adenotonsillar microbioma: an update. *Postgrad Med J.* 2018;94[1113]: 398-403.)

cases of oropharyngeal infections are *Actinomycetes, Neisseria gonorrhoeae, Corynebacterium diphtheriae, Chlamydia pneumonia,* and *Mycoplasma pneumoniae,* which all account for approximately less than 1% of pharyngitis in all patients.[12]

Diagnosis of these other bacterial causes of pharyngitis can be difficult, and often clinical suspicion is necessary to make these diagnoses. *Actinomycetes* is a bacterium that is part of the oral cavity flora; however, it can manifest with a picture of acute infection with suppurative complications in the oral cavity and oropharynx. Typically, an infection is caused in an immunocompromised host, but it can manifest as recurrent tonsillitis in children.[23] Diagnosis of actinomycosis infection requires biopsy and tissue that shows yellow, sulfur granules.[24] This can also mimic a tonsillar mass and adenopathy, which increases suspicion for malignancy in many patients (Figure 19-3). For patients in whom *N. gonorrhoeae* is considered, an adequate sexual history must be obtained. The advent of childhood vaccinations against diphtheria has been monumental in preventing *C. diphtheriae* as a cause of often life-threatening pharyngeal infections. It will manifest with a gray membrane coating the oropharynx that causes respiratory distress often requiring intubation and airway protection. A history of walking pneumonia will likely be a clue to the diagnosis of *Chlamydia* or *Mycoplasma pneumoniae.*

Fungal

Candida albicans represents a normal oral flora in most patients. However, in the immunocompromised, those at the extremes of age, or those receiving chronic antibiotic treatment, this fungus can become pathologic, although

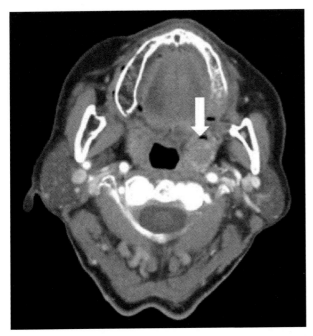

• **Figure 19-3** **Actinomycetes.** Note the left-sided asymmetry and rim enhancement *(arrow).* Biopsy showed sulfur granules and actinomycosis without evidence of malignancy.

nonpredisposed persons can and do develop oral candidiasis.[25] There are four main presentations for infection: (1) pseudomembranous (thrush), (2) erythematous, (3) hyperplastic, and (4) denture-induced stomatitis. In the thrush subtype, there are thick white plaques that can be easily removed from an inflamed mucosal surface. By contrast, the erythematous subtype results in smooth red patches overlying the mucosa of the palatal, lingual, or buccal surfaces. The hyperplastic subtype can appear similarly to pseudomembranous candidiasis; however, the infection cannot be typically scraped from the mucosa. Finally, denture-induced stomatitis can present with localized erythema to the denture-bearing surfaces of the maxilla and palate and fissuring to the corners of the mouth.[26]

History and Examination

The history and physical examination are essential to making an accurate diagnosis. An acute oropharyngeal infection or tonsillitis caused by a bacterium or a virus often manifests with subtle differences, and distinguishing between them is challenging. Acute infections often occur in younger populations, but when they do occur in adults, the organisms are often different and the strains have a tendency to be more resistant to treatment with different disease manifestations.[4,27] Asking whether someone has been exposed to a sick contact may help clue in the physician to an infection but does not necessarily indicate the causative organism. Many of the symptoms of sore throat, fever, fatigue, and dysphagia are overlapping. It is important to ask how long the symptoms have been present and whether episodes are recurrent, because these are key points that may alert the physician to the source of infection and the need for different management. Timing and seasonality of the symptoms also may be helpful in determining a specific organism. GAS and many of the respiratory viruses occur in the winter/early fall, whereas EBV and HIV can occur at any time.

Examination findings often are similar between both bacteria and viruses. Examination findings include erythema of the oropharynx, tonsillar exudates, uvular swelling, and cervical adenopathy. It is important when examining patients who have suspected oropharyngeal infections not to overlook signs of trismus, neck pain, and voice changes, which can indicate complications of pharyngitis.

The importance of differentiating GAS from other causes of oropharyngeal infections is essential because one of the reasons to treat streptococcal pharyngitis is to prevent nonsuppurative complications such as rheumatic fever caused by GAS. Often GAS infections manifest with sore throat without cough.[10] Clinicians have tried to create a set of clinical criteria to help diagnose streptococcal pharyngitis, but its utility is uncertain. These criteria, the Centor criteria, include a 4-point scoring scale based on signs and symptoms suggestive of GAS bacterial pharyngitis. This scoring system has been shown to have a high negative predictive value in some reports (81%) as opposed to its positive predictive value (48%).[5] Some studies show that even patients with all 4

TABLE 19-2	Centor Criteria*	
Modified Centor Criteria		
Fever	1 point	
Absence of cough	1 point	
Anterior cervical adenitis	1 point	
Tonsillar Exudate	1 point	
Age (y)		
2-14 y	1 point	
15-44 y	0 point	
≥ 45 y	−1 point	

*Note the modified version accounts for age.
Data adapted from Weber R. Pharyngitis. *Prim Care Clin Office Pract.* 2014;41:91-98.

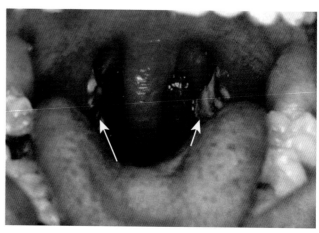

• **Figure 19-4** Bilateral Tonsillar Exudates *(arrows)*. This is an example of mononucleosis with erythema and exudates of the tonsils. (Adapted from Belleza W, Kalman S. Otolaryngologic emergencies in the outpatient setting. *Med Clin N Am.* 2006;90[2]:329-353.)

criteria have less than a 60% chance of having a positive throat culture, which is the gold standard for diagnosis.[1] The utility of a scoring system in making a diagnosis of GAS pharyngitis is that it helps stratify patients into high, medium, or low probability of having the disease. These criteria are used to guide further workup and should be used with additional diagnostic information to confirm GAS.[1,5] The use of these criteria alone can lead to an incorrect diagnosis of GAS and increase the use of unnecessary antibiotics. It is important to note that GAS often manifests differently in children/adolescents and adults, so the criteria do not necessarily apply equally to all patients; however, there is a newer scoring system that accounts for a patient's age (Table 19-2).

For many of the respiratory viral causes of oropharyngeal and tonsillar infections, the history will be slightly different and include symptoms of upper respiratory tract illness such a cough, coryza, and congestion. In more severe viral causes such as EBV and HIV there will be a stronger history of fatigue and systemic symptoms. EBV often affects patients in the second decade of life, with the highest incidence in patients 15 to 24 years old, and it occurs in college students and patients in close contact.[15] A strong suspicion on the part of the physician is often needed to diagnose these viruses because the symptoms initially closely mimic more benign, self-limited diseases.

Examination findings in these more virulent viruses also may be more diffuse and involve organ systems outside of the head and neck. Thus, if there is any suspicion for EBV, CMV, or HIV, a full examination is indicated.

EBV can manifest with bilateral tonsillar hypertrophy and exudates, palatal petechiae, rash, and splenomegaly, which occurs in 15 to 65% of patients (Figure 19-4).[15] HIV can mimic a mononucleosis-like infection in an acute retroviral syndrome. If there is any suspicion for HIV based on the history of the patient, a workup should be performed because after the acute phase, there is a latent period for the virus, in which there are no systemic symptoms for a number of years typically.[16] CMV can cause pharyngitis

with symptoms of vasculitis, liver disease, and fatigue.[18]

An adequate history needs to be taken if *N. gonorrhoeae* is suspected. Systemic symptoms and findings, such as arthritis or genitourinary symptoms such as pain and discharge, can be relevant for patients with pharyngitis and should not be ignored if discussed in the history.

C. diphtheriae is a historical point in developed countries since the advent of vaccination; however, the symptoms should be considered in patients who have not been immunized or are from underdeveloped countries. The oropharynx will be covered with a thick, gray membrane coating the oropharynx. It can be scraped off and causes bleeding and edema of the tissues beneath the membrane. The membrane over the oropharynx is often life threatening because of upper airway obstruction. It is associated with cardiac toxicity and neurotoxicity; thus a full history and examination is mandated.[12]

Diagnosis

Bacterial Causes

Although the diagnosis of acute oropharyngeal infections often can be made on the history and examination, it is important to determine the organism involved. It is essential to rule out GAS to avoid nonsuppurative complications and rheumatic heart disease. Because the symptoms for GAS are nonspecific, and clinical judgment is not an effective mean of accurate diagnosis,[6] different laboratory tests have been created to make this diagnosis.

With the appropriate use of the clinical scoring systems, it can help to guide the next step in treatment. If 2 or 3 of the Centor criteria are met, a rapid antigen detection test (RADT) should be performed. If 4 of the Centor criteria are met, it has been suggested that empiric treatment for GAS can be started or RADT performed.[1] The RADT is a throat swab that is used to detect cell wall carbohydrate antigens via a specific enzyme immunoassay antibody.[10,12] The sensitivities of this test range from 70 to 90%;[1,10,12] however, the specificity of this test is extremely high at greater than 95%.[1,7,10] Thus patients who have a positive RADT and symptoms of pharyngitis should have antibiotic therapy initiated. Patients without any symptoms do not need to be tested because a positive test without symptoms would indicate carrier status as opposed to being acutely infected. The diagnostic ability of the test increases if there is a greater likelihood of the patient having GAS pharyngitis.[7] If an RADT is negative, a throat culture should be sent as a more definitive test. Throat culture is ultimately the gold standard by which diagnosis of GAS pharyngotonsillitis is made. The throat swab for culture needs to be collected from the surface of the pharynx or tonsils because collections from other sites in the oral cavity reduce diagnostic accuracy.[1,10]

When this algorithm is used, the diagnostic sensitivity and specificity are both greater than 95%[1] and it is the most cost-effective management[10] (Figure 19-5)

Throat culture takes 24 to 48 hours to return. Because of the limited morbidity of the disease, risks of antibiotic resistance, and relative accuracy of most recent testing, guidelines released by the Infectious Disease Societies of America have advised against the use of empiric antibiotics and recommend antibiotic therapy only after a positive culture result.[28] The delay in treatment does not affect the rates of nonsuppurative complications such as rheumatic heart disease or poststreptococcal glomerulonephritis.[1,10] Currently the question of whether to treat GAS has been raised

because there are such low rates of rheumatic heart disease and renal involvement after GAS in the developed world.[7]

The algorithm of RADT followed by culture may be more useful in children and unnecessary in adults. Some reports recommend against a throat culture in the face of a negative RADT in adults because the incidence of GAS is lower and the incidence of rheumatic heart disease is minimal.[1]

Other, less common bacterial causes should be considered with throat culture to confirm the diagnosis. *N. gonorrhoeae* can be obtained by a throat culture on Thayer-Martin agar. It should be noted that asymptomatic colonization with *N. gonorrhoeae* can occur, however.[2] Culture of the pseudomembrane of *C. diphtheriae* should be performed on Loeffler or tellurite selective media.[6,12] In lieu of cultures, the nucleic acid amplification test (NAAT) has been deployed for *N. gonorrhoeae* and *Chlamydia trachomatis* testing. Although the U.S. Food and Drug Administration has not yet approved its use, the Centers for Disease Control and Prevention (CDC) does recommend it as a screening tool for these infections, given its increased sensitivity.[29]

Viral Causes

For many of the respiratory viruses that cause acute oropharyngeal and tonsillar infections, no diagnostic test is available. Most of the viral causes of the infection are self-limited; thus it is neither cost effective nor necessary to determine the

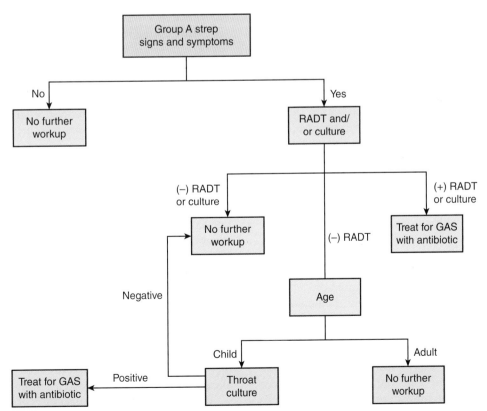

• **Figure 19-5** Algorithm for Workup of Acute Pharyngitis. (Adapted from Kociolek LK, Shulman ST. In the clinic: pharyngitis. *Ann Intern Med.* 2012;157[5]:ITC3-1–ITC3-16.)

organism. However, workup of EBV and HIV warrant special attention.

If EBV is suspected as a cause of acute pharyngotonsillitis, workup with laboratory tests is a necessary part of the evaluation. Because EBV often causes an infectious mononucleosis, workup with a complete blood count (CBC) and differential is necessary. The CBC will often show marked lymphocytosis,[5] which helps suggest EBV mononucleosis as opposed to a left-shifted leukocytosis of bacterial causes of oropharyngeal infections. Some reports indicate that a lymphocyte count of greater than 4.0×10^9 in patients with symptoms strongly suggestive of EBV is a reliable predictor of the infection. It should be still further confirmed with more specific testing, however.[30] Peripheral blood smear with more than 10% atypical lymphocytes also strongly suggests infection with EBV.

Further testing involved antigen/antibody interaction. EBV induces heterophile antibodies against viral antigens that cross-react with antigens from sheep and horse red cells, and these are present in approximately 90% of infected individuals within the first 2 to 3 weeks of illness.[12,15] The reported sensitivity and specificity of the heterophile antibody test is reported as 85 and 94%, respectively.[15] Rapid monospot tests are available for screening of patients with suspected EBV. Children often do not produce heterophile antibodies, so false negative results are more common in this age group.[12] Some reports indicate only 25 to 50% of 12-year-old children will be positive for this antibody.[15] It is important to note that these tests may be negative in patients who present with symptoms early in the viral course, so a negative test does not necessarily rule out an infection with EBV.

The diagnosis of EBV mononucleosis can be made with a combination of clinical presentation, atypical lymphocytosis, and presence of heterophile antibody. The confirmatory test is antibody titers to viral capsid antigens. Immunoglobulin-M (IgM) antibodies are seen within the first 4 to 8 weeks of a primary infection, and if positive, acute infection can be diagnosed. IgG can be present in the blood throughout one's lifetime. However, they are not present early in the infection, so will not help much in the acute setting.

If a patient presents with mononucleosis-type picture, but is EBV negative with a negative heterophile antibody, HIV and CMV infections should be suspected. CMV is often the cause, and is particularly important in pregnant women because of the risk to the fetus. This can be confirmed with testing for IgM and IgG antibodies.[5,18] The CDC recommends that testing begin with a combination immunoassay that detects HIV-1 and HIV-2 antibodies and HIV-1 p24 antigen. All specimens reactive on this initial assay undergo supplemental testing with an immunoassay that differentiates HIV-1 from HIV-2 antibodies. Specimens that are reactive on the initial immunoassay and nonreactive or indeterminate on the antibody differentiation assay proceed to HIV-1 nucleic acid testing for resolution.

Treatment (Medical Versus Surgical)

The treatment of acute oropharyngeal and tonsillar infections depends on the causative organism. Bacterial infections require antibiotics, whereas viral causes are self-limited. Treating oropharyngeal infections and tonsillitis is controversial because increased use of antibiotics has led to the concern of increased resistance among organisms. Thus it is suggested that treatment be started only for culture-proven cases, including GAS.[20] The rationale behind treatment is to prevent complications from the infection and shorten duration of symptoms. Studies of cost effectiveness of treatments indicate that starting empiric antibiotics for symptomatic adult patients was ineffective, and it leads to unnecessary overuse of antibiotics and increased medication side effects.[10]

Medical

GAS is the most common cause of pharyngotonsillitis; thus treatment options have been well studied for this organism. In fact, it is the only commonly occurring organism for which antibiotic therapy is indicated.[19] It has been shown that even bacterial infections are often self-limited, so treatment goals are essentially to avoid complications of the oropharyngeal infection.[1,12] Penicillin used to be the mainstay of antibiotic classes used for management of this organism, and there has yet to be a case of reported penicillin resistance in GAS.[4,6] Initiation of a 10-day course of penicillin dosing 3 or 4 times daily can be used as first-line therapy for penicillin-tolerant patients.[4,6,31] Amoxicillin is often used as a first-line therapy for GAS because of the once-daily dosing regimen. A 10-day course of amoxicillin has been shown to be just as effective as penicillin for GAS eradication in the oropharynx of acutely infected individuals.[1,32] Patients who have EBV and are being treated with antibiotics for a presumed bacterial pharyngitis often can present with a maculopapular rash when given amoxicillin or ampicillin. That can be used as a clue to aid in the diagnosis of EBV.

Oral cephalosporins are a reasonable second option for treatment because they have good coverage against GAS and eradicate the organism completely.[33] In patients who are allergic to penicillin, oral macrolide antibiotics are the best options for coverage of GAS oropharyngitis. The most commonly prescribed macrolides are azithromycin and clarithromycin because they have a lower side effect profile than erythromycin. Duration of treatment with azithromycin is typically only 5 days with once-daily dosing, which makes it an attractive therapy for convenience. The downside of treatment with macrolides is that resistance has been reported with short-term use of the antibiotic, which has not been seen with penicillins.[12,33] It is also a more expensive family of antibiotics. Thus it is typically reserved for penicillin-allergic patients and not used as a first-line therapy.

Treatment for other bacterial causes of pharyngitis can be pursued. In the case of *N. gonorrhoeae* and *C. trachomatis*, the therapy is equivalent to the protocol for genital infection (intramuscular ceftriaxone and oral azithromycin). Although infrequently encountered, *C. diphtheriae* should be treated with contact precautions, erythromycin or penicillin, and antitoxin.[34]

In addition to antibiotic therapy to treat the infectious agent in oropharyngitis, there is a role for adjuvant use of steroids in patients with GAS pharyngitis. Steroid use has been thoroughly studied in adult patients as a single dose during an acute infection. The mechanism of their action is thought to be mediated through an antiinflammatory effect, which helps reduce pain symptoms associated with severe oropharyngeal infections. They can be administered either orally or intramuscularly to help reduce symptoms of pain in acute infections and often lead to a quicker recovery.[35-37] The data on their use is mixed, however, and in GAS pharyngitis only a small clinical improvement can be expected.[38] They also can have unwanted side effects in some patients. Thus the decision regarding their use can be left to the clinical judgment of the physician.

For EBV infections and mononucleosis, the use of steroids is also an area of uncertainty. The data evaluating its efficacy in uncomplicated cases is mixed, and in uncomplicated cases steroids do not provide much therapeutic benefit. However, the most benefit appears to be derived in patients with severe tonsillar hypertrophy causing obstruction. Antivirals have been shown to be ineffective in treating EBV.[12,15] As with other viruses, the diseases are typically self-limited, so steroid treatment is for symptom relief and is not routinely required.

Treatment of oral and oropharyngeal candidiasis focuses on both primary management and preventive therapies for at-risk groups. Among immunocompromised individuals, primary treatment with either fluconazole or nonabsorbed antifungals, such as nystatin, is the mainstay of treatment. Still further, preventive therapy consisting of the same therapeutics is effective in management. This recommendation is appropriate for those undergoing chemotherapy and other iatrogenic immune suppression and individuals suffering from HIV. By contrast, among immunocompromised children and adolescents, primary therapy for the infection is advocated, but prophylactic measures are not well studied to be effective in the population. Finally, those suffering from denture-induced stomatitis should be treated for their primary infection, but prophylaxis and even strict denture hygiene has limited studied benefit.[26]

Surgical

For patients who have recurrent episodes of acute pharyngotonsillitis that continue despite multiple antibiotic courses, there is a surgical option of a tonsillectomy. Other indications for surgical management with tonsillectomy include suppurative complications of a pharyngotonsillitis such as a peritonsillar abscess. The criteria for tonsillectomy in patients with recurrent infection are debated.

However, current recommendations suggest a tonsillectomy for patient with seven episodes of pharyngitis in 1 year, five episodes in 2 consecutive years, and three in 3 consecutive years.[39,40] This is known as the Paradise criteria. However, recent guidelines for tonsillectomy have included some concessions, expanding the indication for tonsillectomy. For example, the American Academy of Otolaryngology–Head and Neck Surgery released updated guidelines for tonsillectomy in the pediatric population, recommending consideration of tonsillectomy for patients with "modifying factors which favor tonsillectomy." These included antibiotic allergies; periodic fevers, aphthous stomatitis, pharyngitis, adenitis (PFAPA) syndrome; or more than one lifetime occurrence of peritonsillar abscess.[41] Much of the debate around this topic is centered around the fact that there is no universal definition for an acute pharyngotonsillitis based on clinical criteria. In the studies used to define these surgical criteria, it was not necessary to document a cause of the infection.[40]

The expected benefit from having a tonsillectomy is a reduction in the frequency and severity of oropharyngeal infections for up to 2 years.[42] This benefit may be underestimated, however, because the study reporting this value included only severe cases of recurrent infection in the surgical arm of their study.[40]

Surgical management is not without risk. A tonsillectomy has the known risks of pain, dehydration, and bleeding that may require an additional surgical procedure to control it. Thus the options for management need to be strongly considered. Often a 12-month observation period is an option before tonsillectomy is performed.

Complications

The complications of acute oropharyngeal infections and tonsillitis can be broken down into two different types of complications: suppurative and nonsuppurative. The suppurative causes occur more frequently, and the nonsuppurative causes are quite rare in the industrialized countries. The rate of all complications has been reduced dramatically with the introduction of antibiotics; however, serious sequelae can occur if these complications are not identified.

Suppurative

The complications often seen with acute pharyngitis are abscesses and deep space neck infections. The complex anatomy and fascial planes of the head and neck create a number of pathways for spread of infection. There are many types of deep space neck infections, but the most common one in both children and adults is a peritonsillar abscess (PTA) (Figure 19-6).[43] A PTA can result in very serious complications, more commonly in males or adults older than 40, which include mediastinitis, extension into other deep neck spaces, and even necrotizing fasciitis.[44] However, the infection of an acute pharyngitis can spread to the parapharyngeal space, the buccal space, masticator space, the retropharyngeal space, the danger space, the prevertebral space, and the carotid space. The infection of an acute pharyngitis can

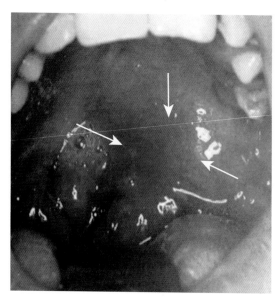

• **Figure 19-6** Left-Side Peritonsillar Abscess Demonstrating Bulging and Erythema of the Soft Palate *(Arrows)* with the Uvula Deviated to the Right. (Adapted from Belleza W, Kalman S. Otolaryngologic emergencies in the outpatient setting. *Med Clin North Am.* 2006;90[2]:329-353.)

directly extend, as well, into the parapharyngeal space, the buccal space, the masticator space, the retropharyngeal space, the danger space, the prevertebral space and the carotid space. Each of these spaces is its own distinct plane, and infection in some of these spaces can be life threatening if not treated appropriately. One series review of the literature from 1994 to 2004 found a mortality rate of 6.1 to 41.7% when life-threatening complications occurred.[45]

Acute pharyngitis is becoming a less frequent cause of these complications since the advent of penicillins, whereas there is an increase in deep space neck infection of odontogenic origin.[8,45] This emphasizes the need for a thorough evaluation of the dental structures during history and physical examination. Similarly, patients with complex medical histories such as diabetes or HIV tend to have atypical complications.[8]

Diagnosis of these complications often can be suspected on history and physical examination. When evaluating for deep space involvement, neck pain, and range of motion, in addition to any trismus or voice changes help raise suspicion for complications. Studies have tried to use clinical data as predictors of who will develop suppurative complications; however, this has not been shown to be useful as a predictive tool.[46]

The diagnosis often relies on imaging with CT scan with contrast enhancement, which has essentially become the standard of care to identify deep space suppurative infections.[8] Imaging is especially important in evaluating for retropharyngeal danger space and prevertebral infections because they can spread into the thoracic cavity. The one exception to that would be for an uncomplicated PTA, which often does not require imaging.

One other suppurative complication for the physician to be aware of is Lemierre syndrome, which results from PTA extension to the tonsillar veins and the internal jugular vein

(Figure 19-7). The spread of infection into the venous system will cause thrombosis in the vein, which leads to septic embolization and respiratory failure.[47] This was a complication that was much more common in the preantibiotic era but does occur still today. The complication is more common in children, with some more recent studies demonstrating rates as high as 14.4 cases per million in adolescents.[48,49] The organism that is classically associated with this syndrome is the anaerobe *Fusobacterium necrophorum,* and in fact it has been hypothesized that the increase in cases is explained by this bacterium's intrinsic resistance to macrolides and fluoroquinolones.[50] However, other organisms and polymicrobial infections can be responsible as well (Figure 19-8).

The diagnosis of these suppurative complications and deep neck infections caused by an acute pharyngitis is important because management often requires procedural or surgical intervention. Intravenous antibiotics with penicillins such as ampicillin/sulbactam or clindamycin are considered first-line antibiotics. Clindamycin provides good anaerobic coverage for the polymicrobial environment of the abscess. Studies analyzing the complications of a deep neck infection found that the only prognostically significant factor contributing to complications was the involvement of more than one neck space, whereas hospital stays were likely to be increased in patients with medical comorbidities, a leukocytosis, and the need for both medical and surgical treatment.[45]

The role of the physician in knowing when to be suspicious for a deep space neck infection cannot be overemphasized. Despite the fact that medical treatments are improving the rates of these complications, they do occur and can have serious sequelae if not diagnosed in a timely manner.

Nonsuppurative

Acute rheumatic fever and glomerulonephritis are the nonsuppurative complications that are most concerning after an acute infection of the oropharynx. It is beyond the scope of this chapter to discuss how to manage these complications or work them up; however, it is essential to be aware of the fact that there are systemic complications. These complications are typically a result of a GAS pharyngitis. The mechanism is due to cross-reactivity and molecular mimicry of the streptococcus antibody within different organs.[51] Traditionally, the nonsuppurative complications of acute pharyngotonsillitis are the reason that this often self-limited disease is treated. With the use of antibiotics some studies have reported 80% reduction in the incidence of acute rheumatic fever when compared to no antibiotics.[10]

Acute rheumatic fever can cause a wide constellation of nonspecific symptoms that include arthritis, carditis, subcutaneous nodules, and chorea. Symptoms usually manifest approximately 2 to 3 weeks after an acute GAS pharyngitis. It is rare in developed countries; however, rheumatic heart disease after an acute GAS oropharyngeal infection is the leading cause of acquired heart disease in many countries,

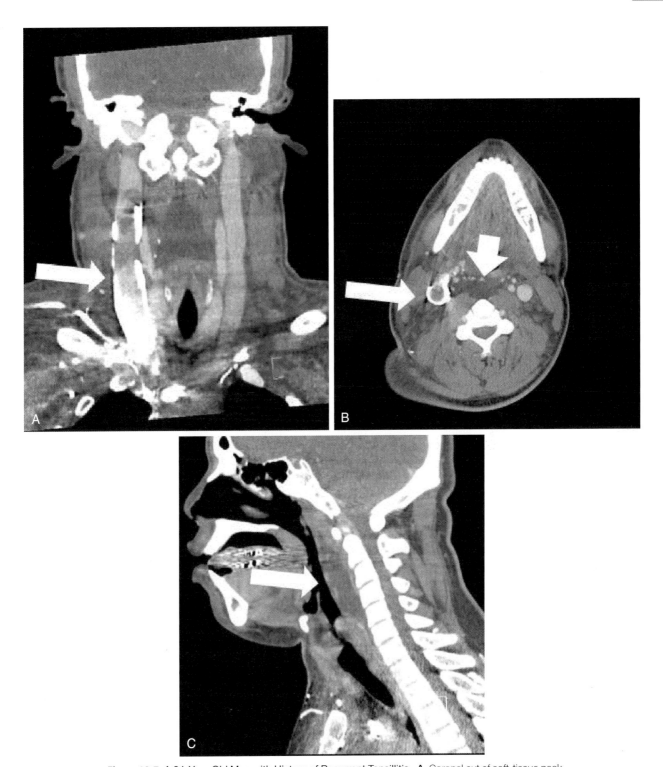

• **Figure 19-7** A 24-Year-Old Man with History of Recurrent Tonsillitis. **A,** Coronal cut of soft-tissue neck CT scan with contrast demonstrating thrombosis of right internal jugular vein *(arrow)* from acute tonsillitis leading to retropharyngeal phlegmon. **B,** Axial cut demonstrating retropharyngeal phlegmon *(short arrow)*, tonsillar edema, and right internal jugular vein thrombosis *(long arrow)*. **C,** Sagittal cut demonstrating retropharyngeal phlegmon *(arrow)*.

such as sub-Saharan Africa, India, and Australia,[10] and it is the leading cause of cardiovascular death in some developing areas of the world.[51] There is little evidence to support the idea the treatment of acute pharyngitis caused by GAS prevents acute glomerulonephritis.[10,12]

Nonsuppurative complications can also occur in conjunction with acute pharyngotonsillar infections not caused by GAS. In EBV infections systemic complications such as splenic rupture can occur and be life threatening. It occurs in approximately 0.5 to 1% of cases of primary EBV infection.[15]

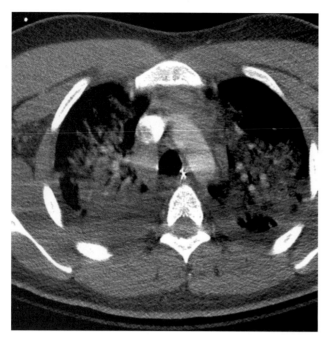

• Figure 19-8 Extensive bilateral airspace opacities consistent with acute respiratory distress syndrome in a male 17-year-old patient presenting with anerobic tonsillitis *(Fusobacterium necrophorum)* and sepsis.

EBV has the potential to cause multiple hematologic complications, such as hemolytic anemia, thrombocytopenia, and hemolytic-uremic syndrome.[15] Superimposed bacterial pharyngitis with EBV pharyngotonsillitis can cause deep space neck abscess.

Awareness of these potential nonsuppurative complications is essential because their management can be complex and involve multiple medical teams. Timely diagnosis is necessary to prevent complications or organ failure as a result of the systemic involvement.

Conclusions

Oropharyngeal and tonsillar infections are responsible for a large percentage of visits to the physician each year. The causative organisms can be bacterial, viral, or both. Although viral causes are more common, the bacterial causes often require a more involved workup because failure to treat them can have more severe consequences. Viral causes are treated with supportive care, but particular care should be taken not to overlook EBV and HIV as potential viral organisms causing pharyngitis. GAS pharyngitis is the most common bacterial cause of oropharyngeal infection. Fast and accurate diagnosis of GAS is essential because starting antibiotic therapy will help prevent both suppurative and nonsuppurative complications. This diagnosis can be facilitated with rapid antigen detection test and confirmed with throat culture. Once the causative organism is identified, prompt initiation of antibiotics with either penicillin or cephalosporin should be started. For recurrent infections or suppurative complications, surgical intervention should be given consideration as well. For a physician, prompt treatment must be weighed

against being too aggressive and increasing antibiotic resistance. This is an area that will continue to make acute pharyngitis and tonsillitis a topic of discussion in the future.

References

1. Kociolek LK, Shulman ST. In the clinic: pharyngitis. *Ann Intern Med.* 2012;157(5):ITC3-1-ITC3-16.
2. Murray PR, Rosenthal KS, Pfaller MA. *Medical Microbiology.* 6th ed. Philadelphia: Mosby/Elsevier; 2009:947.
3. Cirilli AR. Emergency evaluation and management of the sore throat. *Emerg Med Clin North Am.* 2013;31(2):501-515.
4. Mitchell MS, Sorrentino A, Centor RM. Adolescent pharyngitis: a review of bacterial causes. *Clin Pediatr (Phila).* 2011;50(12):1091-1095.
5. Chan TV. The patient with sore throat. *Med Clin North Am.* 2010;94(5):923-943.
6. Murray RC, Chennupati SK. Chronic streptococcal and non-streptococcal pharyngitis. *Infect Disord Drug Targets.* 2012;12(4):281-285.
7. European Society for Clinical Microbiology and Infectious Diseases, Pelucchi C, Grigoryan L, et al. Guideline for the management of acute sore throat. *Clin Microbiol Infect.* 2012;18(suppl 1):1-28.
8. Vieira F, Allen SM, Stocks RMS, Thompson JW. Deep neck infection. *Otolaryngol Clin North Am.* 2008;41(3):459-483, vii.
9. Pfoh E, Wessels MR, Goldmann D, Lee GM. Burden and economic cost of group A streptococcal pharyngitis. *Pediatrics.* 2008;121(2):229-234.
10. Wessels MR. Clinical practice: streptococcal pharyngitis. *N Engl J Med.* 2011;364(7):648-655.
11. Lee KJ. *Essential Otolaryngology Head & Neck Surgery.* New York: McGraw Hill Professional; 2012:1 electronic text (xvii, 1117 p. ill).
12. Bisno AL. Acute pharyngitis. *N Engl J Med.* 2001;344(3):205-211.
13. Weber R. Pharyngitis. *Prim Care.* 2014;41(1):91-98.
14. Patel NA. Pediatric COVID-19: systematic review of the literature. *Am J Otolaryngol.* 2020;41:102573.
15. Luzuriaga K, Sullivan JL. Infectious mononucleosis. *N Engl J Med.* 2010;362(21):1993-2000.
16. Hernandez-Vargas EA, Middleton RH. Modeling the three stages in HIV infection. *J Theor Biol.* 2013;320:33-40.
17. Usatine RP, Tinitigan R. Nongenital herpes simplex virus. *Am Fam Physician.* 2010;82(9):1075-1082.
18. Rafailidis PI, Mourtzoukou EG, Varbobitis IC, Falagas ME. Severe cytomegalovirus infection in apparently immunocompetent patients: a systematic review. *Virol J.* 2008;5:47.
19. Swidsinski A, Göktas O, Bessler C, et al. Spatial organisation of microbiota in quiescent adenoiditis and tonsillitis. *J Clin Pathol.* 2007;60:253-260.
20. Johnston JJ, Douglas R. Adenotonsillar microbiome: an update. *Postgrad Med J.* 2018;94:398.
21. Rufener JB, Yaremchuk KL, Payne SC. Evaluation of culture and antibiotic use in patients with pharyngitis. *Laryngoscope.* 2006;116(10):1727-1729.
22. Martin JM, Green M. Group A streptococcus. *Semin Pediatr Infect Dis.* 2006;17(3):140-148.
23. Melgarejo Moreno P, Meseguer DH, Garrido AM, et al. A correlation between age and *Actinomyces* in the adenotonsillar tissue of children. *B-ENT.* 2006;2(2):95-97.
24. Carinci F, Polito J, Pastore A. Pharyngeal actinomycosis: a case report. *Gerodontology.* 2007;24(2):121-123.

25. Bassiouny A, El-Refai HA, Nabi EA, Fateen AM, Hendawy DS. Candida infection in the tongue and pharynx. *J Laryngol Otol.* 1984;98:609-612.

26. Pankhurst CL. Candidiasis (oropharyngeal). *BMJ Clin Evid.* 2013 Nov 8;2013:1304. PMID: 24209593; PMCID: PMC3821534.

27. Brook I, Foote Jr PA. Comparison of the microbiology of recurrent tonsillitis between children and adults. *Laryngoscope.* 1986;96(12):1385-1388.

28. Shulman ST, Bisno AL, Clegg HW, et al. Clinical practice guideline for the diagnosis and management of group A streptococcal pharyngitis: 2012 update by the Infectious Diseases Society of America. *Clin Infect Dis.* 2012;55:e86-e102.

29. Workowski KA, Boylan GA. Sexually transmitted diseases treatment guidelines, 2015. *MMWR Recomm Rep.* 2015;64(3):1-137.

30. Biggs TC, Hayes SM, Bird JH, Harries PG, Salib RJ. Use of the lymphocyte count as a diagnostic screen in adults with suspected Epstein-Barr virus infectious mononucleosis. *Laryngoscope.* 2013;123(10):2401-2404.

31. Zoorob R, Sidani MA, Fremont RD, Kihlberg C. Antibiotic use in acute upper respiratory tract infections. *Am Fam Physician.* 2012;86(9):817-822.

32. Feder Jr HM, Gerber MA, Randolph MF, Stelmach PS, Kaplan EL. Once-daily therapy for streptococcal pharyngitis with amoxicillin. *Pediatrics.* 1999;103(1):47-51.

33. Shulman ST. Evaluation of penicillins, cephalosporins, and macrolides for therapy of streptococcal pharyngitis. *Pediatrics.* 1996;97(6 Pt 2):955-959.

34. Farizo KM, Strebel PM, Chen RT, et al. Fatal respiratory disease due to *Corynebacterium diphtheriae*: case report and review of guidelines for management, investigation, and control. *Clin Infect Dis.* 1993;16:59-68.

35. O'Brien JF, Meade JL, Falk JL. Dexamethasone as adjuvant therapy for severe acute pharyngitis. *Ann Emerg Med.* 1993;22(2):212-215.

36. Wei JL, Kasperbauer JL, Weaver AL, Boggust AJ. Efficacy of single-dose dexamethasone as adjuvant therapy for acute pharyngitis. *Laryngoscope.* 2002;112(1):87-93.

37. Tasar A, Yanturali S, Topacoglu H, et al. Clinical efficacy of dexamethasone for acute exudative pharyngitis. *J Emerg Med.* 2008;35(4):363-367.

38. Wing A, Villa-Roel C, Yeh B, et al. Effectiveness of corticosteroid treatment in acute pharyngitis: a systematic review of the literature. *Acad Emerg Med.* 2010;17(5):476-483.

39. Oomen KP, Modi VK, Stewart MG. Evidence-based practice: pediatric tonsillectomy. *Otolaryngol Clin North Am.* 2012; 45(5):1071-1081.

40. Darrow DH, Siemens C. Indications for tonsillectomy and adenoidectomy. *Laryngoscope.* 2002;112(8 Pt 2 suppl 100): 6-10.

41. Mitchell RB, Archer SM, Ishman SL, et al. Clinical practice guideline: tonsillectomy in children (update). *Otolaryngol Head Neck Surg.* 2019;160:S1-S42.

42. Ramos SD, Mukerji S, Pine HS. Tonsillectomy and adenoidectomy. *Pediatr Clin North Am.* 2013;60(4):793-807.

43. Baldassari C, Shah RK. Pediatric peritonsillar abscess: an overview. *Infect Disord Drug Targets.* 2012;12(4):277-280.

44. Klug TE, Greve T, Hentze M. Complications of peritonsillar abscess. *Ann Clin Microbiol Antimicrob.* 2020;19:32.

45. Staffieri C, Fasanaro E, Favaretto N, et al. Multivariate approach to investigating prognostic factors in deep neck infections. *Eur Arch Otorhinolaryngol.* 2014;271(7):2061-2067.

46. Little P, Stuart B, Richard Hobbs FD, et al. Predictors of suppurative complications for acute sore throat in primary care: prospective clinical cohort study. *BMJ.* 2013;347:f6867.

47. Ridgway JM, Parikh D, Wright R, et al. Lemierre syndrome: a pediatric case series and review of literature. *Am J Otolaryngol.* 2010;31(1):38-45.

48. Lee WS, Jean SS, Chen FL, Hsieh SM, Hsueh PR. Lemierre's syndrome: a forgotten and re-emerging infection. *J Microbiol Immunol Infect.* 2020;53:513-517.

49. Kuppalli K, Livorsi D, Talati NJ, Osborn M. Lemierre's syndrome due to *Fusobacterium necrophorum*. *Lancet Infect Dis.* 2012;12(10):808-815.

50. Kristensen LH, Prag J. Lemierre's syndrome and other disseminated *Fusobacterium necrophorum* infections in Denmark: a prospective epidemiological and clinical survey. *Eur J Clin Microbiol Infect Dis.* 2008;27:779-789.

51. Chakravarty SD, Zabriskie JB, Gibofsky A. Acute rheumatic fever and streptococci: the quintessential pathogenic trigger of autoimmunity. *Clin Rheumatol.* 2014;33(7):893-901.

20

Laryngitis, Epiglottitis, and Tracheitis

TIMOTHY JOHN O'BRIEN AND DAVIS AASEN

Infections of the larynx and trachea can vary from viral illness, such as the common cold, to life-threatening airway obstruction related to edema from bacterial infections. Both pediatric and adult infections are discussed here.

Anatomy

The larynx is located anteriorly to the fourth, fifth, and sixth cervical vertebrae. It is localized by the neighboring boundaries of the oropharynx superiorly, the hypopharynx posteriorly and inferiorly, and the trachea inferiorly. The larynx is composed of multiple cartilages, one bone (hyoid), and multiple ligaments and muscles. The cartilages include the thyroid, cricoid, epiglottis, and arytenoid cartilages. The laryngeal framework is composed of these cartilages and hyoid bone. The hyoid is not articulated to any other bone, but rather is connected distantly via muscular and ligamentous attachment. The hyoid is analogous to the "wishbone" or furcula of poultry.

The thyroid and cricoid cartilages compose the main framework. The thyroid cartilage has a notch superiorly that makes the protuberance of the Adam's apple. The cricoid cartilage marks the narrowest portion of the adult airway because it is the only complete circular ring of the airway (as opposed to the tracheal rings that are truly arches and not complete circular rings).

The epiglottis is composed of fibroelastic cartilage covered with a mucosal surface that tapers inferior to the petiole of the epiglottis. It has both a lingual surface that is considered within the boundaries of the oropharynx and a laryngeal surface that is part of the larynx. Anterior to the epiglottis is the preepiglottic space, a frequent route for spread of malignancy in this region. The vallecula includes the base of the tongue and the base of the lingual surface of the epiglottis. This is a familiar landmark for guiding the placement of various laryngoscope blades used to facilitate endotracheal intubation in securing a patient's airway during surgery.

Posteriorly along the larynx are the arytenoids, a paired set of pyramid-shaped cartilages that rest on the cricoid cartilage posteriorly. The arytenoids allow for a forward rocking and a rotational motion that leads to the adduction and abduction of the vocal folds. The three functions of the larynx, swallowing, phonation and respiration, all rely on the motion of the vocal cords. The intrinsic muscles of the larynx allow for vocal fold motion of the vocal folds. The true motion is more than just adduction and abduction; instead, it is a complex movement in all three dimensions. The vocal fold on either side is primarily composed of the thyroarytenoid muscle, ligament, and a fibroelastic epithelial layer.

The larynx is divided into three parts: the supraglottis, glottis, and subglottis. The supraglottis involves the tip of the epiglottis down along the aryepiglottic folds down to the false vocal folds (ventricular bands). The glottis is composed of the true vocal fold and posterior commissure.

The subglottis begins at the inferior aspect of the true vocal folds at the junction of the squamous and respiratory epithelium down to the inferior edge of the cricoid cartilage (Figure 20-1).

Supraglottitis (Including Epiglottitis)

Supraglottitis involves the inflammation and edema of the epiglottis and frequently the aryepiglottic folds and arytenoids. An interesting bit of history surrounds the theories of the death of George Washington. Many sources have assigned epiglottitis as the cause of death for the first president of the United States. However, further evaluation of the events surrounding his death raise a peritonsillar abscess or Ludwig angina as other possibilities. Or perhaps the bloodletting of 3.5 L of blood might shift more of the blame for his hastened death to his attending physicians.[1]

Epidemiology and Etiology

The more daunting history of epiglottitis involves pediatric infections during most of the twentieth century. Traditionally, in 75 to 90% of cases, the cause of this infection has been a bacterial infection of *Haemophilus influenzae* type B (Hib).[2] Before the Hib vaccine introduction in the 1980s, the most common age of contracting the disease was between 2 and 5 years. With the reduction of Hib infection with the vaccine, the incidence of the disease in children has decreased dramatically. The vaccine is currently given at 2, 4, and 6 months of age. The incidence of epiglottitis after the first 2 years of the vaccination program dropped 75%.

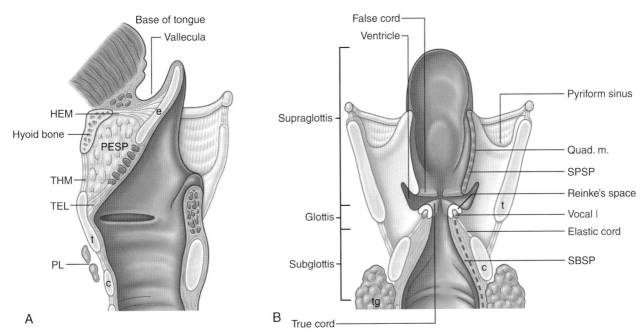

• **Figure 20-1 A,** Midsagittal section of the larynx. Note fenestrations in lower aspect of the epiglottic cartilage. **B,** Coronal section of the larynx. *c,* Cricoid cartilage; *e,* epiglottis; *HEM,* hyoepiglottic membrane; *PESP,* preepiglottic space; *PL,* prelaryngeal (Delphian) lymph nodes; *Quad. m.,* quadrangular membrane; *SBSP,* subglottic space; *SPSP,* supraglottic space; *t,* thyroid cartilage; *TEL,* thyroepiglottic ligament; *tg,* thyroid gland; *THM,* thyrohyoid membrane; *Vocal l,* vocal ligament. (From Gnepp DR. *Diagnostic Surgical Pathology of the Head and Neck.* 2nd ed. Philadelphia: Saunders/Elsevier; 2009.)

By 1996, the incidence of invasive Hib disease in children younger than 5 years had dropped by an astonishing 99%.[3]

Other pathogens such as *Streptococcus pyogenes, Streptococcus pneumoniae, Staphylococcus aureus,* nontypable *H. influenza, Haemophilus parainfluenza, Pseudomonas* species, *Klebsiella* species, *Pasturella,*[4] and *Moraxella catarrhalis* have been implicated. Nontypable *H. influenzae* is the most frequent pathogen in children who have received the vaccine. In adults, the incidence has not changed and has been approximately 1 to 4 per 100,000 per year, Adults are more likely to have the first two streptococcal pathogens listed. There is a slight seasonal variation in nontemperate climates.[5]

There have been additional reports in recent years of supraglottitis from viral pathogens, including COVID. This can be severe enough to require tracheostomy.[6]

Noninfectious causes can often lead to epiglottitis. Trauma to the throat can lead to supraglottitis. A child who has ingested a foreign object and then expelled it may have a delayed onset of edema. Inhaled recreational drugs or other chemicals, gases, or smoke inhalation can all lead to edema of the supraglottis in adult patients.[7] Importantly, supraglottic edema can be related to angioedema or angiotensin-converting enzyme inhibitor use.[8]

Symptoms

Sore throat is the most common symptom of epiglottitis, occurring nearly 100% of the time. A muffled voice, often characterized as a "hot potato" voice, is a classic presentation.

The altered volume of the upper airway from the edema of the supraglottis will change the resonance of the patient's voice, leading to a muffled quality. This voice quality should alert the clinician to the possibility of a severe infection. Frequently, a patient with epiglottitis will be drooling, unable to handle salivary secretions. Cervical lymphadenopathy and fever are also commonly present. When severe airway compromise is present, a child or adult can have stridor or tripod positioning (Figure 20-2). The tripoding is also referred to as the sniffing position; it occurs when a patient is sitting forward with hands on the knees and the neck projected anteriorly with slight extension of the head.

The presence of stridor and positioning is often a sign that the edema is severe and airway compromise is imminent; this is a true medical emergency. It should be noted that a child with epiglottitis has one symptom definitively absent. Cough is not present in epiglottitis, whereas it is the hallmark symptom of laryngotracheobronchitis (croup).

Evaluation

An ill-appearing child with stridor, posturing, and drooling can have the diagnosis made purely based on history and clinical findings. A well-appearing older child, teen, or adult with a sudden onset of muffled voice with sore throat may be more commonly seen in physician offices and emergency departments. However, in a fairly well-appearing patient, a simple oropharyngeal examination can help to differentiate between common acute tonsillitis versus a more inferiorly based and usually more severe infection

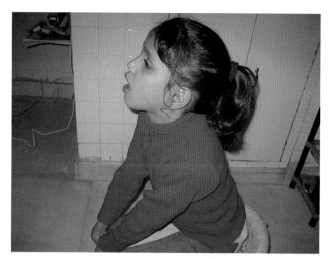

• **Figure 20-2** A Child Assuming the Tripod Position. (From Subramaniam R. Acute upper airway obstruction in children and adults. *Trends Anaesthsia Crit Care.* 2011;1:67-73.)

such as supraglottitis. Acutely hypertrophied tonsils resulting from infection will give the same quality of muffled voice and severe sore throat, but this hypertrophy rarely leads to any sort of concerning airway compromise, except for a possible short-term duration of obstructive sleep apnea. A patient with an acute change of a muffled voice with a sore throat and a normal oropharyngeal examination result should be considered to have a supraglottic process until proved otherwise.

When considering epiglottitis or supraglottitis, the tonsils and oropharynx are normal without exudate or hypertrophy. A lateral neck radiograph may be considered when evaluating the patient; however, this should not be done if it means a delay in properly securing a patient's airway in the operating room with a strong clinical suspicion for epiglottitis. The epiglottitis can be readily seen on a lateral neck radiograph. In supraglottitis, the epiglottis is usually enlarged and thickened; this yields the classic teaching of a "thumbprint sign" (Figure 20-3). A computed tomography (CT) scan of the neck is not necessary for the evaluation of epiglottitis and may actually exacerbate the patient's dyspnea with supine positioning for the examination. A CT scan may be helpful when evaluating deep neck space and parapharyngeal or retropharyngeal abscesses. However, with epiglottitis, having a patient lie supine on the table for a CT scan can often exacerbate dyspnea and it is not usually recommended.

Management

Airway management is the most critical component in the treatment of this infection. Consultation and further evaluation should be obtained from both an anesthesiologist and otolaryngologist when epiglottitis is suspected (Figure 20-4).

This is especially true with children who are suggested to have acute epiglottitis. A child who is tripoding or who has stridor should be handled with extreme caution. When considering all patients with possible airway concern or

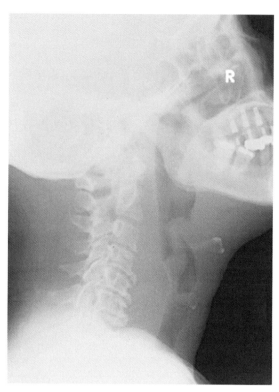

• **Figure 20-3** Lateral Neck Radiograph Reveals a Classic Thumbprint Sign of Epiglottic Edema. (From Sobol SE, Zapata S. Epiglottitis and croup. *Otolaryngol Clin North Am.* 2008;41:551-566. Courtesy M. Bitner, MD, MEd, FACEP.)

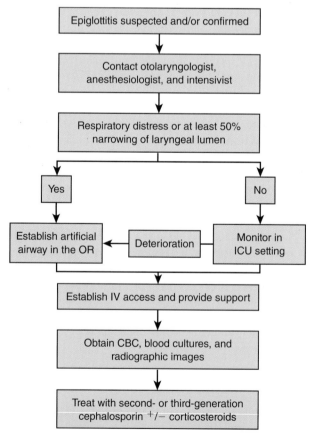

• **Figure 20-4** Algorithm for Treatment of Epiglottitis.

compromise, it is extremely important to have intravenous access for the administration of medications in emergency situations; however, this is often postponed in children with a concerning presentation. Upsetting young children can worsen their already compromised airway and lead to complete obstruction. Intravenous access, attempts at an oropharyngeal examination, or rectal temperature or even obtaining a lateral radiograph is often postponed. Instead, urgent otolaryngologic consultation is obtained for airway stabilization because of imminent acute respiratory failure.

Heliox is often used when airway edema is present as a temporary bridge until the airway is secured with intubation or tracheotomy. Helium mixed with oxygen has a lower viscosity than regular air because the gas mixture is composed of smaller molecules and thus passes through a narrowed region with greater ease.

A child with stridor and positioning has his or her airway secured with intubation in a controlled setting, usually in an operating room. Anesthetic gases are used to breath down the child without any paralytic agents. This leaves the child with spontaneous respiration but sufficiently sedated for laryngoscopy and intubation.

A culture swab can be obtained of the supraglottis at the time of intubation for culture. Inability or difficulty with intubation may necessitate tracheotomy or in an adult patient cricothyroidotomy, or needle catheter jet ventilation. Needle catheter jet ventilation can lead to the development of a pneumothorax if there is also compromise of the egress of the ventilated gases.

Airway stabilization is usually necessary in these severe cases for 24 to 72 hours. Sedated evaluation with laryngoscopy, often at the bedside in the intensive care setting, can be used to visualize and document improvement in supraglottic edema before extubation.

In adults, conservative airway management with vigilant monitoring in the intensive care unit setting is often successful, although intubation is necessary at times. A recent retrospective review at one institution found 11.6% of adults with endoscopy-confirmed epiglottitis required airway intervention supporting this. They found dyspnea, stridor, and a C-reactive protein greater than 100 were associated with need for intervention.[9]

Antibiotics

The standard empiric antibiotic treatment has traditionally been a third-generation cephalosporin, such as ceftriaxone.

Ampicillin-sulbactam also has been used. Metronidazole is often added to provide anaerobic coverage. Intravenous steroids are often given to reduce edema, although no randomized controlled data exist to support or dissuade the usage.

Fortunately, the severe presentation is not nearly as common in the post–Hib vaccine era. However, with a small but growing trend against vaccination, there is a potential for young children to exhibit severe traditional Hib epiglottitis in the future.[10]

Laryngitis (Including Laryngobronchial Tracheitis)

Laryngitis is a global term referring to inflammation of the vocal folds that commonly leads to dysphonia. There are many noninfectious causes for laryngitis. Acute vocal abuse, such as shouting, will often lead to acute inflammation or even hemorrhage that will cause hoarseness. Chronic vocal abuse can lead to nodules, cysts, or polyps. Dysphonia not resolving in an older adult may represent laryngeal cancer, especially in a patient with a significant smoking history. However, infectious causes will be the focus of this section.

Laryngotracheal bronchitis is commonly referred to as croup. Croup is the most common laryngeal inflammatory disease in childhood, and 15% of respiratory disease sick visits to pediatricians are related to croup. There is a seasonal peak in the winter months of nontemperate regions. The most common age is between 6 months and 3 years. This pediatric infection has a high prevalence as a viral infection. The diameter of the subglottis is 4 mm in neonates, approximately 8 mm in children, and approximately 14 mm in adults. Inflammation and edema of the subglottic region, for example with 1 mm of edema circumferentially, will decrease the cross-sectional area by 75% in neonates, by 44% in children, and by less than 25% in adults.[11] The subglottis, being bound by a complete cricoid ring, is often prevented from outward expansion from any edema. The epithelium of the subglottis is loosely adherent to the underlying perichondrium, and there are numerous mucous-secreting glands in this region.[12]

Symptoms

Initial symptoms of croup include a phase of common upper respiratory tract illness symptoms. The child may have a mild cough, low-grade fever, and perhaps rhinitis. As the inflammation and edema progress, the patient may develop hoarseness, dyspnea, stridor, and the classic croupy "seal" or barking cough. Stridor may be inspiratory or biphasic.

The child with croup can be differentiated from the child with epiglottitis. Epiglottitis is usually a rapid onset over a few hours, and the child may be drooling or posturing and have no cough. The child with croup has the classic croup cough, with the symptoms increasing gradually over a few days. The child has a normal supine posture.

In a child with possible croup, lateral and anteroposterior views of the chest and neck may be obtained. The epiglottis is crisp on the lateral view, and the anteroposterior view may have a "steeple sign" (Figure 20-5). This sign is a narrowing of the subglottis and is helpful to differentiate from a supraglottitis. Most children are treated in the outpatient setting.

The need for hospitalization depends on the severity of the dyspnea and lack of improvement with treatment in the emergency room setting. The most common therapy is inhaled humidity, which will loosen any dried mucus and allow for expectoration and thus an improved airway diameter. Nebulized racemic epinephrine can decrease tissue

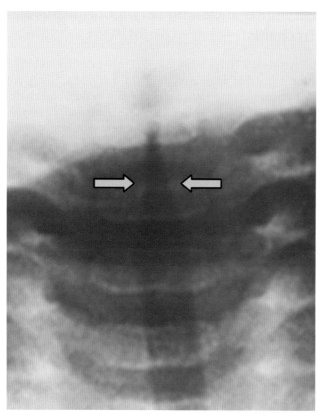

• **Figure 20-5** "Steeple Sign" May be Seen on an Anteroposterior View of a Chest Radiograph. (From Sobol SE, Zapata S. Epiglottitis and croup. *Otolaryngol Clin North Am.* 2008;41:551-566. Courtesy M. Bitner, MD, MEd, FACEP.)

edema and improve symptoms temporarily. Corticosteroids are commonly used in both oral and parenteral forms, the latter being in the emergency department or an inpatient setting. Antipyretics and decongestants are also often used as adjuncts.

Endoscopy as a diagnostic tool or also therapeutic with intubation is not usually necessary and is reserved for those clinically worsening despite medical and inhaled therapies.

Those with severe situations may have developed a secondary bacterial infection that can require cultures and debridement of the airway. Children with recurrent episodes of croup can be referred to an otolaryngologist for a laryngoscopy and bronchoscopy when they are well in between episodes to look for any predisposing anatomic factors, such as subglottic cysts or stenosis. These children might be starting with a narrower airway. Only a small amount of edema would be necessary to give symptoms of croup and therefore might be an explanation of why they are having recurrent episodes. Patients with a history of intubation, even perhaps as a newborn or neonate, are more likely to have a baseline subglottic stenosis present.

Bacterial Tracheitis

Bacterial tracheitis is a unique entity that is rarely seen and can be a highly morbid infection in children; it should be included in the differential diagnosis for an acutely stridulous child. Bacterial tracheitis is associated with a superinfection that leads to thick membranous tracheal secretions that do not clear effectively with coughing. Children will often have a history of symptoms for several days, which might suggest a viral upper respiratory tract infection. After a 2- to 3- day prodrome, the child with bacterial tracheitis would then begin to have a rapid onset of a high fever, respiratory distress, and a toxic appearance. The most common symptoms include cough (85%), stridor (77%), and voice changes (67%).[13] Typical croup therapies are not usually helpful. *S. aureus* has been seen in 33 to 75% of cases. Other bacteria isolated on culture include *H. influenzae,* group A *Streptococcus, S. pneumoniae, Streptococcus* viridans, *Klebsiella* species, *Escherichia coli,* and *Neisseria* species.

A chest radiograph often may reveal subglottic narrowing and haziness along the trachea suggestive of membranous secretions. Bronchoscopy is the gold standard for diagnosis. Bronchoscopy is often necessary as a therapeutic measure in addition to its diagnostic value. Sloughed mucosa often is obstructive of the tracheal lumen and must be debrided with forceps and suction. The secretions should be sent for culture. Frequently, subsequent endoscopic debridements are necessary. The child will often require intubation for 3 to 7 days. Antibiotic coverage with a penicillin or first-generation cephalosporin should be used to treat *S. aureus* infection. Vancomycin might be necessary in a clinical setting in which methicillin-resistant *Staphylococcus aureus* (MRSA) is suggested. A 3 to 4% mortality rate with bacterial tracheitis seems to be improving, and less severe presentations at an older age seem to be the current trend of the disease.

Nonbacterial Tracheitis

As with other parts of the airway, inhalation of noxious fumes, aspiration, or systemic disease can lead to inflammation of the tracheal lumen, leading to respiratory distress. This includes reactions to immunotherapy[14] and viruses such as COVID.[15]

Other Forms of Infectious Laryngitis

Fungal infection of the true vocal folds can commonly occur. This infection is often related to inhaled steroid use, especially in the inhaled steroid powder disk type of inhaler. A patient with hoarseness lasting more than a few weeks, and who is using inhaled corticosteroids, should be referred to an otolaryngologist for a laryngeal evaluation. Treatments for candidal laryngitis usually involving oral fluconazole as topical troches or swish-and-swallow antifungal medications will not sufficiently coat the larynx. Other fungal infections such as blastomycosis, histoplasmosis, and coccidioidomycosis, are also rarely seen infections of the larynx.

References

1. Morens DM. Death of a president. *N Engl J Med.* 1999;341(24):1845-1849.

2. Shah RK, Roberson DW, Jones DT. Epiglottitis in the Hemophilus influenzae type B vaccine era: changing trends. *Laryngoscope.* 2004;114(3):557-560.

3. :>Progress toward elimination of *Haemophilus influenzae* type b invasive disease among infants and children—United States, 1998-2000. *MMWR Morb Mortal Wkly Rep.* 2002;51(11):234-237.

4. Jan L, Boute P, Mouawad F. *Pasteurella multocida* acute epiglottitis. *Eur Ann Otorhinolaryngol Head Neck Dis.* 2021;138(2):100-102.

5. Berger G, Landau T, Berger S, Finkelstein Y, Bernheim J, Ophir D. The rising incidence of adult acute epiglottitis and epiglottic abscess. *Am J Otolaryngol.* 2003;24(6):374-383.

6. Meng X, Han C, Wang Y. Acute epiglottitis caused by COVID-19: a systematic review. *Biomol Biomed.* 2023;23(4):568-574.

7. Sataloff RT. Upper airway distress and crack-cocaine use. *Otolaryngol Head Neck Surg.* 1994;111(1):155.

8. Chan NJ, Soliman AM. Angiotensin converting enzyme inhibitor-related angioedema: onset, presentation, and management. *Ann Otol Rhinol Laryngol.* 2015;124(2):89-96.

9. Vaid P, Farrell E, Donnelly M. Predictors of airway intervention in acute supraglottitis (AS), a recent 7- year experience. *Am J Otolaryngol.* 2021;42(6):103084.

10. Hammer LD, Curry ES, Harlor AD, et al. Increasing immunization coverage. *Pediatrics.* 2010;125(6):1295-1304.

11. Salamone FN, Bobbitt DB, Myer CM, Rutter MJ, Greinwald Jr JH. Bacterial tracheitis reexamined: is there a less severe manifestation? *Otolaryngol Head Neck Surg.* 2004;131(6):871-876.

12. Sobol SE, Zapata S. Epiglottitis and croup. *Otolaryngol Clin North Am.* 2008;41(3):551-566, ix.

13. Casazza G, Graham ME, Nelson D, Chaulk D, Sandweiss D, Meier J. Pediatric bacterial tracheitis: a variable entity—case series with literature review. *Otolaryngol Head Neck Surg.* 2019;160(3):546-549.

14. Tellez-Garcia E, Valdivia Padilla A, Grosu H. Immunotherapy-induced eosinophilic tracheitis. *Cureus.* 2022;14(4):e24130.

15. Ohnishi H, Arakawa Y, Anabuki K, Yokoyama A. Tracheitis associated with COVID-19. *Intern Med.* 2023;62(11):1697-1698.

21

Infections of the Thyroid Gland

JACOB GADY AND ROBERT PIORKOWSKI

The thyroid gland is a critical part of the endocrine system. Its function is crucial for brain, heart and muscle metabolism, and proper bone maintenance. The thyroid gland is highly resistant to infection because of its rich lymphatic system, blood supply, and high iodine content.[1,2] Thyroid infections and abscesses account for approximately 0.7% of surgical pathologic conditions of the thyroid gland.[1-3] The majority of pathologic conditions of the thyroid gland is made up of thyroiditis (granulomatous, De Quervain's, lymphocytic, radiation-induced), autoimmune conditions (Hashimoto), Graves' disease, primary or metastatic neoplasm, hemorrhage into an existing cyst, amiodarone-associated thyrotoxicosis, infarction, amyloidosis, and sarcoidosis. Despite the rarity of these infections, it is important to appreciate thyroid infections can occur. Recently, there has been evidence that coronavirus disease-19 (COVID-19) infections are associated with nonthyroidal illness syndrome, subacute thyroiditis, and thyrotoxicosis.[4]

Thyroid infections occur secondarily to congenital/anatomic abnormalities, disseminated infections in the immunocompromised hosts and, in some cases, they are idiopathic. There is the potential for significant morbidity and even mortality with thyroid infections.[5-9] Considering the age, sex, and comorbidities can also help the clinician determine whether to consider thyroid infections or abscess.

A thyroid infection will manifest with one or more of the following symptoms: (1) acute anterior neck swelling, (2) pain, (3) odynophagia, and (4) pyrexia.[1-3,5-10] Often, these patients have normal thyroid function tests.[1-3,5-12] Transient or permanent hypothyroidism can occur in approximately 2 to 3% of patients and thyrotoxicosis may occur in 5% as a result of the disease or treatment. Most patients will present with a mild to moderate leukocytosis, elevated erythrocyte sedimentation rate, and elevated C-reactive protein.[1,8,10,13]

Ultrasound is usually the first imaging modality of choice. Often it will show a hypoechoic area, or heterogenous area within the gland. If an abscess cavity is visualized, fine-needle aspiration can be attempted to drain the fluid and provide for culture. CT scan with contrast and magnetic resonance imaging can aid in diagnosis as well (Figure 21-1). If congenital anomalies are suspected, direct laryngoscopy and barium studies may show a fistulous tract (Figure 21-2).[1-3,5,8-13]

In some cases, medical management with systemic antibiotics is sufficient, but often surgical intervention is necessary. Absent cultures and sensitivities, empiric antibiotic treatment targets the most common pathogens in thyroid abscesses, such as *Staphylococcus aureus* and *Streptococcus* species.* Less common pathogens include *Klebsiella* species, *Salmonella* species, *Nocardia* species, *Acinetobacter, Hemophilus influenzae, Escherichia coli, Eikenella corrodens,* and fungi. As much as 30% of suppurative thyroiditis is found to be polymicrobial infection.* Surgical intervention includes biopsy, incision and drainage, or open neck surgery depending on the underlying pathologic condition.

Congenital and Anatomic Anomalies Associated With Thyroid Infections

Congenital anomalies leading to thyroid infections may be a result of brachial sinuses, cysts, or fistulas. In particular, brachial pouch anomalies have been associated with neck abscesses and acute suppurative thyroiditis.[20,21] Brachial cysts have no external connection and therefore retain secretions. Brachial sinuses communicate with the skin or pharynx (typically hypopharynx). Branchial fistulas will connect the pharynx to the skin through the intervening tissue, which can be the perithyroid tissues or the thyroid parenchyma itself. Most brachial anomalies arise from the fourth brachial arch and, less commonly, from the third brachial arch.[20-22]

The pyriform sinus is most often involved with brachial arch anomalies. The pyriform sinus is bounded medially by the aryepiglottic fold and laterally by the thyroid cartilage and thyrohyoid membrane. Pyriform sinus fistulas are a remnant of the third and fourth pharyngeal pouch. The pyriform sinus fistula typically courses anterior-inferior through the perithyroid tissues or the thyroid gland substance itself. If the fistulous tract becomes inflamed, the swelling of the adjacent tissues can cause obstruction of the fistulous tract and development of an acute infection.[21-26]

---

*References 2, 3, 8, 10, 13, 14-19.

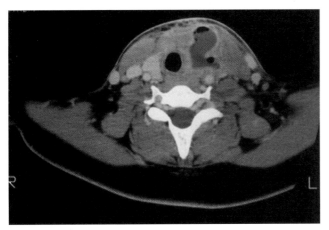

• **Figure 21-1** CT Scan Demonstrating a Recurrent Abscess Arising from the Pyriform Fossa. (From Houghton DJ, Gray HW, MacKenzie K. The tender neck: thyroiditis or thyroid abscess? *Clin Endocrinol.* 1998;48:521-524.)

Fourth brachial arch anomalies are the most common congenital anomaly thought to be related to thyroid abscesses in children and adults. The fourth brachial arch anomalies originate from the apex of the pyriform sinus and pass through the cricothyroid membrane beneath the superior laryngeal nerve. The presentation of both third and fourth brachial arch anomalies will vary with age. Neonates will present with respiratory distress and failure. Young

children (typically ≥8 years) will present with acute-onset neck pain, typically on the left; swelling; suppurative thyroiditis; pyrexia; elevated erythrocyte sedimentation rate; C-reactive protein; and leukocytosis (Figure 21-3).[21-27]

Third brachial arch anomalies originate from the base of the pyriform sinus and pass superior to the superior laryngeal nerve. Third brachial arch anomalies can manifest as neck abscess or acute suppurative thyroiditis. The majority of third brachial arch anomalies occur on the left side and are typically identified in childhood. However, Nicoucar et al.[23] found that patients presenting with acute suppurative thyroiditis were older at the time of diagnosis (≥8 years). These patients present with acute painful neck swelling, and neonates and infants may present with respiratory distress.[23,24-27]

Organisms associated with brachial arch anomaly infections are typically *S. aureus* and *Streptococcus* species. Less common infections were found to have *Klebsiella, E. coli, Pseudomonas aeruginosa, Haemophilus* species, *E. corrodens, Citrobacter* species, and *Proteus* species.[†]

Children and adults with recurrent cervical abscess or suppurative thyroiditis, particularly on the left, should be initially evaluated with direct laryngoscopy, barium swallow, and/or CT scan to rule out a pyriform sinus fistula. CT scan, barium swallow study, or a thyroid scan with technicium-99 will help with the diagnosis. CT scan can demonstrate the location and extent of the pyriform sinus fistula, particularly if performed shortly after a barium swallow

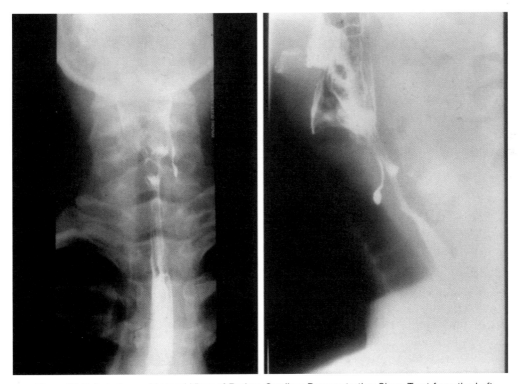

• **Figure 21-2** Anterior and Lateral View of Barium Swallow Demonstrating Sinus Tract from the Left Pyriform Fossa. (From Houghton DJ, Gray HW, MacKenzie K. The tender neck: thyroiditis or thyroid abscess? *Clin Endocrinol.* 1998;48:521-524.)

[†]References 2, 3, 8, 10, 13, 14-19.

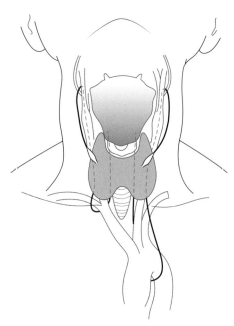

• **Figure 21-3** Path of Fourth Brachial Arch Fistula. (From Nicoucar K, Giger R, Pope HG, Jaecklin T, Dulguerov P. Management of congenital fourth branchial arch anomalies: a review and analysis of published cases. *J Pediatr Surg.* 2009;44:1432-1439.)

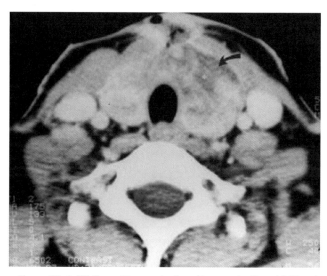

• **Figure 21-4** CT Scan Demonstrating Abscess in Thyroid Gland. (From Parmar H, Hashmi M, Rajput A, Patankar T, Castillo M. Acute tuberculous abscess of the thyroid. *Australas Radiol.* 2002;46: 186-188.)

study (see Figures 21-1 and 21-2). Fine-needle aspiration of abscess or fluid will aid in directing medical therapy and reduce edema on adjacent tissues. Conventional radiographs do not appear to aid in the diagnosis.[5-13]

Treatment remains combined surgical and medical management. Incision and drainage and open neck procedures with or without partial thyroidectomy are typically performed, but endoscopic procedures with cauterization of the fistulous tract have been described. Nicoucar et al.[23] found that of the 64% of patients who initially underwent incision and drainage, 94% required additional surgery, including incision and drainage and open neck surgery. In a series of seven patients that who underwent endoscopic cauterization, four were followed for 18 months and had no evidence of recurrence. Open neck surgery and removal of the fistulous tract is curative and currently is the treatment of choice.[22]

Tuberculosis Infection/Thyroid Infection

There have been multiple case reports describing acute tuberculosis abscesses of the thyroid gland or tuberculosis thyroiditis. Typically, these are associated with tubercular foci elsewhere in the body. However, there have been cases described where other tubercular foci were not identified.[28,29]

These patients will present with acute neck swelling for less than 1 month. There is associated erythema, pain, pyrexia, and often cervical lymphadenopathy on the affected side. Laboratory values are typically euthyroid. There may be a leukocytosis, and typically erythrocyte sedimentation rate and C-reactive protein levels are elevated. These patients should be evaluated with the enzyme-linked immunosorbent assay test for HIV.

Ultrasound evaluation will demonstrate an irregular, cystic-appearing mass with patchy hypodense, nonenhancing areas of the gland involved with the disease process. These patients should also have radiographic examination of their chest, either with chest CT or an anteroposterior chest film. Contrast-enhanced CT scan will sometimes show an abscess in the thyroid gland (Figure 21-4).[28-30]

As with any infection, surgical incision and drainage is often required. The areas of the gland thought to be affected should be removed as well.

Histopathologic evaluation, in addition to Gram stain and culture and sensitivity, should be performed. Histologic evaluation has demonstrated five pathologic varieties of tuberculosis of the thyroid: (1) multiple lesions throughout the gland in association with miliary tuberculosis; (2) a goiter with caseation; (3) cold abscess formation sometimes manifesting on the surface of the gland; (4) chronic fibrosing tuberculosis; and (5) acute abscess formation. Histopathologic evaluation will demonstrate epithelioid cells and multinucleated giant cells with areas of normal thyroid follicles.[30]

Gram stain will be positive for acid-fast bacilli, and culture will be positive for *Mycobacterium tuberculosis*. Most patients respond well to combined surgical therapy and antituberculosis chemotherapy and demonstrate resolution of their disease.

Infections of the Thyroid Gland in the Immunocompromised Host

Infections of the thyroid are rare but can occur, particularly in immunocompromised patients. Aside from congenital anomalies, patients with autoimmune diseases, organ transplant patients on chronic immunosuppressive therapy, patients on chronic corticosteroids, and those with advanced acquired immunodeficiency syndrome are at particular risk. Thyroid infections in the immunocompromised host usually spreads from neighboring tissues or by lymphatics and hematologic spread.[13-20]

Patients will present with anterior neck pain, edema, erythema, odynophagia, and often pyrexia. Bacterial infections are more common than fungal infections and seem to occur more often in patients with a history of thyroid disease. The bacteria species cultured from thyroid infections in immunocompromised patients are similar to those discussed previously in this chapter. Treatment is typically combined antimicrobial agents, incision and drainage, and total or subtotal thyroidectomy.

Approximately 40 cases of fungal thyroid infections in the immunocompromised host have been described in the literature. The fungal species most frequently isolated are *Aspergillus* species, followed by *Candida* species, *Coccidiomycosis* species, *Cryptococcus neoformans,* and *Pseudallescheria boydii*. Patients presenting with fungal thyroid infections may be euthyroid, hypothyroid, or hyperthyroid at presentation. They may have leukocytosis (depending on their underlying disease state), and elevated erythrocyte sedimentation rate and C-reactive protein.[13-20]

Acute infectious thyroiditis should be considered in immunocompromised patients. Clinicians should have a low threshold to perform ultrasound-guided fine-needle aspiration if the clinical presentation suggests thyroid infection but the gland appears structurally normal on imaging. Most pathologic conditions are consistent with hematogenous spread or a focal abscess.

Treatment should include antifungals, such as fluconazole and amphotericin B. Surgical treatment is incision and drainage of any abscess or fluid, and potentially total or subtotal thyroidectomy.

The majority of thyroid gland pathology is not infectious. However, the clinical picture can be confusing and patients may present with symptoms similar to those of an infection. It is therefore important to be aware and understand some of these more common entities, including autoimmune conditions (Hashimoto's thyroiditis), thyroiditis (granulomatous, De Quervain's, lymphocytic, radiation-induced), and Graves' disease.

Hypothyroidism can exist as congenital hypothyroidism resulting from inborn errors of thyroid metabolism and enzymatic defects. Worldwide, iodine deficiency is the leading cause of hypothyroidism. Acquired hypothyroidism can be surgically or radiation induced, secondary (i.e., thyroid-stimulating hormone [TSH] deficiency), or autoimmune. The most common autoimmune hypothyroidism is due to Hashimoto's, thyroiditis.[31,32]

Patients with Hashimoto's thyroiditis may present with a painless, diffusely enlarged, goitrous thyroid gland. These patients are usually females in their fourth to six decade of life. Some patients in the postpartum period can develop autoantibodies similar to those in Hashimoto's thyroiditis. Serum analysis will reveal circulating autoantibodies, including antimicrosomal, antithyroid peroxidase, and antithyroglobulin. In the early stages of the disease patients can develop thyrotoxicosis ("Hashitoxicosis"). Laboratory values demonstrate elevated triiodothyronine (T_3) and thyroxine (T_4), which are being released from the damaged thyroid follicles, and a decrease in TSH. Most patients will present with hypothyroidism, with low T_3 and T_4, and an increase in TSH. There are a wide range of symptoms, including fatigue, cold intolerance, weight gain, myxedema, and alopecia. These patients are managed with thyroid hormone supplementation medications.[31-35]

Subacute granulomatous thyroiditis (De Quervain's thyroiditis) may also manifest with anterior cervical neck pain and thyroid enlargement. This condition seems related to a recent viral infection, particularly upper respiratory tract infections. This disease is seen more commonly in females between their fourth and fifth decade of life. Thyroid tests may reveal thyrotoxicosis, with elevated T_3 and T_4 released from thyroglobulin and thyroid follicles, and low TSH levels. Evaluation with ultrasound will demonstrate thyroid hypoechogenicity, and thyroid scan will demonstrate low thyroid radionuclide uptake. This condition is self-limiting, and these patients rarely develop long-term thyroid dysfunction. It is treated nonsurgically with antiinflammatory medications and systemic corticosteroids for more severe cases.[35-38]

Subacute lymphocytic thyroiditis will often manifest with painless enlargement of the thyroid gland. Like most other thyroid disorders, subacute lymphocytic thyroiditis is commonly found in females in their fourth to sixth decades. This condition is usually self-limiting, but these patients can develop transient hyperthyroidism and hypothyroidism.[34,35,38,39]

Graves' disease is a thyroid disorder most commonly seen in women between the ages of 30 to 60 years old and may be associated with thyroiditis and thyrotoxicosis. Patients will present with either one or a combination of the following: hyperthyroidism, diffuse thyroid enlargement, exophthalmos, and myxedema. Treatment for Graves' disease is typically antithyroid medication, iodine-31 (^{131}I) ablation, and/or surgery. Antithyroid medications are methimazole and propylthiouracil (PTU). Both methimazole and PTU prevent the synthesis of triiodothyronine (T_3) and thyroxine (T_4) by inhibiting the enzyme thyroperoxidase. If the antithyroid medications are ineffective, patients are treated with radioactive ^{131}I or surgery. Surgery is indicated for patients who have failed medical management or those who develop thyrotoxic Graves' disease. Surgery involves subtotal thyroidectomy or near-total thyroidectomy.[34,35,39]

Thyroid dysfunction during COVID-19 infection has been observed in both nonthyroidal illness syndrome and subacute thyroiditis. It is unclear whether this is a direct result of the SARS-CoV-2 infection or the secondary inflammatory and endocrine effects. Patients infected with SARS-CoV-2 have been noted to have decreased reverse T_3 levels and a decline in T_4 and TSH in critically ill patients.[40,41] Some retrospective studies demonstrate 28 to 60% of patients tested with COVID-19 will have evidence of low reverse T_3 (rT_3).[40-42]

There is evidence suggesting subacute thyroiditis or De Quervain's thyroiditis may be associated with COVID-19 infection in some individuals. A prospective study followed 61 survivors of the 2002 SARS epidemic (with no preexisting endocrine diseases) 3 months after recovery and observed that 6.7% of them became biochemically hypothyroid (with one case of primary and three of central hypothyroidism) and 39% had hypocortisolism (two of the patients with hypercortisolism also had transient subclinical thyrotoxicosis). The authors speculated that these effects might be due to SARS-induced reversible hypophysitis or a direct effect of the virus on the hypothalamus.[43,44] The data presenting related to COVID-19 infection is certainly interesting but still being parsed due to the complex nature of this infection.

References

1. Cawich SO, Hassranah D, Naraynsingh V. Idiopathic thyroid abscess. *Int J Surg Case Rep*. 2014;5(8):484-486.
2. Fonseca IF, Avvad CK, Sanchez EG, Henriques JL, Leão LM. Acute suppurative thyroiditis with multiple complications. *Arq Bras Endocrinol Metab*. 2012;56(6):388-392.
3. Jonas NE, Fagan JJ. Internal jugular vein thrombosis: a case study and review of the literature. *Internet J Otorhinolaryngol*. 2007;6:2.
4. Rossetti CL, Cazarin J, Hecht F. COVID-19 and thyroid function: what do we know so far? *Front Endocrinol (Lausanne)*. 2022;13:1041676. Available at: https://doi.org/10.3389/fendo.2022.1041676.
5. Thanos L, Mylona S, KaliorasV, Pomoni M, Batakis N. Potentially life-threatening neck abscesses: therapeutic management under CT guided drainage. *Cardiovasc Intervent Radiol*. 2005;28(2):196-199.
6. Deshmukh HG, Verma A, Siegel LB, et al. Stridor: the presenting feature of a thyroid abscess. *Postgrad Med J*. 1994;70:847-850.
7. Desouza RF, Dilip A, Mervyn C. Thyroid abscess with cutaneous fistula: case report and review of the literature. *Thyroid Sci*. 2008;3(11):1-4.
8. Paes JE, Burman KD, Cohen J, et al. Acute bacterial suppurative thyroiditis: a clinical review and expert opinion. *Thyroid*. 2010;20:247-255.
9. Sioka E, Efthimiou M, Skoulakis C, Zacharoulis D. Thyroid abscess requiring emergency intervention. *J Emerg Med*. 2011;43(6):e455-e456.
10. Houghton DJ, Gray HW, MacKenzie K. The tender neck: thyroiditis or thyroid abscess? *Clin Endocrinol*. 1998;48:521-524.
11. Ilyin A, Zhelonkina N, Severskaya N, Romanko S. Nonsurgical management of thyroid abscess with sonographically guided fine needle aspiration. *J Clin Ultrasound*. 2007;35:333-337.
12. Schweitzer VG, Olson NR. Thyroid abscess. *Otolaryngol Head Neck Surg*. 1981;89(2):226-229.
13. Cespedes C, Duran P, Uribe C, Chahin S, Lema A, Coll M. Thyroid abscess: a case series and literature review. *Endocrinol Nutr*. 2013;60(4):190-196.
14. Echevarria Villegas MP, Franco Vicarioo R, Solano Lopez Q, Landin Vicuna R, Teira Cobo R, Miguel de la Villa F. Acute suppurative thyroiditis and *Klebsiella pneumoniae* sepsis: a case report and review of the literature. *Rev Clin Esp*. 1992;190(9):458-459.
15. Yoshino Y, Inamo Y, Fuchigami T, et al. A pediatric patient with acute suppurative thyroiditis caused by *Eikenella corrodens*. *J Infect Chemother*. 2010;16:353-355.
16. Svenungsson B, Lindberg AA. Acute suppurative salmonella thyroiditis: clinical course and antibody response. *Scand J Infect Dis*. 1981;13(4):303-306.
17. Jacobs A, Gros DAC, Gradon JD. Thyroid abscess due to *Acinetobacter calcoaceticus*: case report and review of the causes of and current management strategies for thyroid abscesses. *South Med J*. 2003;96(3):300-307.
18. Parmar H, Hashmi M, Rajput A, Patankar T, Castillo M. Acute tuberculous abscess of the thyroid. *Australas Radiol*. 2002;46:186-188.
19. Goldani LZ, Zavascki AP, Maia AL. Fungal thyroiditis: an overview. *Mycopathologia*. 2006;161:129-139.
20. McAninch EA, Xu C, Lagari VS, Kim BW. Coccidiomycosis thyroiditis in an immunocompromised host post-transplant: case report and literature review. *J Clin Endocrinol Metab*. 2014;99(5):1537-1542.
21. Suprabha J, Vijay K, Shital P. Acute bacterial thyroid abscess as a complication of septicemia. *Infect Dis Clin Pract*. 2000;9:383-386.
22. Seo JH, Park YH, Yang SW, Kim HY. Refractory acute suppurative thyroiditis secondary to pyriform sinus fistula. *Ann Pediatr Endocrinol Metab*. 2014;9:104-107.
23. Nicoucar K, Giger R, Pope HG, Jaecklin T, Dulguerov P. Management of congenital fourth branchial arch anomalies: a review and analysis of published cases. *J Pediatr Surg*. 2009;44:1432-1439.
24. Pereira KD, Losh GG, Oliver D, Poole M. Management of anomalies of the third and fourth brachial pouches. *J Pediatr Otorhinolaryngol*. 2004;68:43-50.
25. Prasad TRS, Chong CL, Mani A, et al. Acute suppurative thyroiditis in children secondary to pyriform sinus fistula. *Pediatr Surg Int*. 2007;23:779-783.
26. Kubota M, Suita S, Kamimura T, Zaizen Y. Surgical strategy for the treatment of pyriform sinus fistula. *J Pediatr Surg*. 1997;32:34-37.
27. Wang HK, Tiu CM, Chou YH, Change CY. Imaging studies of pyriform sinus fistula. *Pediatr Radiol*. 2003;33:328-333.
28. Miyauchi A, Matsuzuka F, Kuma K, Takai S. Piriform sinus fistula: an underlying abnormality common in patients with acute suppurative thyroiditis. *World J Surg*. 1990;14:400-405.
29. Parmar H, Hashmi M, Rajput A, Patankar T, Castillo M. Acute tuberculosis abscess of the thyroid gland. *Australas Radiol*. 2002;46:186-188.
30. Das DK, Pant CS, Chachra KL, Gupta AK. Fine needle aspiration cytology diagnosis of tuberculous thyroiditis: a report of eight cases. *Acta Cytol*. 1992;36:517-522.
31. Caturegli P, DeRemigis A, Rose NR. Hashimoto thyroiditis: clinical and diagnostic criteria. *Autoimmun Rev*. 2014;13(4-5):391-397.
32. Lorini R, Gastaldi R, Traggiai C, Perucchin PP. Hasthimoto's thyroiditis. *Pediatr Endocrinol Rev*. 2003;1(suppl 2):205-211.
33. Johnson AG, Phillips ME, Thomas RJS. Acute tuberculous abscess of the thyroid gland. *Br J Surg*. 1993;60:667-669.
34. Fink H, Hintze G. Autoimmune thyroiditis (Hashimoto's thyroiditis): current diagnosis and therapy. *Med Klin (Munich)*. 2010;105(7):485-493.
35. Longo MD. *Harrison's Principles of Internal Medicine*. 18th ed. New York: McGraw-Hill; 2011.
36. Kumar V, Abbas AK, Aster JC, Fausto N. *Robbins & Cotran Pathologic Basis of Disease*. 8th ed. Philadelphia: Saunders; 2010.

37. Harach HR, Williams ED. The pathology of granulomatous diseases of the thyroid gland. *Sarcoidosis*. 1990;7(1):19-27.

38. Sheu SY, Schmid KW. Inflammatory disease of the thyroid gland. epidemiology, symptoms and morphology. *Pathologe*. 2003;24(5):339-347.

39. Singer PA. Thyroiditis: acute, subacute, and chronic. *Med Clin North Am*. 1991;75(1):61-77.

40. Kannan CR, Seshadri KG. Thyrotoxicosis. *Dis Mon*. 1997;43(9):601-677.

41. Fliers E, Boelen A. An update on non-thyroidal illness syndrome. *J Endocrinol Invest*. 2021;44:1597-1607. Available at: https://doi.org/10.1007/s40618-020-01482-4.

42. Chen M, Zhou W, Xu W. Thyroid function analysis in 50 patients with COVID-19: a retrospective study. *Thyroid*. 2021;31(1):8-11. Available at: https://doi.org/10.1089/thy.2020.0363.

43. Zou R, Wu C, Zhang S, et al. Euthyroid sick syndrome in patients with COVID-19. *Front Endocrinol (Lausanne)*. 2020;11:566439. Available at: https://doi.org/10.3389/fendo.2020.566439.

44. Leow MKS, Kwek DSK, Ng AWK, Ong KC, Kaw GJL, Lee LSU. Hypocortisolism in survivors of severe acute respiratory syndrome (SARS). *Clin Endocrinol (Oxf)*. 2005;63:197-202. Available at: https://doi.org/10.1111/j.1365-2265.2005.02325.x.

PART 3

Special Topics Related to Head and Neck Infections

22

Neck Infections Related to Vascular Interventions

PATRICK CLYNE THOMPSON AND ANTOINE M. FERNEINI

Although uncommon, infectious complications following vascular interventions in the neck do occur. Because of the wide range of clinical presentation, these complications can mimic other entities, such as a pulseless mass of a pseudoaneurysm. In this chapter, we will briefly discuss complications that can occur after the most common vascular procedures in the neck including carotid endarterectomy and stenting, and superficial thrombophlebitis.

Carotid Endarterectomy and Stenting

In the United States, cerebrovascular disease is the fifth leading cause of mortality, accounting for roughly 163,000 deaths annually.[1] Ischemic-embolic events are the main cause of stroke, with as much as 20% being related to carotid atherosclerotic disease and stenosis.[1-3] Medical therapy is the standard of care for the treatment of low- and moderate-risk carotid stenosis. This therapy includes dietary and lifestyle modifications, along with medical therapy such as aspirin, clopidogrel, and statins. But when surgery is indicated for critical stenosis, carotid endarterectomy (CEA) is the gold standard and has been shown in multiple randomized clinical trials to reduce the risk of stroke and death in both symptomatic and asymptomatic patients.[4-8]

Multiple techniques have been used in the past to close the carotid endarterectomy arteriotomy, but the most common one is the patch angioplasty closure. This technique is proven to decrease the chances of recurrent stenosis and stroke.[9-12] Different materials have been used for the patch angioplasty, including autologous vein, prosthetic material (polytetrafluoroethylene [Dacron]), and bioprosthetic materials such as bovine pericardium.

The use of vein has fallen out of favor because it requires a donor site (usually the groin) and has an increased reported risk of carotid blowout.[13] More than 95% of the patches currently being used are bovine pericardium because it is readily available, is easy to handle, has less needle-hole bleeding, is resistant to thrombosis, has no ultrasound interference, and is theoretically resistant to infection (with a cost and complication rate comparable to prosthetic material).[4]

The most common complications for CEA are perioperative stroke and myocardial infarction, with the latter being the most common cause of death.[1] Patch infection is an uncommon but feared complication[14-17] that can lead to patch rupture or pseudoaneurysm formation. Patch infection usually requires further surgical intervention and carries a high morbidity and mortality.[18]

The incidence of wound and patch infection after CEA is rare and usually limited to case reports. The National Surgical Quality Improvement Program (NSQIP) reported incidence of carotid surgical site infection was only 0.5 to 1%.[1] In fact, only 125 cases of prosthetic graft infection have been reported from 1962 to 2012.[19] One of the largest series on bovine pericardium closure reported that only 3 of 457 cases (0.6%) were complicated with patch infection. In addition, there was no significant difference, in terms of complications, compared with other closure techniques.[4]

The most common bacteria involved in patch infections are gram-positive cocci (staphylococci or streptococci). Other bacteria include *Enterobacter* (four cases), *Pseudomonas* (three cases), *Bacteroides* (three cases), coliforms (three cases), *Proteus* (two cases), and *Enterococcus* and *Corynebacterium* species (one case each).[19]

Of the few reported cases of patch infection, the presentation was often insidious. The most commonly reported symptoms include pseudoaneurysm (33% of cases), local draining sinuses (30%), and neck swelling (24%). Less frequently, it can manifest with signs of a local infection (16%), systemic sepsis (8%), pain (5%), and stroke (3%).[20] Some cases present with a nontender neck mass prompting unnecessary testing and consults (Figure 22-1).

Post-CEA infection has a bimodal distribution, with 39% of the cases developing 2 months postoperatively and 63% developing after 6 months.[18] The early presentation is usually associated with local wound complications, such as a wound infection, hematoma, or dehiscence. Patients with a late infection exhibit a draining sinus tract or a pseudoaneurysm.

Multiple imaging modalities can be used diagnostically, including duplex ultrasound, computed tomography (CT) angiography, magnetic resonance angiography, or the

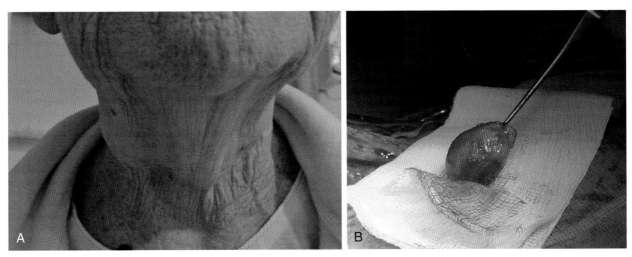

• **Figure 22-1** Carotid Painless Mass Associated with a Patch Infection. **A,** Soft tissue mass in the right anterior triangle. **B,** Intraoperative photograph of the excised encapsulated lesion from the right carotid artery. (From Knight BC, Tait WF. Dacron patch infection following carotid endarterectomy: a systematic review of the literature. *Eur J Vasc Endovasc Surg.* 2009;37:140-148.)

angiogram, which is the traditional gold standard for pseudoaneurysm diagnosis.[21,22]

Duplex ultrasound is noninvasive, cost-effective, and readily available. It facilitates evaluation of the internal carotid artery and its patency. It is also used to visualize the surrounding tissues to identify fluid collections, and it is highly sensitive for detecting pseudoaneurysm formation.[23] It also can be used to detect early signs of patch infection. Although rarely used, Dacron patches can show early ultrasound changes before a clinical infection is apparent. This change appears as a patch corrugation (as early as 11 months before clinical manifestations).[24]

Plain angiography has been traditionally considered the gold standard test; however, it is invasive and has known complications, including groin wound infection and embolic complications (e.g., transient ischemic attack, cerebral vascular accident).[25-27] Plain angiography also has a high false-negative rate, in some cases missing pseudoaneurysm. Diagnostic angiography is not recommended for suspected post-CEA infection.

Because of the low number of cases reported, there is no consensus regarding how to treat CEA patch infections, but patch excision and reconstruction are considered the standard of care. This procedure carries a higher morbidity and major stroke rate than a traditional CEA does (9 to 12% compared with 50% for carotid ligation in the same setting).[15] Carotid ligation is reserved for patients with methicillin-resistant *Staphylococcus aureus* (MRSA) infections, because of the high virulence of this organism or the preoperative presence of internal carotid artery occlusion (seen on ultrasound).

Reconstruction with autologous tissue is recommended, using either a vein patch or bypass or an arterial conduit.[26] When using a vein, there is concern about vein patch blowout after repair on an infected field.[28] These reports are usually anecdotal and underreported in the literature. To improve the outcomes, it is advisable to use the saphenous vein from the groin; however, this results in sacrificing the saphenous vein, which could be used as a conduit for other procedures, and an increased infection rate of the groin incision.

The use of a prosthetic patch or conduit should be avoided at all costs because it carries a high risk of reinfection.[15,29,30] A more conservative approach has been used in some patients in whom comorbidities or overall health status does not allow for lengthy procedures. This approach involves antibiotic treatment for a long period and local debridement of grossly infected tissue (i.e., leaving the patch intact).[20] The use of a muscle flap, mainly sternocleidomastoid, has been described to assist with closure and antibiotic delivery to the infected field.[15,31,32]

The recent availability of cryopreserved human allografts presents another option for revascularization and has been used successfully in a few reported cases.[33-35]

There are reported cases of the use of covered stents on post-CEA infection as temporizing or palliative measures. These cases show good short-term results with no long-term follow-up.[18] At this point, the use of covered stents in these cases is not recommended.

Carotid Stenting

As a primary procedure, carotid artery stenting (femoral or transcarotid) has historically been used for patients with comorbidities that preclude them from having a CEA or patients after radiotherapy to the neck; however, over recent years adoption of transcarotid artery revascularization has increased. There are limited reports of carotid stent infection. Although rare and likely underreported, this complication is serious, with a reported mortality as high as 50%. Early recognition and management improve outcomes. Similar to post-CEA infections, symptoms are nonspecific, ranging from postoperative fever and sepsis to neck swelling or a carotid-cutaneous fistula.[36]

It is unclear how an infection of the stent occurs. The most likely explanation is transient bacteremia that seeds the stent or a primary infection at the time of insertion.

The time of presentation can be insidious, and most cases present late (usually 1 to 2 years after the procedure). One case reported an early infection, with symptoms starting as early as 48 hours after stenting and rapidly progressing to a pseudoaneurysm and rupture, requiring urgent surgery with carotid resection and saphenous vein bypass revascularization.[37] Treatment solely with antibiotics is an option but carries high mortality; therefore, the recommended treatment is resection and revascularization similar to what is done for post-CEA infections.[37]

Carotid Pseudoaneurysm

Only 4% of peripheral aneurysms are carotid aneurysms, and only 0.7% of CEA are complicated with a carotid pseudoaneurysm. Other causes for carotid pseudoaneurysm include infection, patch degeneration,[38-41] central lines, and neck trauma.[39]

Conventional treatment, as explained earlier for CEA infection, is excision and revascularization, with a few reported cases of the use of carotid stents to exclude the pseudoaneurysm in a controlled infection setting with a low virulent organism or after trauma.[42,43]

Thrombophlebitis

Thrombophlebitis is a localized venous disorder that, as its name implies, is defined by an inflammatory reaction of that venous segment.[44] It represents a broad entity, with varying degrees of severity, that are well illustrated in the case of neck veins. Although this inflammation makes the affected vein susceptible to at least two factors of the Virchow triad (endothelial damage and stasis) by its damage and scarring of the vein walls, it is also not necessarily associated with thrombosis.[45] It is important to distinguish between superficial venous thrombophlebitis and deep venous thrombosis or thrombophlebitis, especially in the neck veins. The internal jugular (deep) venous thrombophlebitis carries with it far more dire consequences and requires an aggressive intervention.

Superficial venous thrombophlebitis (SVT) restricts its definition to the superficial veins underlying the skin. In the neck, this would usually imply the external jugular vein; however, it can affect any other vein in the neck as well, especially if the patient was exposed to trauma or infection. SVT can arise in any superficial vein of the body, but is mostly seen in the lower extremities and the external jugular veins.[46] The vast majority of the reported literature and clinical trials regarding SVT relate to lower-extremity disease. The data and management of SVT in the neck are largely extrapolated from these reports. It should be noted that conditions such as valvular reflux and varicosities that have

been reported to be the most common risk factors for SVT generally do not apply.[47]

The reported incidence of SVT in the United States is 125,000 cases per year.[46] There is an increasing incidence with increased age, female sex (with the incidence in men rising from 0.05 per 1000 per year in the third decade to 1.8 per 1000 per year in the eighth decade compared with 0.31 per 1000 per year to 2.2 per 1000 per year in women).[48] SVT will often resolve independently, without intervention or specific medical treatment; therefore, these numbers are likely underreported.

The risk factors and cause for SVT are the three factors of the Virchow triad: endothelial damage, venous stasis, and hypercoagulability. Endothelial damage is probably most applicable to the external jugular vein SVT, because this is a commonly used vein for peripheral intravenous (IV) catheters, particularly in patients with otherwise difficult vascular access. Direct endothelial injury is associated with this puncture and subsequent infusion of medications and other inflammation-inducing solutions. Chemotherapeutic infusions can increase the likelihood of SVT.[46] Infection also may be associated with intravenous catheterization. Organisms such as *S. aureus, Pseudomonas* species, *Klebsiella* species, *Peptostreptococcus* species, *Propionibacterium* species, *Bacteroides fragilis, Prevotella* species, and *Fusobacterium* species have all been implicated in more severe septic thrombophlebitis.[49] Severe infections can develop into suppurative SVT, requiring removal of any foreign body that might be present and the administration of IV antibiotics. Rarely will actual excision of the vein be required to treat this entity.[47]

Regarding venous stasis, varicose veins, usually associated with a saphenous vein reflux, are the most prominent example of venous stasis leading to SVT. This, as mentioned previously, is the most common risk factor for SVT; however, such a mechanism will not usually be present in neck veins given the typical absence of valves and the direct assistance of gravity in draining the head and neck venous blood.

Any number of exposures and conditions may put a patient in a hypercoagulable state, such as pregnancy, oral contraceptives, infections, smoking, prothrombotic conditions, and malignancy. The phenomenon of migratory thrombophlebitis deserves special mention given its association with malignancy. Migratory thrombophlebitis describes the repeated thrombosis and inflammation of superficial veins, most commonly in the lower extremities but possible at varying sites; it was associated with adenocarcinoma in the tail of the pancreas by Trousseau in 1856 (Trousseau syndrome).[46] Other studies have demonstrated that patients with SVT as a first thrombotic episode were more likely to have several hypercoagulable states compared with a control population. Patients with two or more episodes were more likely to have antibodies against anticardiolipin.[50,51]

Diagnosis of SVT is still mostly based on a clinical examination alone. Tenderness, pain, and erythema along the course of the affected vein are the classic symptoms. These symptoms may appear over the course of hours to days, but generally resolve over the course of days to weeks. A palpable nodule or cord will usually indicate the presence of a thrombus in the varicosity or vein, and this may persist for months after initial symptom onset.[46] After the initial inflammation resolves, a brown or bruised discoloration of the area may also persist.

In the case of septic or suppurative thrombophlebitis, patients may have constitutional symptoms such as high-grade fever, in addition to purulent drainage, and sometimes frank abscess. Risk of septic thrombophlebitis increases if peripheral IV catheters are left in place for more than 2 to 3 days.[52] For this reason, peripheral IV catheters should be removed or switched to new locations after the same time period.

Duplex ultrasonography is helpful in diagnosing an SVT. This test is inexpensive, noninvasive, and reliable for determining the location and extent of thrombotic disease. Duplex ultrasound findings in SVT can include surrounding soft tissue edema, vein wall thickening, and increased echogenicity. The affected vein may have evidence of thrombosis, including incompressibility. It is also valuable for assessing for a deep vein thrombosis (DVT). There may be a thrombus extending beyond the limits of the outward inflammatory changes seen on clinical examination. This may be particularly useful if there is concern for disease occurring in proximity to a junction with the deep system. Upper extremity SVT and thrombosis is less likely to progress to DVT compared with lower extremity SVT.[53] One could postulate that the same would hold true for external jugular SVT progression to internal jugular DVT. This could possibly be explained by the reduced impact of venous reflux in the upper extremities and neck; however, no data have confirmed this.

The management of SVT will depend on the clinical severity of the presentation and risk or presence of a concurrent DVT. The mainstay of treatment in most cases will be supportive care with warm or cool compresses and nonsteroidal antiinflammatory drugs (NSAIDs). Most cases will respond to treatment within several days, and complete resolution should occur over 7 to 21 days.[46] A palpable cord or nodule of the thrombosed vein may remain for the next several months.

NSAIDs have been shown to effectively treat the pain and inflammatory symptoms of SVT in addition to reducing extension and recurrence. A randomized controlled trial comparing NSAIDs to placebo demonstrated 15% recurrence or extension, or both, with NSAID treatment compared with 30% for placebo.[54]

Anticoagulation for SVT has been studied with generally favorable results. The same study demonstrating the reduced recurrence and extension with NSAIDs found further reduction with 40 mg of daily subcutaneous enoxaparin and 1.5 mg/kg daily of subcutaneous enoxaparin to 8% and 7%, respectively.[54] Treatment with 2.5 mg of subcutaneous daily fondaparinux, and direct oral anticoagulants, also have been studied and shown to reduce recurrent thrombus and phlebitis. However, enoxaparin has not been shown to reduce DVT incidence and fondaparinux had an absolute risk reduction of 0.3%.[55] Given the generally benign course of SVT and high cost of low-molecular-weight heparin (LMWH) and fondaparinux, anticoagulation has not been found to be cost-effective, and these treatments are usually avoided in favor of NSAIDs in otherwise low-risk patients.[56] The American College of Chest Physicians recommends anticoagulation in SVT for patients at higher risk of thromboembolism, specifically with an affected venous segment greater than 5 cm, proximity less than 3 to 5 cm to the deep system, or positive medical risk factors.[57] It should be noted that all these studies are in patients with lower-extremity SVT, and all conclusions may not necessarily apply to SVT of the neck; however, symptomatic treatment with NSAIDs will usually be acceptable.

For suppurative thrombophlebitis, treatment should consist of immediate removal of any source of infection (especially IV catheters), and initiation of IV antibiotics. Antibiotics should have activity against usual skin flora, such as staphylococci, and may include first-generation cephalosporins or vancomycin in the case of MRSA. Antibiotic treatment should be tailored based on culture and sensitivity testing. The duration of treatment has not been studied, but 2 weeks is usually appropriate. Surgery is rarely required, and is reserved for patients not responding to antibiotics. Surgery frequently entails incision and drainage of any purulent collection with excision of the affected vein segment.[58,59]

Other considerations in the management of SVT should include workup for other hypercoagulable disorders or malignancy. SVT that is recurrent or migratory could suggest malignancy, as seen in Trousseau syndrome. Such patients may warrant further evaluation of the deep venous system with ultrasound, blood testing as part of a hypercoagulable panel, or other imaging such as CT or colonoscopy to screen for malignancy.

Lemierre's syndrome is a rare but dire disease worthy of special mention in the realm of thrombophlebitis of the head and neck. Also known as human necrobacillosis and anaerobic post-anginal sepsis, it is sometimes used to describe a primary infection of the head and neck with *Fusobacterium necrophorum*. Classically, it involves a constellation of findings involving a recent history of pharyngotonsillar disease, evidence of ipsilateral internal jugular vein thrombosis, metastatic lesions in the lungs or other remote site such as the joints, and isolation of the bacterium *F. necrophorum* from blood or other sterile body sites.[60]

Lemierre's syndrome is worthy of mention. André Lemierre, for whom the entity is named, neither discovered the bacteria nor initially described the entity; however, he provided a clear description of this pattern of findings in association with the bacterium in a 20-case series for *The Lancet* in 1920.[61] Although there is little supporting documentation, this syndrome is thought to have been a much more common disease before the introduction of antibiotics in 1940. With penicillin, this syndrome became the "forgotten disease."[60] It is a rare disease, but because of increasing awareness and changing patterns of antibiotic use and resistance, its incidence has been noted to be increasing. Two studies from Denmark estimated the incidence from 1990 to 1995 at 0.8 to 1.5 cases per 1 million people per year, compared with 1998 to 2001 when it rose to 3.6 cases per 1 million people per year.[62,63]

Lemierre first associated the syndrome with the bacterium now known as *F. necrophorum,* a gram-negative, anaerobic, β-hemolytic rod that is part of the normal flora of the human mouth, vagina, and gastrointestinal tract. A review of further cases reports that 57% of cases were associated with *F. necrophorum,* 30% with *Fusobacterium* species, and 3% with *F. nucleatum.*[64] Occasionally, Lemierre's syndrome has been associated with other bacteria such as *Staphylococcus, Streptococcus, Proteus, Eikenella, Bacteroides,* and *Peptostreptococcus* species. In the setting of a recent or ongoing internal jugular vein catheterization, one should suspect skin flora such as *Staphylococcus* species.[65]

Most often this syndrome follows an episode of pharyngitis. No specific mechanism has been confirmed to describe the spread of *Fusobacterium* species to the internal jugular vein; however, it has been shown that *F. necrophorum* activates high-molecular-weight kininogen and factor XI, which leads to activation of the intrinsic pathway of coagulation and can precipitate the characteristic internal jugular vein thrombosis.[66]

Pharyngitis is the most common initial symptom for the disease and occurs in 87% of cases. Patients subsequently manifest more symptoms of infection, including fever, chills, rigors, night sweats, and malaise. These symptoms usually occur 4 to 12 days after the onset of pharyngitis. Local symptoms from the intravascular spread of infection can evolve over the same time frame and often include lateral cervical neck pain, dysphagia, dyspnea, hemoptysis, and arthralgias.[60]

Laboratory workup is not usually used for diagnosis except for cultures showing the characteristic *Fusobacterium* species. However, leukocytosis, thrombocytopenia, and liver and renal function abnormalities may also be present. Septic arthritis, usually of the hip, occurs in up to 27% of cases, and synovial fluid cultures can also show the associated bacteria.[67]

Imaging studies are a crucial part of the diagnosis of Lemierre's syndrome. Routine chest radiographs are usually obtained first because of the pulmonary complaints. These and subsequent chest CT scans can show multiperipheral, nodular, or wedge-shaped pulmonary lesions and possibly empyema. Often these lesions will have a feeding blood vessel.[61,67]

Lateral neck pain will usually prompt evaluation of the cervical vasculature. This is most easily and noninvasively performed with a duplex ultrasound of the jugular veins, which has high specificity and sensitivity for thrombosis of the internal jugular vein. This can be limited in the evaluation of the tissue and vessel adjacent to the mandible, clavicle, and skull base.[60] More often, CT with contrast media is more diagnostic. It has high sensitivity and specificity for jugular vein thrombosis. This can also evaluate the soft tissue of the remaining neck and oropharynx for abscesses and other lesions.[60]

Prolonged antibiotic treatment is the mainstay of therapy for Lemierre's syndrome. Metronidazole, penicillin G, clindamycin, β-lactam and β-lactamase combinations (ampicillin-sulbactam, piperacillin-tazobactam), carbapenems, imipenem, meropenem, and chloramphenicol have demonstrated in vitro activity against *F. necrophorum.*[68,69] Metronidazole is generally considered the drug of choice.[60] If the syndrome is related to a recent IV catheterization, it would be appropriate to start empiric coverage against skin flora such as vancomycin. Culture and sensitivity testing should be done for the most effective and narrow final antibiotic regimen. The duration of treatment may range from 3 to 6 weeks. A longer course (up to 6 weeks) is thought to be sufficient for penetration of infected fibrin clot associated with internal jugular vein thrombosis.[61,68] Antibiotic treatment should be started intravenously, but may be converted to oral once the patient's fever is resolved and oral intake is tolerated.

Therapeutic anticoagulation in this disease has been a controversial point. Theoretically, this should reduce septic thromboembolic complications from the infected thrombus. Clinically, there has been varied reported experience, with some authors reporting heparin anticoagulation to be beneficial, but at least one series of 53 cases claims favorable outcomes with only 21% receiving anticoagulation.[70-72] Ultimately, the patient's clinical course, comorbidities, and bleeding risk should be taken into account. However, in the presence of confirmed thrombosis on radiographic imaging and septic embolic complications, it is not unreasonable to proceed with therapeutic anticoagulation.

Surgical intervention for Lemierre's disease is rarely described with surgical excision of the thrombosed vein. Surgery appears to be most beneficial for incision and drainage of abscess collections within the neck, lung, or other areas with septic embolic complications.[60] Surgical excision of the vein is described mainly for patients with persistent septic complications refractory to medical therapy and anticoagulation.[65] Regarding excision of the internal jugular vein, surgical exploration can be performed with exposure of the internal jugular vein. Surgeons should be wary during exploration and mobilization of structures for friability in the setting of ongoing inflammation and infection. In addition, one should also be mindful that the clot burden may extend further toward the skull base than in more typical cervical vascular surgery procedures, and exploration may require more extensive dissection.

References

1. Enomoto LM, Hill DC, Dillon PW, et al. Surgical specialty and outcomes for carotid endarterectomy: evidence from the National Surgical Quality Improvement Program. *J Surg Res*. 2014;188:339-348.

2. Centers for Disease Control and Prevention, National Center for Health Statistics. National Vital Statistics System, Mortality 2018-2021 on CDC WONDER Online Database, released in 2021. Data are from the Multiple Cause of Death Files, 2018-2021, as compiled from data provided by the 57 vital statistics jurisdictions through the Vital Statistics Cooperative Program.

3. Howell GM, Makaroun MS, Chaer RA. Current management of extracranial carotid occlusive disease. *J Am Coll Surg*. 2009;208:442.

4. Ho KJ, Nguyen LL, Menard MT. Intermediate outcome of carotid endarterectomy with bovine pericardial patch closure compared with Dacron patch and primary closure. *J Vasc Surg*. 2012;55:708-714.

5. The Asymptomatic Carotid Surgery Trial (ACST) Collaborative Group. Prevention of disabling and fatal strokes by successful carotid endarterectomy in patients without recent neurological symptoms: randomized controlled trial. *Lancet*. 2004;363:1491-1502.

6. The Asymptomatic Carotid Atherosclerosis Study Group. Endarterectomy for asymptomatic carotid artery stenosis. *JAMA*. 1995;273:1421-1428.

7. Randomized trial of endarterectomy for recently symptomatic carotid stenosis. Final results of the MRC European Carotid Surgery Trial (ECST). *Lancet*. 1998;351:1379-1387.

8. North American Symptomatic Carotid Endarterectomy Trial Collaborators. Benefit of carotid endarterectomy in patients with symptomatic moderate or severe stenosis. *N Engl J Med*. 1998;339:1415-1425.

9. Bond R, Rerkasem K, Naylor AR, et al. Systematic review of randomized controlled trials of patch angioplasty versus primary closure and different types of patch materials during carotid endarterectomy. *J Vasc Surg*. 2004;40:1126-1135.

10. Eikelboom BC, Ackerstaff RG, Hoeneveld H, et al. Benefits of carotid patching: a randomized study. *J Vasc Surg*. 1988;7:240-247.

11. Rosenthal D, Archie Jr JP, Garcia-Rinaldi R, et al. Carotid patch angioplasty: immediate and long-term results. *J Vasc Surg*. 1990;12:326-333.

12. Muto A, Nishibe T, Dardik H, et al. Patches for carotid artery endarterectomy: current materials and prospects. *J Vasc Surg*. 2009;50:206-213.

13. Beard JD, Mountney J, Wilkinson JM, et al. Prevention of postoperative wound hematomas and hyperperfusion following carotid endarterectomy. *Eur J Vasc Endovasc Surg*. 2001;21:490-493.

14. Naylor AR, Payne D, London NJ, et al. Prosthetic patch infection after carotid endarterectomy. *Eur J Vasc Endovasc Surg*. 2002;23:11-16.

15. El-Sabrout R, Reul G, Cooley DA. Infected postcarotid endarterectomy pseudoaneurysms: retrospective review of a series. *Ann Vasc Surg*. 2000;14:239-247.

16. Asciutto G, Geier B, Marpe B, et al. Dacron patch infection after carotid angioplasty: a report of 6 cases. *Eur J Vasc Endovasc Surg*. 2007;33:55-57.

17. Rockman CB, Su WT, Domenig C, et al. Postoperative infection associated with polyester patch angioplasty after carotid endarterectomy. *J Vasc Surg*. 2003;38:251-256.

18. Mann CD, McCarthy M, Nasim A, et al. Management and outcome of prosthetic patch infection after carotid endarterectomy: a single-center series and systematic review of the literature. *Eur J Vasc Endovasc Surg*. 2012;44:20-26.

19. Naughton PA, Garcia-Toca M, Rodriguez HE, et al. Carotid artery reconstruction for infected carotid patches. *Eur J Vasc Endovasc Surg*. 2010;40:492-498.

20. Knight BC, Tait WF. Dacron patch infection following carotid endarterectomy: a systematic review of the literature. *Eur J Vasc Endovasc Surg*. 2009;37:140-148.

21. Ghandi D. Computerised tomography and magnetic resonance angiography in cervicocranial vascular disease. *J Neuro Ophthalmol*. 2004;24:306-314.

22. Le Blang S, Nunez D. Non-invasive imaging of cervical vascular injuries. *Am J Roentgenol*. 2000;174:1269-1278.

23. Zhou W, Bush R, Lin P, et al. Carotid artery pseudoaneurysms after endovascular stent placement: diagnosis and follow-up duplex ultrasonography. *J Vasc Ultrasound*. 2005;29:28-32.

24. Lazaris A, Sayers R, Thompson M, et al. Patch corrugation on duplex ultrasonography may be an early warning of prosthetic patch infection. *Eur J Vasc Endovasc Surg*. 2005;29:91-92.

25. Lane B, Moseley IF, Stevens JM. The Central Nervous System: The skull and brain: methods of examination: diagnostic approach. In: Grainger RG, Allison D, eds. *Grainger and Allison's Diagnostic Radiology: A Textbook of Medical Imaging*. 3rd ed. Vol 3. London: Churchill Livingstone; 2001:2053–2055.

26. Fayed AM, White CJ, Ramee SR, et al. Carotid and cerebral angiography performed by cardiologists: cerebrovascular complications. *Catheter Cardiovasc Interv*. 2002;55:277-280.

27. Davies KN, Humphrey PR. Complications of cerebral angiography in patients with symptomatic carotid territory ischaemia screened by carotid ultrasound. *J Neurol Neurosurg Psychiatr*. 1993;56:967-972.

28. Tawes RL, Treiman RL. Vein patch rupture after carotid endarterectomy: a survey of the Western Vascular Society members. *Ann Vasc Surg*. 1991;5:71-73.

29. Graver LM, Mulcare RJ. Pseudoaneurysm after carotid endarterectomy. *J Cardiovasc Surg*. 1986;27:294-297.

30. Baker WH, Stern ME. Persistent cerebrovascular symptoms following carotid endarterectomy. In: *Complications in Vascular Surgery*. New York: Grune and Stratton; 1993:275-294.

31. Naylor A, Payne D, London N, et al. Prosthetic patch infection after carotid endarterectomy. *Eur J Vasc Endovasc Surg*. 2002;23:11-16.

32. Zacharoulis D, Gupta S, Seymour P, et al. Use of muscle flap to cover infections of the carotid artery after endarterectomy. *J Vasc Surg*. 1997;25:769-773.

33. Brown KE, Heyer K, Rodriguez H, et al. Arterial reconstruction with cryopreserved human allografts in the setting of infection: a single-center experience with midterm follow-up. *J Vasc Surg*. 2009;49:660-666.

34. Lesèche G, Castier Y, Petit MD, et al. Long-term results of cryopreserved arterial allograft reconstruction in infected prosthetic grafts and mycotic aneurysms of the abdominal aorta. *J Vasc Surg*. 2001;34:616-622.

35. Noel AA, Gloviczki P, Cherry KJ, et al. Abdominal aortic reconstruction in infected fields: early results of the United States cryopreserved aortic allograft registry. *J Vasc Surg*. 2002;35:847-852.

36. Kaviani A, Ouriel K, Kashyap VS. Infected carotid pseudoaneurysm and carotid-cutaneous fistula as a late complication of carotid artery stenting. *J Vasc Surg*. 2006;43:379-382.

37. Son S, Choi NC, Choi DS, et al. Carotid stent infection: a rare but potentially fatal complication of carotid artery stenting. *J Neurointervent Surg*. 2014;7(4):e14.

38. El-Sabrout R, Cooley DA. Extracranial carotid artery aneurysm: Texas Heart Institute experience. *J Vasc Surg.* 2000;31:43-45.

39. Schummer W, Schummer C, Voigt R, et al. Pseudoaneurysm: a rare complication of internal jugular vein cannulation: two case reports in liver transplant patients. *Anasthesiol Intensivmed Notfallmed Schmerzther.* 2003;38:542-554.

40. Naylor AR, Payne D, London NJ, et al. Prosthetic patch infection after carotid endarterectomy. *Eur J Vasc Endovasc Surg.* 2002;23:11-16.

41. Borazjani BH, Wilson SE, Fujitani RM, et al. Postoperative complications of carotid patching: pseudoaneurysm and infection. *Ann Vasc Surg.* 2003;17:156-161.

42. Lin HB, Bush RL, Lumsden AB. Successful stent-graft exclusion of a bovine patch-related carotid artery pseudoaneurysm. *J Vasc Surg.* 2003;38:396.

43. Patel JV, Rossbach MM, Cleveland TJ, et al. Endovascular stent-graft repair of traumatic carotid artery pseudoaneurysm. *Clin Radiol.* 2002;57:308-310.

44. Rodriguez-Peralto JL, Carrillo R, Rosales B, et al. Superficial thrombophlebitis. *Semin Cutan Med Surg.* 2007;26:71-76.

45. Cesarone MR, Belcaro G, Agus G, et al. Management of superficial vein thrombosis and thrombophlebitis: status and expert opinion document. *Angiology.* 2007;58(suppl 1):7S-14S, discussion 14S-15S.

46. Lee JT, Kalani MA. Treating superficial venous thrombophlebitis. *J Natl Compr Canc Netw.* 2008;6:760-765.

47. Cronenwett JL, Johnston KW. *Rutherford's Vascular Surgery.* 8th ed. Philadelphia: Saunders; 2014.

48. Coon WW, Willis PW III, Keller JB. Venous thromboembolism and other venous disease in the Tecumseh community health study. *Circulation.* 1973;48:839-846.

49. Brook I, Frazier EH. Aerobic and anaerobic microbiology of superficial suppurative thrombophlebitis. *Arch Surg.* 1996;131:95-97.

50. Martinelli I, Cattaneo M, Taioli E, et al. Genetic risk factors for superficial vein thrombosis. *Thromb Haemost.* 1999;82:1215-1217.

51. de Godoy JM, Batigalia F, Braile DM. Superficial thrombophlebitis and anticardiolipin antibodies: report of association. *Angiology.* 2001;52:127-129.

52. Maki DG, Ringer M. Risk factors for infusion-related phlebitis with small peripheral venous catheters: a randomized controlled trial. *Ann Intern Med.* 1991;114:845-854.

53. Sassu GP, Chisholm CD, Howell JM, et al. A rare etiology for pulmonary embolism: basilic vein thrombosis. *J Emerg Med.* 1990;8:45-49.

54. Superficial Thrombophlebitis Treated by Enoxaparin Study Group. A pilot randomized double-blind comparison of a low-molecular-weight heparin. a nonsteroidal anti-inflammatory agent, and placebo in the treatment of superficial vein thrombosis. *Arch Intern Med.* 2003;163:1657-1663.

55. Leizorovicz A, Becker F, Buchmuller A, et al. Clinical relevance of symptomatic superficial-vein thrombosis extension: lessons from the CALISTO study. *Blood.* 2013;122:1724-1729.

56. Blondon M, Righini M, Bounameaux H, et al. Fondaparinux for isolated superficial vein thrombosis of the legs: a cost-effectiveness analysis. *Chest.* 2012;141:321-329.

57. Buller HR, Agnelli G, Hull RD, et al. Antithrombotic therapy for venous thromboembolic disease: the Seventh ACCP Conference on Antithrombotic and Thrombolytic Therapy. *Chest.* 2004;126:401S-428S.

58. Khan EA, Correa AG, Baker CJ. Suppurative thrombophlebitis in children: a ten-year experience. *Pediatr Infect Dis J.* 1997;16:63-67.

59. Villani C, Johnson DH, Cunha BA. Bilateral suppurative thrombophlebitis due to Staphylococcus aureus. *Heart Lung.* 1995;24:342-344.

60. Wright WF, Shiner CN, Ribes JA. Lemierre syndrome. *South Med J.* 2012;105:283-288.

61. Riordan T. Human infection with Fusobacterium necrophorum (Necrobacillosis), with a focus on Lemierre's syndrome. *Clin Microbiol Rev.* 2007;20:622-659.

62. Hagelskjaer LH, Prag J, Malczynski J, et al. Incidence and clinical epidemiology of necrobacillosis, including Lemierre's syndrome, in Denmark 1990-1995. *Eur J Clin Microbiol Infect Dis.* 1998;17:561-565.

63. Hagelskjaer Kristensen L, Prag J. Lemierre's syndrome and other disseminated Fusobacterium necrophorum infections in Denmark: a prospective epidemiological and clinical survey. *Eur J Clin Microbiol Infect Dis.* 2008;27:779-789.

64. Karkos PD, Asrani S, Karkos CD, et al. Lemierre's syndrome: a systematic review. *Laryngoscope.* 2009;119:1552-1559.

65. Leon Jr LR, Patel J, Labropoulos N, et al. Excision of internal jugular vein for catheter-related thrombophlebitis. *Ann Vasc Surg.* 2006;20:117-119.

66. Holm K, Frick IM, Bjorck L, et al. Activation of the contact system at the surface of Fusobacterium necrophorum represents a possible virulence mechanism in Lemierre's syndrome. *Infect Immun.* 2011;79:3284-3290.

67. Riordan T, Wilson M. Lemierre's syndrome: more than a historical curiosa. *Postgrad Med J.* 2004;80:328-334.

68. Bondy P, Grant T. Lemierre's syndrome: what are the roles for anticoagulation and long-term antibiotic therapy? *Ann Otol Rhinol Laryngol.* 2008;117:679-683.

69. Kowalsky SF, Echols RM, McCormick EM. Comparative serum bactericidal activity of ceftizoxime/metronidazole, ceftizoxime, clindamycin, and imipenem against obligate anaerobic bacteria. *J Antimicrob Chemother.* 1990;25:767-775.

70. Armstrong AW, Spooner K, Sanders JW. Lemierre's syndrome. *Curr Infect Dis Rep.* 2000;2:168-173.

71. Bach MC, Roediger JH, Rinder HM. Septic anaerobic jugular phlebitis with pulmonary embolism: problems in management. *Rev Infect Dis.* 1988;10:424-427.

72. Goldhagen J, Alford BA, Prewitt LH, et al. Suppurative thrombophlebitis of the internal jugular vein: report of three cases and review of the pediatric literature. *Pediatr Infect Dis J.* 1988;7:410-414.

23

Head, Neck, and Orofacial Infections in Pediatric Patients

GABRIEL M. HAYEK AND DAVID SHAFER

The pediatric patient population has constant exposure to pathogens through mechanisms ranging from a toddler's attempt at ingesting various fomites to exposures to pathogens at day care facilities and schools. The growing child's immune system is under a seemingly constant threat, and when functioning correctly, it can ward off many of its assailants before signs of clinical infection. On occasion, the combination of a portal of entry, a sufficient number of pathogens, and a susceptible host manifests as a clinical infection. The clinician must determine the infection's nature and severity and render the appropriate treatment. The clinician should be familiar with the more commonly encountered infections. Whereas full textbooks are devoted to infectious diseases in the pediatric population, this chapter aims to familiarize the clinician with a summary of the more commonly encountered infections affecting the head and neck region.

Bacterial Infections

Skin Infections

Impetigo

Impetigo is a superficial infection limited to the epidermis resulting from group A streptococcal species and *Staphylococcus aureus*. The infection is usually the result of colonization of skin or nasal passages. Impetigo is highly contagious and often spreads in childcare centers and schools, with a peak incidence in children 2 to 5 years of age.

Impetigo manifests in bullous and nonbullous forms. The nonbullous type accounts for 70% of reported cases.[1] Small vesicles arise and are surrounded by erythema. The oozing from these lesions produces the honey-colored crusting characteristic of this infection (Figure 23-1). The bullous form can give rise to larger lesions filled with clear or sometimes dark fluid, resulting from *S. aureus* exotoxins A and B (which the clinician can culture from intact vesicles). Topical treatments such as mupirocin are usually effective in eliminating nonbullous forms, whereas antibiotic resistance in some regions and bullous forms of impetigo

may require oral antibiotics (cephalexin or clindamycin) for resolution.

Erysipelas

Erysipelas is a superficial infection of the dermis and upper lymphatics that often manifests in the pediatric population. The most common cause is streptococcal species of typical skin flora (β-hemolytic *Streptococcus* species). Group B streptococcal species (particularly in neonates exposed during vaginal birth to a mother positive for group B *Streptococcus*) and staphylococcal species (including methicillin-susceptible [MSSA] and methicillin-resistant [MRSA] *S. aureus*) also can be a cause. The bacteria's portal of entry is often via insect bites, scratches, or abrasions; this leads to abundant organisms that produce an exotoxin, causing the manifestations of erysipelas. Although lesions in the extremities often result from compromise of skin integrity, this is not always the case in facial infections.[2] The patient often exhibits fever, malaise, leukocytosis, and skin signs. These signs include an erythematous region with sharp demarcations, warmth on palpation (rubor), and edema/induration. Hematologic assays show positive titers for anti-streptolysin O (ASO), but it can take 10 days to obtain adequate levels to be evident on assays. In one study, it was positive in only 40% of cases of erysipelas.[3] For this reason, ASO levels are of low clinical significance in cases of erysipelas. Outpatient treatment regimens include β-lactamase penicillins, cephalosporins, and clindamycin, which are usually effective against streptococcal and staphylococcal species.[3] A patient with constitutional symptoms may require admission for parenteral antibiotics. Although the patient will often begin to feel better within a few days of antibiotic administration, skin manifestations may take longer to resolve.

Methicillin-Resistant and Methicillin-Sensitive *Staphylococcus aureus*

S. aureus, particularly community-acquired methicillin-resistant *S. aureus* (CA-MRSA), has been increasing over the past two decades. San Francisco General Hospital saw a

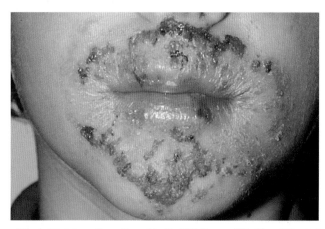

• **Figure 23-1** Impetigo. (From Neville BW, Damm DD, Allen CM, et al [eds]. *Oral and Maxillofacial Pathology*. 4th ed. St Louis: Elsevier; 2016.)

rise in prevalence of CA-MRSA from 7 to 29% over 6 years (1993 to 1999).[4] A large percentage (34%) of the U.S. population are asymptomatic carriers of *S. aureus* and less than 1% carry the more troublesome methicillin-resistant strain.[5] As this trend continues, abscess formation resistant to multiple antibiotics will continue to plague pediatric clinics. The infections caused by these bacteria often result in abscess formations that are commonly loculated. Appropriate drainage (and obtaining cultures) with specific attention to breaking up loculations is required. Copious irrigation and drain placement (if necessary) is advised. Cultures should drive the antibiotic regimen. Clindamycin, doxycycline, and trimethoprim-sulfamethoxazole (TMP-SMX; Bactrim) have been efficacious in treating CA-MRSA, although increasing rates of resistance to these regimens are present in various regions. Hospital-acquired MRSA can be treated with vancomycin, daptomycin, tigecycline, or linezolid while awaiting culture data that allow for specific antibiotic tailoring.

Bite Wounds

Domestic animal and human bites are the bite wounds most commonly encountered in the head and neck region. Children are most at risk for bites to the face, whereas adults typically sustain extremity injuries. The patient's immunization status (especially regarding tetanus) requires verification with any bite wound. Tetanus immunoglobulin and toxoid should be administered to patients without prior immunization for tetanus. If the patient has not received a tetanus booster within the 5 years preceding the injury, the patient should receive the tetanus toxoid vaccine. In addition, the animal's immunization status should be verified for an up-to-date rabies vaccination, because this diagnosis carries a 100% mortality rate and is avoidable with proper prophylaxis.

Cat Bites

Cat bites represent approximately 5 to 10% of animal bite wounds.[6] Cat bites are usually puncture wounds without significant loss of tissue. They are prone to infection because of bacteria such as *Pasteurella multocida* and *Pasteurella septica*. The bite wound should be irrigated copiously with sterile normal saline or dilute povidone-iodine solution. Small puncture wounds should be left open to heal by secondary intention.

Dog Bites

Approximately 20% of the 4.5 million Americans bitten by a dog annually seek treatment.[7] Although any breed may cause a bite wound, the more devastating injuries occur from breeds that many consider aggressive; therefore, universal prevention should be taught and practiced in any home with a domesticated animal.[8] Dog bites or attacks can result in significant tissue loss and devastating lacerations with resultant cosmetic deformities despite the best efforts of a well-trained surgeon. These wounds require copious irrigation, debridement of macerated skin margins and compromised tissues, and primary closure with close postoperative monitoring for infection. *Pasteurella canis, P. multocida,* and *Capnocytophaga canimorsus* are a few of the bacteria responsible for dog bite infections.

Human Bites

Human bites require aggressive washout (debridement) like other bite wounds. Although HIV and hepatitis transmission through a bite wound is unlikely, it is not impossible. Human bite wounds can become infected, and they are often polymicrobial. Cultures of a wound can produce aerobic staphylococcal and streptococcal species (skin flora), *Eikenella corrodens,* and various gram-negative organisms such as *Pseudomonas* or *Proteus* species (oral flora).

An antibiotic prescription after a bite wound is recommended and should provide coverage for the previously mentioned organisms. Amoxicillin-clavulanate (Augmentin) or cefuroxime for the penicillin-allergic yet cephalosporin-tolerant patient is the recommended antibiotic, providing broad coverage. Patients allergic to penicillins and cephalosporins require treatment with clindamycin plus a fluoroquinolone or TMP-SMX. A 7-day course of either regimen should suffice. Patients admitted to the hospital and unable to take oral antibiotics can be given intravenous ceftriaxone, ampicillin-sulbactam, cefoxitin, or clindamycin with a fluoroquinolone.

Acne

Various forms of acne exist, and differentiation is paramount to the treatment. Acne is prevalent in moderate to severe forms in up to 20% of the adolescent population as part of pubertal growth.[9] Sebaceous glands enlarge and increase sebum production because of increased androgen levels. Acne vulgaris develops within the sebaceous follicles, where the glands drain into follicular canals. These areas, called *comedones,* are dilated follicular sacs filled with keratin, lipids, and bacteria. Blackheads are open comedones, with the visualization of the obstructing "plug," whereas whiteheads are closed comedones with a minute opening. The bacterium most often responsible for these lesions is *Propionibacterium acnes.* Mild disease consists of comedones, as outlined earlier, whereas the number of papules and pustules present defines increased severity to moderate or severe disease. Further worsening of the inflammation can result in severe acne, characterized by large, painful lesions. Severe acne may be nodulocystic acne or, occasionally, acne conglobata. Treatment is based on the severity and ranges from topical treatments (6 to 8 weeks) of retinoid, benzoyl peroxide, or both. Acne of increased severity often requires regimens of oral antibiotics (usually tetracycline, doxycycline, or TMP-SMX) or isotretinoin. No widely accepted evidence supports the idea that ingesting certain foods exacerbates acne, but recent studies suggest that diets with high glycemic loads may aggravate acne.[10]

Acne can manifest in neonates, most often as closed comedones. Up to 20% of neonates will develop one or more comedones in the first few months of life.[11] It results from hypertrophic sebaceous glands and does not usually require treatment, because it will resolve spontaneously over a few months. Acne that develops after the age of 1 year is termed *infantile acne;* it most often consists of papules and pustules with lesions lasting several months. Topical benzoyl peroxide and tretinoin are usually efficacious in resolving this problem. Occasionally, oral antibiotics are required; erythromycin is the antibiotic of choice because tetracyclines are contraindicated in the pediatric population.

Intraoral Bacterial Infection

Acute Necrotizing Ulcerative Gingivitis and Periodontitis

Colloquially known as *trench mouth,* acute necrotizing ulcerative gingivitis is relatively rare in North America but shows increased incidence in developing countries. It often manifests with malodorous breath, a gray pseudomembranous slough on the gingival mucosa, and blunting or obliteration of the interdental papilla. In addition, patients may have a rapid onset of pain and can have systemic symptoms such as fever, malaise, and dehydration owing to poor oral intake.[12] The bacteria most often responsible include *Prevotella intermedia, Fusobacterium* species, *Treponema denticola,* and other oral spirochetes.[13] Predisposing factors include poor nutritional status, smoking, and immune compromise. The treatment includes mechanical debridement, improved and vigilant oral hygiene, and antibiotics (penicillin, metronidazole).

Aggressive Localized Periodontitis

Aggressive localized periodontitis, formerly known as *juvenile periodontitis,* primarily affects the first molars and incisors. By definition, it is localized to the "first molar/incisors with interproximal attachment loss on at least two permanent teeth, one of which is a first molar, and involving no more than two teeth other than first molars and incisors."[14] It occurs in less than 1% of adolescents and most

commonly manifests at the onset of puberty. Black male teenagers exhibit the highest predilection for this disease. The associated bone loss occurs at threefold to fourfold the rate of chronic periodontitis. *Aggregatibacter actinomycetemcomitans* and *Porphyromonas gingivalis* appear to have a role because of the association of these bacteria with these defects seen in adolescents.[15,16]

Odontogenic Abscess

The oral flora involved in abscesses of odontogenic origin is similar to that in adults. At birth, the oral cavity is sterile and uncolonized. However, within the first few days of life, it begins to become colonized with *Streptococcus salivarius* and subsequently the other bacteria that comprise those found in the adult population (e.g., *Staphylococcus, Actinomyces, Nocardia, Bacteroides* species).[17] The eruption of dentition allows the anaerobic bacteria to populate the gingival sulci and *Streptococcus mutans* and *Streptococcus sanguinis* (responsible for a large portion of dental caries) to colonize the enamel. Untreated dental caries that progresses to the pulp creates a portal of entry into the root apices, alveolus, maxilla, mandible, and surrounding spaces as the disease progresses. Infections in a child's submandibular and lingual spaces are infrequent, but necessitate the close attention of the treating team to ensure that the smaller, developing airway is not compromised (Figure 23-2). Incision and drainage is the treatment for an abscess, along with extraction or treatment of the offending tooth. Patients with developing, partially erupted third molars risk developing pericoronitis and associated abscesses (most notably the adjacent pterygomandibular space). Impacted teeth that impede proper oral hygiene should be extracted, preferably before developing infections or complications. Of note, azithromycin is now the first-line recommended antibiotic in patients with a penicillin allergy, given the black box warning associated with clindamycin.

Osteomyelitis

An entire chapter (Chapter 18) in this book is devoted to osteomyelitis. However, it is essential to note that pediatric osteomyelitis mainly affects the axial skeleton's long bones. It rarely affects the skull or bones of the facial skeleton. Although osteomyelitis is extraordinarily rare, patients who complain of persistent pain in an area after an extraction (with or without purulence) should have the appropriate workup to rule out this destructive, infectious process.

Chronic Nonbacterial Osteomyelitis

Chronic nonbacterial osteomyelitis is also known as chronic recurrent multifocal osteomyelitis (CRMO). The rheumatic literature describes this pathologic condition as an autoinflammatory bone disease. The discussion here is merely to avoid confusion because it is a noninfectious process that occurs mainly in the pediatric population and is often confused with infectious osteomyelitis. The new nomenclature will help to prevent future confusion.

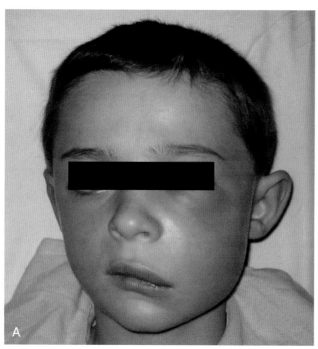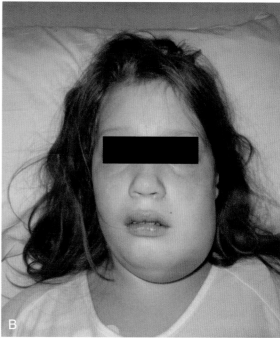

• **Figure 23-2 A,** Left canine space infection of maxillary odontogenic origin. **B,** Left submandibular space infection of mandibular odontogenic origin. (**A,** Courtesy Dr. Brian Alpert. **B,** Courtesy Dr. George Kushner.)

Viral Infections

Human Papillomavirus

As a papovavirus, human papillomavirus (HPV) is a DNA virus that can give rise to oral papillomas. These lesions can manifest on the face's epidermis or any intraoral mucosal site. Intraorally, the lesions primarily involve the hard and soft palate and uvula. The lesions are usually isolated; although they can be large, they are commonly smaller than 1 cm. Lesions are sessile or pedunculated masses amenable to excision and should undergo histopathologic analysis (Figure 23-3). There are more than 100 subtypes of HPV.

Subtype 16 is related to neoplastic changes and oral cancer, accounting for over 90% of such cases.[18] An HPV vaccine is now available and recommended as part of the standard vaccine series.

Pediatric patients with HPV that may result from sexual abuse should be appropriately questioned sensitively and reported to the appropriate authorities for further investigation to ensure the patient's safety.

Parvovirus B19

A single-stranded DNA virus, parvovirus B19 causes erythema infectiosum, also known as *fifth disease*, which is

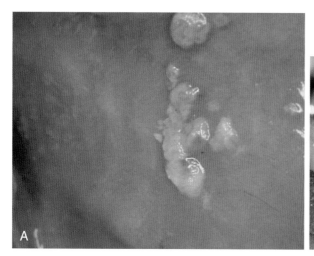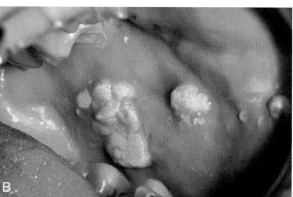

• **Figure 23-3 A,** Condyloma on buccal mucosa. **B,** Multiple exophytic and somewhat papillary nodules of the lip, buccal mucosa, and gingiva. (**A,** From Newman MG, Takei HH, Klokkevold PR, et al [eds]. *Carranza's clinical periodontology.* 11th ed. St Louis: Saunders; 2012. **B,** From Neville BW, Damm DD, Allen CM, et al [eds]. *Oral and maxillofacial pathology.* 4th ed. St Louis: Saunders; 2016.)

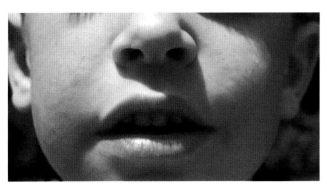

• **Figure 23-4** Erythema Infectiosum *(Fifth Disease)* Caused by Parvovirus B19. (Courtesy Centers for Disease Control and Prevention, Atlanta, GA.)

notable for its "slapped cheek" appearance in children affected by the virus (Figure 23-4). It most often manifests in children aged 5 to 15 years and lasts 1 to 3 weeks before fading. More troublesome is the aplastic anemia crisis that this virus can precipitate in a small subset of patients. Rarely, a patient's symptoms manifest as a pure red cell aplasia caused by inadequate host response to the infection. This disease is often self-limiting, and supportive care, including transfusion, should be administered as necessary. Finally, fetal infection can lead to anemia, hydrops fetalis, or miscarriage.

Molluscum Contagiosum

Molluscum contagiosum results from a poxvirus and is a viral infection of the epithelium. It gives rise to multiple 2- to 3-mm papules, each with a central depression. These papules are often located on the face, extremities, and trunk and generally spare the mucous membranes and palmar surfaces. The diagnosis is usually made based on clinical appearance alone. Treatment of the disease may require topical agents (a wide variety are used depending on the affected area), though immunocompetent patients usually resolve spontaneously. Although single lesions typically last only 2 to 3 months, autoinoculation causes persistent infection and usually lasts 6 to 12 months.

Coxsackie Virus

Coxsackie virus, which causes hand, foot, and mouth disease, is common in children younger than 10 years. Transmission is by respiratory droplet and is highly communicable. Generalized symptoms of fever and sore throat develop shortly before oral vesicular lesions. These 2- to 3-mm vesicles might not be seen intact, but may appear as ulcerations if the vesicles have already sloughed the superficial layer. Following the appearance of oral lesions, cutaneous lesions manifest in approximately three-fourths of all cases, most commonly on the palmar surfaces of the hands and feet. Coxsackie virus A 16 is the most widely implicated, but other A and B strains have been isolated. Diagnosis is clinical, and only treatment of symptoms is required, as the disease is self-limiting.

Paramyxovirus

Measles most often begins with fever, cough, coryza, and conjunctivitis. Koplik's spots typically manifest on the second day of illness and are usually found on the buccal mucosa, but can be found on other mucosal surfaces. The maculopapular rash then begins at the face and ears and descends with the lesions often coalescing and covering the body within an additional 48 hours. The rash will then fade in the same order that it appeared. Serious complications that may result from the disease include pneumonia and encephalitis. Diagnosis is based on clinical examination, although polymerase chain reaction or specific antibody testing can be confirmatory. The live-attenuated measles, mumps, and rubella vaccine given to children at 2 years of age (and often revaccination at an older age in grade or middle school) has caused a sharp decline in cases.

Primary and Secondary Herpetic Gingivostomatitis

Herpes simplex virus 1 exhibits a seroprevalence in the United States of approximately 60%.[19] Luckily, not all infected have manifestations of primary herpetic gingivostomatitis. Herpes simplex virus 1 causes this disease; initially, it can cause ulcerations on any mucosal surface. Recurrence of the illness manifests in the keratinized mucosa of the hard palate, gingiva, and the vermilion and surrounding tissues. Primary gingivostomatis lesions, along with fever, malaise, and cervical lymphadenopathy, are usually seen in the pediatric population. The lesions are multiple small erythematous ulcerations that remain present for 7 to 10 days. Resolution of the lesions occurs without intervention, and the virus then enters a dormant phase in the nerve tissue and can return later as a secondary or recurrent herpes simplex infection.

Fungal Infections

Oral Candidiasis

Thrush (oral candidiasis) is a superficial candidal infection of the mucous membranes of the oral cavity. It affects approximately 5% of immunocompetent newborns and a more significant percentage of immunocompromised newborns. It is uncommon to develop thrush after 1 year, except when the child is currently taking antibiotics. The infection manifests as a white, wipeable plaque. Once wiped away, the underlying mucosa is erythematous or ulcerated. Minor infections may resolve without treatment. When indicated, treatment usually consists of nystatin oral rinse. Occasionally, in breast-fed infants, the mother should also be treated and given oral fluconazole. Persistence after 1 year of age in the absence of antibiotics, or persistent disease in an infant who is refractory to the treatments rendered, necessitates further workup for underlying immunologic disorders.

Tinea Capitis

Tinea capitis, or *ringworm* as it is colloquially known, is a disease that mainly affects prepubescent children.[20] The *Trichophyton* and *Microsporum* genera mainly cause these cutaneous fungal infections. They manifest on the scalp with inflammation, resulting in scaling and hair loss. This hair loss often results in a "black-dot" pattern in which the hair shaft is broken at the level of the scalp (however, this only holds true for individuals with black hair, the "dot" pattern being dependent on hair color). These lesions can result in hair loss (with permanent alopecia if significant scarring occurs) and can also lead to pustules or abscess formation. First-line therapy for tinea capitis in children is griseofulvin and terbinafine. Griseofulvin has a long history of use in treating tinea capitis, but requires a long duration of therapy (6 to 12 weeks), whereas terbinafine treatment only requires 2 to 6 weeks with similar efficacy.[21]

Although thrush and tinea capitis infections comprise the bulk of fungal pediatric diseases encountered, deep fungal infections can manifest in immunocompromised patient populations, such as patients undergoing chemotherapy.[22] These diseases, such as blastomycosis, coccidioidomycosis, and histoplasmosis, are systemic and rarely present with isolated features to the head or neck region.

Parasitic Infections

Lice and Scabies

Various parasites can inhabit the scalp (e.g., Bott flies), but are uncommon in most patient populations. In developed countries, the main parasites affecting pediatric populations are scabies and pediculosis (i.e., lice). Pediculosis affects an estimated 6 to 12 million children annually in the United States.[23] Head lice are approximately 1 to 3 mm long. Females lay up to 300 eggs, which are a yellow-white color, that hatch and mature into an adult in approximately 20 days.[24] Lice cannot jump or fly; therefore, transmission can occur only with proximity from one host to the next. The main presentation is pruritus caused by a delayed hypersensitivity reaction, but prolonged infection can result in anemia, which can be profound. Treatment is with topical permethrin (1%) shampoo. There are newer treatments available, but these are costly and resistance patterns are not yet known. Noninsecticidal agents including dimethicone and isopropyl myristate have shown promising results. Nonpharmacologic management with heat and wet combing are options, but studies show mixed results.

Another common parasite encountered is scabies, which manifests as intense pruritus. Scalp scabies occurs mainly in infants and children. The crusted lesions are usually not limited to the scalp; they may also be present on the face, palms, and soles of the feet. The diagnosis is mainly clinical, along with microscopic examination for mites, eggs, or feces. Transmission occurs by skin-to-skin contact or close quarters, such as bed-sharing. Treatment options include topical permethrin

5% cream (usually the first line of treatment) or two doses of oral ivermectin (200 μg/kg/dose) given 14 days apart.

In both of these infections, it is imperative to rule out additional close contacts as carriers, and that peripheral fomite that may harbor organisms that could cause reinfection (e.g., bedding, clothing) are also treated with washing (hot water at 130°C [266°F]) and drying in a hot dryer. Placing items in a sealed bag for 2 weeks is also effective.

Tickborne Infections (Bacterial and Parasitic)

Depending on geographic location, children with a tick may be at risk for various diseases, such as Lyme disease, Rocky Mountain spotted fever (RMSF), babesiosis, and tularemia. These diseases are grouped here based on their mode of infection, comprising both bacterial (Lyme disease, RMSF, ehrlichiosis, and tularemia) and parasitic (babesiosis) diseases. The ticks often require many hours of attachment to transmit the disease; therefore, timely removal is crucial. Sometimes, the patient (or the patient's parents) might not recall a tick bite despite diagnosing a tickborne infection. Hard ticks (Ixodidae) will feed for days if left undisturbed, and removal within the first 24 hours of attachment may help prevent contracting Lyme disease. In the head and neck, the scalp provides good coverage or camouflage for a tick and requires careful inspection for a residing tick in any patient or child who is at risk for tickborne infections. In addition, some patients affected by one tickborne infection will have multiple infections resulting from a single tick bite.[25] This section will discuss the two most common tickborne illnesses in the United States: Lyme disease and RMSF.

Lyme Disease (Vector: *Ixodes scapularis*; Pathogen: *Borrelia burgdorferi*)

A typical or classic case involving this bacterial infection will manifest with erythema migrans—a large, flat, red rash with central clearing, causing the lesion to appear like a target (or "bull's-eye") with the central cleared portion as the site of the tick bite. Of patients with erythema migrans, 80% will have a single lesion, whereas others will have multiple lesions.[26] Erythema migrans can resolve without antibiotics; however, the patient remains at risk for disease progression to further stages. A generalized rash, fever, headache, and myalgias may be present. Arthralgias and neurologic symptoms also can be identified, including meningitis, encephalitis, ascending weakness like that of Guillain-Barré, or cranial nerve VII paralysis (Bell's palsy). Heart block (first, second, or third degree) can also manifest as a sign of disseminated Lyme disease. An erythema migrans lesion in a patient who lives in or has visited a region with known endemic disease is essentially diagnostic. Serologic testing may confirm the diagnosis, but even this is unreliable. The treatment regimens depend on the stage of the disease, with doxycycline or ceftriaxone often used. Amoxicillin or erythromycin is the treatment of choice for children younger than 8 years. Disseminated or late disease requires parenteral antibiotics, requiring a prolonged treatment of 1 to 2 months. Consultation with an infectious disease specialist is appropriate in these cases.

Rocky Mountain Spotted Fever (Vector: *Dermacentor variabilis;* Pathogen: *Rickettsia rickettsii*)

The bacterial infection known as RMSF includes high fevers and a maculopapular rash that can appear as multiple small lesions that begin peripherally at the extremities (usually at the wrists and ankles) and spread centrally. However, up to 15% of patients with RMSF never exhibit a rash formation.[27] Headaches, myalgia, and malaise are also common in the presentation of this tickborne illness. Less common symptoms include seizures, encephalopathy, confusion, thrombocytopenia, and hyponatremia. Treatment for life-threatening manifestations of RMSF is doxycycline and chloramphenicol (even in children).

Babesiosis, tularemia, Q-fever, Colorado tick fever, and ehrlichiosis are other, less prevalent tickborne diseases with a low incidence; however, they can manifest with Lyme disease or RMSF.

Infections Based on Anatomic Site (Varying Etiology)

Pharyngitis and Tonsillitis

A "sore throat" is a common complaint with an exhaustive list of possible precipitating factors. Examination of the oropharynx in these patients may show erythema in varying severity. Examining the tonsillar bed will identify hypertrophy or exudates (Figure 23-5). Pharyngitis may be part of a constellation of symptoms associated with a systemic infection, and inspection for rhinorrhea, conjunctivitis, and cough may direct the practitioner to consider a viral cause for the pharyngitis or tonsillitis (rhinovirus, influenza virus, parainfluenza virus, adenovirus, coxsackievirus, and respiratory syncytial virus are among the possibilities). An assay for group A *Streptococcus* (GAS) with a rapid strep test or additional cultures can help elucidate the infection's nature. The peak incidence for acute *Streptococcus* tonsillitis is at 5 to 6 years of age. The Centor criteria help identify patients who are at risk for GAS consisting of (1) body temperature greater than 38.1°C (100.5°F), (2) absence of cough, (3) tonsillar exudates, and (4) cervical lymphadenopathy.[28] Patients with fewer than two of these criteria require no additional test, whereas two or more factors indicate the need for a rapid strep test and possible throat culture, depending on the result of the rapid strep assay. Other bacteria implicated in tonsillitis and pharyngitis include *Neisseria gonorrhoeae, Arcanobacterium haemolyticum, Mycoplasma pneumoniae,* and *Chlamydophila pneumoniae.* Treating GAS pharyngitis/tonsillitis is vital to avoid rare, severe complications, including scarlet fever, rheumatic fever, and acute glomerulonephritis. Proven bacterial infections require treatment with antibiotics tailored to the culture and sensitivities.

Concerning signs and symptoms of a patient with a complicated "sore throat" include stridor or other respiratory distress, dysphagia or inability to handle oral secretions, or a palpable mass or discrete swelling. Infection of the tonsil can lead to the accumulation of purulence between the tonsil and the tonsillar capsule, resulting in a peritonsillar abscess; this is the most common complication of acute tonsillitis requiring aspiration or incision and drainage (depending on severity). After drainage, the patient should respond well to the antibiotic regimen prescribed, usually penicillin (erythromycin or azithromycin if the patient is allergic to penicillin). Extension beyond the peritonsillar region into the lateral or posterior pharyngeal space requires hospital admission, incision, drainage, and intravenous antibiotics.

Infections of the Sinuses

The maxillary sinuses are not pneumatized until approximately age 4 years, the sphenoid sinus becomes distinct by

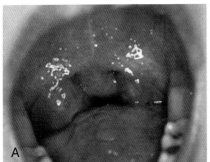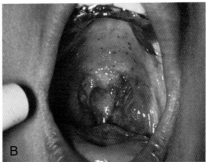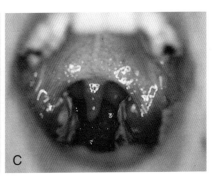

• **Figure 23-5** Pharyngotonsillitis. This common syndrome has several causative pathogens and a wide spectrum of severity. **A,** The diffuse tonsillar and pharyngeal erythema seen here is a nonspecific finding that can be produced by a variety of pathogens. **B,** This intense erythema, seen in association with acute tonsillar enlargement and palatal petechiae, is highly suggestive of group A β-streptococcal infection, although other pathogens can produce these findings. **C,** This picture of exudative tonsillitis is most commonly seen with either group A streptococcal or Epstein-Barr virus infection. (From Zitelli BJ, McIntire SC, Nowalk AJ [eds]. *Atlas of Pediatric Physical Diagnosis.* 6th ed. Philadelphia: Saunders; 2012. **B,** Courtesy Michael Sherlock, Lutherville, MD.)

age 5, and the frontal sinuses begin to develop at age 7 and continue to develop into the late teenage years. These sinuses drain through small ostia, which can become obstructed with surrounding edematous mucosa, thus preventing adequate drainage and creating an environment where bacteria can flourish. These conditions can result in sinusitis.

Sinusitis manifests in acute and chronic forms. Acute sinusitis follows a recent upper respiratory tract infection (often viral). The paranasal sinuses can then become secondarily infected with bacteria. Acute sinusitis lasts up to 4 weeks. *Moraxella catarrhalis, Streptococcus pneumoniae,* and *Haemophilus influenzae* are the more common bacteria associated with acute sinusitis. Patients with acute sinusitis complain of headache, mucopurulent nasal discharge, pressure sensation in the areas overlying the sinuses involved, pain in the maxillary teeth, and soft tissue swelling adjacent to the sinus involved. Patients predisposed to sinusitis include those with immunocompromise, cystic fibrosis, nasal polyps, anatomic defects (clefting), ciliary dysfunction, allergic rhinitis, and smokers. The diagnosis is often made based on clinical examination alone. Plain films such as a panoramic or Water's view may show sinus opacification indicative of current disease. A complicated case with soft tissue swelling or abscess formation warrants further workup that can include imaging, but usually, sinusitis in and of itself is not an indication for CT.

Subacute sinusitis (4 to 12 weeks of symptoms) and chronic sinusitis (>12 weeks of symptoms) involve different bacteria.[29] The significant bacteria responsible for chronic sinusitis are *Pseudomonas aeruginosa,* GAS, *S. aureus,* and anaerobes such as *Bacteroides* and *Fusobacterium* species. Imaging, including CT scans of chronic sinus disease, will demonstrate thickening of the affected sinus mucosa (or even complete opacification of the affected sinus) (Figure 23-6).

Treatment for uncomplicated sinusitis consists of antibiotic therapy. First-line agents are amoxicillin-clavulanate, TMP-SMX, and azithromycin, adding metronidazole or clindamycin when anaerobic infection is suspected. Because of the increased risk of severe complications, including intracranial extension of infection or osteomyelitis of the adjacent frontal bone (Pott's puffy tumor), frontal sinusitis is often treated with parenteral antibiotics initially. Once there is clinical improvement, oral therapy begins. In addition, children with orbital cellulitis without an obvious dental or skin source should be evaluated for sinus disease because infection of the paranasal sinuses can lead to periorbital swelling or cellulitis. This process is also often treated initially with parenteral antibiotics, including ceftriaxone. Mucolytics such as guaifenesin may help to thin the secretions and improve drainage. Local vasoconstrictors like oxymetazoline (ages six years and up) or phenylephrine (ages two years and up with appropriate dose formulation) may help to open the ostium and allow for drainage. However, patients should be counseled on the risk of developing rhinitis medicamentosa with prolonged use. Refractory,

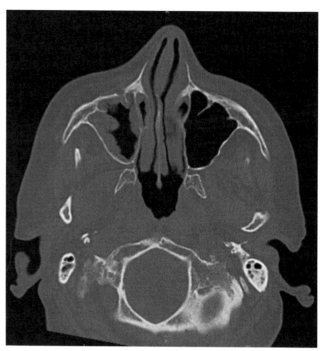

• **Figure 23-6** Noncontrasted axial CT image demonstrating right maxillary chronic sinusitis with evident mucosal thickening.

chronic sinusitis, or recurrent acute sinusitis (four or more episodes within 1 year) might not respond to medical therapy alone, and treatment with sinus surgery may be required (e.g., functional endoscopic sinus surgery) for surgical drainage, including enlargement of ostia.

Dacryocystitis

Acute infection of the nasolacrimal sac is a common problem in the infant population. Swelling in the medial canthal region noted at birth is often not infection but rather distention caused by amniotic fluid that has no port for egress because of a blockage of the nasolacrimal duct or the valve of Hasner. Digital massage can often lead to the resolution of this swelling. If there is no resolution, surgery involving probing and cannulation of the ducts with stents may be indicated. More troubling is the newborn or infant with medial orbital edema with overlying erythema that is concerning for orbital cellulitis or dacryocystitis. The swelling of the medial canthal region develops with extreme tenderness and erythema overlying the edematous region. Bacteria associated with these infections are upper respiratory tract organisms such as *Streptococcus* and *Staphylococcus* species. The practitioner should have a low threshold for admission and intravenous antibiotics (cefuroxime or similar) to prevent disease progression, such as orbital cellulitis.

Conjunctivitis

Conjunctivitis may be infectious or noninfectious. Noninfectious causes include allergies, foreign bodies (including contact use or overuse), and chemical conjunctivitis. Infectious causes are usually due to bacterial or viral sources. Bacterial conjunctivitis accounts for half to three-fourths of all infectious conjunctivitis, with the most common bacteria isolated from these cases being *S. aureus, Staphylococcus epidermidis, S. pneumoniae, M. catarrhalis, Pseudomonas, Haemophilus, Neisseria, Chlamydia,* and *Bartonella* species.

Symptoms and signs associated with bacterial conjunctivitis include unilateral or bilateral hyperemia, tearing, drainage, or discharge, notably in the morning, that could result in "gluing" of the eyes on awakening. Involvement of preauricular lymph nodes with notable adenopathy in a sexually active youth (possibly present with concomitant urethritis) is concerning for *Neisseria* or *Chlamydia* species conjunctivitis. Exposure to felines in patients with conjunctivitis with preauricular and submandibular adenopathy concerns for *Bartonella* species as the infectious agent. (*Bartonella* species is one of the more common causes of Parinaud oculoglandular syndrome.)

Bacterial conjunctivitis is usually treated based on examination, although most cases are self-limiting. Any cultures obtained can help to guide antibiotic therapy. Usually, warm compresses and topical antibiotics successfully treat bacterial conjunctivitis. Chronic and severe cases (with increased discharge) should have cultures taken to guide therapy. Any discovery of bacteria associated with sexually transmitted diseases should raise concern for abuse, and appropriate reporting should occur. *Neisseria* or *Chlamydia* species infection warrants systemic, topical antibiotic therapy.

Adenovirus, enterovirus, and Coxsackie virus are most often associated with conjunctivitis. The process usually begins as a unilateral conjunctivitis that can spread to the contralateral eye. Patients often complain of a foreign body sensation and more generalized viral symptoms of fever, sore throat, and preauricular adenopathy. In some cases, subconjunctival hemorrhage is present. Viral conjunctivitis is also a diagnosis based on clinical impression. If herpes simplex virus is suspected (because of an ipsilateral facial vesicular rash), prompt referral to an ophthalmologist for a corneal examination to determine its possible involvement is paramount. Otherwise, treatment for viral conjunctivitis is supportive, and the affected child should be kept from contact with others (e.g., school, day care) for several days to 1 week as the symptoms resolve.

Ophthalmia neonatorum (conjunctivitis within the first month of life) is usually associated with normal skin flora (*Streptococcus* and *Staphylococcus* species), but vertical transmission of chlamydia, gonorrhea, or herpes simplex virus is possible. Erythromycin ointment is placed on newborns at birth to help prevent this vertical transmission. However, some centers use povidone-iodine to control ophthalmia neonatorum, and up to 5 to 10% of infants develop chemical conjunctivitis (which manifests in the first 24 hours of life).[30]

Airway Infections

The practitioner may encounter airway infections focused on the head and neck, including bacterial tracheitis, croup, and epiglottitis. Bacterial tracheitis is an uncommon infection that predominantly affects children 8 years of age and younger. The typical patient exhibits cough, inspiratory stridor with prolonged inspiration, fever, and purulent secretions in the airway, depending on the patient's ability to mobilize these secretions. Causative agents include *S. aureus, H. influenzae,* and β-hemolytic streptococcal species. Patients frequently have a history of a preceding upper airway viral infection. Direct laryngoscopy allows differentiation between epiglottitis and tracheitis depending on the findings noted on examination. A lateral radiograph of the neck will display no distinct findings, and the epiglottis will appear normal (in contrast to epiglottitis with the "thumb sign"). Treatment includes protection of the airway (with intubation in a controlled setting), debridement of the pseudomembranes if present, and broad-spectrum antibiotics (e.g., ceftriaxone tailored to aspirate cultures return).

Epiglottitis has declined significantly with the increased immunization against *H. influenzae* (specifically type B). These patients exhibit high fever, stridor owing to upper airway obstruction, and a muffled voice. The patient may posture by leaning forward and have tongue protrusion to maintain airway patency. Lateral films may demonstrate a "thumb" sign with edema of the epiglottis. This condition, like bacterial tracheitis, is treated by immediate airway control with intubation, preferably in a controlled setting, followed by supportive care.

Croup commonly affects the upper airway and manifests with a barking cough typically preceded by nonspecific upper airway symptoms. It typically affects children between the ages of 6 months and 3 years. As the airway swelling continues, breathing becomes more difficult for the patient. The pathophysiology is related to the parainfluenza virus, but influenza, adenovirus, and respiratory syncytial virus can also be at fault. Treatment modalities include racemic epinephrine and oral dexamethasone (up to 0.6 mg/kg). Close monitoring is required until there is no longer a concern for airway obstruction.

Otitis Externa

Otitis externa usually manifests as inflammation of the external auditory canal, usually with rapid onset. The patient will often complain of fullness, pain, or itching. The most common bacteria associated with otitis externa are *P. aeruginosa, S. epidermidis,* and *S. aureus.* A 10-day course of steroids with or without antibiotics (both topical) is often successful in treating this condition; immunocompromised patients may require oral antibiotics in addition to the topical regimen prescribed.

Otitis Media

Pelton[31] showed that the cluster of cloudy tympanic membrane (TM), bulging TM, and TM with impaired mobility correlated with acute otitis media; therefore, assessment of position and mobility is essential. Common bacterial pathogens include *S. pneumoniae, H. influenzae,* and *M. catarrhalis.* Viral infections also have been implicated (respiratory syncytial virus, rhinovirus, adenovirus, influenza). Although many practitioners will prescribe antibiotics for acute otitis media, this has contributed to antibiotic resistance; attempting to prescribe more prudently and allowing many patients to resolve without intervention is increasingly common. According to guidelines by the American Academy of Pediatrics and the American Academy of Family Physicians, children with a suspected diagnosis of acute otitis media at younger than 6 months of age require antibiotics; those with a likely diagnosis and ages 6 months to 2 years should also take antibiotics; and those older than 2 years of age have the option for observation, but only if follow-up is sure and there is no severe illness (e.g., high fever, severe pain). Follow-up visits must be performed to ensure resolution, especially in the developing patient who may have an undiagnosed effusion that can impair hearing and speech development. Treatment for patients who are not allergic to penicillin should be amoxicillin unless *M. catarrhalis* or a β-lactamase–producing organism is suspected, in which case amoxicillin-clavulanate is the treatment of choice. The dosing regimen is high (90 mg/kg/day for amoxicillin). Azithromycin or clarithromycin are the treatment options of choice in the penicillin-allergic patient.

Cervical Lymphadenitis

Cervical lymphadenitis has multiple possible causes in pediatric patients. The pediatric facial/head/neck surgeon will often be a consulting clinician during the treatment of this process. Familiarity with the anatomy of this region is essential, including the superficial and deep cervical chains, jugulodigastric, submaxillary, and the regions they each drain. Infectious agents causing cervical lymphadenitis include viral agents (adenovirus, Coxsackie virus, HIV, cytomegalovirus, and Epstein-Barr virus being the most notable), bacterial (e.g., *Staphylococcus, Streptococcus, Mycobacterium, Bartonella* species), fungal (e.g., histoplasmosis, *Candida* species), and parasitic (e.g., toxoplasmosis). The treatment team should attempt to elucidate other signs and symptoms that may point to the cause of the lymphadenitis. A definitive swelling with fluctuance (by examination or imaging such as ultrasound or CT) will often require drainage and cultures, including aerobic, anaerobic, acid-fast, and fungal. Of course, the practitioner must consider congenital lesions in the pediatric population when dealing with swelling in this region (e.g., thyroglossal duct cysts, branchial cleft cysts, cystic hygromas). In addition, any neck swelling that persists beyond 6 to 8 weeks requires a reassessment of the history and physical and consideration and workup for underlying disorders.[32]

Antibiotic Considerations in Pediatric Populations

Antibiotic use in pediatric populations requires the practitioner to be aware of the contraindications of classes of antibiotics in some of the pediatric populations, as well as the appropriate weight-based dosing regimens. Dosing regimens are weight-based (milligrams per kilogram, up to a maximum daily dose, usually the equivalent of the adult dosing regimen). Occasionally (e.g., amoxicillin dosing for acute otitis media), the regimen may exceed that of a typical adult dosing regimen, depending on the child's weight. Prescribers should avoid fluoroquinolones in children younger than 18 years because of the effects on developing cartilage, which can result in arthropathy. According to the American Academy of Pediatrics, the only indications for their use in patients younger than 18 years are complicated urinary tract infections, pyelonephritis, and postexposure anthrax treatment.[33] Prescribers should also avoid tetracycline antibiotics in the pediatric population because of the permanent discoloration it causes on the developing dentition. The clinical crowns of the aesthetic, anterior teeth develop until the age of 8 years, and for this reason, should be avoided until this age unless clinical judgment in cases such as RMSF requires appropriate dosing of doxycycline.[34,35] Prescribers should be aware of side effects with any medication. This knowledge of prescribed medications should include possible drug–drug interactions, as unwanted and deleterious side effects can be of more significant concern in pediatric populations because of drug-related pharmacokinetic changes.

References

1. Larru B, Gerber J. Cutaneous bacterial infections caused by *Staphylococcus aureus* and *Streptococcus pyogenes* in infants and children. *Pediatr Clin North Am.* 2014;61:457-478.
2. Vary J, O'Connor K. Common dermatologic conditions. *Med Clin North Am.* 2014;98:445-485.
3. Leppard BJ, Seal DV, Colman G, Hallas G. The value of bacteriology and serology in the diagnosis of cellulitis and erysipelas. *Br J Dermatol.* 1985;112:559-567.
4. Niami TS, LeDell KH, Como-Sabetti K, et al. Comparison of community and health care associated methicillin-resistant *Staphylococcus. JAMA.* 2003;290:2976-2984.
5. Kuehnert MJ, Kruson-Moran D. Prevalence of *Staphylococcal aureus* nasal colonization in the United States, 2001-2002. *J Infect Dis.* 2006;193:172-179.
6. Ellis R, Ellis C. Dog and cat bites. *Am Fam Phys.* 2014;90:239-243.
7. Gilchrist J, Sacks JJ, White D, Kresnow MJ. Dog bites: still a problem? *Inj Prev.* 2008;14:296-301.
8. Sacks JJ, Sinclair L, Gilchrist J, Golab GC, Lockwood R. Breeds of dogs involved in fatal human attacks in the United States between 1979 and 1998. *J Am Vet Med Assoc.* 2000;217:836-840.
9. Bhate K, Williams HC. Epidemiology of acne vulgaris. *Br J Dermatol.* 2013;168:474-485.
10. Bowe WP, Joshi SS, Shalita AR. Diet and acne. *J Am Acad of Derm.* 2009;63:124-141.
11. Kliegman R, Stanton B, St Geme J, Shor N. Acne. In: *Nelson Textbook of Pediatrics.* 20th ed. Philadelphia: Saunders; 2015.
12. Hodgdon A. Dental and related infections. *Emerg Med Clin North Am.* 2013;31:465-480.
13. Loesche WJ, Syed SA, Langhorn BE, et al. The bacteriology of acute necrotizing ulcerative gingivitis. *J Periodontol.* 1982;53:223-230.

14. Lang N, Bartold PM, Cullinan M, et al. Consensus report: aggressive periodontitis. *Ann Periodontol.* 1999;4:53.

15. Newman MG, Takei HH, Klokkevold PR, Carranza FA. Acute gingival infections. In: *Carranza's Clinical Periodontology.* 11th ed. St. Louis: Saunders; 2012:97-103.

16. Song HJ. Periodontal considerations for children. *Dent Clin North Am.* 2012;57:17-37.

17. Socransky SS, Manganiello SD. The oral microbiota of man from birth to senility. *J Periodontol.* 1971;42:485-496.

18. Palmer O, Grannum R. Oral cancer detection. *Dent Clin North Am.* 2011;55:537-548.

19. Xu F, Sternberg M, Kottiri BJ, et al. Trends in herpes simplex virus type 1 and type 2 seroprevalence in the United States. *JAMA.* 2006;296:964-973.

20. Elewski E. Tinea capitis: a current perspective. *J Am Acad Dermatol.* 2000;42:1-20.

21. Tey HL, Tan AS, Chan YC. Meta-analysis of randomized, controlled trials comparing griseofulvin and terbinafine in the treatment of tinea capitis. *J Am Acad Dermatol.* 2011;64:663-670.

22. Marcoux D, Jafarian F, Joncas V, et al. Deep cutaneous fungal infections in immunocompromised children. *J Am Acad Dermatol.* 2009;61:857-864.

23. Centers for Disease Control and Prevention. *Head Lice: Epidemiology and Risk Factors.* Available at: http://www.cdc.gov/parasites/lice/head/epi.html. Accessed September 14, 2015.

24. Gunning K, Pippitt K, Kiraly B, Sayler M. Pediculosis and scabies: a treatment update. *Am Fam Phys.* 2012;86:535-541.

25. Hersh MH, Ostfeld RS, McHenry DJ, et al. Co-infection of blacklegged ticks with *Babesia microti* and *Borrelia burgdorferi* is higher than expected and acquired from small mammal hosts. *PLoS One.* 2014;9(6):e99348. Available at: http://journals.plos.org/plosone/article?id=10.1371/journal.pone.0099348. Accessed March 5, 2015.

26. Shapiro E. Lyme disease. *N Engl J Med.* 2014;370:1724-1731.

27. Adams J. Tick-borne diseases. In: *Emergency Medicine.* 2nd ed. Philadelphia: Saunders; 1518-1525.

28. Centor RM, Witherspoon JM, Dalton HP, et al. The diagnosis of strep throat in adults in the emergency room. *Med Decis Making.* 1981;1:239-246.

29. Brook I. Acute and chronic bacterial sinusitis. *Infect Dis Clin North Am.* 2007;21:427-448.

30. David M, Rumelt S, Weintraub Z, et al. Efficacy comparison between povidone iodine 2.5% and tetracycline 1% in prevention of ophthalmia neonatorum. *Ophthalmology.* 2011;118:1454-1458.

31. Pelton SI. Otoscopy for the diagnosis of otitis media. *Pediatr Infect Dis J.* 1998;17:540-543.

32. Healy CM, Baker CJ Cervical lymphadenitis. *Feigin and Cherry's Textbook of Pediatric Infectious Diseases.* 7th ed. Philadelphia: Saunders; 2014:175–189.

33. Committee on Infectious Disease. The use of systemic fluoroquinolones. *Pediatrics.* 2006;118:1287-1292.

34. Grossman ER, Walchek A, Freedman H. Tetracyclines and permanent teeth: the relation between dose and tooth color. *Pediatrics.* 1971;47:570-576.

35. Kline JM, Weitholter JP, Kline VT, Confer J. Pediatric antibiotic use: a focused review of fluoroquinolones and tetracyclines. *US Pharm.* 2012;37:56-59.

24

Infections in Critically Ill Patients

ELIZABETH RODERICK AND NISHANT D. MERCHANT

Health Care–Associated Infections

All patients admitted to the hospital are at risk of developing a health care–associated infection (HCAI), formerly known as nosocomial infections. Studies from high-income countries demonstrated that 5 to 15% of hospitalized patients acquire HCAIs, but the critically ill population is at an increased risk with a rate of HCAI of 9 to 37%.[1-3] Although intensive care units (ICUs) account for a fraction of total beds in most U.S. hospitals, more than 20 to 80% of all HCAIs are acquired in ICUs[3,4] because these patients are critically ill and immunocompromised. ICU-acquired infections account for substantial morbidity, mortality, and expense.[5] The risk of HCAI increases with the length of patient stay in the ICU and patients become more exposed to resistant pathogens.[6]

This chapter discusses the common types of HCAI in the critically ill, hospitalized patient. Strategies for managing and preventing these infections are presented as are its sequelae of sepsis and septic shock.

Presentation of Health Care–Associated Infections

Many different potential findings in the critically ill patient suggest development of an HCAI. Patients can present with a fever[7], tachycardia, tachypnea, leukocytosis, hyperglycemia, thrombocytosis, hypotension, hypoxia, alteration of mental status, ileus, diarrhea, and other potential clues that an infection is brewing. As the infection causes a systemic effect, the patient will go on to develop sepsis or septic shock, which is often the cause for admission into the ICU or prolongation of stay.

Sepsis and Septic Shock

Despite advances in medicine and critical care, the incidence of sepsis in ICUs continues to rise. Sepsis is life-threatening organ dysfunction caused by a dysregulated host response to infection. Organ dysfunction is defined by the 2016 Surgical Critical Care Medicine (SCCM)/European Society of Critical Care Medicine (ESICM) as an increase of two or more points in the Sequential Organ Failure Assessment (SOFA) score.[8,9] Septic shock, a type of vasodilatory or distributive shock, is defined as sepsis that has circulatory, cellular, and metabolic abnormalities, which leads to vasopressor requirement to maintain a mean arterial pressure (MAP) of 65 mm Hg or greater, despite fluid resuscitation, and a lactate level above 2 mmol/L. The definitions of systemic inflammatory response syndrome (SIRS) and severe sepsis have fallen out of favor. There is now an emphasis on rapid identification and treatment of sepsis to improve outcomes. The qSOFA and National Early Warning Score (NEWS) were created to aid in rapid identification of septic patients[10,11]. qSOFA score comprises three components: respiratory rate of 22 breaths/min or greater, altered mentation, and systolic blood pressure of 100 mm Hg or less. A score of 2 or greater is associated with poor outcomes because of sepsis. NEWS is an aggregate scoring system derived from six physiologic parameters, including respiration rate, oxygen saturation, systolic blood pressure, pulse rate, level of consciousness or new confusion, and temperature. The aggregate score represents the risk of death from sepsis and indicates the urgency of the response with a score of 0 to 4 associated with a low risk, 5 to 6 with medium risk, and 7 or more associated with high risk. The qSOFA score has been demonstrated to have limited applicability for sepsis identification in the ICU and caution must be taken when using this scoring system alone in the identification of sepsis.[12]

Initial Resuscitation

Treatment of sepsis and septic shock often requires the placement of invasive catheters to provide aggressive treatment and monitoring—namely, central venous access, urinary catheterization, arterial catheterization for hemodynamic monitoring, and endotracheal intubation with mechanical ventilation. Pulmonary artery catheterization is rarely performed in patients with suspected sepsis. The primary goal during the initial resuscitation is the rapid restoration of perfusion and the early administration of antibiotics. Goals during the first 6 hours of resuscitation include:
- Central venous pressure of 8 to 12 mm Hg
- MAP of 65 mm Hg or greater

- Urine output of 0.5 mL/kg/h or greater
- Central venous (superior vena cava) or mixed venous oxygenation saturation of 70 or 65%, respectively
- Targeting resuscitation to normalize serum lactate

Because of profound vasodilation during the inflammatory response, patients with sepsis will need aggressive fluid resuscitation using balanced crystalloids or normal saline given at 30 mL/kg started by 1 hour and completed in the first 3 hours after presentation. This is often followed by vasopressor therapy if they progress to shock. Norepinephrine is the initial vasopressor of choice, with vasopressin as a second agent at a fixed dose of 0.04 units (U)/hour when increasing doses of norepinephrine are needed to maintain MAP. Dynamic parameters such as respiratory changes in the vena caval diameter, radial artery pulse pressure, aortic blood flow peak velocity, left ventricular outflow tract velocity-time integral, and brachial artery blood flow velocity, in addition to maneuvers such as the passive leg raise are used to assess fluid responsiveness. The most recent Surviving Sepsis Guidelines suggest trending lactate until the value has normalized.[13] Some patients will experience adrenal insufficiency and require stress-dose steroids to maintain hemodynamic stability[14].

Etiology of Health Care–Associated Infections

Several factors contribute to the high incidence of these infections in the hospital and the associated poor patient outcomes.

- Critically ill patients have more chronic comorbid illnesses, more wounds, and more severe physiologic derangements, making it difficult for them to resist opportunistic organisms.
- The high frequency of indwelling devices among patients in the ICU provides a portal of entry for microorganisms and infection.
- The use and maintenance of devices necessitate frequent contact with health care personnel, which predisposes patients to colonization and infection with HCAI pathogens.
  - Improper hand hygiene and fomites contribute to this factor.[5,15,16]
- Multidrug-resistant (MDR) pathogens are being isolated with increasing frequency in ICUs.

The most common and clinically important infections in the ICU are often associated with the supportive devices that critically ill patients often require. These include catheter-associated urinary tract infections (UTIs), ventilator-associated pneumonia, and intravascular catheter-related bloodstream infections (BSIs). Other common HCAIs that cause serious morbidity and potential mortality are *Clostridioides difficile* infection (CDI) and surgical-site infection (SSI), which are also preventable HCAIs. These types of infections are not only the most common, but are also to some extent preventable.[6,17,18]

As the pathogens continue to develop and demonstrate resistance, prevention is the best approach to reduce its

impact on the critically ill population.[19,20] Many common HCAI pathogens make up the ESKAPE group, which also have an increased rate of resistance. These organisms are the gram-negative (*K. Pneumoniae, A. baumannii, P. Aeruginosa,* and *Enterobacter* spp.) and gram-positive (*Enterococcus faecium* and *S. aureus*), with gram-negative organisms being responsible for 10 to 14% of the infections.[21,22]

Diagnosis

Cultures from different sources as clinically appropriate should be obtained before initiating antimicrobial therapy if there is no significant delay in the start of treatment (>45 minutes). At least two sets of blood cultures (aerobic and anaerobic) should be obtained before antimicrobial therapy. At least one should be drawn percutaneously, and one drawn from each vascular access device. Routine laboratory tests should be sent, including complete blood count, chemistry panel, liver enzymes, bilirubin, coagulation studies, and an arterial blood gas. Imaging studies to identify a source of infection should be performed promptly. A chest radiograph should be part of the imaging workup, with CT scanning possibly needed to identify a source of sepsis. In patients who are extremely ill and hemodynamically unstable, it is important to optimize treatment and resuscitation before proceeding with diagnostics if it requires traveling out of the ICU. Often the diagnosis of sepsis is made empirically at the bedside based on patient presentation or retrospectively when data such as blood cultures return positive or that the patient has a good clinical response to the administration of antibiotics.

Antimicrobial Therapy

Administration of effective intravenous antimicrobials within the first hour of recognition of septic shock can improve patient outcomes. Initial empiric therapy that has activity against all likely organisms and that penetrates tissues in adequate concentrations based on source of infection should be chosen. The antibiotic regimen should be reassessed daily for potential deescalation as laboratory and diagnostic information is finalized. Ideally, combination empirical therapy should not be administered for more than 3 to 5 days. Duration of therapy is typically 3 to 8 days, although longer courses are certainly appropriate for specific clinical situations.[23] Antiviral therapy should be initiated as early as possible in patients with severe sepsis or shock of viral origin. Antimicrobials should not be used in patients with inflammatory states or hypotension determined to be of noninfectious cause, although this may be a diagnosis of exclusion and patients often receive antibiotics over the course of the diagnostic workup.

Source Control

A specific anatomic location of infection, possibly requiring emergent intervention for source control, should be sought and diagnosed or excluded. When source control in a severely septic patient is required, the effective intervention with the least physiologically damaging insult should be used (e.g., percutaneous rather than surgical drainage of an abscess). If intravascular access devices are thought to be a possible source of infection, the catheter should be removed. Addressing the source of infection is often the key to controlling sepsis and the inflammatory cascade; however, once the cascade has been set into motion, patients can have profound metabolic derangements, even after the source of infection is identified and treated. Care at this point is supportive to maintain the goals of resuscitation and reestablish homeostasis.

The challenge of critical care lies not only in the initial resuscitation and maintenance of adequate oxygenation and perfusion, but also in the subsequent management of patients after sepsis has resolved. The interventions performed to support patients through an acute episode are commonplace in the ICU, but vigilance and appropriate stewardship over intravascular devices, endotracheal tubes, and antibiotics are essential to minimize the opportunities for HCAIs.

Catheter-Associated Urinary Tract Infection[24]

Epidemiology

UTI used to be the most common HCAI, but a point prevalence study from 2015 demonstrated that the rates of UTIs are decreasing. It is now the fifth most common HCAI.[25] Although many individual catheter-associated UTIs (CAUTIs) do not cause severe morbidity and mortality or increase hospital cost significantly, the cumulative effect of these frequent infections is significant[3,26,27,28] because they make up 75% of UTIs in the hospital.[29] In the United States, CAUTIs are the cause of HCAI bacteremia 20% of the time and pneumonia 50% of the time, which has an attributed mortality of 15 to 25%.[30-33]

Risk Factors

Approximately 12 to 16% of adult hospital inpatients will have an indwelling urinary catheter during their hospitalization. The duration of catheterization is an important risk factor for catheter-associated bacteriuria and UTI as each day that the catheter remains increases the risk of acquiring a CAUTI by 3 to 7% and is therefore is a major target of prevention efforts.[34,35] Other risk factors include:[36,37]
- Female sex
- Older age
- Diabetes mellitus
- Absence of systemic antibiotics
- Catheter insertion outside of the operating room
- Bacterial colonization of the drainage tubing or bag
- Errors in catheter care (e.g., errors in sterile technique, not maintaining a closed drainage system)

CAUTI can be extraluminal or intraluminal to the catheter. Extraluminal infection occurs by entry of bacteria into the bladder along the biofilm that forms around the catheter in the urethra.[38] This biofilm protects the pathogens from antibiotics and host defense[39] and are often the source of gram-positive infections.[40] Intraluminal infection results from urinary stasis caused by drainage failure, or because of contamination of the urine collection bag with subsequent ascending infection and are often the source of gram-negative infections.[40] Extraluminal infection is more common than intraluminal infection and therefore speaks to the preventable nature of these infections and the focus on early removal and hygiene. Based on the organisms that frequently cause CAUTI, the patient's perineal flora and the provider's hand flora would be the likely sources.

The causative pathogens in catheter-associated bacteriuria and UTI commonly include *Escherichia coli* and other Enterobacteriaceae, but *Pseudomonas aeruginosa,* enterococci, staphylococci, and fungi are also significant causes. Some of these organisms associated with catheter-related bacteriuria may lack some of the virulence factors that allow the usual uropathogens to adhere to the uroepithelium, but they take advantage of access to the bladder via the catheter. An example of such an organism is *Candida* species, which almost never cause UTI in the absence of an indwelling catheter.[41]

Clinical Presentation

Symptoms of CAUTI are often subtle, especially in critically ill patients, and do not necessarily refer to the urinary tract. Fever is the most common symptom, although it is nonspecific. Localizing symptoms can include flank or suprapubic discomfort, costovertebral angle tenderness, and catheter obstruction. In the ICU, more often the findings are nonspecific, such as fever, leukocytosis, malaise, altered mental status, hypotension, metabolic acidosis, or respiratory alkalosis.[42] Patients who recently had a catheter removed may experience dysuria, frequent urination, or urgency as well.

Diagnosis

CAUTI is diagnosed by laboratory evaluation of a urine sample from a patient with an indwelling catheter or a patient who is no longer catheterized but had an indwelling urinary catheter within the previous 48 hours. The Infectious Diseases Society of America (IDSA) guidelines define catheter-associated bacteriuria as follows:
- Symptomatic bacteriuria (UTI)—Culture growth of 10^3 colony-forming units (cfu)/mL or greater of bacteria in the presence of symptoms or signs compatible with UTI, without other identifiable source in a patient with indwelling urethral, indwelling suprapubic, or intermittent catheterization. Symptoms include fever and suprapubic or costovertebral angle tenderness. Otherwise unexplained systemic symptoms include altered mental status, hypotension, or evidence of SIRS.
- Asymptomatic bacteriuria—Culture growth of 10^5 cfu/mL or greater of bacteria in the absence of symptoms compatible

with UTI in a patient with indwelling urethral, indwelling suprapubic, or intermittent catheterization.

These definitions are different from those used by the Centers for Disease Control and Prevention (CDC) National Health Safety Network, which were created for surveillance purposes, and not specifically for clinical care. The CDC uses the same definition for asymptomatic bacteriuria, but defines CAUTI as the presence of fever, suprapubic tenderness, urinary urgency, urinary frequency, dysuria, or costovertebral angle pain in a patient with urine culture bacterial counts of 10^5 cfu/mL or greater, where an indwelling urinary catheter has been in place for more than 2 consecutive days. Of those patients with bacteriuria, 10 to 25% develop symptoms of UTI.

If the diagnosis is based on nonspecific signs and symptoms, the evaluation should rule out the possibility of other infections before attributing the findings to a UTI. Certain findings, such as pyuria and the appearance or smell of the urine, are particularly nonspecific and should not be used to diagnose a UTI when found in isolation. Pyuria is frequently found in catheterized patients with bacteriuria, whether they have symptoms or not, and odorous or cloudy urine has not been demonstrated to be indicative of either bacteriuria or a UTI that requires treatment.

Urine culture must be obtained using an aseptic technique by either obtaining a clean catch, replacing the Foley catheter before obtaining a sample, or with proper cleansing of the side port if the Foley cannot be removed.

Treatment

Antimicrobial selection should be based on the culture results when available. Patients who are septic or otherwise seriously ill warrant prompt treatment before the availability of culture data. In such cases, empiric antibiotics should be tailored to results of past cultures, use of prior antimicrobial therapy, hospital or community patterns of antimicrobial resistance, and any allergies of the patient. Urine Gram stain, if available, can also guide empiric antibiotic choice. If Gram stain is not available, empiric therapy should provide coverage against gram-negative bacilli. Gram-negative bacilli can be treated empirically with a third-generation cephalosporin or a fluoroquinolone. If *P. aeruginosa* is suspected, treatment with a fluoroquinolone, fourth-generation cephalosporin, or β-lactam with β-lactamase inhibitor can be administered. If an extended-spectrum β-lactamase–producing organism is suspected (usually based on prior cultures), treatment options are generally limited to carbapenems. Gram-positive cocci on urine Gram stain may represent enterococci or staphylococci, and empiric management with vancomycin is generally appropriate until further susceptibility information is available. Duration of treatment can vary depending on isolated pathogens and host comorbidities; however, 3 to 14 days of therapy for a CAUTI is generally appropriate based on IDSA guidelines.[43]

- 3-day regimen for women 65 years or younger without upper urinary symptoms and Foley removed.

- 5-day regimen of levofloxacin in patients who are not severely ill may be considered.
- 7 days is the recommended duration to treat CAUTI with resolution of symptoms; otherwise extend treatment to 10 to 14 days.

Candiduria is a common finding in patients with indwelling bladder catheters, particularly in those who are taking antibiotics or are diabetic. Most patients with candiduria are asymptomatic, and this merely represents colonization. Progression to candidemia is uncommon, and therefore in patients with long-term catheterization, it is often not treated.

The optimal approach to catheter management in the setting of UTIs is unclear, especially in critically ill patients in whom the need for fluid calculations and immobility are factors. Minimization of the use of indwelling catheters, when possible, is preferred. In general, patients who no longer require catheterization should have the catheter removed and receive appropriate antimicrobial therapy. If long-term catheterization is needed and intermittent catheterization is not feasible, the original indwelling catheter should be replaced at the initiation of antibiotic therapy. Catheter replacement is associated with fewer and later relapses than retaining the original catheter, because biofilm penetration of most antibiotics is poor. Complications of CAUTIs that can be avoided with proper detection and treatment include involvement of the upper urinary tract, leading to pyelonephritis and bacteremia.

Prevention

In October 2008, the Centers for Medicare and Medicaid Services stopped reimbursing hospitals for CAUTIs. Although this decision has led to increased vigilance regarding catheter placement and removal, and some institutions have seen a decline in incidence, CAUTIs and the reimbursement changes have created a cost burden on hospitals across the United States. In 2014, a panel sponsored by the Society for Healthcare Epidemiology of America released recommendations on the prevention of CAUTIs. The guidelines stress the importance of the judicious use of urethral catheters only for appropriate indications, expertise and sterile technique in catheter placement, continual reassessment for the need for the catheter, and maintenance of a closed drainage system that is sterile with unobstructed flow. Antimicrobial agents have a limited role in the prevention of CAUTI, and there is no clear benefit to using prophylactic antibiotics during catheterization to reduce the risk of infection.

Ventilator-Associated Pneumonia[44]

Epidemiology

Hospital-acquired pneumonia (HAP) and ventilator-associated pneumonia (VAP) are now cited as the most common hospital-acquired infection. It is a serious problem, with an estimated incidence of 10 to 25% and an all-cause mortality of 25 to 50%. Patients with VAP have a prolonged ventilator course by 7 to 11 days, hospital length of stay by 11 to 13 days, and additional cost of approximately $40,000.[45,46]

Definitions of pneumonia, HAP, and VAP have remained unchanged since 2005 as stated by the American Thoracic Society (ATS) and IDSA.[47] Pneumonia is defined as a new lung infiltrate with clinical evidence of infection; this would include fever, leukocytosis, hypoxia, and/ or purulent sputum. HAP is defined as pneumonia acquired 48 hours after admission and VAP is pneumonia acquired after 48 hours of mechanical ventilation.

The primary route of infection of the lungs is through microaspiration of organisms that have colonized the oropharyngeal tract. Pathogens can also come from the gastrointestinal (GI) tract. Approximately 45% of healthy persons aspirate during sleep, and an even higher proportion of severely ill patients aspirate frequently. Although often regarded as partially protective, the presence of an endotracheal tube still allows aspiration of oropharyngeal material or bacteria of GI origin. Depending on the number and type of microorganisms that reach the lower respiratory tract, pneumonia may develop.

HAP can be caused by a wide variety of pathogens and can be polymicrobial. Common pathogens include aerobic gram-negative bacilli (e.g., *E. coli, Klebsiella pneumoniae, Enterobacter* species, *P. aeruginosa, Acinetobacter* species) and gram-positive cocci (e.g., *Staphylococcus aureus,* methicillin-resistant *S. aureus* [MRSA], *Streptococcus* species). HAP and VAP owing to viruses or fungi are significantly less common, except in the immunocompromised patient. There are few data regarding the extent to which pathogens that cause VAP differ from those in nonintubated patients with HAP.

Risk Factors

Risk factors for the development of HAP coexist with mechanical ventilation. The risk factors include age older than 70 years, underlying chronic lung disease, immunosuppression, previous thoracoabdominal surgery, depressed level of consciousness, malnutrition, enteral nutrition, and supine positioning. The frequency of MDR bacteria causing HAP is increasing, especially among patients in ICUs. Risk factors for infection with MDR pathogens include:[20]

- Receipt of antibiotics within the preceding 90 days
- Current hospitalization of 5 days or longer
- High frequency of antibiotic resistance in the community or in the specific hospital unit
- Immunosuppressive disease, therapy, or both
- Severe septic shock

Clinical Presentation

VAP typically manifests with a new or progressive pulmonary infiltrate and one or more of the following findings: fever, purulent tracheobronchial secretions, leukocytosis, or increased respiratory rate. These symptoms and signs can develop gradually or suddenly. Patients with VAP are typically unable to provide any history because they are sedated or their ability to communicate is impaired by the endotracheal or tracheostomy tube. The few patients who are able to convey symptoms often report dyspnea or chest congestion. On auscultation, patients typically have diffuse, asymmetric rhonchi. The rhonchi are often accompanied by focal findings, such as crackles and decreased breath sounds. Bronchospasm (wheezing and increased expiratory time) and hemoptysis also can be present. Again, these pulmonary signs are often accompanied by systemic abnormalities, such as fever, encephalopathy, or sepsis.

Patients with VAP may exhibit deterioration in respiratory parameters, as identified during routine assessment of the mechanical ventilator. This may even be the initial sign of a developing VAP. Respiratory findings include increased respiratory rate, decreased tidal volumes, increased minute ventilation, and decreased oxygenation. Many patients will require more ventilatory support or inspired oxygen to maintain previous levels of oxygenation.

Diagnosis

Diagnostic evaluation is required when VAP is suspected, because clinical features alone can be nonspecific. The goal is to confirm VAP and to identify the likely pathogen so that the appropriate treatment can be initiated. After physical examination, the evaluation proceeds with a chest radiograph. A normal chest radiograph excludes VAP, whereas an abnormal radiograph in a patient with suspected VAP should prompt the collection of respiratory tract secretions. An abnormal chest radiograph for a patient with VAP can include alveolar infiltrates, air bronchograms, and silhouetting of adjacent solid organs. Patients with VAP will have an abnormal chest radiograph in addition to clinical signs of infection. These patients should have their respiratory tract sampled and specimens sent for Gram stain and culture to confirm the diagnosis and to guide therapy. Chest computed tomography (CT) without contrast is not routine but may be useful in identifying a target lobe for sampling or in those with a previous diagnosis of pneumonia to evaluate for new or progressive changes. Ultrasound also may be used, although VAP diagnosis with this modality is user dependent and whether it leads to improved outcomes over conventional chest imaging is unknown.

Empiric antibiotic therapy is indicated for all cases of suspected VAP; ideally, it should be initiated after the collection of respiratory samples because antibiotic administration before specimen collection can reduce the sensitivity of the microscopic analysis and culture. It is only unless the clinical suspicion is low and the microscopic analysis of lower respiratory tract samples is negative that antibiotic coverage would not be started. Occasionally, severe illness or delay in sampling requires that empiric antibiotic therapy be initiated before diagnostic sampling.

Lower respiratory tract sampling is indicated for all patients who are suspected of having VAP and have an abnormal chest radiograph. There are a variety of methods available to sample material from the airways and alveoli, including nonbronchoscopic (i.e., blind) and bronchoscopic techniques. Nonbronchoscopic lower respiratory tract sampling includes tracheobronchial aspiration or mini–bronchoalveolar lavage (mini-BAL). Tracheobronchial aspiration is performed by advancing a catheter through the endotracheal tube until resistance is met and then applying suction. Mini-BAL is performed by advancing a catheter through the endotracheal tube until resistance is met, infusing sterile saline through the catheter, and then aspirating. Nonbronchoscopic sampling can be performed by a respiratory therapist without clinician supervision, and therefore reduces the cost, allows specimens to be obtained quickly, and facilitates serial sampling, if necessary. Bronchoscopic sampling is performed using either BAL or a protected specimen brush (PSB). BAL involves the infusion and aspiration of sterile saline through a flexible bronchoscope that is introduced through the endotracheal tube and then advanced into a bronchial segmental orifice. A PSB is a brush that is contained within a protective sheath. It is designed to minimize the likelihood that the brush will be contaminated during bronchoscopy. The procedure involves placing the bronchoscope tip next to a bronchial segmental orifice, pushing the sheath through the bronchoscope, and then advancing the brush out of the sheath and into the airway. Specimens are collected by brushing the airway wall, withdrawing the brush into the sheath, and then removing the sheath from the bronchoscope. Bronchoscopic sampling and nonbronchoscopic sampling have been compared in the setting of suspected VAP.[48] The evidence indicates that bronchoscopic sampling does not improve mortality, length of hospital stay, duration of mechanical ventilation, or length of ICU stay.[49] However, it minimizes airway contamination of the alveolar samples and provides an accurate assessment of the alveolar cell population. Bronchoscopic sampling can lead to a narrower antimicrobial regimen and more rapid deescalation of antimicrobial therapy, which could possibly reduce antibiotic resistance.

The respiratory specimens obtained should be sent for Gram stain and culture. This can be used to semiquantitate cell types and to characterize the morphology of bacteria. The presence of abundant neutrophils is consistent with VAP, and the bacterial morphology may suggest a likely pathogen. Gram stain analysis may decrease the incidence of inappropriate antimicrobial therapy and improve diagnostic accuracy when correlated with culture results.

Quantitative or semiquantitative cultures of respiratory samples are both acceptable, with the choice depending largely upon availability. Quantitative cultures can be performed on bronchoscopic or nonbronchoscopic specimens. VAP is supported when an established threshold of bacterial growth is exceeded. Only bacteria that are pulmonary pathogens should be counted. For example, *Staphylococcus epidermidis,* enterococci, and most gram-positive bacilli should not be counted, because they rarely cause pneumonia, and may represent a contaminant. Thresholds of 10^6 colony-forming units (cfu)/mL for samples obtained by tracheobronchial aspiration, 10^4 cfu/mL for samples obtained by BAL, or 1000 cfu/mL for samples obtained by PSB are acceptable for diagnosis. Generally, quantitative cultures derived from nonbronchoscopic specimens tend to have a lower specificity than do quantitative cultures derived from bronchoscopic specimens; however, this is balanced by a higher sensitivity, resulting in comparable diagnostic accuracy.

The final diagnosis of VAP is made when a patient who has been on mechanical ventilation for 48 hours or longer develops a new or progressive infiltrate, with clinical signs of pneumonia, and the respiratory specimens are positive (i.e., increased neutrophils are seen in the microscopic analysis and growth of a pathogen in culture exceeds the predefined threshold). VAP cannot be confirmed or excluded until the culture results are complete, which generally takes 2 to 3 days. At that time, the patient should be reevaluated to determine whether additional diagnostic evaluation or changes in management are warranted. These decisions are based on the culture results and the patient's response to empiric therapy.

Differential Diagnosis

There are many reasons for patients to have changes in ventilatory status with abnormal chest radiographs, so that in addition to pursuing a diagnosis of VAP, other diagnoses should be considered, including:

- Aspiration pneumonitis
- Pulmonary embolism
- Acute respiratory distress syndrome
- Pulmonary hemorrhage
- Pulmonary contusion
- Infiltrating tumor
- Radiation pneumonitis
- Drug reactions, most notably antineoplastic medications
- Vasculitis

Treatment

Patients with negative cultures who have not improved may not have VAP; therefore, other diagnoses or sites of infection should be sought. Patients with negative cultures who have improved might not have VAP, and antimicrobial therapy should be discontinued. Patients with positive cultures who have not improved probably have VAP, but they may be receiving inappropriate antimicrobial therapy, have a complication of the VAP (e.g., abscess, empyema), have another source of infection, or have a second diagnosis. The antimicrobial regimen should be adjusted, and potential causes for failing to improve should be sought. Patients with positive cultures who have improved after antibiotic treatment likely have VAP; the antimicrobial therapy should therefore be narrowed according to the culture results.

Antibiotic therapy significantly improves survival for patients with HAP, VAP, or health care–associated pneumonia. Establishing the diagnosis of VAP in such patients can be difficult, especially those in whom clinical, radiologic, and microbiologic findings can be due to other causes besides pneumonia. This difficulty in diagnosis can lead to overtreatment and therefore increase the risk of superinfection and antibiotic toxicity. Antimicrobial selection should be based on risk factors for MDR pathogens, including any recent antibiotic therapy, the flora specific to the hospital or ICU, the presence of underlying diseases, and available culture data. Once the results of cultures are available, therapy should be narrowed on the basis of the susceptibility pattern.

In critically ill patients who have been receiving antibiotics before the onset of pneumonia, and in institutions where drug-resistant pathogens are frequent, coverage of MRSA, *P. aeruginosa,* and antibiotic-resistant gram-negative bacilli such as *Acinetobacter* species and *Legionella* species should be considered. If MRSA is a frequent HCAI pathogen in the institution, linezolid or vancomycin is a necessary first choice for staphylococcal coverage, but it should be discontinued if MRSA is not isolated.

Although combination antimicrobial therapy for HAP caused by gram-negative pathogens (especially *Pseudomonas* species) is commonly administered, there is no conclusive evidence to support this practice. The best rationale for the use of combination therapy is that it provides a greater spectrum of activity when there is risk for MDR pathogens (e.g., if the pathogen is resistant to one agent, then it may be susceptible to the other). Other commonly cited reasons for combination therapy include the potential for synergistic efficacy and the potential to reduce the emergence of resistance. However, it is not clear that two agents offer improved outcomes for treating gram-negative pneumonia. Patients who have diabetes mellitus, renal disease, or structural lung disease or who have been recently treated with glucocorticoids may require coverage for *Legionella* species (using azithromycin or a fluoroquinolone). HAP and VAP caused by *Legionella* species are also more common in hospitals where the organism is present in the hospital water supply. Patients who have aspirated or had recent abdominal surgery may warrant coverage for anaerobes (using clindamycin, β-lactam–β-lactamase inhibitor, or a carbapenem).

Guidelines have been created for antibiotic regimens and empiric coverage of HAP and VAP in patients with no known risk factors for MDR pathogens; however, the growing emergence of MDR pathogens makes most ICU patients susceptible to MDRs by virtue of meeting ICU admission criteria and requiring mechanical ventilation. It is common for ICUs with high acuity to adopt protocols for empiric coverage of these organisms. The following is an example of empiric antibiotic coverage for VAP:[21]

- Vancomycin IV to cover gram-positive bacteria, including MRSA, dosing based on renal function

Plus
- Cefepime for gram-negative coverage (2 g IV q8h) with severe infection and CrCl > 60 mL/min

Plus
- Tobramycin (5–7 mg/kg IV once daily) for double coverage of gram-negative and *Pseudomonas* species

The choice of a specific agent for empiric therapy should be based on knowledge of the prevailing pathogens (and susceptibility patterns) within a specific institution or ICU, often guided by a committee, including multidisciplinary staff members (e.g., pharmacy, infectious diseases, internal medicine, and critical care), as is the case with this regimen.

When the cause of VAP has been identified on the basis of reliable microbiologic methods, treatment regimens should be simplified and directed to that pathogen. The choice of agent should be dictated by the results of susceptibility testing. It is important to avoid broad-spectrum therapy once a pathogen has been identified, to minimize any selective process. Patients who are improving clinically, hemodynamically stable, and able to take oral medications can be switched to oral therapy. If the pathogen has been identified, the choice of antibiotic for oral therapy is based on the susceptibility profile for that organism. If a pathogen is not identified, the choice for oral therapy is either the same antibiotic as the intravenous antibiotic or an agent in the same drug class that achieves adequate lung penetration when administered orally.

The duration of therapy should be based on the clinical response. Procalcitonin levels, though not helpful in the diagnosis of VAP, may be useful in making the decision to discontinue antibiotic therapy, though further research is required.[50] The standard duration of therapy in the past was 14 to 21 days in part because of a concern for difficult to treat pathogens (e.g., *Pseudomonas* species). However, it is generally accepted that a shorter course can significantly reduce the amount of antimicrobial drugs used in hospitals where the emergence of resistant pathogens is a concern while providing adequate treatment for VAP. It is currently recommended that if a patient has improved after 48 to 72 hours and a pathogen is isolated, antimicrobial therapy should be tailored on the basis of the susceptibility pattern, and be continued to complete a total course of 7 days. Depending on the specific patient, if *P. aeruginosa* were the isolated pathogen, a 15-day regimen may be warranted, and for up to 21 days for MRSA, again, depending on the extent of infection and clinical course.[51] If the patient has not improved and a resistant pathogen is suspected, therapy should be changed to provide coverage for MDR pathogens until a specific pathogen is identified, in which case pathogen-directed treatment should be chosen on the basis of the susceptibility pattern. In addition, failure to improve at 72 hours should prompt a search for infectious complications, other diagnoses, or other sites of infection.

Prevention

Mechanical ventilation and endotracheal intubation is a risk factor for the development of pneumonia and at times an unavoidable intervention for adequate support of the critically ill patient. Thus, there are steps that should be taken to minimize the risk of VAP in the ICU. These steps include head-of-bed positioning, maintaining patients in a semirecumbent or upright position (>45 degrees), oral hygiene and the use of chlorhexidine mouthwash, subglottic drainage to avoid pooling of secretions, maintaining endotracheal cuff pressures at 30 cm H_2O to decrease aspiration of secretions, using noninvasive ventilation when possible, and considering extubation daily. Other strategies include maximizing patients before extubation with spontaneous breathing trials and minimal sedations to decrease the need for reintubation. The implementation of VAP preventive measures into bundles is an effective strategy to ensure combined interventions and to minimize the risk of this common HCAI.

Catheter-Related Bloodstream Infections[52]

Epidemiology

The variety and number of intravascular devices used for vascular access in the U.S. health care system has greatly increased in the last 30 years. They are a common, standard means of administering treatment and monitoring hemodynamics in critically ill patients. Infections, however, can and do result from the use of these devices, and they cause significant morbidity, mortality, and financial cost each year. This is especially true in the ICU, where approximately 48% of patients or more have a central venous catheter in place. In 2017, the CDC reported 24,265 central line–associated BSIs reported by 3576 U.S. acute care hospitals. In part the result of increased awareness and preventive measures, this was a 19% decrease in incidence compared to that in 2015.[53] There are two variations of BSI that require clarification: catheter-related BSI (CRBSI) and central line-associated BSI (CLABSI). CRBSI is the clinical definition used when diagnosing or treating patients. It defines the catheter as the cause of the BSI. As now recommended by the CDC, the Joint Commission, and the Agency for Healthcare Research and Quality, the risk of central venous catheter (CVC)-related BSI is expressed as catheter-associated BSIs per 1000 CVC days. All health care–associated BSIs that cannot be reasonably linked to a site of local infection are attributed to the patient's CVC. The implication of this definition is that the true risk of CVC-related BSI is overestimated, given that some BSIs are secondary from unrecognized sites of infection or may be due to other intravascular devices.[25]

Risk Factors

Although the difference between CLABSI and CRBSI are somewhat difficult to discern, the risk factors, diagnosis, and treatment remain the same. Common risk factors for BSIs include total parenteral nutrition, granulocytopenia, chemotherapy, burns, infection at another site, or bone marrow transplant. The size of the catheter, number of lumens, location, type, function, duration of use, emergent placement, skill of the provider placing the line, and handwashing all play a role in the development of a BSI as well.

Clinical Presentation

Local signs of infection, such as phlebitis or inflammation at the insertion site, are uncommon initial manifestations of catheter infection. Catheter-related BSI should be suspected when bacteremia occurs in the setting of a CVC with no other apparent source of infection. Fever is the most sensitive clinical manifestation, although it is nonspecific. Other clinical signs of BSI include hemodynamic instability, altered mental status, catheter dysfunction, and signs of sepsis that start abruptly after catheter use. Patients can also develop complications from BSIs as well, including suppurative thrombophlebitis, endocarditis, osteomyelitis, or hematologic spread of infection to other sites. Clinical improvement shortly after catheter removal can suggest CRBSI, but routine catheter removal is not necessary without microbiologic confirmation of infection.

Diagnosis

Diagnosis of CRBSI requires establishing the presence of bacteremia and that the BSI is related to the catheter. Confirmation of CRBSI can be made on blood cultures obtained before initiating antibiotics in patients with suspected CRBSI. Ideally, paired peripheral and central blood cultures should be obtained. One of the following criteria must be met:

- Culture of the same organism from both the catheter tip and at least one percutaneous blood culture
- Culture of the same organism from at least two blood samples (one from a catheter hub and the other from a peripheral vein or second lumen) that meet criteria from quantitative blood cultures or differential time to positivity

Quantitative blood cultures that indicate CRBSI require a bacterial colony count from the catheter hub sample that is threefold to fivefold greater than that from a peripheral blood sample or second lumen. Semiquantitative cultures demonstrating greater than 15 cfu/mL of the same microbe from the insertion site, hub site, and peripheral blood culture also support a diagnosis of CRBSI. *Differential time to positivity* refers to growth from the catheter hub sample at least 2 hours before growth detected from the peripheral vein sample. Sensitivity and specificity for differential time to positivity are approximately 85 and 91%, respectively.[54]

Catheter cultures should be performed when a catheter is removed for a suspected catheter-related BSI; however, there is no role for routine catheter cultures in the absence of clinical suspicion of infection. Blood cultures positive for *S. aureus*, coagulase-negative staphylococci, or *Candida* species should increase suspicion for CRBSI when no other source of infection is identified.

Treatment

Empiric antibiotics should be initiated for patients with suspected BSI after blood cultures are obtained. The choice of antibiotics for CRBSI depends on clinical circumstances, including severity of illness and general risk factors for infection. According to a report from the CDC National Healthcare Safety network from 2011 to 2017, *Enterobacteriaceae* was the most commonly reported pathogen in CRBSI except in the ICU, where the most commonly reported pathogen group was *Candida*.[55] However, given that coagulase-negative *Staphylococcus* species and *S. aureus* remain common BSI pathogens, and isolates are often resistant to methicillin, vancomycin is considered appropriate empiric coverage. Daptomycin can be used as an alternative in institutions in which MRSA has an increased minimum inhibitory concentration of vancomycin greater than 2 µg/mL.[5] Situations in which antibiotic therapy is not required include:

- Positive tip culture in the absence of clinical signs of infection
- Positive blood cultures from a catheter with negative cultures from a peripheral vein
- Phlebitis without infection

Additional empiric coverage for gram-negative organisms depends on the circumstances and the severity of illness. For example, if CRBSI is suspected in a patient with neutropenia or sepsis, empiric therapy should include coverage for gram-negative bacilli. If CRBSI from *Candida* species is suspected, empiric therapy with echinocandins should be given for patients with certain risk factors, including total parenteral nutrition, prolonged use of broad-spectrum antibiotics, hematologic malignancy, bone marrow or solid organ transplant, femoral catheterization, or colonization by *Candida* species at multiple sites. Fluconazole is appropriate antifungal coverage for patients without azole exposure in the previous 3 months.

When the results of cultures become available, antibiotic therapy should be tailored. Patients who have received vancomycin for empiric treatment and have CRBSI because of methicillin-susceptible *S. aureus* should be switched to oxacillin or nafcillin. Duration of antibiotic treatment depends on the clinical circumstances, the isolated pathogen, and susceptibility profiles. In cases of coagulase-negative *Staphylococcus* BSI, treatment for 5 to 7 days is sufficient if the catheter is removed. The treatment for *S. aureus* is variable: for hematologic complications such as endocarditis, patients should be treated for 4 to 6 weeks. The absence of hematologic complications calls for a shorter duration of therapy, approximately 14 days. The antibiotic choice for *S. aureus* would be dependent on methicillin resistance. A 7- to 14-day course of treatment is recommended for *Enterococcus* species using ampicillin with or without aminoglycoside, or vancomycin, linezolid, or daptomycin for ampicillin-resistant organisms. Gram-negative bacilli require treatment with a third- or fourth-generation cephalosporin, carbapenems, β-lactam–β-lactamase, with or without an aminoglycoside for a 7- to 14-day course.

In general, catheter removal is recommended. Cases in which catheter removal could be optional include infection with coagulase-negative *Staphylococcus* species, in which case

antibiotic therapy should be extended to 10 to 14 days.[56] Another circumstance in which catheter removal may be optional is infection with *Enterococcus* species in a patient with a long-term catheter. Salvage of the catheter may be attempted in the setting of uncomplicated CRBSI that involves long-term catheters and uncommon pathogens other than *S. aureus*, *P. aeruginosa*, fungi, or mycobacteria. Systemic and antimicrobial lock therapy may be given via the catheter for the duration of the therapy depending on the organism. The efficacy of antibiotic lock therapy remains uncertain, and there are concerns regarding antimicrobial resistance and fungal infection.

Regardless of pathogen, catheter removal is recommended in cases of complicated infections, which include severe sepsis, hemodynamic instability, endocarditis, evidence of another site of infection, suppurative thrombophlebitis, osteomyelitis, or bacteremia that persists at least 72 hours after initiation of antimicrobial therapy. After catheter removal, antibiotics should be continued for 4 to 6 weeks for complicated BSI, possibly longer for osteomyelitis. Guidewire exchange is generally not advised, but is acceptable in circumstances in which catheter removal is necessary for CRBSI, but there is a high risk for mechanical complications or bleeding for catheter reinsertion. If catheter removal is not possible, antibiotics should be administered through the colonized catheter.

Prevention

Through adherence to best practices, BSIs are thought to be largely preventable. These prevention measures are emphasized in guidelines from the Healthcare Infection Control Practices Advisory Committee, the CDC, and work groups from professional organizations representing an array of medical disciplines. Adherence to hand hygiene recommendations and aseptic technique during catheter insertion and dressing changes remain the most important measures for the prevention of catheter-associated infections. Other preventive measures include:

- Appropriate site selection
- Barrier precautions
- Changing catheter administration kits at appropriate intervals
- Ensuring proper catheter-site and catheter hub care
- Removal and replacement of lines in less than 48 hours if placed emergently
- Ensuring catheter removal when no longer needed
- Catheter-related bundles and checklists[57,58,59–61]

Determinants of Infection Risk

Three major determinants of CRBSI risk exist: location of catheter placement, duration of catheter placement, and type of catheter. All types of catheters are associated with a risk of both local and CRBSI, including peripheral IV catheters, peripherally inserted central catheters (PICCs), arterial catheters for hemodynamic monitoring, CVCs, and pulmonary artery catheters.

The risk of infection for peripheral venous catheters is higher when they are placed in the lower extremity versus upper extremity and higher in the wrist or upper arm compared with the hand. Site selection for CVCs is also important; CRBSI is more common with catheters placed in the femoral region, compared with the internal jugular vein. The site with the lowest risk of infection is the subclavian line; however, the inability to place it with ultrasound guidance or limited operator experience may not make this the overall safest site.

The duration of the catheter is also a risk factor for CRBSI for both venous and arterial catheters. For peripheral venous catheters, most hospitals have a policy for replacement at regular intervals, commonly every 4 days or earlier if there are signs of phlebitis or malfunction.

The risk of infection with central venous and pulmonary artery catheters increases over time; however, a defined period to change the catheters routinely has not been established. Given the lack of consensus, and the other potential complications of central line placement, routine replacement of CVCs is not currently recommended. Indications for catheter replacement include purulence at the insertion site, hemodynamic instability suspected to be due to CRBSI, or confirmed CRBSI by culture. Again, guidewire exchanges are not advised because this approach increases the risk of BSI versus selecting a new site.

Arterial catheters, primarily used for hemodynamic monitoring, are ubiquitous in ICUs and are often overlooked as possible sources of infection. These catheters are among the most heavily manipulated catheters in the ICU and operating room. Some studies show the risk of arterial CRBSI to be comparable to that with traditional multilumen CVCs.[25] The risk of infection increases after 4 to 6 days. Given the limited number of arterial access sites, routine replacement of these catheters is not recommended.

PICCs have been associated with lower rates of BSI than have centrally inserted catheters; however, many initial studies were conducted among outpatients. Studies among inpatients have demonstrated infection rates comparable to those of other CVCs.[62]

Many hospitals have adopted checklists to standardize procedures when placing catheters. These bundles are a collection of interventions, similar to those for VAP, adherence to which has shown reductions in CRBSIs. Ultimately the only way to ensure prevention of a line infection is not to have a line. Devices should be assessed for necessity daily and removed if no longer deemed necessary. This decreases morbidity and mortality associated with CRBSIs and decreases subsequent financial impact.

Clostridioides Difficile Colitis[63]

Epidemiology

CDI is one of the most common hospital-acquired infections and is the leading cause of hospital-associated infectious diarrhea. It is a growing cause of morbidity and mortality, especially among elderly patients. Colonization of the intestinal tract occurs via the fecal-oral route by the ingestion of spores. Most often, C. difficile colonizes the human intestinal tract after the normal gut flora has been disrupted by antibiotic therapy. Once introduced into the altered intestinal tract, the organism creates exotoxins that bind to epithelial cells of the large intestine. The toxins A and B disrupt the cytoskeleton of the cells, causing fluid shifts and creating an inflammatory response, leading to diarrhea and colitis. The dysregulation caused by the toxins can be variable, ranging from a mild case of focal colitis, to severe sepsis, toxic megacolon, multiple organ dysfunction, and death.

Patients are at increased risk of developing diarrhea while in the hospital, and the majority of ICU patients have diarrhea at some point during their ICU stay. Most episodes of diarrhea are noninfectious; however, infectious causes of diarrhea in the ICU are concerning because of the increased likelihood of complications and the potential ease of transmission. C. difficile was identified in 1978 as the causative agent for 15 to 25% of antibiotic-associated diarrhea and colitis. Since its recognition, the incidence and severity of health care–associated C. difficile–associated diarrhea have been steadily increasing.

Risk Factors

The risk factors for CDI encompass three general categories. These include changes in the intestinal mucosa or immune system, host factors, and environmental causes. Changes in the intestinal mucosa or immune system can be due to medications, procedures, or radiation. Medications include the previously mentioned antibiotics, where the majority of hospitalized patients with CDI will have had antibiotic exposure within the previous 30 days. The earliest cases of CDI were largely attributed to clindamycin, which, in addition to fluoroquinolones and cephalosporins, remains the most common antibiotic class implicated in the development of CDI. Virtually all antibiotics, including metronidazole and vancomycin, can predispose patients to CDI. Chemotherapeutic agents and radiation treatment also change the immune system and can upset the GI flora, allowing the overgrowth of C. difficile and toxin production. GI prophylaxis is standard in most ICUs, yet some studies have shown proton pump inhibitors and H2-blockers to be associated with an increased risk of CDI. Studies are conflicting, however, and a direct cause and effect relationship has not been established.[64-67] Other disruptions in the GI tract have been implicated in the development of CDI, including abdominal surgery, nasogastric tubes, and enemas.

Host factors that are associated with an increased CDI risk include age older than 65 years, multiple comorbidities, peripartum women and children, inflammatory bowel disease, HIV (likely because of associated antibiotic use), and chronic kidney disease requiring hemodialysis, presumably because of frequent contact with the health care environment. Previous episodes of CDI also put patients at risk for repeat infection, especially if they require ongoing antibiotic treatment for other infections.

Finally, environmental factors can put patients at risk for development of CDI. Patients become infected primarily from spores present on the hands of health care workers, thus making hand hygiene a priority among all hospital staff members. The length of stay in the hospital also increases the risk of CDI, because the longer patients are admitted, the more likely they will be exposed to spores and antibiotics.

Clinical Presentation

The clinical manifestations of CDI can range from asymptomatic carrier to mild or moderate diarrhea, to fulminant colitis leading to sepsis or death. Approximately 20% of adults in hospitals are *C. difficile* carriers who do not have diarrhea, but do shed *C. difficile* in their stool. Watery diarrhea is the cardinal clinical symptom of CDI, often 10 to 15 times a day, with associated lower abdominal pain, distention, nausea, and loss of appetite. Melena and hematochezia are rarely seen in CDI. Low-grade fevers and leukocytosis are common findings in patients with *C. difficile*–associated diarrhea. Severe abdominal pain, without diarrhea, can indicate toxic megacolon with ileus, especially if accompanied by fever greater than 38.5°C (101.3°F) and profound leukocytosis, but this is a rare manifestation.

Fulminant colitis can manifest as severe lower or diffuse abdominal pain, diarrhea, distention, high fever, hypovolemia, and lactic acidosis. Recognition of deterioration toward fulminant colitis is essential because it can progress to toxic megacolon or colonic perforation, sepsis, and death. Timely recognition and surgical intervention can be potentially lifesaving.

Diagnosis

The definition of CDI includes the presence of diarrhea (three or more unformed stools in less than 24 hours), a stool test result that is positive for the presence of toxigenic *C. difficile* or its toxins, or endoscopic or histopathologic findings demonstrating pseudomembranous colitis. Rarely, a patient will have an ileus and colonic distention without significant diarrhea. Confirming the diagnosis in these patients can prove difficult without the appropriate sample.

Generally, testing for *C. difficile* or its toxins should be performed only on unformed stool. Testing stool from asymptomatic patients does not change clinical indications for treatment and is not recommended, nor is it recommended to test stool for evidence of cure. There are a variety of methods to detect toxigenic *C. difficile* in stool, each with advantages and limitations. These methods include:
- Polymerase chain reaction
- Enzyme immunoassays (EIAs) for *C. difficile* glutamate dehydrogenase
- EIA for *C. difficile* toxins A and B
- Cell culture cytotoxicity assay
- Selective anaerobic culture

Polymerase Chain Reaction

Polymerase chain reaction (PCR) testing is becoming more common. This sensitive and specific molecular test can rapidly detect the *C. difficile* toxins A and B gene in a stool sample and is highly accurate. Results from PCR can be available in 1 hour. Given the high sensitivity of PCR and the possibility for false-positive test results, this test is sometimes paired with an enzyme immunoassay for confirmation.

Enzyme Immunoassay for *Clostridioides difficile* Glutamate Dehydrogenase

Glutamate dehydrogenase (GDH) antigen is an enzyme that is produced by *C. difficile* bacteria. The detection of GDH does not distinguish between toxigenic and nontoxigenic strains. These EIA tests were initially not very sensitive and therefore were often used as an initial screening tool, paired with other tests to confirm positive results. The testing has improved over time, and newer tests have a sensitivity of 85 to 95%, with a specificity of 89 to 99%. GDH antigen testing results are usually available in less than 1 hour.

Enzyme Immunoassay for *Clostridioides difficile* Toxins A and B

Most *C. difficile* strains produce both toxins A and B, although some produce only one. The sensitivity for EIA for toxins is variable (63 to 94%), but it is highly specific (up to 99%). There is a higher false-negative rate because of the amount of toxin needed to be detected for the test to be positive. This testing has become popular in hospitals across the United States because it is easy to use and cost effective.

Cell Culture Cytotoxic Assay

Cell culture cytotoxic assay is the gold standard for the diagnosis of *C. difficile*. A sample is added to a layer of cultured cells, and the presence of toxin is detected by the cytotoxic effect on fibroblasts. The cytotoxicity assay is more sensitive than EIAs but is labor intensive and can take up to 2 days for results.

Selective Anaerobic Stool Culture

Stool culture is the most sensitive diagnostic test and is most often used for epidemiologic studies; however, it is not clinically practical because of the length of time to obtain results.

Adjunctive Diagnostic Tools

Diagnostic imaging is generally nonspecific in CDI, and although abdominal radiographs may show colonic dilation, or a CT scan can confirm colitis, the diagnosis of CDI is finalized with laboratory testing or endoscopy.

Pseudomembranous colitis is essentially pathognomonic for CDI, but can be diagnosed only by visualization of pseudomembranes on sigmoidoscopy or colonoscopy, or by histopathologic examination. Unfortunately, direct visualization using any of these techniques will detect pseudomembranes in only 51 to 55% of CDI cases diagnosed by combined clinical and laboratory criteria with both a positive stool culture and a positive stool cytotoxin test.

Treatment

Treatment for CDI should include supportive therapy with fluid and electrolyte replacements. If possible, the inciting antimicrobial agents should be discontinued, because these can increase the risk of recurrence. When severe or complicated CDI is suspected, initiating empiric therapy is appropriate. For almost 30 years, metronidazole and vancomycin had been the mainstays of treatment for CDI. Metronidazole was the drug of choice for an initial episode of mild to moderate CDI with a dosage of 500 mg orally (PO) three times per day for 10 to 14 days and vancomycin 125 mg PO four times per day for 10 days was the drug of choice for initial episodes of severe CDI. Vancomycin orally (or via rectal enemas in the case of ileus or GI surgery), with or without metronidazole intravenously, is the appropriate regimen for the treatment of severe, complicated CDI. For a severe manifestation, the vancomycin dosage is increased to 500 mg four times per day or 500 mg per 100 mL of normal saline rectally every 6 hours. The metronidazole dosage is also increased to 500 mg intravenously (IV) every 8 hours. In patients with hemodynamic instability requiring vasopressor support, a combination of intravenous metronidazole and oral vancomycin is recommended. Oral vancomycin is not absorbed systemically and achieves appropriate therapeutic levels in the colon. Intravenous forms of vancomycin, therefore, have no role in the treatment of CDI. Intravenous metronidazole, however, is excreted via the biliary system with exposure across the intestinal mucosa. Fecal concentrations reach therapeutic levels, making intravenous administration useful in patients with an ileus or in whom oral therapy is not feasible. Administration of both agents does not have any synergistic effect, but it is recommended in acutely ill patients as a way to get antibiotics to the colon as quickly as possible.

The IDSA and Society for Healthcare Epidemiology of America (SHEA) released updated clinical practice guidelines in 2021. These were based on a review of four noninferiority random controlled trials between 2011 and 2018 that demonstrated that fidaxomicin had increased sustained response to CDI 4 weeks after end of therapy as compared with standard vancomycin and comparable initial clinical cure rates while having a more narrow spectrum of coverage, low side effect profile, and less frequent dosing. Fidaxomicin 200 mg twice daily for 10 days is now the preferred regimen in initial CDI episodes. Caution should be exercised in patients with congestive heart failure.[68]

In patients who become severely ill (e.g., lactic acidosis, hemodynamic instability, worsening abdominal pain), surgical consultation should be obtained and colectomy should be considered. Checking the trend in the serum lactate level and peripheral white blood cell count can provide information that can aid in surgical decision-making. In the event that surgical intervention is necessary, subtotal colectomy with ileostomy and preservation of the rectum is performed.

Relapse or reinfection occurs in 10 to 25% of treated *C. difficile* cases. The clinical presentation may be similar to or more severe than the initial presentation. For CDI recurrence—both first and subsequent episodes—fidaxomicin 200 mg given twice daily for 10 days is preferred. Bezlotoxumab, a human monoclonal antibody, may be administered as an adjunct to treatment in recurrent episodes (dose 10 mg/kg IV). As the administration of fidaxomicin remains cost prohibitive in many institutions, the previously described metronidazole and vancomycin regimens for both initial and recurrent episodes remain acceptable alternatives.[68]

There are numerous investigations into adjunctive therapies for CDI. These therapies include intravenous immunoglobulin, probiotics, human monoclonal antibodies, bacteriotherapy using fecal transplant, and new antibiotics.

Prevention

The approach for preventing transmission of CDI in the hospital is to decrease patients' risk of exposure and prevent transmission to other patients. Decreasing the risk of CDI must involve a degree of antimicrobial stewardship, because the first line of defense against CDI is healthy intestinal flora. Strategies to interrupt transmission include proper and consistent hand hygiene and contact precautions, including gloves and gowns for health care workers. If possible, patients should have single rooms or be cohorted, with each patient provided a dedicated commode if possible. Contact precautions should be maintained while the patient is symptomatic with diarrhea. Identification and removal of environmental sources of infection is important, as is cleaning with chlorine-containing agents or sporicidal agents in areas of contamination.

Surgical Site Infection[69]

SSI, defined as an infection related to a surgical procedure that occurs near the surgical site within 30 days after surgery or up to 90 days when an implant is involved, are common and associated with significant morbidity and mortality and increased length of hospital and ICU stays. According to the CDC, 2 to 4% of those undergoing surgical procedures in the United States will develop a surgical site infection.[70]

Risk Factors

Risk factors for impaired wound healing such as cigarette smoking, older age, vascular disease, obesity, malnutrition, diabetes, and immunosuppressive therapy are also risk factors for SSI. Other risk factors include recent or remote infection at the surgical site, recent surgery, and recent hospitalization. Wound edema, proximity to other open or contaminated wound sites, and the degree of contamination of the surgical wound at the time of surgery also have been shown to increase risk of SSI.

Diagnosis

Superficial Surgical Site Infection

These infections are diagnosed by evaluation of the skin surrounding the wound for erythema, induration, warmth, drainage with or without odor, purulence, wound breakdown, and pain. Some patients may also have systemic signs such as fever and leukocytosis.

Deep Incisional Surgical Site Infection

These infections involve the fascia and/or muscle and may manifest with a fluctuant mass or similar signs and symptoms as superficial SSIs.

Organ and Space Surgical Site Infection

Patients typically present with fever, malaise, pain, tenderness, sometimes without overlying skin changes. These infections include abscesses or empyemas.

Necrotizing Infections

These infections can often be lethal and are considered a surgical emergency. They can manifest as early as 24 hours after surgery, commonly with sepsis. Peri-incisional pain is often severe and out of proportion to the expected degree of pain. There also may be skin discoloration, blistering, and devitalization with copious dishwater drainage. Laboratory analysis will reveal gross abnormalities with leukopenia or leukocytosis, hyponatremia, and other evidence of end-organ failure. The common causative organisms include group A *Streptococcus* and clostridia.

Imaging

Although diagnosis is made primarily on physical examination, especially for superficial infections, the clinician should have a low threshold for obtaining cross-sectional imaging in those with findings concerning for systemic infection for evaluation of involvement of underlying tissues or the organ space. Ultrasound is useful for superficial infections, whereas CT scans are better used for deeper infections.

Prevention

Risk of SSI can be reduced through a number of preventive factors. Elective surgery should be avoided in those with an active infection. Perioperative antibiotics should be administered within 1 hour of surgical incision, should be selected to target probably antimicrobial contaminants, and should be discontinued within the first two postoperative days.[71] If

there is hair in the surgical field, it should be clipped, not shaved. Proper skin preparation and maintenance of sterile conditions and good surgical technique such as gentle traction, effective hemostasis, removal of devitalized tissue, obliteration of dead space, and wound closure without tension can decrease risk. Normothermia and euglycemia should be targeted.

Treatment

Antibiotics

Samples for cultures should be obtained directly from the specific site of infection in the open wound, taking care not to sample the surrounding skin because this will make it difficult to discern colonization versus infection. Antibiotics should be initiated and tailored to culture results.

Surgical Management

Once the diagnosis of superficial/deep incisional SSI is made, the wound should be opened, infected fluid should be drained, and necrotic and devitalized tissue should be debrided. Deep tissue should be sent for culture. Deep SSI may require operative exploration or percutaneous drainage.

References

1. Allegranzi B, Storr J, Dziekan G, et al. The first global patient safety challenge "clean care is safer care": from launch to current progress and achievements. *J Hosp Infect.* 2007;65(suppl 2):115-123.
2. Vincent JL. Nosocomial infections in adult intensive-care units. *Lancet.* 2003;361(9374):2068-2077.
3. Nuvials X, Palomar M, Alvarez-Lerma F, et al. Health-care associated infections: patient characteristics and influence on the clinical outcome of patients admitted to ICU—Envin-Helics registry data. *Intensive Care Med Exp.* 2015;3(suppl 1):A82.
4. Fridkin SK, Welbel SF, Weinstein RA. Magnitude and prevention of nosocomial infections in the intensive care unit. *Infect Dis Clin North Am.* 1997;11(2):479-496.
5. Sydnor ER, Perl TM. Hospital epidemiology and infection control in acute-care settings. *Clin Microbiol Rev.* 2011;24(1):141-173.
6. Magill SS, Edwards JR, Bamberg W, et al. Emerging Infections Program healthcare-associated infections and antimicrobial use prevalence survey team multistate point-prevalence survey of health care-associated infections. *N Engl J Med.* 2014;370(13):1198-1208.
7. O'Grady N P, et al. Society of Critical Care Medicine and the Infectious Diseases Society of America Guidelines for Evaluating New Fever in Adult Patients in the ICU. *Crit Care Med.* 2023;51(11):1570–1586. doi:10.1097/CCM.0000000000006022.
8. Singer M, Deutschman CS, Seymour CW, et al. The Third International Consensus definitions for sepsis and septic shock (sepsis-3). *JAMA.* 2016;315(8):801-810.
9. Shankar-Hari M, Phillips GS, Levy ML, et al. Developing a new definition and assessing new clinical criteria for septic shock: for the Third International Consensus definitions for sepsis and septic shock (sepsis-3). *JAMA.* 2016;315(8):775-787.
10. Vincent J L, et al. The SOFA (Sepsis-related organ failure assessment) score to describe organ dysfunction/failure. On behalf of

the working group on sepsis-related problems of the European society of intensive care medicine. *Intensive Care Med.* 1996;22:707–710.

11. Smith G B, et al. The ability of the National Early Warning Score (NEWS) to discriminate patients at risk of early cardiac arrest, unanticipated intensive care unit admission, and death. *Resuscitation.* 2013;84:465–470.

12. Raith EP, Udy AA, Bailey M, et al. Prognostic accuracy of the SOFA Score, SIRS Criteria, and qSOFA Score for in-hospital mortality among adults with suspected infection admitted to the intensive care unit. *JAMA.* 2017;317(3):290-300.

13. Evans L, Rhodes A, Alhazzani W, et al. Surviving sepsis campaign: international guidelines for management of sepsis and septic shock 2021. *Crit Care Med.* 2021;49:e1063.

14. Lemieux S M, Levine A R Low-dose corticosteroids in septic shock: Has the pendulum shifted? *Am J Health Syst Pharm.* 2019;76(8):493–500.

15. Askarian M, Yadollahi M, Assadian O. Point prevalence and risk factors of hospital acquired infections in a cluster of university-affiliated hospitals in Shiraz, Iran. *J Infect Public Health.* 2012;5(2):169-176.

16. Tagoe DN, Desbordes KK. Investigating potential sources of transmission of healthcare-associated infections in a regional hospital, Ghana. *Int J Appl Basic Med Res.* 2012;2(1):20-24.

17. Magill SS, Hellinger W, Cohen J, et al. Prevalence of healthcare-associated infections in acute care hospitals in Jacksonville, Florida. *Infect Control Hosp Epidemiol.* 2012;3(3):283-291.

18. Magill SS, Wilson LE, Thompson DL, et al. Emerging infections program hospital prevalence survey team reduction in the prevalence of healthcare-associated infections in US acute care hospitals, 2015 vs 2011. *Open Forum Infect Dis.* 2017;4(suppl 1):S49.

19. Cai Y, Venkatachalam I, Tee NW, et al. Prevalence of healthcare-associated infections and antimicrobial use among adult inpatients in Singapore acute-care hospitals: results from the First National Point Prevalence Survey. *Clin Infect Dis.* 2017;64(suppl 2):S61-S67.

20. Cassini A, Plachouras D, Eckmanns T, et al. Burden of six healthcare-associated infections on European population health: estimating incidence-based disability-adjusted life years through a population prevalence-based modelling study. *PLoS Med.* 2016;13(10):e1002150.

21. Sievert DM, Ricks P, Edwards JR, et al. National Healthcare Safety Network (NHSN) Team and Participating NHSN Facilities. Antimicrobial-resistant pathogens associated with healthcare-associated infections: summary of data reported to the National Healthcare Safety Network at the Centers for Disease Control and Prevention 2009–2010. *Infect Control Hosp Epidemiol.* 2013;34(1):1-14.

22. Boucher HW, Talbot GH, Bradley JS, et al. Bad bugs, no drugs: no ESKAPE! An update from the Infectious Diseases Society of America. *Clin Infect Dis.* 2009;48(1):1-12.

23. Kalil AC, Metersky ML, Klompas M, et al. Management of adults with hospital-acquired and ventilator-associated pneumonia: 2016 Clinical Practice Guidelines by the Infectious Diseases Society of America and the American Thoracic Society. *Clin Infect Dis.* 2016;63:e61.

24. Patel P K, et al. Strategies to prevent catheter-associated urinary tract infections in acute-care hospitals: 2022 Update. *Infection Control & Hospital Epidemiology.* 2023;44(8):1209–1231. doi:10.1017/ice.2023.137.

25. Magill SS, O'Leary E, Janelle SJ, et al. Emerging Infections Program Hospital Prevalence Survey Team. Changes in prevalence of health care-associated infections in U.S. hospitals. *N Engl J Med.* 2018;379(18):1732-1744.

26. Foxman B. Epidemiology of urinary tract infections: incidence, morbidity, and economic costs. *Dis Mon.* 2003;49(2):53-70.

27. Tenke P, Mezei T, Böde I, Köves B. Catheter-associated urinary tract infections. *Eur Urol Suppl.* 2017;16(4):138-143.

28. Saint S. Clinical and economic consequences of nosocomial catheter-related bacteriuria. *Am J Infect Control.* 2000;28:68.

29. Chenoweth CE, Gould CV, Saint S. Diagnosis, management and preventions of catheter associated urinary tract infection. *Infect Dis Clin North Am.* 2014;28:105-119.

30. Nicolle E. Urinary catheter associated infections. *Infect Dis Clin North Am.* 2012;26:13-27.

31. Bryan CS, Reynolds KL. Hospital-acquired bacteremic urinary tract infection: epidemiology and outcome. *J Urology.* 1984; 132(3):494-498.

32. Paradisi F, Corti G, Mangani V. Urosepsis in the critical care unit. *Crit Care Clin.* 1998;14(2):165-180.

33. Maki DG, Tambyah PA. Engineering out the risk for infection with urinary catheters. *Emerg Infect Dis.* 2001;7(2):342-347.

34. McGuckin M. *The Patient Survival Guide: 8 Simple Solutions to Prevent Hospital and Healthcare-Associated Infections.* New York: Demos Medical Publishing; 2012.

35. Lo E, Nicolle LE, Coffin SE, et al. Strategies to prevent catheter-associated urinary tract infections in acute care hospitals: 2014 update. *Infect Control Hosp Epidemiol.* 2014;35:464-479.

36. Stamm WE. Catheter-associated urinary tract infections: epidemiology, pathogenesis, and prevention. *Am J Med.* 1991;91(3): S65-S71.

37. Leelakrishna P, Karthik Rao B. A study of risk factors for catheter associated urinary tract infection. *Int J Adv Med.* 2018;5(2):334-339.

38. Trautner BW, Darouiche RO. Role of biofilm in catheter-associated urinary tract infection. *Am J Infect Control.* 2004; 32:177.

39. Roilides E, Simitsopoulou M, Katragkou A, Walsh TJ. How biofilms evade host defenses. *Microbiol Spectr.* 2015;3(3):1-10.

40. Magi DG, Tambyah PA. Engineer out of the risk of infection with urinary catheter. *Emerg Infect Dis.* 2001;7:342-347.

41. Fisher J F, et al. Candida urinary tract infection: pathogenesis. *Clin Infect Dis.* 2011;52(6):S437–S451. doi:10.1093/cid/cir110.

42. Tambyah PA, Maki DG. Catheter-associated urinary tract infection is rarely symptomatic: a prospective study of 1,497 catheterized patients. *Arch Intern Med.* 2000;160:678-682.

43. Hooton TM, Bradley SF, Cardenas DD, et al. Diagnosis, prevention and treatment of catheter-associated urinary tract infection in adults: 2009 international clinical practice guidelines from the Infectious Diseases Society of America. *Clin Infect Dis.* 2010; 50(5):625-663.

44. Klompas M, et al. Strategies to prevent ventilator-associated pneumonia, ventilator-associated events, and nonventilator hospital-acquired pneumonia in acute-care hospitals: 2022 Update. *Infection Control & Hospital Epidemiology.* 2022;43(6):687–713. doi:10.1017/ice.2022.88.

45. Muscedere JG, Day A, Heyland DK. Mortality, attributable mortality, and clinical events as end points for clinical trials of ventilator-associated pneumonia and hospital-acquired pneumonia. *Clin Infect Dis.* 2010;51(suppl 1):S120-S125.

46. Kollef MH, Hamilton CW, Ernst FR. Economic impact of ventilator-associated pneumonia in a large matched cohort. *Infect Control Hosp Epidemiol.* 2012;33:250-256.

47. American Thoracic Society (ATS) and Infectious Diseases Society of America (IDSA). Guidelines for the management of adults with

hospital-acquired, ventilator-associated, and healthcare-associated pneumonia. *Am J Respir Crit Care Med*. 2005;171:388-416.

48. Martin-Loeches I, Deja M, Koulenti D, et al. Potentially resistant microorganisms in intubated patients with hospital-acquired pneumonia: the interaction of ecology, shock and risk factors. *Intensive Care Med*. 2013;39(4):672-681.

49. Chastre J, Fagon JY. Ventilator-associated pneumonia. *Am J Respir Crit Care Med*. 2002;165(7):867-903.

50. Luyt CE, Combes A, Trouillet JL, Chastre J. Value of the serum procalcitonin level to guide antimicrobial therapy for patients with ventilator-associated pneumonia. *Semin Respir Crit Care Med*. 2011;32(2):181-187.

51. Khilnani GC, Zirpe K, Hadda V, et al. Guidelines for antibiotic prescription in intensive care unit. *Indian J Crit Care Med*. 2019;23(suppl 1):S1-S63.

52. Buetti N, et al. Strategies to prevent central line-associated bloodstream infections in acute-care hospitals: 2022 Update. *Infection Control & Hospital Epidemiology*. 2022;43(5):553–569. doi:10.1017/ice.2022.87.

53. Centers for Disease Control and Prevention. Vitals signs: central line-associated blood stream infections—United States, 2001, 2008, and 2009. *MMWR Morb Mortal Wkly Rep*. 2011;60:243-248.

54. Safdar N, Fine JP, Maki DG. Meta-analysis: methods for diagnosing intravascular device-related bloodstream infection. *Ann Intern Med*. 2005;142(6):451-466.

55. Novosad SA, Fike L, Dudeck MA, et al. Pathogens causing central-line-associated bloodstream infections in acute-care hospitals—United States, 2011-2017. *Infect Control Hosp WEpidemiol*. 2020;41:313-319.

56. Al Mohajer M, Darouiche RO. Sepsis syndrome, bloodstream infections, and device-related infections. *Med Clin North Am*. 2012;96:1203-1223.

57. Mermel LA. Prevention of intravascular catheter-related infections. *Ann Intern Med*. 2000;132:391-402.

58. Maki DG, Kluger DM, Crnich CJ. The risk of bloodstream infection in adults with different intravascular devices: a systematic review of 200 published prospective studies. *Mayo Clin Proc*. 2006;81:1159-1171.

59. Mermel LA, McCormick RD, Springman SR, et al. The pathogenesis and epidemiology of catheter-related infection with pulmonary artery Swan-Ganz catheters: a prospective study utilizing molecular subtyping. *Am J Med*. 1991;91:197S.

60. Gil RT, Kruse JA, Thill-Baharoziam MC, et al. Triple- vs. single-lumen central venous catheters: a prospective study in a critically ill population. *Arch Intern Med*. 1989;149:1139.

61. O'Grady NP, Alexander M, Dellinger EP, et al. Guidelines for the prevention of intravascular catheter-related infections. Centers for Disease Control and Prevention. *MMWR Recomm Rep*. 2002;51(RR-10):129.

62. Safdar N, Maki DG. Risk of catheter-related bloodstream infection with peripherally inserted central venous catheters used in hospitalized patients. *Chest*. 2005;128:489-495.

63. Johnson S, et al. Clinical Practice Guideline by the Infectious Diseases Society of America (IDSA) and Society for Healthcare Epidemiology of America (SHEA): 2021 Focused Update Guidelines on Management of Clostridioides difficile Infection in Adults. *Clin Infect Dis*. 2021;73(5):e1029–e1044. doi:10.1093/cid/ciab549.

64. Cadle RM, Mansouri MD, Logan N, et al. Association of proton-pump inhibitors with outcomes in *Clostridium difficile* colitis. *Am J Health Syst Pharm*. 2007;64(22):2359-2363.

65. Linsky A, Gupta K, Lawler EV, et al. Proton pump inhibitors and risk for recurrent *Clostridium difficile* infection. *Arch Intern Med*. 2010;170(9):772-778.

66. Howell MD, Novack V, Grgurich P, et al. Iatrogenic gastric acid suppression and the risk of nosocomial *Clostridium difficile* infection. *Arch Intern Med*. 2010;170(9):784-790.

67. Tawam D, Baladi M, Jungsuwadee P, Earl G, Han J. The positive association between proton pump inhibitors and *Clostridium difficile* infection. *Innov Pharm*. 2021;12(1):10.24926/iip.v12i1.3439. Available at: https://doi.org/10.24926/iip.v12i1.3439.

68. Johnson S, Lavergne V, Skinner AM, et al. Clinical practice guideline by the Infectious Diseases Society of America (IDSA) and Society for Healthcare Epidemiology of America (SHEA): 2021 focused update guidelines on management of *Clostridioides difficile* infection in adults. *Clin Infect Dis*. 2021;73(5):e1029-e1044.

69. Calderwood M S, et al. Strategies to prevent surgical site infections in acute-care hospitals: 2022 Update. *Infection Control & Hospital Epidemiology*. 2023;44(5):695–720. doi:10.1017/ice.2023.67.

70. Berríos-Torres SI, Umscheid CA, Bratzler DW, et al. Centers for Disease Control and Prevention guideline for the prevention of surgical site infection, 2017 [published correction appears in *JAMA Surg*. 2017;152(8):803]. *JAMA Surg*. 2017;152(8):784-791. Available at: https://doi.org/10.1001/jamasurg.2017.0904.

71. Rosenberger LH, Politano AD, Sawyer RG. The surgical care improvement project and prevention of post-operative infection, including surgical site infection. *Surg Infect (Larchmt)*. 2011;12(3):163-168.

25

Head, Neck, and Orofacial Infections in Immunocompromised Patients

KEVIN C. LEE, STEVEN HALEPAS, AND ELIE M. FERNEINI

The progression toward a clinical infection rests on the outcome of a complex interplay between a pathogen and its host. For the infection to manifest, it often requires some physical or chemical imbalance to tip the scale in favor of the pathogen. This chapter reviews relevant host defenses and how defects in these systems can influence the risk of infection in the head and neck region.

Host Response to Infection

The first impediment to infection is the epithelial barrier that covers the surface and lines cavities in the head and neck area. Epithelial cells adhere to each other via tight junctions that aid in the prevention of passive intrusion by microorganisms and small molecules. In addition, excretory products from cells within the lining epithelium aid in aggregation and clearance of presenting pathogens. Nonspecific surface products such as saliva, tears, sweat, and sebum help to clear the epithelial surface via dilution and washout. More specifically, surface defense is afforded by products such as immunoglobulin A (IgA) and lysozyme, which have direct microbicidal activity. Next in line to stem the invasion of microbes are the complement cascade, phagocytic cells of the immune system (neutrophils, eosinophils, macrophage–monocytes), and the release of chemical mediators that aid in the recruitment of the adaptive immune response.

Compared with the innate immune response, the adaptive response is the more complex and specific system and is divided into humoral and cellular immunity. Within the cellular immune response, a microbial antigen is presented to T lymphocytes by antigen-presenting cells, which selects certain populations to proliferate. The subset of T lymphocytes that is involved in antigen recognition and downstream signaling are called *helper T lymphocytes*. This clonal expansion leads to immunologic memory for a pathogen and confers improved defense in the setting of a repeated presentation. Other subsets of T lymphocytes aid in identifying and eliminating non-self or infected cells and help to regulate the immune system. (See Chapter 1 for an expanded discussion of this topic.)

Humoral immunity refers to immunoglobulin elaboration and the complement cascade, which help in identifying pathogens and marking them for elimination. B cells, which are responsible for immunoglobulin synthesis, also maintain a memory for recently identified antigens and can quickly respond in the setting of a repeat encounter.

Etiology of Deficiency

Immunodeficiency relates to any failing of the immune system in its ability to produce a normal response to a pathogen. A deficit in host immunity can occur anywhere along the complex series of interactions that compose the immune response. These defects can be classified as either primary, in which there is an inherited or intrinsic flaw in the immune system, or secondary, in which the immune system is adversely affected by an infectious agent, pharmacologic therapy, or metabolic state.

Primary Immunodeficiency States

Primary immunodeficiency (PID) includes a complex group of more than 150 immunologic deficits with many various clinical manifestations. When compared with their immunocompetent counterparts, patients with PID are at increased risk of infection, autoimmune diseases, and some malignancies.[1] The prevalence of PID in the United States is estimated to be between 1 in 500 and 1 in 1200 people.[2] More than half of the known PID diseases primarily affect the humoral immune response,[3] and any or all of the immunoglobulins can be deficient. The most common infections seen in cases of immunoglobulin deficiency are bacterial sinopulmonary infections, including sinusitis, bronchitis, pneumonia, and otitis media.[4] When there is a primary defect in the cellular immune response, there is an elevated risk of infection with salmonella and nontuberculoid mycobacterial infections, and infections with opportunistic pathogens, including *Pneumocystis jiroveci*, *Cryptosporidium parvum*, and *Candida* spp.[5] Finally, defects in complement and phagocyte function increase the risk of infections by encapsulated bacteria, including *Streptococcus pneumoniae* and *Haemophilus influenzae*.[1,6] There also can be defects in both cellular and humoral immunity. Examples of conditions in which there is a primary defect in both cellular and humoral immunity include Wiskott-Aldrich syndrome, DiGeorge's syndrome, and ataxia telangiectasia. These patients are particularly susceptible to opportunistic infections, but the most common infectious presentations are candidiasis, diarrhea, respiratory infection, and failure to thrive.[7]

PID prevention consists of early detection and management of an acute infection. When the infection is present, it should be treated in a timely and aggressive fashion. It is important to note that in some cases of immunoglobulin deficiency, the serologic markers used to identify a pathogen might not be effective. Currently, there are no definitive recommendations for antibiotic prophylaxis for surgical procedures that go beyond perioperative dosing in select cases; therefore, one should consider involving the patient's primary care provider, immunologist, and pulmonologist in the perioperative planning.

Secondary (Acquired) Immunodeficiency States

Of particular importance to ancillary providers are the acquired immunodeficiency states in which the underlying immunodeficiency may be the result of the treatment of another condition, a side effect of therapy, or a consequence of an unrelated but uncontrolled disease process. These acquired immune deficits can disrupt any pathway of the normal immune response, and the specific pathway involved determines how the deficiency will manifest. Some of these secondary deficiencies may be reversible, and priority should be given to restoring normal immune function whenever a fulminant infection is present.

Pathway of Deficiency

In addition to classifying immunodeficiency states as either primary or secondary, the specific pathway affected can be used to better understand and anticipate the potential infections that one may be vulnerable to.

Granulocyte Disorders

Granulocyte disorders can be qualitative or quantitative; however, management considerations are similar. Some conditions that lead to qualitative dysfunction include some hematologic disorders, diabetes mellitus, uremia associated with renal failure, liver failure, burns, chronic infection, and some pharmacotherapies. As mentioned elsewhere in this chapter, the specific qualitative dysfunction can include dysfunction of diapedesis, chemotaxis, phagocytosis, and production of reactive oxygen species.

Granulocytopenia was first correlated with increased risk of infection as early as the 1960s.[8] The demonstrated risk was found to start at neutrophil counts less than 1000/mm³, and was greatest at counts less than 100/mm³. In fact, between 48 and 60% of neutropenic patients who become febrile have an established or occult infection, and between 16 and 20% of patients with profound neutropenia (neutrophil count <100/mm³) have bacteremia.[8,9] In addition, the duration of neutropenia also has been linked to increased morbidity and mortality. In early studies of neutropenia in patients receiving chemotherapy for cancer, the probability of acquiring a bacterial or fungal infection approached 100% when the duration of neutropenia was greater than 3 weeks.[10] Patients in whom the duration of neutropenia is less than 7 to 10 days are considered to be at low risk, compared with those in whom the duration is greater than 15 days (high risk).[11]

The causes of granulocytopenia are numerous and include disease states such as hematologic malignancies or malnutrition, suppression from select pharmacotherapies, trauma, or radiation therapy. Observation that morbidity and mortality significantly increased when febrile neutropenic patients went untreated led to the recommendation to start early empiric antibiotic therapy.[12] It has even been demonstrated in a large meta-analysis study that antibiotic prophylaxis in the early afebrile period of neutropenia reduces the rate of all-cause and infection-related mortality. The number needed to treat for each instance was 34 and 48, respectively.[13] Febrile neutropenia is a medical emergency. Patients should be hospitalized and observed closely with extensive exposure history, review of systems, and physical examination. Another management strategy that has evolved to combat serious infections in neutropenic patients is the administration of hematopoietic growth factors, including granulocyte- and granulocyte-macrophage-colony–stimulating factors (G-CSF and GM-CSF). Although initially tried as adjuncts to empiric antibiotics, G-CSF and GM-CSF appear to have benefit only in preventive strategies in which the aim is to limit the degree and duration of neutropenia.[10]

Humoral Immunodeficiency

Humoral or soluble factors of the immune system include immunoglobulins and complement. Defective immunoglobulin production is the most common cause of primary immunodeficiency and accounts for more than half of all cases of immunodeficiency.[14] In general, humoral immunodeficiencies do not manifest until after the first 6 months of life because of conferred protection from circulating maternal antibodies. These humoral immunodeficiencies range from total lack of serum immunoglobulins (Bruton's agammaglobulinemia) to conditions in which levels of immunoglobulins are normal, although, they are deficient in their function. A variety of primary humoral immunodeficiencies are the result of genetic defects, such as common variable immunodeficiency, X-linked infantile agammaglobulinemia, hyper-IgM syndrome, and selective IgA deficiency.[14] These patients are subject to recurrent sinopulmonary infections with encapsulated organisms such as *H. influenzae* and *S. pneumoniae*.[14] A second, more heterogenous group of patients are also humorally immunodeficient. In this group, there is an acquired hypogammaglobulinemia because of increased catabolism, accelerated protein loss, or pharmacologic inhibition.[15,16] The most common conditions in this category include nephrotic syndrome; protein-losing enteropathies such as intestinal lymphangiectasia[17] and Crohn's disease;[18] cytomegalovirus, Epstein-Barr virus, and rubella; corticosteroid or anticonvulsant treatment; burns;[19] and some malignancies (chronic lymphocytic leukemia[20] and multiple myeloma).[21] This group of patients, like those with genetic defects that result in humoral immunodeficiency, is also subject to recurrent sinopulmonary infections.

As with immunoglobulins, complement factors can be deficient in multiple ways. Complement deficiencies are grouped into where the deficiency lies in the complement cascade. Complement deficiencies, in general, increase a patient's risk of infection, but also predispose patients to developing autoimmune diseases. Early deficiencies (C1, C2, and C4) and C3 deficiency increase the risk of infection from pyogenic bacteria and predispose patients to developing a systemic lupus erythematosus–like syndrome and vasculitis or glomerulonephritis, respectively.[14] Late complement deficiencies (C5 to C9) increase the risk of infection with encapsulated bacteria, but do not increase the risk of developing an autoimmune condition.[14]

Cellular Immunodeficiency

It is generally understood that the humoral immune response predominates in the clearance of soluble antigens and extracellular microorganisms and that the cellular immune response has a main role in the eradication of intracellular pathogens, including some bacteria, parasites, and viruses.[22] Despite this distinction, both immune responses are coordinated largely through the assistance of T cells.[22] In particular, CD4 T cells have the potential to activate phagocytes to eliminate microorganisms contained in their phagosomes, and CD8 T cells aid in the elimination of any cell harboring microbes or foreign proteins in their cytoplasm.[23] Of all primary immunodeficiencies, deficiencies of T lymphocytes can be the most severe because they have roles in the antigen-specific and antigen-independent immune responses.[24] Some clinical manifestations of T cell deficiency include opportunistic infections, recurrent bacterial and viral infections, autoimmune hemolytic anemia, lymphoid hepatitis and dermatitis, and Hodgkin lymphoma.[24] In addition to falling into the category of primary immunodeficiencies, T cell dysfunction is also found in lymphoproliferative malignancies; chronic viral infections, including cytomegalovirus, HIV, and Epstein-Barr virus; and with some immunosuppressive therapies such as corticosteroids, cyclophosphamide, cyclosporine, and tacrolimus.[25]

Nonneoplastic Conditions Associated With Acquired Immunodeficiency

As described in other textbooks, immunodeficiency is most practically divided into subgroups based on the principal cause for the deficiency. With this in mind, numerous immune defects arise from conditions unrelated to a malignant or neoplastic process.

Splenectomy

The spleen is a solid organ with several immune-modulating properties. Normally, the spleen is responsible for processes such as fetal hematopoiesis, filtering of microorganisms and erythrocytes, elaboration of IgM and immune synthesis, acting as a cellular reservoir for platelets and granulocytes, and iron metabolism.[26] More controversially, the spleen also has a role in the complement cascade with production of properdin, opsonin, and tuftsin, which stimulates interleukin-1 (IL-1) production and facilitates phagocytosis.[26] Hence, the loss of the spleen can have far-reaching effects on host response to specific organisms. Functional hyposplenism or asplenia, commonly associated with sickle cell disease, also can be present in other conditions such as celiac disease, sarcoidosis, systemic lupus erythematosus, ulcerative colitis, amyloidosis, and bacterial endocarditis.[26] After undergoing splenectomy, patients are weakly responsive to foreign polysaccharides and are uniquely susceptible to organisms with polysaccharide capsules,[27] such as *H. influenzae*, *S. pneumoniae*, and *Neisseria meningitidis*, and can even develop osteomyelitis from species of *Salmonella*.[28]

Of specific interest is how to manage traumatic injuries with high potential for infection and chemoprophylaxis for elective procedures on patients who are asplenic. *Capnocytophaga canimorsus*, found in the saliva of 16 to 24% of dogs and 17% of cats, can lead to overwhelming postsplenectomy infection.[29,30] As a result, it is widely accepted that splenectomized patients receive immediate prophylactic antibiotics after an animal bite.[31,32] For bite wounds, a commonly used regimen is amoxicillin-clavulanate (Augmentin) for 3 to 5 days after the injury, although this does not substitute for proper wound management. Splenectomized patients should also receive prophylactic antibiotics for any febrile episode.[33] In the case of fever, ceftriaxone with or without vancomycin is reasonable, which covers *S. pneumoniae*, *H. influenzae*, *N. meningitidis*, and capnocytophaga.[33] Similarly, antibiotic prophylaxis in the form of penicillin V, amoxicillin, or clindamycin can be used for head and neck procedures in which there will be contamination from highly colonized surfaces and secretions.[34]

Diabetes Mellitus

Immune compromise caused by the physiologic derangements in diabetes mellitus has been studied extensively. The primary source for the increased risk and difficulty controlling infection appears to be hyperglycemia.[35,36] Blood glucose in the range of 198 to 270 mg/dL and greater appears to be able to cause immunologic dysfunction.[37] By itself, hyperglycemia has significant effects on innate and cellular immunity. Neutrophils have poor adherence, impaired chemotaxis, and decreased ability to produce reactive oxygen species as part of their oxidative burst.[38,39] Indeed, in the hypoxic environment of some infections there is a decreased expression of genes involved in encoding enzymes that take part in glycolysis, oxidative metabolism, and mitochondrial function.[40] In addition, monocytes and macrophages may have elevated catabolism of proinflammatory cytokines and increased production of matrix metalloproteases.[41,42] Phagocytosis by host immune cells also has been found to be significantly compromised. Patients with diabetes have an elevated cytosolic Ca^{++} content,[43] which can decrease adenosine triphosphate production and reduce phagocytic ability of neutrophils.[44] Phagocytosis is also impaired through the effect of hyperglycemia on complement and Fc receptor–mediated identification of pathogens.[45]

Fortunately, many of the immune defects related to hyperglycemia can be alleviated through tight glycemic control.[46] In studies involving cardiothoracic surgery, goal blood glucose of less than 200 mg/dL was found to significantly decrease the incidence of deep sternal wound infections in patients with diabetes[46] and improved neutrophil phagocytosis.[47] The findings of increased risk of postsurgical infection go beyond cardiothoracic surgery as well. In a study of a variety of elective procedures, it was found that patients with blood glucose measurements greater than 220 mg/dL on postoperative day 1 had a 2.7-fold greater risk of infection than did patients whose blood glucose was maintained at less than 220 mg/dL.[48] In general, there is no strong indication for prophylactic antibiotics in routine surgery for patients with good glycemic control; however, strong consideration should be given for antibiotic prophylaxis in patients with poor glycemic control.

In addition to increased susceptibility to infections that are found in normal immunocompetent and nondiabetic hosts, patients with diabetes are also at risk for infections that are relatively unique to immunocompromised individuals. Rhinocerebral mucormycosis is an acute fungal infection with high mortality (15 to 34%).[49] It is highly aggressive and stems from the nasal or oral mucosa with rapid extension to the orbit and central nervous system via the paranasal sinuses. Growth of the fungus is enabled by the glucose-rich and acidic environment of the diabetic nasal and oral cavities. Intranasal or palatal necrotic lesions are pathognomonic,[50] and orbital involvement leads to ocular pain, proptosis, and ophthalmoplegia (Figure 25-1). Definitive diagnosis is made based on frozen section and demonstration of branching hyphae. Treatment consists of correcting the underlying metabolic derangement, discontinuation of all immunosuppressive agents, and early surgical debridement. Antifungal treatment with amphotericin B should also be instituted as early as possible, with broad-spectrum triazoles being used as an equally successful alternative.[49] Hyperbaric oxygen therapy, although not yet proved

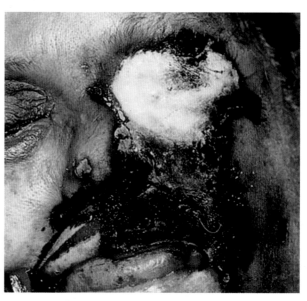

• **Figure 25-1** Black Necrotic Lesions Involving the Nose, Hard Palate, Left Cheek, and Left Orbit Consistent with Rhinocerebral Mucormycosis in a Patient with Diabetes. (From Tryfon S, et al. Rhinocerebral mucormycosis in a patient with latent diabetes mellitus: a case report. *J Oral Maxillofac Surg.* 2002;60:328-330.)

successful in large trials, has the potential to limit fungal growth, improve healing, augment neutrophil function, and aid in reversing lactic acidosis.[51]

Malignant or invasive otitis externa is another infection that is unique to patients with diabetes. Approximately 90% of cases are associated with diabetes,[49] with diabetic microangiopathy being a significant predisposing factor.[52] It is a severe infection of the external auditory canal with extension into the adjacent soft tissues and eventual involvement of the skull base. *Pseudomonas aeruginosa* is the causative organism in virtually all cases.[53] Presenting symptoms include severe otalgia, otorrhea, hearing loss, and occasionally temporomandibular joint pain. Advanced disease involvement of cranial nerves VII, IX, X, and XI can lead to palsies and is an indicator of a poor prognosis.[52] On physical examination, there is often intense cellulitis of the external auditory canal and polypoid granulation tissue at the junction between bone and cartilage.[54,55] Evaluation of suspected malignant or invasive otitis externa should include computed tomography or magnetic resonance imaging, culture of any drainage, and biopsy of the site of infection to aid in ruling out other invasive diseases (Figure 25-2). The standard for treatment is systemic antipseudomonal antibiotics for 6 to 8 weeks. In advanced disease, hospitalization, surgical debridement, and an extended course (>12 weeks) of parenteral antibiotics may be necessary.[52]

Alcohol Abuse and Liver Disease

Alcohol alone, and in conjunction with other states that commonly coexist with alcohol abuse (e.g., malnutrition), can have a profound negative influence on the immune system. Function[56] and production[57] of phagocytic cells

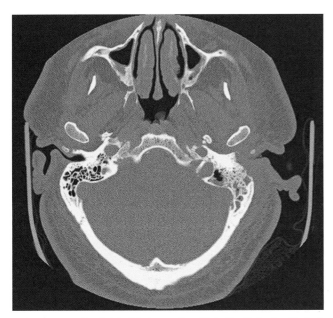

• **Figure 25-2** An Axial CT Scan of a Diabetic Patient with Left Malignant Otitis Externa Showing Bony Erosion of the Posterior External Auditory Canal and Mastoid Cortex. (From Carfrae MJ, Kesser BW. Malignant otitis externa. *Otolayrngol Clin North Am.* 2008; 41(3):537-549.)

and T cell subpopulations, respectively, can be impaired. Specifically, CD4 cell count numbers rivaling those found in acquired immunodeficiency virus (AIDS) have been found in patients with chronic alcoholism and protein calorie malnutrition.[58]

Renal Disease

Immune deficits in chronic renal disease can result from the uremic state, from the underlying condition that led to renal failure, or directly from the interventions used to manage chronic kidney disease.[59] In 1961, Schreiner was the first to note unique susceptibility to infections in patients with renal failure.[59] Since then, additional observations such as poor response to vaccination and prolonged skin graft survival have confirmed that renal disease greatly impairs host defenses.[60,61,62] Renal disease can cause impairments to both cell-mediated and humoral immune responses, albeit in largely different methods. Except in nephrotic syndrome, in which a patient may lose significant quantities of IgG in his or her urine, humoral immunity remains largely intact.[63] The depressed cell-mediated immunity in renal failure appears to be multifactorial. Fc-mediated phagocytosis and monocyte-dependent antigen presentation have been shown to be reproducibly impaired in uremic states. In addition, a suppressor molecule found in uremic patients has been shown in studies to downregulate the mitogenic responses of normal lymphocytes.[27] Finally, the proinflammatory cytokines tumor necrosis factor, IL-6, and IL-10 are increased, which produces a catabolic state. Many of these abnormalities do not improve with dialysis, and may even be exacerbated, because of complement activation by dialysis membranes and

consumption of immune products.[64] There is a general consensus that perioperative antibiotic prophylaxis is successful in many surgical procedures; however, there is no universal guideline for use of routine antibiotic prophylaxis for outpatient or office procedures in the setting of renal failure. Both surgical site and vascular access infections can have devastating consequences in patients with severe chronic renal disease. Consultation with a nephrologist may be warranted on an individual basis for indications and dosing of antibiotics when warranted.

Intravenous Drug Abuse

Infections are a common cause of morbidity and mortality in the context of intravenous drug abuse (IVDA). Compared with the repeated violation of skin and mucosal barriers and injection of nonscrutinized substances, any immune defect that directly results from IVDA probably plays a minor role in the contraction of infection. Most immune deficits in intravenous drug abusers are in natural killer and antibody-dependent cellular cytotoxicity.[65] In treatment of infections in IVDA patients, it is important to consider coverage with broad-spectrum antibiotics, at least initially, because the IVDA patient may have had many prior infections treated with typical antibiotic therapy. As with other infections in immunocompromised hosts, there is a role for culture and sensitivity. It is also essential to consider the possibility of hematogenous spread of the infection to distant sites, including cardiac valves and joints, that is not uncommon.[66,67]

Malnutrition

Malnutrition is known to be associated with multiple forms of immunodeficiency, with different specific nutritional deficiencies having variable effects on the immune system. For example, protein-calorie malnutrition and pyridoxine, folate, and vitamin A deficiencies can lead to insufficiency of the cell-mediated immune response.[27] In addition, protein-calorie malnutrition and zinc deficiency can result in thinning of skin or epidermolysis. The generalized malnutrition of kwashiorkor can also cause impaired chemotactic response and microbicidal activity of neutrophils[68] and low levels of IgA.[27]

It is crucial to note that malnutrition is often not a primary diagnosis in these patients, and that it often accompanies other chronic illnesses and conditions, such as diabetes mellitus, chronic renal failure, depression, alcoholism, chronic gastrointestinal conditions, and chemotherapy.

Aging

Increased susceptibility to infection in older patients is the result of a combination of age-related effects on skin and mucous membranes, accumulation of illness, and immunosenescence. Although routine aging is thought to contribute heavily to skin changes seen in older people, accumulation of actinic damage from ultraviolet light seems to account for the majority of these alterations.[69] Regarding its function as a barrier, skin changes in aging include thinning of dermis, loss of elasticity, and decreased water content. The number and size of sweat glands also diminish,[70] and sebum production from sebaceous glands decreases at a rate of 23% per decade in men and 32% per decade in women starting in adolescence.[71] This decrease in physiochemical defense also has a significant role in increased susceptibility to infection in the aging population, as lipid-rich sebum prevents water loss and inhibits growth of certain fungi and bacteria.[69] Finally, aged skin shows a reduced quantity of dermal blood vessels. The significance of this finding is that older skin has diminished nutrient exchange, impaired thermoregulation, lower skin surface temperature, and decreased pericyte synthetic activity.[69]

Not only is there a baseline change in skin structure and function, but wound healing is also affected. In the short term, dehiscence of surgical wounds is notably higher with increasing age.[72] This finding, however, is short-lived. Two weeks after wounding, age does not seem to adversely affect collagen synthesis.[73] Interestingly, the visual quality of scarring on microscopic evaluation has even been shown to be superior in older subjects.[74]

Organ Transplant Recipients

Since the first successful solid organ transplant in 1954, there have been many improvements in surgical technique and maintenance therapy. With these improvements, it is increasingly likely that providers outside transplant centers will encounter transplant recipients. Before transplant, patients suffer from immune suppression related to their pretransplant disease. With transplantation, the premorbid condition may improve; however, immunosuppression related to the medications used in preventing graft rejection can lead to significant immunocompromise. Medications used in prevention of graft rejection fall into four categories: corticosteroids, antibodies, antimetabolites, and calcineurin inhibitors. The effects of corticosteroids on the immune system are broad and described elsewhere in this chapter. Antibodies used in rejection prevention are monoclonal or polyclonal antibodies that bind to B and T cell receptors. The target cells are then eliminated from the circulation via opsonization, lysis, or apoptosis.[75] Antimetabolites act by interfering with different phases of cellular reproduction. Finally, calcineurin inhibitors block calcineurin phosphatase activity, which is responsible for cytokine expression.[76]

Generally, only the universal guidelines for surgical antibiotic prophylaxis should be in effect for transplant recipients.[76,77] Moreover, there is no indication for expanding coverage to include specific atypical or opportunistic organisms.[77] Transplant recipients are usually administered long-term antibiotic prophylaxis (for *Pneumocystis jiroveci*, candida, cytomegalovirus), and this should be continued through the perioperative period.[76] After 6 months, graft recipients receiving maintenance doses of immunosuppressive therapy and with good graft function are at risk of the same infections as the general population and rarely contract an opportunistic infection.[78] In this regard, elective head and neck surgery should be delayed until maintenance therapy has been instituted and acceptable graft function has been achieved.[77]

Collagen Vascular Disease

Collagen vascular diseases as a group have the potential to significantly impede normal immune function, which is often compounded by therapies used in its treatment. Systemic lupus erythematosus (SLE), scleroderma, rheumatoid arthritis (RA), and polymyositis are some of the more well-known and well-studied forms of collagen vascular disease. As a mark of their influence on the immune response, infections are a main cause of morbidity and mortality in patients with SLE.[79,80]

SLE greatly influences both humoral and cellular aspects of the immune response. In SLE, there is commonly a reduced number of complement proteins and receptors[81,82] and a reduced number of immunoglobulins.[83] Neutrophils show abnormalities in chemotaxis, phagocytosis, cytokine production, and oxidative metabolism.[81,82] Monocytes also have defective phagocytosis and oxidative metabolism because of autoantibodies against Fc gamma receptors and decreased tumor necrosis factor-α.[82,84] To inhibit the immune response further, both SLE and the corticosteroids used in treatment of SLE reduce the number and activity of T helper (T_h) cells, predisposing patients with SLE to infection by intracellular pathogens.[85] At present, there is conflicting evidence regarding how to objectively account for the degree of increased risk of infection in patients with SLE, but some suggest that the SLE disease activity index is a predictive factor for hospitalization.[86]

In contradistinction to SLE, scleroderma and polymyositis lead to increased risk of infection by their local influence on specific tissues. In cases of significant esophageal involvement, there is an increased incidence of aspiration pneumonia.[87] Similarly, in patients with significant Raynaud phenomenon, there is an increased risk of superinfection when there is digital ischemia and ulceration.[88]

Finally, pharmacotherapeutic immunosuppression seems to play the most important role in the immunodeficiency found in patients with RA. In a large series, it was found that variables most closely associated with infection included cumulative methotrexate dose and duration of steroid therapy. Patients with collagen vascular disease present a unique problem when considering prophylactic antibiotics for certain routine procedures. SLE and, to a different extent, RA are not only associated with increased risk of infection because of immunosuppression; they can lead to other conditions that predispose patients to developing specific infections. With SLE, there is a significantly increased risk of developing cardiac valvular disease, and in RA, total joint replacement may be one aspect of therapy. Recently, in a joint statement the American Dental Association and American Academy of Orthopedic Surgeons proclaimed that routine antibiotic prophylaxis is no longer indicated for total prosthetic joints.[89] In this statement, there was reference to an increased odds ratio for prosthetic joint infection in patients with some forms of immunocompromise, including those receiving immunosuppressive therapy or with RA. However, it was questioned whether this odds ratio was clinically significant.[89] To date, there is still no conclusive evidence that supports the use of antibiotic prophylaxis in SLE; however, given the increased risk of infection in patients with SLE, many sources, including the Lupus Foundation of America, continue to recommend antibiotic prophylaxis before dental treatment and surgical procedures.[90] In the setting of the speculation regarding antibiotic prophylaxis for prosthetic joints in immunosuppressed individuals with SLE and RA, a conclusion should be decided on a case-by-case basis in conjunction with the patient's other providers.

Corticosteroid Use

Corticosteroids are synthetic analogues to endogenous hormones produced in the adrenal cortex. Despite some of their well-known systemic side effects (e.g., atrophy, poor wound healing),[91] they are often used for management of specific pulmonary and rheumatologic diseases and for induction and maintenance of immunosuppression in transplant patients. Corticosteroids have numerous actions on the immune system, although their primary avenue for influence appears to be that of inhibition of the production of specific T cell cytokines that promote T_h1 differentiation and promote cellular immunity[92,93] and suppression of antibody and complement binding.[75] Even a single steroid dose can cause significant lymphocytopenia and monocytopenia because of the redistribution of cells out of the circulation.[94] At high doses, steroids can impair neutrophil adherence to endothelium[95] and inhibit reactive oxygen species elaboration in phagocytes, thus permitting continued growth of microorganisms intracellularly.[94]

The risk of infectious complications from steroid use is related to dose and duration of treatment. In a large meta-analysis including 71 trials, it was found that the rate of infection was 12.7% in patients undergoing steroid treatment compared with 8.0% in the control group.[96] Furthermore, the rate of infectious complication was not increased in patients who received a cumulative dose less than 700 mg of prednisone equivalent, or less than 10 mg of prednisone per day.[96] Total time of exposure to steroid therapy also has been correlated with incidence of infection, with a cumulative duration of less than 21 days leading to a decreased risk.[94] At this time there is no definitive role for prophylactic antibiotic administration in patients being treated with long-term, low-dose corticosteroids; however, strong consideration should be given to the use of prophylactic antibiotics in the setting of high-dose steroids or when a large microbial inoculum is anticipated.[48] For transplant recipients receiving corticosteroids, there are specific guidelines found elsewhere for antibiotic prophylaxis targeting specific opportunistic pathogens.

HIV and AIDS

HIV is characterized by infection and destruction of CD4 T cells. Untreated HIV can lead to opportunistic infections or malignancy. Two major variants of the virus exist, with HIV-1 being the more virulent and more ubiquitous.[27] In 2012, there was an estimated 35.3 million people living with HIV,[97] owing to the increased efficacy and availability of antiretroviral therapy. In the United States, more than 50,000 new infections occur annually. Among those living with HIV, approximately 18% are unaware of it.[92] At diagnosis, approximately one third of patients have CD4 counts less than 200/mm³.[98]

The immunologic defects in HIV/AIDS are numerous. As mentioned previously, at the root of the profound immune compromise in AIDS is CD4 T cell depletion. This depletion is due to direct cytotoxicity during the viral replicative cycle, anergy, superantigen stimulation of T cell subpopulations, induction of apoptosis via gene cross-linking, and cellular immunity-related cytotoxicity.[27]

Classically, most opportunistic infections in HIV occur when CD4 cell counts are less than 200/mm³. Recent studies, however, show that some of these opportunistic infections (i.e., esophageal candidiasis, Kaposi's sarcoma, pulmonary tuberculosis [TB]) have been found in patients with CD4 counts greater than 200/mm³.[99] Some premorbid conditions that increase the risk of AIDS-defining illness in patients with CD4 counts greater than 500/mm³ include intravenous drug use, advanced age, and HIV viral loads greater than 10,000 copies/mL.[99] At CD4 cell counts greater than 750/mm³, incidence of opportunistic infections appear to decline, leading one to think that immune recovery approaches completion at this level.[99]

Of particular note, a common presenting sign or symptom of infection in an HIV-positive patient is an enlarged lymph node. Enlarged cervical lymph nodes in HIV-positive individuals should be investigated because they may represent infection with *Mycobacterium tuberculosis* or *Pneumocystis jiroveci*, lymphoma, Kaposi's sarcoma, or other processes.[100] Of the HIV-positive patients with cervical lymphadenopathy, approximately 40% will have benign reactive lymphadenopathy,[100] and 20 to 30% may be associated with TB.[100] The first method of surgical diagnosis should be a fine-needle aspiration, which is successful at obtaining a definitive diagnosis in more than 50% of instances.[100] Circumstances in which there should be higher suspicion for a cause other than benign reactive lymphadenopathy include a node larger than 2 cm and growing; onset associated with an episode of low CD4 count; asymmetric, unilateral, or localized lymphadenopathy; unexplained constitutional symptoms; associated mediastinal lymphadenopathy; or hepatosplenomegaly.[100]

Another presentation of increased incidence and related to the head and neck is that of rhinosinusitis. The maxillary and ethmoid sinuses are the most frequently involved,[100] and patients may complain of fever, facial pain, nasal congestion, and mucopurulent nasal drainage. The increased susceptibility to sinusitis is thought to be due to local and systemic immune compromise and impaired mucociliary clearance times. As with sinusitis in the general population, the most common causative agents in sinusitis in patients with HIV are *S. pneumoniae, H. influenzae,* and *Moraxella catarrhalis* in acute sinusitis and *Staphylococcus* species, *Pseudomonas* species, and anaerobes in chronic sinusitis. However, under circumstances in which the CD4 count is less than 50 cells/μL, the absolute neutrophil count is less than 600 cells/μL, or there are unilateral symptoms with or without fever, one should consider invasive fungal sinusitis as the cause.[100]

Neoplastic Conditions Associated With Acquired Immunodeficiency

With malignancy, and to a lesser extent with benign neoplasm, there may be immune system compromise from breakdown of cutaneous or mucosal barriers, immunosuppression because of a chemotherapeutic regimen, or as a consequence of the disease process itself. Secondary immunodeficiency often accompanies hematologic malignancies such as chronic lymphocytic leukemia and multiple myeloma. In these situations, immune compromise is a consequence of both bone marrow overcrowding and impaired clearance function of the neoplastic cells. For solid cancers, malignancy itself can play a role in infection susceptibility, although the most profound immunosuppression is often seen with cancer treatments. Nonliquid cancers can compromise immunity by invading the bone marrow, disrupting mucosal barriers, and reducing tissue perfusion through thrombosis or mass effect. Malignant cells themselves are sometimes recognized as antigenic and can prompt a host inflammatory response in an attempt to clear them. Although this response is typically insufficient for cure, it is the basis of ongoing investigation into immunotherapy treatments. Both cancer effects and treatment sequelae of chemotherapy and radiotherapy can lead to episodes of profound neutropenia. As mentioned earlier, the incidence of infection drastically increases as the neutrophil count falls to less than 1000/mm^3, with significant risk of bacteremia at less than 100/mm^3.[13] One intervention to combat the degree and duration of neutropenia when possible is the use of G-CSF and GM-CSF, which has been found to be cost effective in cases of neutropenia with fever or documented infection.[101] These growth factors are often used in cytotoxic chemotherapy-induced neutropenia.

Prevention and Management of Infection in the Immunocompromised Host

Immunity works to defend against infection; however, it also plays a crucial role in wound healing. Macrophages are important in locally promoting angiogenesis and fibroblast proliferation. Patients who are cytopenic or who have any compromise in vascularity such as after radiation will effectively experience delayed ability or inability to heal. Open or persistent surgical wounds can further predispose to postoperative infection which the immunodeficient host is ill-equipped to battle. The primary steps in prevention of the immunocompromised host are similar to those used in preventing infection in the immunocompetent host. Meticulous surgical technique, careful tissue manipulation, debridement of nonviable tissue, and elimination of dead space are of prime importance in preventing infections at surgical sites. In addition, although there is a lack of definitive evidence for antibiotic prophylaxis for specific immunodeficient conditions, multidisciplinary consultation and the patient's history of illness may be useful in the decision-making process.

Every effort should be made to correct or medically optimize patients before elective surgery. Despite the heterogony of conditions, there are often a few universal steps that can be taken to optimize immunodeficient patients for elective procedures. Scheduling procedures around chemotherapy cycles may be prudent if the degree of immunosuppression is expected to be severe. Bloodwork is regularly obtained in patients being treated with adjuvant cytotoxic therapy and should be reviewed by the surgeon. In addition, other objective metrics such as the HIV-positive patients' absolute neutrophil count and the diabetic patients' glycosylated hemoglobin levels will help in making an educated assessment of risk for infectious complication. If delaying the procedure will not necessarily result in improved immunity it is important to counsel patients on their risk for infection based on their level of immune compromise. Some surgeons recommend obtaining primary closure over dental extraction sites to reduce the bacterial exposure during the healing process. This practice has not been proven to reduce the risk of postoperative complication in the radiated or immunocompromised host.

Conversely, there are steps that can be taken to optimize patients from a head and neck surgery perspective before a planned immunosuppressive therapy regimen. For example, oral mucositis is a well-documented adverse effect of some chemotherapeutic regimens; therefore, steps to optimize oral health should be considered before any induction chemotherapy.[96] Similarly, extraction of hopeless or chronically infected teeth is routinely performed as a clearance before cancer or transplant surgery to avoid subsequent odontogenic infection.

In the setting of overt infection in an immunocompromised individual, culture and sensitivity testing should be considered. Until results are returned, interval broad-spectrum coverage to include pathogens to which the individual is most susceptible should be initiated. Attention should also be given to the setting of treatment, with consideration for inpatient monitoring based on both the severity of infection and the degree of immune compromise.

References

1. Bonilla FA, Bernstein IL, Khan DA, et al. Practice parameter for the diagnosis and management of primary immunodeficiency. *Ann Allergy Asthma Immunol.* 2005;94(5 suppl 1):S1-S63.

2. Boyle JM, Buckley RH. Population prevalence of diagnosed primary immunodeficiency diseases in the United States. *J Clin Immunol.* 2007;27:497-502.

3. Modell V, Gee B, Lewis DB, et al. Global study of primary immunodeficiency diseases (PI)-diagnosis, treatment, and economic impact: an updated report from the Jeffrey Modell Foundation. *Immunol Res.* 2011;51:61-70.

4. Fried AJ, Bonilla FA. Pathogenesis, diagnosis, and management of primary antibody deficiencies and infections. *Clin Microbiol Rev.* 2009;22:396-414.

5. Notarangelo LD. Primary immunodeficiencies. *J Allergy Clin Immunol.* 2010;125(suppl 2):S182-S194.

6. Ram S, Lewis LA, Rice PA. Infections of people with complement deficiencies and patients who have undergone splenectomy. *Clin Microbiol Rev.* 2010;23:740-780.

7. Younger EM, Epland K, Zampelli A, et al. Primary immunodeficiency diseases: a primer for PCPs. *Nurse Pract.* 2015;40:1-7.

8. Bodey GP, Buckley M, Sathe YS, et al. Qualitative relationships between circulating leukocytes and infections in patients with acute leukemia. *Ann Intern Med.* 1966;64:328-339.

9. Lucas KG, Brown AE, Armstrong D. The identification of febrile, neutropenic children with neoplastic disease at low risk for bacteremia and complications of sepsis. *Cancer.* 1996;77:791-798.

10. Chanock SJ, Pizzo PA. Fever in the neutropenic host. *Infect Dis Clin North Am.* 1996;10:777-796.

11. Rubin M, Hathorn JW, Pizzo PA. Controversies in the management of febrile neutropenic cancer patients. *Cancer Invest.* 1988;6:167-184.

12. Pizzo PA. Evaluation of fever in the patient with cancer. *Eur J Cancer Clin Oncol.* 1989;25(suppl 2):S9.

13. Grafter-Gvili A, Fraser A, Paul M, et al. Antibiotic prophylaxis for bacterial infections in afebrile neutropenic patients following chemotherapy. *Cochrane Database Syst Rev.* 2012;(1):CD004386.

14. Sleasman JW, Virella G. Primary immunodeficiency diseases. In: Virella G, ed. *Medical Immunology.* 6th ed. New York: Informa Healthcare; 2007.

15. Ochs HD, Smith CIE, Puck JM. *Primary Immunodeficiency Diseases.* London: Oxford University Press; 2014.

16. Waldman TA, Nelson DA. Inherited immunodeficiencies. In: Frank MM, Austen KF, Claman HN, Unanue ER, eds. *Samter's Immunologic Diseases.* Vol. 1. Toronto: Little, Brown and Co.; 2001.

17. Strober W, Wochner RD, Carbone PP, et al. Intestinal lymphangiectasia. *J Clin Invest.* 1967;46:1643.

18. Elson CO, James SP, Graeff AS, et al. Hypogammaglobulinemia due to abnormal suppressor T-cell activity in Crohn's disease. *Gastroenterology.* 1984;86:569.

19. Shirani KZ, Vaughan GM, McManus AT, et al. Replacement therapy with modified immunoglobulin G in burn patients: preliminary kinetic studies. *Am J Med.* 1984;76:175.

20. Cooperative Group for the Study of Immunoglobulin in Chronic Lymphocytic Leukemia. Intravenous immunoglobulin for the prevention of infection in chronic lymphocytic leukemia. *N Engl J Med.* 1988;319:902.

21. Walchner M, Wick M. Elevation of CD8+ CD11b+ Leu–8– T cells is associated with the humoral immune deficiency in myeloma patients. *Clin Exp Immunol.* 1997;109:310.

22. Farber DL, Virella G. Cell-mediated immunity. In: Virella G, ed. *Medical Immunology.* 6th ed. New York: Informa Healthcare; 2013.

23. Abbas AK, Lichtman AH. Effector mechanisms of cell-mediated immunity. In: Abbas AK, Lichtman AH, eds. *Basic Immunology: Functions and Disorders of the Immune System.* 2nd ed. Philadelphia: Saunders; 2009.

24. Fischer A. T-lymphocyte immunodeficiencies. *Immunol Allergy Clin North Am.* 2000;20:113-127.

25. Vartivarian S, Bodey G. Infection associated with malignancy. In: Gorbach SL, Bartlett JG, Blacklow NR, eds. *Infectious Diseases.* 2nd ed. Philadelphia: WB Saunders; 2003.

26. Sumaraju V, Smith LG, Smith SM. Infectious complications in asplenic hosts. *Infect Dis Clin North Am.* 2001;15:551-565.

27. Sleasman JW, Virella G. AIDS and other acquired immunodeficiency diseases. In: Virella G, ed. *Medical Immunology.* 6th ed. New York: Informa Healthcare; 2013.

28. Sickle Cell Association of America. *Research and Screening.* Available at: https://www.sicklecelldisease.org/2021/10/22/scdaa-news-advisory-salmonella-and-sickle-cell-disease/. Accessed February 12, 2015.

29. Mirza I, Wolk J, Toth L, et al. Waterhouse-Friederichsen syndrome secondary to *Capnocytophaga canimorsus* septicemia and demonstration of bacteremia by peripheral blood smear. *Arch Pathol Lab Med.* 2000;124:859-863.

30. Westwell AJ, Spenser MB, Kerr KG. DF-2 bacteria following cat bites. *Am J Med.* 1987;83:1170.

31. Brigden ML. Detection, education and management of the asplenic or hyposplenic patient. *Am Fam Physician.* 2001;63:499-506.

32. Howell JM, Woodward GR. Precipitous hypotension in the emergency department caused by *Capnocytophaga canimorsus* sp nov sepsis. *Am J Emerg Med.* 1990;8:312-314.

33. Rubin LG, Schaffner W. Care of the asplenic patient. *N Engl J Med.* 2014;371:349-356.

34. Stanley AC, Christian JM. Sickle cell disease and perioperative considerations: review and retrospective report. *J Oral Maxillofac Surg.* 2013;71:1027-1033.

35. Harrison GA, Schultz TZ, Schaberg SJ. Deep neck infection complicated by diabetes mellitus. *Oral Surg Oral Med Oral Pathol.* 1983;55:133-137.

36. Sugata T, Fujita Y, Myoken Y, et al. Cervical cellulitis with mediastinitis from an odontogenic infection complicated by diabetes mellitus: report of a case. *J Oral Maxillofac Surg.* 1997;55:864-869.

37. McMahon MM, Bistrain BR. Host defenses and susceptibility to infection in patients with diabetes mellitus. *Infect Dis Clin North Am.* 1995;9:1-9.

38. Mattson J, Cerutis D. Diabetes mellitus: a review of the literature and dental implications. *Compendium.* 2001;22:757-772.

39. Naghibi M, Smith R, Baltch A, et al. The effect of diabetes mellitus on chemotactic and bactericidal activity of human polymorphonuclear leukocytes. *Diabetic Res Clin Pract.* 1987;4:27-35.

40. Bouche C, Serdy S, Kahn CR, et al. The cellular fate of glucose and its relevance in type 2 diabetes. *Endocr Rev.* 2004;25:807-830.

41. Campbell MJ. A light and electron microscope study of blood vessels from the gingival tissues of non-diabetic and diabetic patients. *Aust Dent J.* 1971;16:235-239.

42. Lalla E, Lamster IB, Schmidt AM. Enhanced interaction of advanced glycation end-products with their cellular receptor for RAGE: implications for the pathogenesis of accelerated periodontal disease in diabetes. *Ann Periodontol.* 1998;3(1):13-19.

43. Rapaport Y, Himelfarb MZ, Zikk D, et al. Cervical necrotizing fasciitis of odontogenic origin. *Oral Surg Oral Med Oral Pathol.* 1991;72:15-18.

44. Alexiewicz J, Kumnar D, Smogorzewski M, et al. Polymorphonuclear leukocytes in non-insulin dependent diabetes mellitus: abnormalities in metabolism and function. *Ann Intern Med.* 1995;123:919-924.

45. Saiepour D, Sehlin J, Oldenborg PA. Hyperglycemia-induced protein kinase C activation inhibits phagocytosis of C3b- and immunoglobulin g-opsonized yeast particles in normal human neutrophils. *Exp Diabesity Res.* 2003;4:125-132.

46. Zerr K, Furnary A, Grunkmeier G, et al. Glucose control lowers the risk of wound infection in diabetics after open heart operations. *Ann Thorac Surg.* 1997;63:356.

47. Rassias A, Marrin C, Arruda J, et al. Insulin infusion improves neutrophil function in diabetic cardiac surgery patients. *Anesth Analg.* 1998;88:1101.

48. Gupta S, Koirala J, Khardori R, et al. Infections in diabetes mellitus and hyperglycemia. *Infect Dis Clin North Am.* 2007;21: 617-638.

49. Tierney MR, Baker AS. Infection of head and neck in diabetes mellitus. *Infect Dis Clin North Am.* 1995;9:195.

50. Kajs-Wyllie M. Hyperbaric oxygen therapy for rhinocerebral fungal infection. *J Neurosci Nurs.* 1995;273:174-181.

51. Rubin Grandis J. The changing face of malignant necrotizing external otitis: clinical, radiological, and anatomic correlations. *Lancet Infect Dis.* 2004;41:34-39.

52. Rubin J, Yu VL. Malignant external otitis: insights into pathogenesis, clinical manifestations, diagnosis, and therapy. *Am J Med.* 1988;85:391-398.

53. Joshi N, Caputo GM, Weitekamp MR, et al. Primary care: infections in patients with diabetes. *N Engl J Med.* 1999;341: 1906-1912.

54. Handzel O, Halperin D. Necrotizing malignant external otitis. *Am Fam Physician.* 2003;682:309-312.

55. Macgregor RR. Alcohol and immune defense. *JAMA.* 1986; 256:1474.

56. Roselle GA, Medenhal CL, Chedid A, et al. Alcohol modulation of immune function: clinical and experimental data. *Alcohol Clin Exp Res.* 1995;19:551-554.

57. Gordon NC, Connelly S. Management of head and neck infections in the immunocompromised patient. *Oral Maxillofac Surg Clin North Am.* 2003;15:103-110.

58. Pesanti EL. Immunologic defects and vaccination in patients with chronic renal failure. *Infect Dis Clin North Am.* 2001; 15(3):813-832.

59. Schreiner GE, Maher JF, eds. *Uremia: Biochemistry, Pathogenesis, and Treatment.* Springfield, IL: Charles C Thomas; 1961.

60. Dammin GJ, Couch NP, Murray JE. Prolonged survival of skin homografts in uremic patients. *Ann N Y Acad Sci.* 1957;64: 967-976.

61. Rytel MW, Dailey MP, Schiffman G, et al. Pneumococcal vaccine immunization of patients with renal impairment. *Proc Soc Exp Biol Med.* 1986;182:468-473.

62. Nohr C. Non-AIDS immunosuppression. In: Wilmore DW, Cheung LY, Harken AH, et al., eds. *Scientific American Surgery, section VII, subsection 3.* New York: Web MD; 1998.

63. Van Der Meer JWN. Defects in host defense mechanisms. In: Rubin RH, Young LS, eds. *Clinical Approach to Infection in the Immunocompromised Host.* 3rd ed. New York: Plenum; 1988.

64. Brown SM, Stimmel B, Taub RN, et al. Immunologic dysfunction in heroin addicts. *Arch Intern Med.* 1974;134:1001.

65. Chandrasekar PH, Narula AP. Bone and joint infection in intravenous drug abusers. *Rev Infect Dis.* 1986;8:904.

66. Saravolatz LD, Burch KH, Quinn EL, et al. Polymicrobial infective endocarditis: an increasing clinical entity. *Am Heart J.* 1978;95:163.

67. Douglas SD, Schopfer K. Analytical review: host defense mechanisms in protein-energy malnutrition. *Clin Immunol Immunopathol.* 1976;5:1-5.

68. Thomas DR, Burkemper N. Preface: aging skin and wound healing. *Clin Geriatr Med.* 2013;29:xi-xx.

69. Fenske NA, Lober CW. Structural and functional changes of normal aging skin. *J Am Acad Dermatol.* 1986;15:571-585.

70. Plewig G, Koigman AM. Proliferative activity of the sebaceous glands of the aged. *J Invest Dermatol.* 1978;70:314.

71. Mendoza Jr CB, Postlethwait RW, Johnson WD. Incidence of wound disruption following operation. *Arch Surg.* 1970;101: 396-398.

72. Kurban R, Bhawan J. Histological changes in skin associated with aging. *J Dermatol Surg Oncol.* 1990;16:908-914.

73. Horan MA, Ashcroft GS. Ageing, defense mechanisms and the immune system. *Age Aging.* 1997;26:15S-19S.

74. Mukherjee S, Mukherjee U. A comprehensive review of immunosuppression used for liver transplantation. *J Transplant.* 2009; 2009:701464.

75. Littlewood K. The immunocompromised adult patient and surgery. *Best Pract Res Clin Anaesthesiol.* 2008;22(3):585-609.

76. Whiting J. Perioperative concerns for transplant recipients undergoing non-transplant surgery. *Surg Clin North Am.* 2006;86:1185-1194.

77. Rubin RH. Infection in organ transplant recipients. In: Rubin RH, Young LS, eds. *Clinical Approach to Infection in the Compromised Host.* 3rd ed. New York: Plenum; 1981.

78. Cervera R, Khamashta MA, Font J, et al. Morbidity and mortality in systemic lupus erythematosus during a 5-year period: A multicenter prospective study of 1,000 patients. European Working Party on Systemic Lupus Erythematosus. *Medicine.* 1999;78:167-175.

79. Gladman DD, Hussian F, Ibanez D, et al. The nature and outcome of infection in systemic lupus erythematosus. *Lupus.* 2002; 11:234-239.

80. Bouza E, Moya JG, Munoz P. Infections in systemic lupus erythematosus and rheumatoid arthritis. *Infect Dis Clin North Am.* 2001;15:335-361.

81. Petri M. Infection in systemic lupus erythematosus. *Rheum Dis Clin North Am.* 1998;24:423-456.

82. Cronin M, Balow J, Tsokos G. Immunoglobulin deficiency in patients with systemic lupus erythematosus. *Clin Exp Rheum.* 1988;7:359.

83. Boros P, Muryoi T, Spiera H, et al. Autoantibodies directed against different classes of Fc gamma R are found in sera of autoimmune patients. *J Immunol.* 1993;150:2018-2024.

84. Hellmann DB, Petri M, Whiting-O'Keefe Q. Fatal infections in systemic lupus erythematosus: the role of opportunistic organisms. *Medicine.* 1987;66:341-348.

85. Petri M, Genovese M. Incidence and risk factors for hospitalizations in systemic lupus erythematosus: a prospective study of the Hopkins lupus cohort. *J Rheumatol.* 1992;19:1559-1565.

86. Marie I, Hachulla E, Hatron PY, et al. Polymyositis and dermatomyositis: short term and long term outcome, and predictive factors of prognosis. *J Rheumatol.* 2001;28:2230-2237.

87. Mitchell H, Bolster MB, Leroy EC. Scleroderma and related conditions. *Med Clin North Am.* 1997;81:129-149.

88. Sollecito T, Abt E, Lockhart P, et al. The use of prophylactic antibiotics prior to dental procedures in patients with prosthetic joints. *J Am Dent Assoc.* 2014;146(1):11-18.

89. Lockhart P, Loven B, Brennan M, et al. The evidence base for the efficacy of antibiotic prophylaxis in dental practice. *J Am Dent Assoc.* 2007;138:458-474.

90. Newell-Price J, Bertagna X, Grossman AB, et al. Cushing's syndrome. *Lancet.* 2006;367:1605-1617.

91. Hannaman MJ, Ertl M. Patients with immunodeficiency. *Med Clin North Am.* 2013;97:1139-1159.

92. Kovalovsky D, Refojo D, Holsboer F, et al. Molecular mechanisms and Th1/Th2 pathways in corticosteroid regulation of cytokine production. *J Neuroimmunol.* 2000;109:23-29.

93. Klein NC, Go CH, Cunha BA. Infections associated with steroid use. *Infect Dis Clin North Am.* 2001;15(2):423-432.

94. Goulding NG, Euzger HS, Butt SK, et al. Novel pathways for glucocorticoid effects on neutrophils in chronic inflammation. *Inflamm Res.* 1998;3:S158-S165.

95. Stuck AE, Minder CE, Frey FJ. Risk of infectious complications in patients taking glucocorticoids. *Rev Infect Dis.* 1989;11:954.

96. McKenna SJ. Immunocompromised host and infection. In: Topazian R, Goldberg M, Hupp J, eds. *Oral and Maxillofacial Infections.* 4th ed. Philadelphia: Saunders; 1994.

97. Abrosioni J, Calmy A, Hirschel B. HIV treatment for prevention. *J Int AIDS Soc.* 2011;14:28.

98. Zanoni B, Gandhi R. Update on opportunistic infections in the era of effective antiretroviral therapy. *Infect Dis Clin North Am.* 2014;28:501-518.

99. Mocroft A, Furrer HJ, Miro JM, et al. The incidence of AIDS-defining illnesses at a current CD4 count >/= 200 cells/mL in the post-combination retroviral therapy era. *Clin Infect Dis.* 2013;57:1038-1047.

100. Kim TB, Pletcher SD, Goldberg AN. Head and neck manifestations in the immunocompromised host. In: Flint PW, Haughey BH, Lund VJ, et al., eds. *Cummings Otolaryngology Head and Neck Surgery.* 5th ed. Philadelphia: Mosby; 2010.

101. Greenberg PL, Cosler LE, Ferro SA, Lyman GH. The costs of drugs used to treat myelodysplastic syndromes following National Comprehensive Cancer Network Guidelines. *J Natl Compr Canc Netw.* 2006;6(9):942-953.

26

Infection in the Craniomaxillofacial Trauma Patient

LANCE DAVIS THOMPSON, BABER N. KHATIB, AND R. BRYAN BELL

The oral cavity, in the setting of trauma, is unique among other anatomic areas prone to injury. Arguably no other structure in the body has a higher incidence of open fracture than the mandible. To add to this risk, consider that one must introduce calories into the same cavity that directly communicates with the fractured bones. This wound healing environment or surgical site would be unimaginable for an open tibial fracture. It goes without saying that the perfusion and healing ability of the oral, head, and neck structures make treating these injuries much more forgiving. The tenuous and exposed nature of these injuries likely explains our overtreatment with antibiotics when looking at the literature.

There have been considerable historical changes in the management of traumatic injuries that have contributed to lower rates of infection and improved outcomes. Guidelines for frontal sinus trauma, for example, previously involved exenteration of the sinus,[1] but have now shifted to the preservation of the sinus mucosa in uncomplicated cases.[2] As more data become available, time-limited laceration repair has long passed the "6-hour golden period"[3] and the duration of antibiotic therapy after reduction and rigid fixation of maxillofacial fractures has declined significantly.[4] Improved protocols for antibiotic prophylaxis and debridement have also allowed for earlier and more comprehensive reconstruction of high-velocity injuries. Prompt diagnosis and management with antibiotics decreased the infectious complications of facial injuries in each successive conflict during times of war in the twentieth century.[5] Although some domains of infection in oral, head, and neck trauma patients are limited by a lack of randomized, controlled outcome data, many of the new trends described are bolstered by pooled data from large multicenter trials.

Principles

Classification of Maxillofacial Trauma Wounds

Surgical wounds are classified by level of contamination as established by the Centers for Disease Control and Prevention.[6]

Common wounds encountered in maxillofacial trauma involve a spectrum of bacterial invasion that can be classified as clean-contaminated (class II), contaminated (class III), or infected (class IV). An example of a clean-contaminated wound is that which occurs during the repair of closed fractures. Noninfected open fractures and soft tissue wounds are considered contaminated at the time of repair. Infected traumatic wounds occur because of bacterial infection or environmental debris being present at the time of repair.[7] An algorithm for wound debridement, irrigation, and antibiotic prophylaxis exists and depends on accurate classification at the time of surgical intervention. The majority of maxillofacial trauma management is categorized as clean-contaminated.[8]

Epidemiology of Infections in Maxillofacial Trauma

The collateral blood supply to the face is extensive and allows for treatment of contaminated fractures without infection after routine open reduction and internal fixation. Composite soft and hard tissue injury, however, with loss of periosteal blood supply may predispose fractures to healing complications because of contracture, infection, or fibrosis.[9] It is no surprise that the oropharyngeal flora is a frequent contaminant of traumatic wounds in the head and neck. Head and facial trauma account for 36 and 24% of presenting injuries, respectively, according to the National Trauma Data Bank. Facial fractures can be subdivided by prevalence, with midfacial trauma being most common (72%), followed by the mandible (24%) and frontobasal and supraorbital bone fractures.[10] Because these injuries commonly require operative management, reducing the burden of postoperative infection is an important goal in improving outcomes.

Bacterial Flora

Postoperative wound infections of the head and neck are usually polymicrobial and have been examined in multiple studies to show gram-positive (*Staphylococcus* and

Streptococcus) and gram-negative (*Escherichia, Klebsiella, Serratia, Proteus,* and *Pseudomonas*) organisms, aerobic and anaerobic bacteria, and fungi.[7] Saliva harbors numerous bacterial species, with anaerobes approximately 5 times more common than aerobes. Nevertheless, intraoral lacerations do not commonly become infected. Wounds of the head and neck that become infected are often contaminated with biofilms, which are typically resistant to antimicrobial therapy alone. Commonly, mechanical disruption by drainage or debridement is required for successful treatment, in addition to therapeutic doses of antimicrobials; this is especially true of osteomyelitis.[11] Wound management and prophylaxis should be directed toward the mechanism of injury, because the environmental pathogens can also become embedded within wounds. A frequent example is road burn injuries, which may be contaminated with *Bacillus* species.[12] Contamination with *Clostridium tetani* has high mortality in unimmunized patients, and prophylaxis should be established in traumatized patients. Indications for prophylaxis with tetanus immunoglobulin are described later.

Risk Factors

A number of risk factors may predispose trauma patients to infection, including presence and types of fractures, delay in treatment, and treatment method.[8] Delay in treatment has been the focus of many studies with respect to antibiotic prophylaxis. Patients with multiple traumatic fractures and open facial fractures have been found more likely to develop an infection and may warrant additional antibiotic prophylaxis.[13]

Timing of Repair

There is considerable historical controversy over the so-called *golden period* for laceration repair, with time periods ranging from 3 to 24 hours to avoid infectious complications.[3] Current evidence suggests that there is no supporting evidence for the effects of delayed wound closure on infection rates after laceration repair.[3] Lacerations in the head and neck may in fact afford greater flexibility in delayed closure when compared with extremity wounds.[14,15] Earlier repair may also facilitate a more acceptable cosmetic outcome in facial wounds. The repair of maxillofacial fractures is often delayed several days after the injury, whether by availability of resources or comorbid conditions. Fracture mobility is thought to contribute to a correlation between treatment delay and surgical wound infection.[8] However, the evidence for the association between treatment delay and increased or decreased risk of infection is equivocal.[16] Despite the paucity of prospective, controlled, randomized data with appropriate statistical analysis, there have been numerous guidelines proposed to quantify the effects of treatment delay.[12] A recent literature review has identified the commonly reported complications from delayed treatment to include infection, including abscess and osteomyelitis, wound dehiscence, delayed or nonunion, and need for revision surgery, among others.[16] The benefits of

delayed treatment also have been identified, in allowing for a single anesthetic in the extensively injured patient,[17] more complex imaging,[17] and resolution of soft tissue edema in zygomatic complex fractures[18] and of diplopia in orbital fractures.[19] In general, it is advisable to minimize the time between injury and definitive repair of facial fractures and the time spent in the hospital to avoid nosocomial infection by colonization of hospital-acquired bacteria. The goal to timing of repair is to achieve open reduction and internal fixation within 1 to 3 days of injury for uncomplicated mandibular fracture and between 1 and 14 days for uncomplicated midfacial fractures. Highly comminuted or displaced fractures are generally stabilized with intermaxillary fixation (IMF) in the emergency department on initial assessment to avoid gross mobility of bony segments. High-velocity injuries, such as those that occur with gunshot wounds or other degloving injuries, are generally washed and repaired on the day of injury. Some trauma services have a "direct to OR" policy for the most severe or life-threatening injuries. Therefore, complex facial wounds that are characterized by massive contamination or tissue loss are often repaired within hours of occurrence.

Patient-Specific Implants

There has been a significant increase in the use of patient-specific implants in the orthognathic and oncologic realms in the recent past, and this has also bled into the craniomaxillofacial (CMF) trauma world as well. Using virtual surgical planning, surgeons can more readily recreate the symmetric facial heights, projections, volumes, and contours. The use of patient-specific hardware also has been stated to aid in reduction of the fractures, especially those with difficult access, such as mandibular subcondylar fractures and naso-orbito-ethmoidal fractures.[20]

Prevention

Systemic Wound Management

Optimizing systemic conditions in patients after injury is important for successful wound healing. This is especially critical in the multisystem trauma patient with a prolonged hospitalization and need for resuscitation. For example, mild hypothermia can lead to threefold higher infection rates and leads to increased intraoperative blood loss.[12] Nutritional goals for the trauma patient include maximizing tissue perfusion and oxygen delivery to the wound bed. Patients receiving parenteral nutrition are often at risk for impaired wound healing secondary to essential fatty acid deficiencies. Supplementation with lipids is important for trauma patients, especially those with preexisting poor nutritional status. Malnutrition is best evaluated with a complete history and physical examination and includes unintentional weight loss, cachectic appearance, or history of malabsorption.[7] In addition, fluid supplementation exceeding the amount normally given for optimization of blood pressure and urine output has been shown to increase oxygenation in surgical patients.[12]

Cross-Infection

An important consideration in the prevention of iatrogenic infections is avoidance of glove perforations associated with manipulation of bone, metal, deep cavities, and confined spaces.[21] In maxillofacial surgery, this has been traditionally noted with wire penetration and arch bar placement.[22] Methods of fracture reduction that reduce or obviate the need for IMF with wires, such as bone-anchoring screws or manual reduction, significantly reduce this risk.[23,24] Double-gloving will also reduce the incidence of bacterial or viral cross-contamination by reducing perforations of the inner glove,[25] but it has not been shown to reduce the dexterity of the operator.[21,26]

Debridement

Debridement of the traumatic wound involves the removal of nonviable tissue to reduce the incidence of wound infection or in management of an established infection.[27] This is especially important in the multiply wounded patient with both hard and soft tissue trauma or in the patient with necrotizing infection of the soft tissues. Early debridement is required in necrotizing fasciitis, because rapid infectious spread along avascular tissue planes causes fascial necrosis and loss of skin perforators.[28] Irrigation of the wound also decreases bacterial load, depending on the type and pressure of irrigation. Traditionally, antiseptics such as dilute povidone-iodine or hydrogen peroxide have been used for wound irrigation, but data have shown that these delay wound healing because of cytotoxic effects on fibroblasts and keratinocytes.[29] Instead, it is now recommended to irrigate with sterile normal saline for noninfected wounds[30,31] and to reserve irrigation with antiseptics (e.g., povidone-iodine) for localized treatment of infected or dehisced wounds.[32] High-pressure irrigation is indicated in cases of obvious contamination by environmental debris or with bite wounds.[12] Multiple retrospective and prospective studies have established that shaving is no longer recommended before the repair of scalp lacerations.[14,33] It is thought that microabrasions created during shaving actually increase the risk of infection and that shaving should be performed only for reasons other than prevention of postoperative wound infection.[34] Routinely shaving the scalp for either laceration repair or elective coronal incisions is not advised. The risk of infection in either of these settings is low. Retention of foreign bodies following penetrating trauma can delay healing, especially if of porous or organic composition. Unlike metallic implants, environmental foreign bodies can be difficult to localize with imaging, delaying diagnosis until prolonged inflammation and infection are realized.[35] Wound infection caused by contaminated, retained foreign bodies can be persistent despite antibiotics and can progress beyond superficial skin infections to involve adjacent tissue spaces. Suction-assisted pulse irrigation with sterile saline is the preferred method of mechanical debridement during initial debridement, followed by mechanical scrubbing with "brown and bubbly" dilute hydrogen peroxide and water for highly contaminated wounds.

Prophylaxis

Guidelines for surgical antibiotic prophylaxis have been established by extensive systematic reviews that break down injury patterns as soft tissue versus operative CMF fractures.[36] For soft tissue injuries, the recommendations are based on mechanism of injury and location. For bite injuries, animal or human, and through-and-through injuries, the recommendation is for a 5-day course of amoxicillin/clavulanate. For those with penicillin allergy, the recommendation is for the use of clindamycin or clindamycin–trimethoprim-sulfamethoxazole, respectively. For extraoral lacerations that are high risk, a 5-day course of cephalexin is recommended and those with soil contamination should receive amoxicillin-clavulanate. Again, those who are penicillin allergic can receive clindamycin. For those with intraoral lacerations the recommendation is for a 5-day course of amoxicillin and clindamycin for penicillin allergic patients.

For those with an operative CMF fracture, the following recommendations are put forth: Clean-contaminated injuries receive cefazolin or cefuroxime plus metronidazole or ampicillin-sulbactam.[37] Clindamycin is recommended for patients who are allergic to penicillin. These recommendations are based on well-conducted cohort, case control, and limited randomized controlled studies, and are appropriate for most maxillofacial trauma surgeries. Preoperative antibiotics should be administered within 60 minutes before surgical incision, dosing should be weight based, and administration generally should not extend beyond 24 hours postoperatively. Certain circumstances, such as in immunocompromised patients, severely contaminated wounds, delayed wound closure, open fractures and joint wounds, those at risk for endocarditis, and high-velocity gunshot wounds, warrant additional postinjury prophylaxis.[38] Analyses of combat-related injuries with risk factors for early infection or sepsis also meet the criteria for postinjury prophylaxis.[31] Antibiotic administration cannot be used in place of surgical management of the infected traumatic wound.[12]

Postoperative Antibiotics (BCR)

Prolonged postoperative antibiotic administration ($\geq$5 days) after the operative management of maxillofacial trauma has not demonstrated a benefit in reducing the incidence of infection. Antibiotics have been shown effective only within the first 24 hours after treatment.[13,32] However, increasing severity of trauma may warrant additional antibiotic prophylaxis and should be evaluated on a case-by-case basis. The duration and type of antibiotic therapy have not been elucidated in the literature thus far (Table 26-1).[39-61]

TABLE 26-1   Summary of Antibiotic Prophylaxis Recommendations for the Prevention of Infections in Orofacial, Head, and Neck Trauma*

Indication	Recommendation	Grade
Lacerations—intraoral	Unclear[39]	1C
Lacerations—ear and nose	Antibiotics while packing is in place (nasal, aural)[40]	1B
Lacerations—face (uncomplicated)	Topical antibiotics for the first 48 h,[41] no systemic antibiotics indicated[42]	1C
Ocular/periorbital trauma ocular burn or abrasion	Levofloxacin 500 mg PO or IV daily, postinjury, and continued for 7 days or until retinal evaluation[43] Erythromycin or bacitracin ophthalmic ointment, 1 drop qid or prn for relief[43]	1C
Penetrating neck trauma (sub-platysmal and esophageal)	Broad-spectrum antibiotics for 7-14 days[44,45]	1C
Bite wounds (especially from humans and cats)	Amoxicillin/clavulanate in adults and children, 3-5 days,[46] or clindamycin + ciprofloxacin, cefuroxime axetil, doxycycline, moxifloxacin, or azithromycin for adults, clindamycin + TMP-SMX or azithromycin for children, azithromycin for pregnant patients	1B
Puncture wounds	Tetanus and antipseudomonal prophylaxis[29]	1B
Tooth avulsion	In adults, tetracycline for 1 wk after replantation; in children, penicillin V[47]	1C
Maxillofacial fractures—open, high-velocity, foreign body, or with fixation	Perioperative antibiotics (within 2 h of, and during, surgery)[43,48] to 24 h postoperatively[49,50] cefazolin IV 2 g q8h, clindamycin IV 600 mg q8h, or ceftriaxone IV 1 g q12h[5] adjust for extensive soft tissue injury[43,48]	1B
Mandible fracture—condyle	None indicated[51]	1B
Mandible fracture— simple/compound ± teeth in the line of fracture	Antibiotics from admission to 24 h postoperatively[51] or 48 h postoperatively[51]	1C
Midface fracture—maxilla	None indicated[51]	1B
Midface fracture—zygoma	None indicated[51,52]	1B
Midface fracture—Le Fort pattern	Antibiotics from admission to 24 h postoperatively[53]	1B
Orbit fracture	Antibiotics from admission to 24 h postoperatively with concern for orbital cellulitis[54-56]	1B
Cranial base—temporal bone	Unclear,[57] or consider prophylaxis with concern for CSF fistula[58,59]	1C
Cranial base frontal sinus	Perioperative antibiotics (within 2 h of, and during, surgery) to 48 h postoperatively, avoid >48 h surgical delay[60]	1B

*Grading is based on the GRADE framework[61] as follows: 1A = strong recommendation, high-quality evidence; 1B = strong recommendation, moderate-quality evidence; 1C = strong recommendation, low-quality evidence. Dosing amounts are based on an average 70-kg adult, and unless explicitly stated, they do not take pregnancy, allergy, or other patient-specific factors into account. Compound injuries, preexisting infection, and other comorbidities may necessitate more frequent or prolonged antibiotic use than suggested here.

Soft Tissue Injury

Lacerations

Lacerations of the head and neck are not frequently associated with infection, because of the increased vascularity of this area compared with other locations.[62] Scalp and face wounds nevertheless constitute a majority of lacerations seen in the emergency department. Infection rates for scalp, face, and ear and nose wounds have been reported as 1.7, 3.9, and 3.6%, respectively.[63] However, age, diabetes, jagged and stellate wound edges, visible contamination, and foreign body involvement are all associated with higher infection rates and warrant additional attention to the need

for wound management and prophylaxis.[14] Most common bacterial agents from laceration wound cultures are *Staphylococcus epidermidis* (47.5%) and methicillin-resistant coagulase-negative staphylococci (15%) according to a retrospective study in Korea.[64] Prevention of wound dehiscence is made more challenging because of the variable depth and shape of facial soft tissue wounds in association with numerous muscles of facial expression.[65] Aggressive management is sometimes advocated because of the potential poor cosmetic outcomes associated with wound infection, especially in children and in bite wounds. A prospective multicenter trial has found no correlation between infection and either delay in wound closure or in method of closure, including in facial lacerations. In the same study, history of diabetes, wound contamination, and wound length greater than 5 cm were all significant risk factors for wound infection. In the latter high-risk cases, antibiotic prophylaxis and closer follow-up may be warranted.[15] Timely closure of lacerations is still important, because delays can result in soft tissue swelling and distortion of anatomic landmarks that might predispose the wound to premature dehiscence, exposure, and ultimately infection.[66] Primary closure generally leads to more rapid healing and a better cosmetic outcome than secondary closure does. A meta-analysis has shown that in addition to equally acceptable cosmesis, resorbable (versus nonresorbable) suture use has not been found to influence wound infection rates significantly.[67] Nonsterile glove use is also not associated with adverse outcomes when closing wounds, when compared with sterile gloves.[68] All patients with contaminated wounds should receive the tetanus vaccine if they have not had primary tetanus-diphtheria vaccination and a booster within 5 years. Those without primary immunization should receive both tetanus immune globulin and the vaccine. Otherwise, most lacerations do not require prophylaxis as described previously, but it may be indicated for patients with animal or human bites, excessive wound contamination, vascular insufficiency (e.g., peripheral artery disease), or immunodeficiency. The use of stents, bolsters, or nasal packing may warrant antibiotic prophylaxis until they are removed.[40] It is advisable to perform primary closure on even the most contaminated facial wounds. Although the incidence of infection may be slightly higher than that of healing by secondary intent, the cosmetic benefits of primary wound closure outweigh the ensured risk of facial scarring resulting from delayed wound closure. Recent advances in wound care include implementation of growth factors (e.g., Regranex, a recombinant human platelet–derived growth factor [rhPDGF]),[69] collagen-forming biodegradable gel,[70] galvanotaxic stimulation attracting cells,[71] topical insulin with zinc,[72] low-level laser therapy,[73] tissue glues (cyanoacrylate, fibrin tissue glue), ligating clips (Clearon, Ethistrips), and nanoparticle therapies.[74,75]

Intraoral

Lacerations in the mouth are often considered to be contaminated because of mucosal involvement, but as with other lacerations of the head and neck, they are not often associated with infection. Larger wounds, wounds contaminated with environmental debris, and lacerations that penetrate through both facial skin and oral mucosa ("through and through") may warrant particular care, because they may require significant debridement or multiple layers of closure. Unfortunately, there are few guidelines for the use of antibiotic prophylaxis for all intraoral lacerations; Mark and Granquist[39] found only one randomized controlled trial of such injuries treated within 24 hours of arrival to the emergency department, but did not demonstrate a benefit for prophylaxis because of inadequate sample size. Therefore, it is recommended that antibiotic use should be guided by individual clinician judgment.[39]

Ear

Because of its anatomic location, the external ear is susceptible to laceration in the setting of head trauma. Shear forces can separate the perichondrium from the cartilage, causing a hematoma to form in the subperichondrial space. Because the cartilage is avascular, disruption of its blood supply can lead to necrosis and infection, especially with prolonged exposure of cartilage. Auricular hematoma requires prompt incision and drainage and placement of bolster dressings to prevent recurrence. Bolster dressings, in addition to antistaphylococcal prophylaxis, can help prevent long-term complications, such as cauliflower ear. Auricular cellulitis and chondritis may require similar management. In addition to local wound care, leech therapy has been used for improvement of local tissue perfusion.[76] Precautions also must be taken with traumatic tympanic membrane rupture, because bacteria entering the inner ear can cause infection and subsequent permanent hearing loss, otitis media, or mastoiditis. Ear protection is advised along with otic drops of ofloxacin.[77]

Neck

Aerodigestive tract injury may involve esophageal or laryngeal perforation in addition to disruption of other neck structures. The diagnosis of aerodigestive injury and prevention of infection should be prioritized in selective management through physical examination with esophagoscopy or esophagography as needed.[45] Esophageal injury is particularly worrisome because morbidity is high because of bacterial contamination of the wound.[78] In a 10-year multicenter study of perforating esophageal injuries, Asensio et al[79] showed that cervical injuries are more common (67%) than thoracic or abdominal esophageal injuries, and that timely diagnosis and repair (within 13 hours) of esophageal injury are most critical for reducing complication rate and therefore morbidity and mortality.[79] A review of cervical esophageal injuries from seven studies found a mortality rate of approximately 6%, less than the 21 to 27% mortality in other segments—likely because of containment of contaminated tissue by the fascial layers of the neck.[44] The significantly greater complication rate of patients with esophageal injuries is attributed to infection, such as abscess or mediastinitis.[79] Repair should include irrigation, debridement, layered primary closure, and establishing drainage, along with antibiotic prophylaxis.[43,44] Traumatic esophageal and combined tracheoesophageal injuries are frequently associated with other injuries that might also contribute to infectious complications.[80] There are no conclusive data regarding the change in infectious complications secondary to the now fewer number of selective neck explorations performed in the management of penetrating neck injuries.[43,81]

Eye

The eye is an immunologically privileged organ, and many portions of it are relatively avascular; it is especially susceptible to infection with traumatic contamination. Posttraumatic endophthalmitis may follow penetrating eye injury with or without presence of an intraocular foreign body. Infection is frequently due to contamination by gram-positive, coagulase-negative staphylococci or streptococci, but may also involve other bacteria or may be polymicrobial. Because of the poor outcomes of endophthalmitis in trauma, especially in association with intraocular foreign body, broad-spectrum antibiotics should be considered while the patient is awaiting definitive management. Moxifloxacin (400 mg) or levofloxacin (500 mg) offers coverage for the most common microbes implicated in endophthalmitis, and each is able to reach the aqueous and vitreous humors.[31,82] These regimens also should be considered for corneal abrasion. The periorbita also may be affected in ocular or orbital trauma, resulting in preseptal cellulitis, orbital cellulitis, or cavernous sinus thrombosis. Necrotizing fasciitis should be included in the differential diagnosis of penetrating wound infections; it requires urgent operative debridement and broad-spectrum antibiotics.[28] As part of the maxillofacial trauma triage, prevention of further injury to the globe includes irrigation with a balanced salt solution, conservative debridement, initiation of antibiotic therapy, the use of a Fox shield if needed, and prompt referral to the ophthalmology service for primary closure of ocular wounds.[43]

Bite

Bite wounds can be characterized as penetrating, crush, or avulsion injuries and are all heavily contaminated by the oral flora of the offending organism. In a minority of cases, isolated pathogenic organisms may originate from the patient's own skin flora or secondary invaders at the time of the bite injury.[83] The most common bacterial species isolated from human bite wounds is *Eikenella corrodens,* whereas cat and dog bites are often contaminated with *Pasteurella* species. However, the bacteriology of bite wounds is diverse, and up to 7% of infected wounds are not culturable.[83] Late wound infection can also occur, and prophylaxis against rabid animals is an important preventive measure. Wounds involving cartilage exposure, as in the ear and nose, and those involving crush injuries involving tissue ischemia are more prone to the development of infection.[46,84] It is important to meticulously examine penetrating wounds for occult neurovascular injury. Long-term sequelae of meningitis have been reported because of missed diagnosis of intracranial injury in pediatric bite traumas, because neurologic injury can be difficult to detect in the acute setting.[85] Treatment of bite wounds involves high-pressure irrigation with normal saline solution. Primary debridement and closure of such wounds in the head and neck have been well established, although the need for antibiotic prophylaxis is debated. It is more uniformly supported for cat and human bites compared with dog bites. The authors prescribe prophylactic antibiotics if it is not possible to completely debride wounds or for concern of poor cosmetic outcome if infection does occur.[46] Of note, children are affected by dog bites in the head and neck

region much more frequently than adults. In one 20-year review, more than one fifth of dog bite patients were children 5 years old or younger.[86] This is likely due to their height and underdeveloped situational awareness.

Burn

Topical therapy rather than systemic antibiotics guides prevention of infection in patients with burns. Silver sulfadiazine cream alternating with mafenide acetate cream has been described as an effective combination after primary debridement of the wound. However, wounds that are possibly colonized or presently infected should have antibiotic coverage against pseudomonas.[31] Interestingly, after the initial thermal insult, burn wounds are essentially sterile and then are colonized with a patient's environment, gut, and nasopharyngeal tract.[87] Also, the use of topical antibiotic creams has increased the rate of fungal colonization.[87]

Hard Tissue Injury

Dentoalveolar

Dentoalveolar trauma can lead to infection by interruption of intact mucosa or of alveolar integrity, leading to contamination by a heterogeneous oral flora. In alveolar fractures, concomitant mucosal exposure or fracture instability after splinting can lead to prolonged wound infection. Fracture of both buccal and lingual alveolar cortices and the development of full-thickness mucoperiosteal flaps may contribute to the devitalization of the wound area and promote infection.[88] With tooth injuries, the greatest risk of infection is related to tooth avulsion. Replantation of avulsed permanent teeth is often the treatment of choice, but it involves the introduction of bacteria and foreign material into the tooth socket, depending on the amount of posttraumatic debridement. In cases of intrusion or luxation, infection can be controlled with endodontic therapy and either spontaneous eruption or orthodontic extrusion.[89] Posttraumatic infection involving teeth is generally related to the incidence of pulpal necrosis, which more commonly affects permanent teeth with closed apices. Either endodontic therapy or systemic antibiotic prophylaxis with penicillin or tetracycline is used to manage posttraumatic infection.[88] In immature teeth, topical antibiotics such as minocycline or doxycycline, 1 mg diluted in 20 mL of saline, have been successful in promoting pulpal revascularization and periodontal health when applied before replantation. Systemic penicillin or tetracycline antibiotics also can be used as prophylaxis, although unlike with topical antibiotics, comprehensive clinical studies have not demonstrated their value.[47]

Mandible

Posttraumatic mandibular infections are a result of delayed treatment without antibiotic prophylaxis or the early or late complications of operative management. The incidence of infection is an area of active research, as a significant proportion of facial trauma involves mandible fractures.[90] Because of its association with the alveolus, teeth, and oral mucosa, the mandible's propensity for infection is much higher than other bones in the facial skeleton. The overall postoperative infection rate for mandibular fractures, including the incidence of wound dehiscence, is approximately 20%.[4] In general, infection accounts for one third of complications in the mandible. Although most infections are superficial, some may cause debilitating injury in the form of malunion, nonunion, or osteomyelitis.[91] The mandibular angle is the most common site of fracture and of postoperative infection, whereas condylar fractures have the lowest infection rate.[51,92] Patient-related factors such as teeth in the fracture line, substance abuse, and poor systemic or nutritional health are found to be significant predictors of increased infectious risk.[50,92-94] Furthermore, the use of intraoperative IMF wires to aid in fixation of mandible fractures contributes to cross-infection caused by glove perforations.[22,26] In suitable cases of isolated mandibular fractures, manual reduction simplifies accurate fixation while reducing disease transmission.[23] Maxillomandibular bone-anchoring screws also reduce the need for manipulation of metal wires.[24] Placement of fixation plates at the superior border of the fracture or near the mucosal incision is implicated in inflammation, reduced mucosal blood supply, and eventual wound dehiscence. Avoiding wound dehiscence is ultimately guided by watertight closure of the mucosa and oral antibiotic rinses to avoid infection of the wound margin and subsequent hardware inoculation.[91]

In the acute period after a mandibular fracture, infections are typically related to compromised soft tissues or teeth left in the fractures that may result in osteomyelitis.[95] Late infections occurring in the weeks after operative management may be due to inadequate fixation or infected teeth in the fracture line, which may be treated by local incision and drainage or tooth removal as necessary. Wound dehiscence or superficial purulence may also be treated with antiseptic wound irrigation, such as povidone-iodine.[4] Complications of infectious cause may arise from preoperative, perioperative, and postoperative oral hygiene, alcoholism, metabolic disturbances, tobacco use, prolonged time between injury and definitive treatment, poor patient compliance with treatment, and fracture severity.[95-97] In general, greater infectious complications may be found more often when there are teeth in the line of fracture (25%) than when they are not (15%).[4] Although, a large prospective study of 253 patients with mandibular fractures in third molar removal found a postoperative infection rate of 6.95% and no association between the removal of tooth in line of fracture and the rate of infection.[98] However, a systemic review recommends that teeth in the line of the fracture should be removed if they impair adequate reduction of the bony segments, are involved in an infected fracture, are mobile because of fracture or periodontal disease, have associated

drainage, there is periapical radiolucency, or are involved in infected fracture.[99,100] Teeth that prevent adequate fixation and those that are associated with periodontal or alveolar damage should be managed with extraction at the time of repair.[101] In addition, conditions such as atrophic mandible increases risks of infection by approximately 10 to 20%.[102] Decreased bone height correlates to increased incidence of nonunion, malunion, recurrent fractures, hardware failure, postoperative infection, and osteomyelitis.[95]

The role of antibiotics in these situations is unclear, but prudent use of local or systemic antibiotics may be necessary to prevent further wound complications.[103] A number of studies have demonstrated that preoperative antibiotics do not decrease incidence of postoperative infections or intensive care unit and hospital length of stay.[95] Limiting antibiotic exposure only to intraoperative antibiotic prophylaxis for patients undergoing transoral open-reduction internal-fixation (ORIF) for treatment of open mandibular fractures was not associated with an increased risk of infection.[104] However, in cases of radiographic or clinical evidence of nonunion, screw loosening, plate exposure, or osteomyelitis, surgical retreatment is required.[105] Culture of the wound, drainage, and debridement of fibrous tissue or nonvital bone should precede stabilization with repeated fixation.[106] Antibiotic therapy should be initiated on presentation of a mandibular fracture and continued until at least the time of intervention.[107,108] This protocol is frequently cited in the literature, with the exception of isolated mandibular condyle fractures, for which there is no clear indication for antibiotic prophylaxis at all.[108,109] The majority of recent evidence suggests that increased duration of postoperative antibiotic therapy does not reduce infection rates.[92,110,111] Studies have determined that a range of zero[110] to 48 hours[51] is an effective time period for postoperative antibiotic administration. In addition, a prospective randomized trial has shown recently that prophylaxis beyond 24 hours does not significantly influence infection rates.[4] This is true even for open reduction and internal fixation of compound mandibular fractures, where a prospective study has found no difference between only two postoperative doses of antibiotic prophylaxis compared with longer durations of 5 to 7 days.[112] In addition, treatment delay has been found to be unrelated to the rate of postoperative complications, including risk of infection.[92,93,107,109] It is important to note that because few randomized controlled studies exist, further studies are needed to define the risks of treatment delay, presence of teeth in the fracture line, and oral hygiene with the incidence of infection.[113] Management should consider the individualized nature of each fracture with regard to mandibular biomechanics.[114]

Midface

Unlike mandibular fractures, maxillary and zygoma fractures rarely become infected; they do not warrant postoperative antibiotic prophylaxis.[51] The rate described for postoperative zygoma fracture infection is 1.5%, and infection is more likely to occur with an intraoral approach than with a skin approach.[52] Other studies looking more comprehensively at midfacial trauma have reported infection rates of 9[13] and 4.3%.[53] In general, repair of these fractures frequently involves mucosal surfaces and may also involve cartilage exposure and coverage. Nasal trauma can lead to disruption of the mucoperichondrium, allowing hematoma formation adjacent to the cartilaginous nasal septum. The hematoma must be evacuated by incision of the septal mucosa with a Killian or L-shaped incision and drainage, followed by placement of nasal packing and antibiotic prophylaxis.[115] If the hematoma persists, nasal septal abscess can form with bacterial colonization (typically *Staphylococcus aureus*), which can spread and cause sepsis, orbital, or cranial infections. Abscess formation can lead to rapid necrosis of the cartilage because of the release of bacterial collagenases, resulting in a posttraumatic saddle-nose deformity. In children, such a defect can influence future growth of midfacial projection; therefore, it is especially important to evaluate the septum in children with nasal trauma.[116] As in mandibular trauma, a randomized prospective placebo-controlled trial of Le Fort and zygomatic fractures has shown no difference in infection rates with antibiotic prophylaxis beyond the immediate postoperative period (24 hours) compared with a more prolonged course (5 days).[53] Le Fort level fractures or naso-orbito-ethmoidal complex fractures may present with cerebrospinal fluid (CSF) leaks (rhinorrhea), for which antibiotic prophylaxis is also not recommended (see Cranial Base section).

Orbit

Orbital cellulitis resulting from trauma or orbital fracture repair is a relatively rare occurrence. Infection of the orbital space can lead to sequelae of compression, such as optic neuritis, atrophy, and blindness. Cranial spread of bacteria can lead to cavernous sinus thrombosis and meningitis.[117] It is thought that orbital wall fractures can result in contamination of the wound by paranasal sinus mucosa and warrant treatment as compound fractures with prophylaxis.[55,56] Although there are no clear guidelines regarding the need for antibiotics after orbital trauma, a prospective randomized controlled trial has found that the orbital wound infection rate is not affected by antibiotic prophylaxis greater than 24 hours after surgical repair. The overall infection rate after orbital repair has been found to be 5%.[117] Often, infections are associated with preexisting soft tissue lacerations in the infraorbital tissues, sinusitis, or implanted foreign bodies. A history of penetrating trauma should consider the possibility of occult foreign body and the risk of bacterial inoculation, leading to orbital cellulitis or abscess.[118] Surgical intervention includes orbital decompression with subperiosteal approach or via the paranasal sinuses.[54] Consultation with the ophthalmology service is recommended for close monitoring of ocular changes. Warning signs include pain or edema out of proportion for the expected course. Worsening of visual acuity that occurs several days after the trauma should tip off the provider that further investigation may be warranted.

Nose

Although the nose is the most frequently broken CMF bone, it typically carries a low risk of needing further interventions. Nasal septal hematomas from maxillofacial trauma are a relatively rare occurrence with a suspected incidence of 0.8 to 1.6%, but these are thought to be highly underreported. However, if left untreated, they can lead to significant complications such as septal necrosis or superinfection. Inadequate treatment of an infection in this region can lead to invasion of adjacent structures, including retrograde spread into the meninges and intracranial abscess formation.[119] The bacterial flora of the nose differs from that of the oral cavity, and, thus, the antibiotics used should be tailored accordingly. The national incidence of MRSA colonization within the nasal passages is 32.4%.[120]

Cranial Base

Evidence of skull base fracture can be seen in maxillofacial trauma as CSF otorrhea or rhinorrhea, displacement of cranial bones on imaging, or pneumocephalus. Pneumocephalus is sometimes viewed as evidence of occult CSF leak when it is otherwise difficult to detect in the acute setting.[121] Risk of meningitis is increased with open skull base traumas, where the intracranial space communicates with surrounding tissues of the pharynx or skin. Surgical management of anterior skull base trauma, for example, necessarily includes ensuring drainage via patent ducts or obliteration of mucosal tissues harboring infectious microorganisms. A current literature review of randomized controlled trials shows no clear evidence supporting antibiotic prophylaxis of anterior skull base injuries, regardless of whether a CSF leak is present.[57] In fact, alteration of the normal wound site flora with antibiotics can paradoxically create an infectious environment, and many posttraumatic CSF fistulas close spontaneously (85% within the first week).[122] Surgical intervention should be performed in cases of clear dural disruption, contamination, or failure of lumbar drainage and other more conservative measures to lower the risk of long-term meningitis.

Frontal Sinus

Frontal sinus trauma is particularly worrisome because of the anatomic location near the meninges and brain. Fractures can result in short-term, intracranial infections, as well as long-term infectious sequelae because of obstruction of the nasofrontal outflow tract. Traditionally, treatment of these fractures involved exenteration of the sinus to prevent mucus collection and subsequently became more conservative, with preservation of the supraorbital rims.[9] Management has continued to become more conservative, with the goal of protecting intracranial structures, reestablishing normal forehead contour, and preventing infectious complications.[59]

Currently established guidelines for treatment are based on patency of the frontonasal duct, comminution and displacement of the posterior table, and significance of brain injury or dural embarrassment.[123] Patients with severely displaced and comminuted frontal sinus fractures with significant posterior table involvement, dural lacerations, persistent CSF leak, or brain injury often benefit from cranialization. Those without posterior table involvement, however, benefit from sinus obliteration. Otherwise, sinus function is preserved in patients with repair of the disrupted anterior table.[2,59,123] This protocol allows for sinus preservation in the majority of patients with frontobasilar injury with minimization of short- and long-term infectious sequelae. The foramina of Breschet, which provide venous drainage for the sinus into the subdural venous system, can become a pathway for bacterial infiltration.[124] Obstruction of the duct may then lead to recurrent sinusitis, meningitis, encephalitis, brain abscess, frontal sinus abscess, or osteomyelitis.[125] Late complications, or those occurring 6 months after the initial injury, can also include mucocele, mucopyocele, or both. Mucoceles are slow-growing lesions that obliterate the sinus space and eventually erode through thin posterior bone, usually a result of failure to reestablish frontonasal drainage.[124,126] For complex frontal sinus injuries with dural embarrassment, timing of surgical repair (cranialization or obliteration) before 48 hours has elapsed from the time of injury is associated with significantly reduced risk of infection.[60]

Temporal

Temporal bone fractures are implicated in the development of posttraumatic meningitis, especially when there is evidence of CSF rhinorrhea (13%) versus CSF otorrhea (6%). Historically, antibiotic prophylaxis has not been recommended in the treatment of fractures even with CSF fistulae; however, the presence of concurrent infection may independently raise the risk of meningitis by 20%. Instead, operative closure of CSF fistula is recommended after 7 to 10 days of conservative management. Initial management includes CSF diversion by placement of a lumbar drain for 5 to 7 days.[9] Most leaks, however, will undergo early spontaneous closure.[58,125] A Cochrane review of multiple prospective randomized trials and retrospective cohort studies has indicated that current evidence does not support antibiotic prophylaxis for the prevention of meningitis in patients with basilar skull fractures regardless of CSF leakage.[57] In fact, proliferation of opportunistic infections after prophylaxis caused by disruption of normal bacterial flora has been demonstrated in multiple cases. Therefore, it has been recommended to reduce postoperative antibiotic use to only higher-risk cases, such as those with operative delay, external CSF drainage catheters, or concurrent soft tissue infection.[60,127] It has also been argued that the data from the Cochrane review is misinterpreted and that cases with CSF fistulas of the temporal bone and skull base should have continued antibiotics.[128] The authors believe the final recommendation should be left to clinical judgment.

Osteomyelitis

The development of osteomyelitis is an uncommon but debilitating consequence of maxillofacial trauma. It is not often possible to distinguish the causative agent, although immune status, fracture contamination, and fracture mobility have been cited as possible causes.[129] If left unresolved, these causes lead to acute osteomyelitis contiguous with the area of injury.[130] One study of more than 1400 mandible fractures found that a majority of osteomyelitis cases of the mandible were associated with nonunion.[106] Other documented clinical features include intense pain, intermittent fevers, paresthesia or anesthesia of the mental nerve, sequestra, trismus, lymphadenopathy, and dental pain.[131] Although treatment for osteomyelitis has traditionally involved high doses of parenteral antibiotics for long periods (6 weeks), it has been demonstrated that oral antibiotics are as efficacious as parenteral forms—with less cost and concern for intravenous access—and that type and duration of antibiotic should be individualized to the patient's clinical picture.[132] Hyperbaric oxygen therapy also has been used with some success after debridement and sequestrectomy.[133] Removal of necrotic and infected bone, teeth, and soft tissues remains a mainstay in the treatment of osteomyelitis.

High-Velocity Projectile

The hallmark of high-velocity injury, or commonly gunshot wound (GSW), is the presence of tissue damage far outside the area immediately surrounding the projectile. Terminal ballistic characteristics determine the size of the temporary and permanent wound cavities, which may be contaminated by foreign particles and the bacteria carried by them. Soft-point bullets, for example, are far more likely to fragment and contaminate a deceptively larger area than the entry wound.[134] Because of this, high-velocity injuries are often categorized as contaminated or infected instead of clean-contaminated.[135] Nosocomial infections are more common in these patients, as they tend to be more severely injured.[48] Treatment algorithms for high-velocity wounds emphasize early surgical debridement and irrigation as necessary, primary reconstruction of hard and soft tissues if possible, and establishment of drainage. Delayed closure of wounds will result in scar contracture, making later definitive repair much more difficult. Furthermore, involvement of the oral cavity and the sinus are associated with statistically higher rates of head and neck infections, even in the setting of antibiotic use. In comparison, GSWs to the face without oral cavity, sinus involvement, or need for multiple surgeries have low infection rates and may not benefit from antibiotics.[136] Still, antibiotic prophylaxis plays a major role in the prevention of infection, because debridement can be difficult with enlarged temporary and permanent wound cavities.[48,137] Prophylactic antibiotics are used to prevent localized infection from progressing to osteomyelitis and possible sepsis.[138] Antibiotic administration is highly recommended for both high-energy and low-energy GSWs, although there is a wide variability in standard antibiotic treatment practices by administration route or usage.[139] Recommended antibiotics include benzyl penicillin, oral fluoroquinolone, intravenous cephalosporins (first or third generation), aminoglycoside, and/or gentamicin.[140] Prompt administration of antibiotics is advised for indicated situations but should never be used as a substitute for surgical debridement in soft tissue injury.[141,142] Some surgeons prefer conservative debridement to preserve anatomic landmarks, which can be facilitated in part because of the availability of antibiotics.[135]

Alternatively, aggressive debridement and early reconstruction with free tissue transfer in cases of severe composite tissue injury is preferred at this institution.[143] Complication related to infection of hardware fixation for GSW remains rare because of the robust blood supply of the face.[144]

Hardware Removal

Fixation plates used for repair of maxillofacial fractures can become infected and may necessitate incision and drainage of sterile abscesses or removal of hardware. In general, mandibular hardware necessitates more frequent removal than hardware placed in the midface; this is thought to be due to greater tensile and compressive forces found in the mandible.[145] Plates that lie directly under the mucoperiosteum along the external oblique line or the mandibular body are also more prone to masticatory trauma.[92] The removal rate of titanium plates ranges from 3 to 32% in the literature, and a large portion of removals are cited to be due to infection.[23,146,147] If there is bony union after fracture treatment, any infection, exposure, pain, or other morbidity associated with existing hardware should be treated with hardware removal.[148] Most hardware complications requiring removal occur within the first year.[149]

Summary

Employing a systemic approach to maxillofacial trauma can mitigate the risk of infection and allow for decreased morbidity in addition to decreased health care costs. Practicing evidence-based medicine reduces unnecessary exposure and helps prevent reduced antibiotic sensitivity. In an era of research and development for new medications and antibiotics, surgical principles remain foundational. It is essential that we continue to reevaluate protocols and techniques to ensure an up-to-date standard of care. Advances in this area will continue to redefine medical and surgical management after maxillofacial trauma.

References

1. Reidel-Schenke H. Ueber die Stirnhöhlen und ihre Erkrankungen. *Ueber die Stimhohlen und ihre Erkrankungen.* 1898:16. Available at: https://cir.nii.ac.jp/crid/1130000796864377088. Accessed August 2, 2023.
2. Bell RB. Management of frontal sinus fractures. *Oral Maxillofac Surg Clin North Am.* 2009;21(2):227-242. Available at: https://doi.org/10.1016/j.coms.2008.12.003.
3. Zehtabchi S, Tan A, Yadav K, Badawy A, Lucchesi M. The impact of wound age on the infection rate of simple lacerations repaired in the emergency department. *Injury.* 2012;43(11):1793-1798. Available at: https://doi.org/10.1016/j.injury.2012.02.018.
4. Schaller B, Soong PL, Zix J, Iizuka T, Lieger O. The role of postoperative prophylactic antibiotics in the treatment of facial fractures: a randomized, double-blind, placebo-controlled pilot clinical study. Part 2: Mandibular fractures in 59 patients. *Br J Oral Maxillofac Surg.* 2013;51(8):803-807. Available at: https://doi.org/10.1016/j.bjoms.2013.08.008.
5. Petersen K, Hayes DK, Blice JP, Hale RG. Prevention and management of infections associated with combat-related head and neck injuries. *J Trauma.* 2008;64(3):S265-S276. Available at: https://doi.org/10.1097/ta.0b013e318163d2a6.
6. Mangram AJ, Horan TC, Pearson ML, Silver LC, Jarvis WR. Guideline for prevention of surgical site infection, 1999. *Am J Infect Control.* 1999;27(2):97-134. Available at: https://doi.org/10.1016/s0196-6553(99)70088-x.
7. Holt GR. Essential tissue healing of the face and neck. *JAMA.* 2009;302(2):200. Available at: https://doi.org/10.1001/jama.2009.993.
8. Adalarasan S, Mohan A, Pasupathy S. Prophylactic Antibiotics in maxillofacial fractures. *J Craniofac Surg.* 2010;21(4):1009-1011. Available at: https://doi.org/10.1097/scs.0b013e3181e47d43.
9. Perry M. Maxillofacial trauma—Developments, innovations and controversies. *Injury.* 2009;40(12):1252-1259. Available at: https://doi.org/10.1016/j.injury.2008.12.015.
10. Gassner R, Tuli T, Hächl O, Rudisch A, Ulmer H. Craniomaxillofacial trauma: a 10 year review of 9543 cases with 21067 injuries. *J Craniomaxillofac Surg.* 2003;31(1):51-61. Available at: https://doi.org/10.1016/s1010-5182(02)00168-3.
11. Ray JM, Triplett RG. What is the role of biofilms in severe head and neck infections? *Oral Maxillofac Surg Clin North Am.* 2011;23(4):497-505. Available at: https://doi.org/10.1016/j.coms.2011.07.002.
12. Lieblich SE. Infection in the patient with maxillofacial trauma. In: *Oral and Maxillofacial Trauma.* St. Louis: Elsevier; 2013:790-807. Available at: https://doi.org/10.1016/b978-1-4557-0554-2.00032-0.
13. Lauder A, Jalisi S, Spiegel J, Stram J, Devaiah A. Antibiotic prophylaxis in the management of complex midface and frontal sinus trauma. *Laryngoscope.* 2010;120(10):1940-1945. Available at: https://doi.org/10.1002/lary.21081.
14. Hollander JE, Singer AJ, Valentine SM, Shofer FS. Risk factors for infection in patients with traumatic lacerations. *Acad Emerg Med.* 2001;8(7):716-720. Available at: https://doi.org/10.1111/j.1553-2712.2001.tb00190.x.
15. Quinn JV, Polevoi SK, Kohn MA. Traumatic lacerations: what are the risks for infection and has the 'golden period' of laceration care disappeared? *Emerg Med J.* 2013;31(2):96-100. Available at: https://doi.org/10.1136/emermed-2012-202143.
16. Hurrell MJL, Batstone MD. The effect of treatment timing on the management of facial fractures: a systematic review. *Int J Oral Maxillofac Surg.* 2014;43(8):944-950. Available at: https://doi.org/10.1016/j.ijom.2014.03.003.
17. Weider L, Hughes K, Ciarochi J, Dunn E. Early versus delayed repair of facial fractures in the multiply injured patient. *Am Surg.* 1999;65(8):790-793. Available at: https://doi.org/10.1177/000313489906500818.
18. Hollier LH, Sharabi SE, Koshy JC, Stal S. Facial trauma. *J Craniofac Surg.* 2010;21(4):1051-1053. Available at: https://doi.org/10.1097/scs.0b013e3181e5701c.
19. Tang DT, Lalonde JF, Lalonde DH. Delayed immediate surgery for orbital floor fractures: less can be more. *Can J Plast*

Surg. 2011;19(4):125-128. Available at: https://doi.org/10.1177/229255031101900402.

20. Hong HK, Kim DG, Choi DH, Seo A, Chung HY. Nasoethmoid orbital fracture reconstruction using a three-dimensional printing-based craniofacial plate. *Arch Craniofac Surg.* 2022;23(6):278-281. Available at: https://doi.org/10.7181/acfs.2022.00913.

21. Tanner J, Parkinson H. Double gloving to reduce surgical cross-infection. *Cochrane Database Syst Rev.* 2006;(3):CD003087. Available at: https://doi.org/10.1002/14651858.cd003087.pub2.

22. Pigadas N, Avery CME. Precautions against cross-infection during operations for maxillofacial trauma. *Br J Oral Maxillofac Surg.* 2000;38(2):110-113. Available at: https://doi.org/10.1054/bjom.1999.0145.

23. Bell RB, Wilson DM. Is the use of arch bars or interdental wire fixation necessary for successful outcomes in the open reduction and internal fixation of mandibular angle fractures? *J Oral Maxillofac Surg.* 2008;66(10):2116-2122. Available at: https://doi.org/10.1016/j.joms.2008.05.370.

24. Cornelius CP, Ehrenfeld M. The use of MMF screws: surgical technique, indications, contraindications, and common problems in review of the literature. *Craniomaxillofac Trauma Reconstr.* 2010;3(2):55-80. Available at: https://doi.org/10.1055/s-0030-1254376.

25. Mischke C, Verbeek JH, Saarto A, Lavoie MC, Pahwa M, Ijaz S. Gloves, extra gloves or special types of gloves for preventing percutaneous exposure injuries in healthcare personnel. *Cochrane Database Syst Rev.* 2014;(3):CD009573. Available at: https://doi.org/10.1002/14651858.cd009573.pub2.

26. Khosla A, Padhye M, Girotra C, Gupta K. Efficacy of double gloving technique in major and minor oral surgical procedures: a prospective study. *Ann Maxillofacial Surg.* 2011;1(2):112. Available at: https://doi.org/10.4103/2231-0746.92771.

27. Shvyrkov MB. Erratum to "Facial gunshot wound debridement: debridement of facial soft tissue gunshot wounds" [*J Craniomaxillofac Surg.* 41 (2013) e8-e16]. *J Craniomaxillofac Surg.* 2013;41(5):e77. Available at: https://www.sciencedirect.com/science/article/abs/pii/S1010518212001060?via%3Dihub.

28. Lazzeri D, Lazzeri S, Figus M, et al. Periorbital necrotising fasciitis. *Br J Ophthalmol.* 2009;94(12):1577-1585. Available at: https://doi.org/10.1136/bjo.2009.167486.

29. García-Gubern CF, Colon-Rolon L, Bond MC. Essential concepts of wound management. *Emerg Med Clin North Am.* 2010;28(4):951-967. Available at: https://doi.org/10.1016/j.emc.2010.06.009.

30. Fernandez R, Griffiths R. Water for wound cleansing. *Cochrane Database Syst Rev.* 2012;(2):CD003861. Available at: https://doi.org/10.1002/14651858.cd003861.pub3.

31. Hospenthal DR, Murray CK. Preface: guidelines for the prevention of infections associated with combat-related injuries: 2011 update. *J Trauma.* 2011;71(2):S197-S201. Available at: https://doi.org/10.1097/ta.0b013e318227ac23.

32. Mottini M, Wolf R, Soong PL, Lieger O, Nakahara K, Schaller B. The role of postoperative antibiotics in facial fractures. *J Trauma Acute Care Surg.* 2014;76(3):720-724. Available at: https://doi.org/10.1097/ta.0000000000000123.

33. Horgan MA, Kernan JC, Schwartz MS, Kellogg JX, McMenomey SO, Delashaw JB. Shaveless brain surgery: safe, well-tolerated and cost effective. *Skull Base.* 1999;9(4):253-258. Available at: https://doi.org/10.1055/s-2008-1058134.

34. Sebastian S. Does preoperative scalp shaving result in fewer postoperative wound infections when compared with no scalp shaving? A systematic review. *J Neurosci Nurs.* 2012;44(3):149-156. Available at: https://doi.org/10.1097/jnn.0b013e31825106d2.

35. Ruskin JD, Delmore MM, Feinberg SE. Posttraumatic facial swelling and draining sinus tract. *J Oral Maxillofac Surg.* 1992;50(12):1320-1323. Available at: https://doi.org/10.1016/0278-2391(92)90235-r.

36. Caruso DP, Aquino VM, Tannyhill RJI. Algorithmic approach to antibiotic prophylaxis for traumatic craniomaxillofacial injuries. *J Craniofac Surg.* 2022;33(4):1082. Available at: https://doi.org/10.1097/SCS.0000000000008432.

37. Bratzler DW, Dellinger EP, Olsen KM, et al. Clinical practice guidelines for antimicrobial prophylaxis in surgery. *Am J Health Syst Pharm.* 2013;70(3):195-283. Available at: https://doi.org/10.2146/ajhp120568.

38. Abubaker AO. Use of prophylactic antibiotics in preventing infection of traumatic injuries. *Oral Maxillofac Surg Clin North Am.* 2009;21(2):259-264. Available at: https://doi.org/10.1016/j.coms.2008.12.001.

39. Mark DG, Granquist EJ. Are prophylactic oral antibiotics indicated for the treatment of intraoral wounds? *Ann Emerg Med.* 2008;52(4):368-372. Available at: https://doi.org/10.1016/j.annemergmed.2007.12.028.

40. Patel KG, Sykes JM. Management of soft-tissue trauma to the face. *Oper Tech Otolaryngol Head Neck Surg.* 2008;19(2):90-97. Available at: https://doi.org/10.1016/j.otot.2008.05.004.

41. Waterbrook AL, Hiller K, Hays DP, Berkman M. Do topical antibiotics help prevent infection in minor traumatic uncomplicated soft tissue wounds? *Ann Emerg Med.* 2013;61(1):86-88. Available at: https://doi.org/10.1016/j.annemergmed.2012.08.002.

42. Medel N, Panchal N, Ellis E. Postoperative care of the facial laceration. *Craniomaxillofac Trauma Reconstr.* 2010;3(4):189-200. Available at: https://doi.org/10.1055/s-0030-1268516.

43. Petersen K, Colyer MH, Hayes DK, Hale RG, Bell RB. Prevention of infections associated with combat-related eye, maxillofacial, and neck injuries. *J Trauma.* 2011;71(2):S264-S269. Available at: https://doi.org/10.1097/ta.0b013e318227ad9a.

44. Brinster CJ, Singhal S, Lee L, Marshall MB, Kaiser LR, Kucharczuk JC. Evolving options in the management of esophageal perforation. *Ann Thorac Surg.* 2004;77(4):1475-1483. Available at: https://doi.org/10.1016/j.athoracsur.2003.08.037.

45. Bagheri SC, Khan HA, Bell RB. Penetrating neck injuries. *Oral Maxillofac Surg Clin North Am.* 2008;20(3):393-414. Available at: https://doi.org/10.1016/j.coms.2008.04.003.

46. Stefanopoulos PK. Management of facial bite wounds. *Oral Maxillofac Surg Clin North Am.* 2009;21(2):247-257. Available at: https://doi.org/10.1016/j.coms.2008.12.009.

47. Andersson L, Andreasen JO, Day P, et al. International Association of Dental Traumatology guidelines for the management of traumatic dental injuries. Part 2. Avulsion of permanent teeth. *Dent Traumatol.* 2012;28(2):88-96. Available at: https://doi.org/10.1111/j.1600-9657.2012.01125.x.

48. Petersen K, Riddle MS, Danko JR, et al. Trauma-related infections in battlefield casualties from Iraq. *Ann Surg.* 2007;245(5):803-811. Available at: https://doi.org/10.1097/01.sla.0000251707.32332.c1.

49. Hospenthal DR, Murray CK, Andersen RC, et al. Guidelines for the prevention of infections associated with combat-related injuries: 2011 update: endorsed by the Infectious Diseases Society of America and the Surgical Infection Society. *J Trauma Acute Care Surg.* 2011;71(2):S210. Available at: https://doi.org/10.1097/TA.0b013e318227ac4b.

50. Hindawi YH, Oakley GM, Kinsella CR, Cray JJ, Lindsay K, Scifres AM. Antibiotic duration and postoperative infection rates in mandibular fractures. *J Craniofac Surg.* 2011;22(4):1375-1377. Available at: https://doi.org/10.1097/scs.0b013e31821c9498.

51. Andreasen JO, Jensen SS, Schwartz O, Hillerup Y. A systematic review of prophylactic antibiotics in the surgical treatment of

maxillofacial fractures. *J Oral Maxillofac Surg.* 2006;64(11):1664-1668. Available at: https://doi.org/10.1016/j.joms.2006.02.032.

52. Knepil GJ, Loukota RA. Outcomes of prophylactic antibiotics following surgery for zygomatic bone fractures. *J Craniomaxillofac Surg.* 2010;38(2):131-133. Available at: https://doi.org/10.1016/j.jcms.2009.03.015.

53. Soong PL, Schaller B, Zix J, Iizuka T, Mottini M, Lieger O. The role of postoperative prophylactic antibiotics in the treatment of facial fractures: a randomised, double-blind, placebo-controlled pilot clinical study. Part 3: Le Fort and zygomatic fractures in 94 patients. *Br J Oral Maxillofac Surg.* 2014;52(4):329-333. Available at: https://doi.org/10.1016/j.bjoms.2014.01.010.

54. Simon GJB, Bush S, Selva D, McNab AA. Orbital cellulitis: a rare complication after orbital blowout fracture. *Ophthalmology.* 2005;112(11):2030-2034. Available at: https://doi.org/10.1016/j.ophtha.2005.06.012.

55. Dhariwal DK, Kittur MA, Farrier JN, Sugar AW, Aird DW, Laws DE. Post-traumatic orbital cellulitis. *Br J Oral Maxillofac Surg.* 2003;41(1):21-28. Available at: https://doi.org/10.1016/s0266-4356(02)00259-0.

56. Newlands C, Baggs PR, Kendrick R, et al. Orbital trauma. *BMJ.* 1999;319(7208):516. Available at: https://doi.org/10.1136/bmj.319.7208.516a.

57. Ratilal BO, Costa J, Pappamikail L, Sampaio C. Antibiotic prophylaxis for preventing meningitis in patients with basilar skull fractures. *Cochrane Database Syst Rev.* 2015;(4):CD004884. Available at: https://doi.org/10.1002/14651858.CD004884.pub4.

58. Brodie HA, Thompson TC. Management of complications from 820 temporal bone fractures. *Otol Neurotol.* 1997;18(2):188.

59. Bell RB, Chen J. Frontobasilar fractures: contemporary management. *Atlas Oral Maxillofac Surg Clin.* 2010;18(2):181-196. Available at: https://doi.org/10.1016/j.cxom.2010.08.003.

60. Bellamy JL, Molendijk J, Reddy SK, et al. Severe infectious complications following frontal sinus fracture. *Plast Reconstr Surg.* 2013;132(1):154-162. Available at: https://doi.org/10.1097/prs.0b013e3182910b9b.

61. Guyatt GH, Oxman AD, Vist GE, et al. GRADE: an emerging consensus on rating quality of evidence and strength of recommendations. *BMJ.* 2008;336(7650):924-926. Available at: https://doi.org/10.1136/bmj.39489.470347.AD.

62. Ardeshirpour F, Shaye DA, Hilger PA. Improving posttraumatic facial scars. *Otolaryngol Clin North Am.* 2013;46(5):867-881. Available at: https://doi.org/10.1016/j.otc.2013.06.006.

63. Lammers RL, Hudson DL, Seaman ME. Prediction of traumatic wound infection with a neural network-derived decision model. *Am J Emerg Med.* 2003;21(1):1-7. Available at: https://doi.org/10.1053/ajem.2003.50026.

64. Shin SH, Woo SS, Lee JH, et al. Analysis and management of pathogens isolated from patients with complicated facial lacerations and abrasions. *Int Wound J.* 2023;20(1):85-91. Available at: https://doi.org/10.1111/iwj.13842.

65. Key SJ, Thomas DW, Shepherd JP. The management of soft tissue facial wounds. *Br J Oral Maxillofac Surg.* 1995;33(2):76-85. Available at: https://doi.org/10.1016/0266-4356(95)90204-x.

66. Kretlow J, McKnight A, Izaddoost S. Facial Soft tissue trauma. *Semin Plast Surg.* 2010;24(4):348-356. Available at: https://doi.org/10.1055/s-0030-1269764.

67. Al-Abdullah T, Plint AC, Fergusson D. Absorbable versus nonabsorbable sutures in the management of traumatic lacerations and surgical wounds. *Pediatr Emerg Care.* 2007;23(5):339-344. Available at: https://doi.org/10.1097/01.pec.0000270167.70615.5a.

68. Perelman VS, Francis GJ, Rutledge T, Foote J, Martino F, Dranitsaris G. Sterile versus nonsterile gloves for repair of uncomplicated lacerations in the emergency department. *Ann Emerg Med.* 2004;43(3):362-370. Available at: https://doi.org/10.1016/j.annemergmed.2003.09.008.

69. Margolis DJ, Bartus C, Hoffstad O, Malay S, Berlin JA. Effectiveness of recombinant human platelet-derived growth factor for the treatment of diabetic neuropathic foot ulcers. *Wound Repair Regen.* 2005;13(6):531-536. Available at: https://doi.org/10.1111/j.1524-475X.2005.00074.x.

70. Hess CT. *Clinical Guide to Skin and Wound Care.* Philadelphia: Lippincott Williams & Wilkins; 2012.

71. Kloth LC, McCulloch JM. Promotion of wound healing with electrical stimulation. *Adv Wound Care.* 1996;9(5):42-45.

72. Chen X, Liu Y, Zhang X. Topical insulin application improves healing by regulating the wound inflammatory response. *Wound Repair Regen.* 2012;20(3):425-434. Available at: https://doi.org/10.1111/j.1524-475X.2012.00792.x.

73. Hopkins JT, McLoda TA, Seegmiller JG, David Baxter G. Low-level laser therapy facilitates superficial wound healing in humans: a triple-blind, sham-controlled study. *J Athl Train.* 2004;39(3):223-229.

74. Tocco I, Zavan B, Bassetto F, Vindigni V. Nanotechnology-based therapies for skin wound regeneration. *J Nanomater.* 2012;2012:4.

75. Chhabra S, Chhabra N, Kaur A, Gupta N. Wound healing concepts in clinical practice of OMFS. *J Maxillofac Oral Surg.* 2017;16(4):403-423. Available at: https://doi.org/10.1007/s12663-016-0880-z.

76. Sclafani AP, Mashkevich G. Aesthetic reconstruction of the auricle. *Facial Plast Surg Clin North Am.* 2006;14(2):103-116. Available at: https://doi.org/10.1016/j.fsc.2006.01.004.

77. Eagles K, Fralich L, Stevenson JH. Ear trauma. *Clin Sports Med.* 2013;32(2):303-316. Available at: https://doi.org/10.1016/j.csm.2012.12.011.

78. Bell RB, Osborn T, Dierks EJ, Potter BE, Long WB. Management of penetrating neck injuries: a new paradigm for civilian trauma. *J Oral Maxillofac Surg.* 2007;65(4):691-705. Available at: https://doi.org/10.1016/j.joms.2006.04.044.

79. Asensio JA, Chahwan S, Forno W, et al. Penetrating esophageal injuries: multicenter study of the American Association for the Surgery of Trauma. *J Trauma.* 2001;50(2):289-296. Available at: https://doi.org/10.1097/00005373-200102000-00015.

80. Weiman DS, Walker WA, Brosnan KM, Pate JW, Fabian TC. Noniatrogenic esophageal trauma. *Ann Thorac Surg.* 1995;59(4):845-850. Available at: https://doi.org/10.1016/0003-4975(95)00008-9.

81. Osborn TM, Bell RB, Qaisi W, Long WB. Computed tomographic angiography as an aid to clinical decision making in the selective management of penetrating injuries to the neck: a reduction in the need for operative exploration. *J Trauma.* 2008;64(6):1466-1471. Available at: https://doi.org/10.1097/ta.0b013e3181271b32.

82. Yeh S, Colyer MH, Weichel ED. Current trends in the management of intraocular foreign bodies. *Curr Opin Ophthalmol.* 2008;19(3):225-233. Available at: https://doi.org/10.1097/icu.0b013e3282fa75f1.

83. Abrahamian FM, Goldstein EJC. Microbiology of animal bite wound infections. *Clin Microbiol Rev.* 2011;24(2):231-246. Available at: https://doi.org/10.1128/cmr.00041-10.

84. Simpson WR. Physiological principles of therapy in head and neck cutaneous wounds. *Laryngoscope.* 1977;87(5):792-816. Available at: https://doi.org/0.1002/lary.5540870514.

85. Froind S, Parra AS, Segal N. Delayed diagnosis of intracranial injury due to a dog bite: a case report and review of the literature. *Int J Pediatr Otorhinolaryngol.* 2013;77(9):1400-1402. Available at: https://doi.org/10.1016/j.ijporl.2013.06.032.

86. Piccart F, Dormaar J, Coropciuc R, Schoenaers J, Bila M, Politis C. Dog bite injuries in the head and neck region: a 20-year review. *Craniomaxillofac Trauma Reconstr.* 2019;12(3):199-204.

87. Ladhani HA, Yowler CJ, Claridge JA. Burn wound colonization, infection, and sepsis. *Surg Infect.* 2021;22(1):44-48.

88. Olynik CR, Gray A, Sinada GG. Dentoalveolar trauma. *Otolaryngol Clin North Am.* 2013;46(5):807-823. Available at: https://doi.org/10.1016/j.otc.2013.06.009.

89. AlKhalifa JD, AlAzemi AA. Intrusive luxation of permanent teeth: a systematic review of factors important for treatment decision-making. *Dent Traumatol.* 2014;30(3):169-175. Available at: https://doi.org/10.1111/edt.12104.

90. Iida S, Kogo M, Sugiura T, Mima T, Matsuya T. Retrospective analysis of 1502 patients with facial fractures. *Int J Oral Maxillofac Surg.* 2001;30(4):286-290. Available at: https://doi.org/10.1054/ijom.2001.0056.

91. Lamphier J, Ziccardi V, Ruvo A, Janel M. Complications of mandibular fractures in an urban teaching center. *J Oral Maxillofac Surg.* 2003;61(7):745-749. Available at: https://doi.org/10.1016/s0278-2391(03)00147-2.

92. Gutta R, Tracy K, Johnson C, James LE, Krishnan DG, Marciani RD. Outcomes of mandible fracture treatment at an academic tertiary hospital: a 5-year analysis. *J Oral Maxillofac Surg.* 2014;72(3):550-558. Available at: https://doi.org/10.1016/j.joms.2013.09.005.

93. Biller JA, Pletcher SD, Goldberg AN, Murr AH. Complications and the time to repair of mandible fractures. *Laryngoscope.* 2005;115(5):769-772. Available at: https://doi.org/10.1097/01.mlg.0000157328.10583.a7.

94. Kambalimath HV, Agarwal SM, Kambalimath DH, Singh M, Jain N, Michael P. Maxillofacial injuries in children: a 10 year retrospective study. *J Maxillofac Oral Surg.* 2012;12(2):140-144. Available at: https://doi.org/10.1007/s12663-012-0402-6.

95. Panesar K, Susarla SM. Mandibular fractures: diagnosis and management. *Semin Plast Surg.* 2021;35(4):238-249. Available at: https://doi.org/10.1055/s-0041-1735818.

96. Shridharani SM, Berli J, Manson PN, Tufaro AP, Rodriguez ED. The role of postoperative antibiotics in mandible fractures: a systematic review of the literature. *Ann Plast Surg.* 2015;75(3):353. Available at: https://doi.org/10.1097/SAP.0000000000000135.

97. Odom EB, Snyder-Warwick AK. Mandible fracture complications and infection: the influence of demographics and modifiable factors. *Plast Reconstr Surg.* 2016;138(2):282e. Available at: https://doi.org/10.1097/PRS.0000000000002385.

98. Fernandes IA, Souza GM, Silva de Rezende V, et al. Effect of third molars in the line of mandibular angle fractures on postoperative complications: systematic review and meta-analysis. *Int J Oral Maxillofac Surg.* 2020;49(4):471-482. Available at: https://doi.org/10.1016/j.ijom.2019.09.017.

99. Hosgor H, Coskunses FM, Akin D. Evaluation of the prognosis of the teeth in the mandibular fracture line. *Craniomaxillofac Trauma Reconstr.* 2021;14(2):144-149. Available at: https://doi.org/10.1177/1943387520952673.

100. Khavanin N, Jazayeri H, Xu T, et al. Management of teeth in the line of mandibular angle fractures treated with open reduction and internal fixation: a systematic review and meta-analysis. *Plast Reconstr Surg.* 2019;144(6):1393. Available at: https://doi.org/10.1097/PRS.0000000000006255.

101. Shetty V, Freymiller E. Teeth in the line of fracture: a review. *J Oral Maxillofac Surg.* 1989;47(12):1303-1306. Available at: https://doi.org/10.1016/0278-2391(89)90729-5.

102. Ellis E, Price C. Treatment protocol for fractures of the atrophic mandible. *J Oral Maxillofac Surg.* 2008;66(3):421-435. Available at: https://doi.org/10.1016/j.joms.2007.08.042.

103. Koshy J, Feldman E, Chike-Obi C, Bullocks J. Pearls of mandibular trauma management. *Semin Plast Surg.* 2010;24(4):357-374. Available at: https://doi.org/10.1055/s-0030-1269765.

104. Gaal A, Bailey B, Patel Y, et al. Limiting antibiotics when managing mandible fractures may not increase infection risk. *J Oral Maxillofac Surg.* 2016;74(10):2008-2018. Available at: https://doi.org/10.1016/j.joms.2016.05.019.

105. Yamamoto MK, D'Avila RP, Luz JG de C. Evaluation of surgical retreatment of mandibular fractures. *J Craniomaxillofac Surg.* 2013;41(1):42-46. Available at: https://doi.org/10.1016/j.jcms.2012.05.008.

106. Mathog RH, Toma V, Clayman L, Wolf S. Nonunion of the mandible: an analysis of contributing factors. *J Oral Maxillofac Surg.* 2000;58(7):746-752. Available at: https://doi.org/10.1053/joms.2000.7258.

107. Ellis E. Management of fractures through the angle of the mandible. *Oral Maxillofac Surg Clin North Am.* 2009;21(2):163-174. Available at: https://doi.org/10.1016/j.coms.2008.12.004.

108. Morris LM, Kellman RM. Are prophylactic antibiotics useful in the management of facial fractures? *Laryngoscope.* 2013;124(6):1282-1284. Available at: https://doi.org/10.1002/lary.24364.

109. Chole RA, Yee J. Antibiotic prophylaxis for facial fractures: a prospective, randomized clinical trial. *Arch Otolaryngol Head Neck Surg.* 1987;113(10):1055-1057. Available at: https://doi.org/10.1001/archotol.1987.01860100033016.

110. Miles BA, Potter JK, Ellis E. The efficacy of postoperative antibiotic regimens in the open treatment of mandibular fractures: a prospective randomized trial. *J Oral Maxillofac Surg.* 2006;64(4):576-582. Available at: https://doi.org/10.1016/j.joms.2006.01.003.

111. Lovato C, Wagner JD. Infection rates following perioperative prophylactic antibiotics versus postoperative extended regimen prophylactic antibiotics in surgical management of mandibular fractures. *J Oral Maxillofac Surg.* 2009;67(4):827-832. Available at: https://doi.org/10.1016/j.joms.2008.06.093.

112. Singh RP, Carter LM, Whitfield PH. Antimicrobial prophylaxis in open reduction and internal fixation of compound mandibular fractures: a collaborative regional audit of outcome. *Br J Oral Maxillofac Surg.* 2013;51(5):444-447. Available at: https://doi.org/10.1016/j.bjoms.2012.08.019.

113. Kyzas PA. Use of antibiotics in the treatment of mandible fractures: a systematic review. *J Oral Maxillofac Surg.* 2011;69(4):1129-1145. Available at: https://doi.org/10.1016/j.joms.2010.02.059.

114. Bobrowski AN, Sonego CL, Chagas OL. Postoperative infection associated with mandibular angle fracture treatment in the presence of teeth on the fracture line: a systematic review and meta-analysis. *Int J Oral Maxillofac Surg.* 2013;42(9):1041-1048. Available at: https://doi.org/10.1016/j.ijom.2013.02.021.

115. Ehrlich A. Nasal septal abscess: an unusual complication of nasal trauma. *Am J Emerg Med.* 1993;11(2):149-150. Available at: https://doi.org/10.1016/0735-6757(93)90109-o.

116. Alshaikh N, Lo S. Nasal septal abscess in children: from diagnosis to management and prevention. *Int J Pediatr Otorhinolaryngol.* 2011;75(6):737-744. Available at: https://doi.org/10.1016/j.ijporl.2011.03.010.

117. Zix J, Schaller B, Iizuka T, Lieger O. The role of postoperative prophylactic antibiotics in the treatment of facial fractures: a randomised, double-blind, placebo-controlled pilot clinical study. Part 1: Orbital fractures in 62 patients. *Br J Oral Maxillofac Surg.*

2013;51(4):332-336. Available at: https://doi.org/10.1016/j.bjoms.2012.08.008.

118. Lane KA, Bilyk JR. Current concepts in the management of idiopathic orbital inflammation. In: *Oculoplastics and Orbit*. Berlin: Springer; 2010:47-65. Available at: https://doi.org/10.1007/978-3-540-85542-2_3.

119. Henry M, Hern HG. Traumatic injuries of the ear, nose and throat. *Emerg Med Clin North Am*. 2019;37(1):131-136. Available at: https://doi.org/10.1016/j.emc.2018.09.011.

120. Kuehnert MJ, Kruszon-Moran D, Hill HA, et al. Prevalence of *Staphylococcus aureus* nasal colonization in the United States, 2001–2002. *J Infect Dis*. 2006;193(2):172-179. Available at: https://doi.org/10.1086/499632.

121. Hardt N, Kuttenberger J, eds. *Craniofacial Trauma*. Berlin: Springer; 2010. Available at: https://doi.org/10.1007/978-3-540-33041-7.

122. Bell RB, Dierks EJ, Homer L, Potter BE. Management of cerebrospinal fluid leak associated with craniomaxillofacial trauma. *J Oral Maxillofac Surg*. 2004;62(6):676-684. Available at: https://doi.org/10.1016/j.joms.2003.08.032.

123. Bell RB, Dierks EJ, Brar P, Potter JK, Potter BE. A protocol for the management of frontal sinus fractures emphasizing sinus preservation. *J Oral Maxillofac Surg*. 2007;65(5):825-839. Available at: https://doi.org/10.1016/j.joms.2006.05.058.

124. Guy WM, Brissett AE. Contemporary management of traumatic fractures of the frontal sinus. *Otolaryngol Clin North Am*. 2013;46(5):733-748. Available at: https://doi.org/10.1016/j.otc.2013.07.005.

125. Doonquah L, Brown P, Mullings W. Management of frontal sinus fractures. *Oral Maxillofac Surg Clin North Am*. 2012;24(2):265-274. Available at: https://doi.org/10.1016/j.coms.2012.01.008.

126. Park CM, Stoffella E, Gile J, Roberts J, Herford AS. Osteoplasty flap technique for repair of latent (30-year) post-traumatic frontal sinus mucocele: case report and review of the literature. *J Oral Maxillofac Surg*. 2012;70(9):2092-2096. Available at: https://doi.org/10.1016/j.joms.2011.10.015.

127. Castro B, Walcott BP, Redjal N, Coumans JV, Nahed BV. Cerebrospinal fluid fistula prevention and treatment following frontal sinus fractures: a review of initial management and outcomes. *Neurosurg Focus*. 2012;32(6):E1. Available at: https://doi.org/10.3171/2012.3.focus1266.

128. Diaz RC, Cervenka B, Brodie HA. Treatment of temporal bone fractures. *J Neurol Surg Part B Skull Base*. 2016;77(5):419-429.

129. Lukošiūnas A, Kubilius R, Sabalys G, Keizeris T, Sakavičius D. An analysis of etiological factors for traumatic mandibular osteomyelitis. *Medicina*. 2011;47(7):380. Available at: https://doi.org/10.3390/medicina47070054.

130. Pincus D, Armstrong M, Thaller S. Osteomyelitis of the craniofacial skeleton. *Semin Plast Surg*. 2009;23(2):73-79. Available at: https://doi.org/10.1055/s-0029-1214159.

131. Prasad KC, Prasad SSC, Mouli N, Agarwal S. Osteomyelitis in the head and neck. *Acta Otolaryngol*. 2007;127(2):194-205. Available at: https://doi.org/10.1080/00016480600818054.

132. Spellberg B, Lipsky BA. Systemic antibiotic therapy for chronic osteomyelitis in adults. *Clin Infect Dis*. 2011;54(3):393-407. Available at: https://doi.org/10.1093/cid/cir842.

133. Taher AAY. Osteomyelitis of the mandible in Tehran, Iran. *Oral Surg Oral Med Oral Pathol*. 1993;76(1):28-31. Available at: https://doi.org/10.1016/0030-4220(93)90288-f.

134. von See C, Rana M, Stoetzer M, Wilker C, Rücker M, Gellrich NC. A new model for the characterization of infection risk in gunshot injuries: technology, principal consideration and clinical implementation. *Head Face Med*. 2011;7(1):18. Available at: https://doi.org/10.1186/1746-160x-7-18.

135. Santucci RA, Chang YJ. Ballistics for physicians: myths about wound ballistics and gunshot injuries. *J Urol*. 2004;171(4):1408-1414. Available at: https://doi.org/10.1097/01.ju.0000103691.68995.04.

136. Biaggi-Ondina AP, Deramo P, Kothamasu VS, Kim BW, Wainwright DJ. Infections and antibiotic usage in facial gunshot wounds. *Plast Reconstr Surg Glob Open*. 2020;8(suppl 9):63. Available at: https://doi.org/10.1097/01.GOX.0000720616.05710.e0.

137. Motamedi MHK. Primary treatment of penetrating injuries to the face. *J Oral Maxillofac Surg*. 2007;65(6):1215-1218. Available at: https://doi.org/10.1016/j.joms.2007.03.001.

138. Atesalp AS, Yildiz C, Başbozkurt M, Gür GE. Treatment of type IIIa open fractures with Ilizarov fixation and delayed primary closure in high-velocity gunshot wounds. *Mil Med*. 2002;167(1):56-62. Available at: https://doi.org/10.1093/milmed/167.1.56.

139. Nguyen MP, Como JJ, Golob JF, Reich MS, Vallier HA. Variation in treatment of low energy gunshot injuries: a survey of OTA members. *Injury*. 2018;49(3):570-574. Available at: https://doi.org/10.1016/j.injury.2018.01.027.

140. Baum GR, Baum JT, Hayward D, MacKay BJ. Gunshot wounds: ballistics, pathology, and treatment recommendations, with a focus on retained bullets. *Orthop Res Rev*. 2022;14:293-317. Available at: https://doi.org/10.2147/ORR.S378278.

141. Omid R, Stone MA, Zalavras CG, Marecek GS. Gunshot wounds to the upper extremity. *J Am Acad Orthop Surg*. 2019;27(7):e301. Available at: https://doi.org/10.5435/JAAOS-D-17-00676.

142. Stefanopoulos PK, Pinialidis DE, Hadjigeorgiou GF, Filippakis KN. Wound ballistics 101: the mechanisms of soft tissue wounding by bullets. *Eur J Trauma Emerg Surg*. 2017;43(5):579-586. Available at: https://doi.org/10.1007/s00068-015-0581-1.

143. Gelesko S, Bui TG, Park ES, Dierks EJ, Bobek SL, Bell RB. A protocol for computer planning and intraoperative imaging as an aid to reconstruction of gunshot wounds to the face. *J Oral Maxillofac Surg*. 2013;71(9):e7-e8. Available at: https://doi.org/10.1016/j.joms.2013.06.013.

144. Chaiyasate K, Gupta R, Boudiab EM, et al. Comprehensive treatment and reconstructive algorithm for functional restoration after ballistic facial injury. *Plast Reconstr Surg Glob Open*. 2022;10(7):e4453. Available at: https://doi.org/10.1097/GOX.0000000000004453.

145. Islamoglu K, Coskunfirat OK, Tetik G, Ozgentas HE. Complications and removal rates of miniplates and screws used for maxillofacial fractures. *Ann Plast Surg*. 2002;48(3):265-268. Available at: https://doi.org/10.1097/00000637-200203000-00006.

146. Rallis G, Mourouzis C, Papakosta V, Papanastasiou G, Zachariades N. Reasons for miniplate removal following maxillofacial trauma: a 4-year study. *J Craniomaxillofac Surg*. 2006;34(7):435-439. Available at: https://doi.org/10.1016/j.jcms.2006.07.001.

147. Thorén H, Snäll J, Kormi E, Lindqvist C, Suominen-Taipale L, Törnwall J. Symptomatic plate removal after treatment of facial fractures. *J Craniomaxillofac Surg*. 2010;38(7):505-510. Available at: https://doi.org/10.1016/j.jcms.2010.01.005.

148. Hernandez Rosa J, Villanueva NL, Sanati-Mehrizy P, Factor SH, Taub PJ. Review of maxillofacial hardware complications and indications for salvage. *Craniomaxillofac Trauma Reconstr*. 2016;9(2):134-140.

149. Bakathir AA, Margasahayam MV, Al-Ismaily MI. Removal of bone plates in patients with maxillofacial trauma: a retrospective study. *Oral Surg Oral Med Oral Pathol Oral Radiol Endod*. 2008;105(5):e32-e37. Available at: https://doi.org/10.1016/j.tripleo.2008.01.006.

27

Infections Following Head and Neck Reconstruction

AMIR AZARI, ELIE M. FERNEINI, AND R. BRYAN BELL

Surgery of the oral cavity, mandible, midface, cranium, cutaneous tissues, and scalp have benefited from technological advancements in reconstruction during the past few decades, especially regarding the use of free vascularized flaps. However, flap, donor site, and remote infections are important causes of reconstruction failure; in addition, the incidence of these complications can be high, depending on risk exposures discussed in this chapter. In general, the surgical infection rate for head and neck reconstruction varies widely among institutions, with reported values such as 4,[1] 20,[2] and 39%.[3] Infection is an especially common problem in the postoperative course of head and neck cancer reconstruction, requiring readmissions, additional surgical procedures, and prolonged hospital stays.[2,4] Postreconstruction complications are among the most frequently reported causes of morbidity despite antibiotic prophylaxis;[5-8] therefore, they warrant careful attention to risk classification and prevention.

Limitations of the Literature

Unfortunately, much of the literature guiding the prevention of surgical site infections (SSIs) is retrospective. Potential risk factors are numerous, and although many have been identified, studies are often incomparable because of differences in wound infection definitions, surgical indications, resection and reconstructive donor sites, and inclusion or exclusion of donor or recipient site infections.[9] Successful modalities in facial reconstruction are often reported as case series that are generally biased toward positive results. Ultimately, the goal of this chapter lies in optimizing outcomes, while considering institutional and surgeon preferences.

Disease Characteristics

To some extent, the infection risk in head and neck surgery is related to the defect being reconstructed. Clean, uncontaminated head and neck procedures (typically those that do not violate mucosal barriers) are thought to have low postoperative infection rates,[10] which could influence reconstruction outcomes. However, one recent retrospective review counters this assumption by describing no statistically significant difference between flap and donor site infections in clean-contaminated versus clean procedures.[11] Nevertheless, the stage of disease and extent of the ablative defect generally portend a greater chance of wound infection because of increased reconstruction complexity.[12]

Health Status

Higher American Society of Anesthesiology (ASA) physical status has been cited as a general factor in increased infection risk,[13] especially in relation to age. It is likely that comorbid conditions that increase with age have a greater role in the development of site infections than age itself.[14] This conclusion has been corroborated in large studies that have shown no significant increase in reconstructive complications considering age alone.[15-18] In a sample of 10 patients older than 90 years who underwent free flap reconstruction, only one donor site and one recipient site infection was noted.[19] Nevertheless, wound infections and pneumonia remain the most common sources of infection in patients older than 80 years who have undergone head and neck reconstruction.[20]

Other patient characteristics, such as smoking, dental health, and presence of infections other than SSIs have been implicated as risk factors in some studies, but not in others.[3,14] Trials and retrospective reviews conducted involving reconstruction of oral cavity tumor ablations demonstrate varying significance of diabetes, ASA score, and duration of surgery.[14,21,22] There is some agreement that dental health and intraoperative dental extraction are not related to increases in SSIs.[3] Other risk factors associated with higher risk of postoperative infections include need for postoperative transfusions and higher T and N stage on patients with cancer. There was also a correlation between the increase in surgery duration, hospitalization, and intensive care unit stay with higher risk of infection.[23]

Transfusion

Allogenic blood transfusions are relatively common in patients undergoing head and neck free flap reconstruction, and have been implicated as a risk factor for SSIs in some studies. Transfusion is often a function of surgical complexity and patient comorbidity, and is difficult to isolate as an independent factor for wound infection.[24] Operative blood loss is the relevant predisposing factor, especially in relation to patients with higher T stages; reports have described the extent of blood loss as a significant contributor to SSIs.[6,13,21,25] Furthermore, institutions may have threshold criteria for transfusion, especially for free vascularized flaps. Studies have shown that flap outcomes are adversely affected by transfusion,[26] and patient outcomes improve with fewer units being transfused. This result includes fewer wound infections reported in those who received 0 to 2 units of blood compared with greater than 3 units in a review of 167 patients.[27] A dose-response relationship has been suggested, with each additional unit of leukocyte-depleted red cells increasing the number of postoperative complications.[28] Authors of another review of 129 free flaps suggested lowering the threshold criteria for transfusion to 25% hematocrit, reduced from the traditional 30%.[26]

Radiation and Chemotherapy

Tissue scarring and fibrosis related to prior radiation or chemotherapy increases the complexity of primary and secondary reconstruction. Radiation therapy leads to fibroblast dysfunction, collagen disrepair, and prolonged wound healing, all of which contribute to an increased risk for wound infection in reconstruction.[29-31] Because of the variation of radiation doses, protocols, and timing in relation to surgery, there is little consensus in the literature regarding the extent or significance of this risk.[25] Some studies suggest that radiation therapy is a risk factor in the development of SSIs,[30] but not for flap loss.[32,33] On the other hand, one prospective study found that previous neck dissection was strongly correlated with wound infection, as well as flap loss and need for revision.[34] It has been postulated that these complications are caused by the alteration of anatomy, ligation, or prior injury of potential recipient vessels.[34] It follows that distortions of anatomy, whether by previous surgery or radiation, can mask the detection of occult infections and require careful attention to signs and symptoms of wound breakdown.

Free vascularized flaps avoid complications associated with fibrotic changes in the recipient bed, and can be used to mitigate the risk of wound dehiscence in cases with prior radiation.[22] However, it is important to recognize that the effects of radiation therapy extend up to 6 months after the last radiation dose, with increased levels of transforming growth factor-β1 implicated in infection and wound disruption; this process will affect both free tissue transfers and pedicled flaps.[35] When combined with hardware implantation for fixation purposes, radiation has been associated with double the number of plate infections and increased

risk of fracture, exposure, or nonunion.[36,37] Patients who undergo radiation therapy as part of their treatment for head and neck cancer are at increased susceptibility for osteoradionecrosis (ORN), which has potentially deleterious effects on outcomes of subsequent reconstruction. In the irradiated patient, free flap reconstruction has been shown to be most advantageous in introducing nonirradiated tissue and an independent blood supply, both of which can be compromised with local flaps.[32]

Chemotherapy complicates surgery further in modifying the normal immunologic response to bacteria by reducing immune cell chemotaxis, opsonization, and agglutination, lysis of bacteria, and destruction of bacterial toxins.[9] A prospective trial of wound infections with and without previous chemotherapy found the incidence to be 65 versus 41%, respectively.[9]

Mucosal Involvement

Data from hypopharyngeal tumor removal suggest that opening of the aerodigestive tract is an independent risk factor for wound infection, although the true risk is frequently confounded by increased surgical complexity, preoperative or postoperative chemoradiation, and comorbidities of heavy drinking or smoking.[5,6] Opening of the oral mucosa has been cited as less likely to predispose patients to infection compared with opening the oropharynx, although this may be due to less frequent communication with the neck wound than any property of the oral mucosa.[24] In the oropharynx, direct exposure to the aerodigestive mucosa with establishment of adequate tumor margins may expose the reconstruction site to polymicrobial flora within the oral cavity.[14] Similar exposure by proximity can occur in skull base reconstruction, which must include separation of the contaminated aerodigestive mucosa from the dura, thereby avoiding occult infection.[38] Unsurprisingly, open wounds created by flap exposures (especially pharyngocutaneous fistulas) are considered worrisome, because they signify a persistent underlying infectious risk.[39]

Overall, it is clear that reconstruction of cutaneous wounds not involving mucosal surfaces is less prone to bacterial contaminants. Cutaneous defects offer the advantage of ready sterility and access, shorter insetting time, and easier postoperative monitoring, all of which may contribute to a lesser infection rate. Therefore, it is not surprising that patients with cutaneous defects experience shorter hospital stays and fewer complications.[16]

Osteomyelitis

Osteomyelitis of the craniofacial skeleton presents difficulty in reconstructing intricate contours of the face that have usually already been disturbed by previous surgical manipulation. In general, defects left after debridement of this infected tissue lend themselves toward reconstruction with vascularized flaps, in consideration of possible secondary infection of alloplastic materials.[40] Nevertheless, alloplastic materials in reconstruction of calvarial, lateral skull base, temporal bone, orbit, midface, and mandibular defects allow for customized and prefabricated reconstructions.[40]

Reconstruction Options

Free Flap

The major types of flaps used in head and neck reconstruction include the fibula, radial forearm, anterolateral thigh, latissimus dorsi, scapula, iliac crest, and jejunum. Refinements in surgical technique and widespread use of these flaps have allowed for more complex and successful reconstructions than in the past. Improved outcomes from an independent vascular supply relative to nonvascularized bone grafts and pedicled flaps in an irradiated field include fewer cerebrospinal fluid leaks, site infections, and meningitis rates,[41] regardless of recipient site in the craniofacial skeleton.[42]

The literature provides conflicting reports[43,44] regarding the infectious complication rates of various flaps, as flap choice is often guided by institutional or surgeon preference and reconstructive requirements. In a large retrospective cohort, the type of microvascular free flap was not found to significantly influence complication rate.[16] In other smaller cohorts, the opposite has been found,[30] including greater postoperative infections associated with iliac crest compared with fibula flaps.[44]

Donor site infections are a significant consideration in harvesting the vascularized flap and include wound dehiscence with subsequent tendon exposure, cellulitis, or abscess formation[45] (Figure 27-1). The skin paddle site is typically covered by a split-thickness skin graft from a third surgical site, which contributes to the infectious risk. Negative-pressure dressings have been proposed to facilitate graft success, although they may be associated with an increase in infectious complications.[46] Adjunct allograft materials[47] and full-thickness skin grafts from the neck[48] also have been used with no significant increased infectious risk. There is no

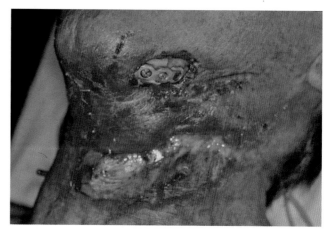

• **Figure 27-2** Infected Recipient Site with Fibular Osteocutaneous Free Flap Failure. The previously operated, radiated, soft tissue and vessel-depleted neck offers perhaps the most significant reconstructive challenge anywhere in the body, with an increased infection rate contributing to a higher risk of flap failure.

significant difference reported in donor site infections between osteocutaneous and soft-tissue flaps[49] or between osteocutaneous and osseous flaps.[45] As long as the vascular pedicle remains patent, infections of the graft generally will not lead to total flap failure (Figure 27-2).

There is evidence that case volume also plays a role in treatment outcomes. The majority of hospitals in which surgeons perform head and neck cancer surgeries are low-volume centers, performing approximately six cases per year.[50] One study found a significantly lower incidence (by 44%) of mortality in higher volume centers after flaps needing rescue, although this was not associated with an increased rate of overall complications.[50]

Pedicle Flaps

The complication rates for both local and free flaps have been reported as 27%, with infection accounting for 7%, in a review of 77 patients.[51] Although infectious complications of pedicled versus free flaps have not been found to be significantly different, the recipient site and type of flap used are viewed as independent risk factors to complications, perhaps because of the increased operating time and added complexity.[14] For example, in skull base surgery, selected use of pedicled flaps (temporalis muscle, pericranial) in limited defect sizes has been reported to be very predictable, with shorter operative time and hospital stay, and complication rates similar to those for free flaps.[52] Successful reconstruction of defects involving violation of the dura has been reported to be less contingent on the type or origin of the flap, but on appropriate dural repair and coverage with well-vascularized tissue.[51]

Nonvascularized Bone Grafts

To promote optimal healing, nonvascularized autogenous grafts should be kept away from mucosal or other

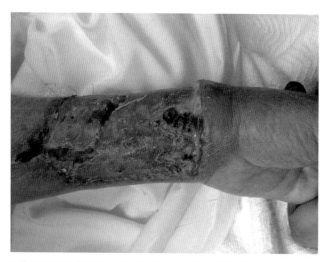

• **Figure 27-1** Infected Radial Forearm Free Flap Donor Site with Exposed Tendon.

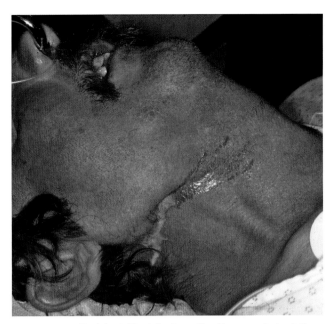

• **Figure 27-3** Recipient Site Infection after Nonvascularized Bone Graft Reconstruction of a Continuity Defect of the Mandible. Continuity mandibular defects greater than 6 cm should be reconstructed with microvascular free tissue transfer.

contaminated surfaces and protected by watertight sutures. In one review, the most common indicator of infection and most common cause of graft failure was wound dehiscence[53] (Figure 27-3). Bone extrusion following dehiscence can then hasten or compound the inflammatory response and graft resorption.[54] One method to avoid this problem includes a staged procedure, with secondary reconstruction through an extraoral approach. Reports from this method indicate a lower infection and loss rate of the graft at 3% and donor site morbidity at 2% with harvesting at the posterior iliac crest.[55] Reconstruction using allogenic bone grafts avoids many of the potential complications of donor sites compared with vascularized flaps, and is generally less time consuming and less resource intensive.

Some surgeons have advocated the use of nonvascularized bone grafts for reconstruction of oncologic defects,[56] but this approach has largely been abandoned in the free flap era, given the reliability of vascularized free tissue transfer and the need for postoperative radiation in many head and neck cancer patients. If nonvascularized bone grafts are used to reconstruct oncologic defects because of poor recipient sites for the vascular pedicle or other reasons, the general principles of osteosynthesis must be followed strictly to prevent mobility, nonunion, and infection. Sites of composite resections are less favorable for this type of reconstruction, as dead space from tissue loss may persist. Thus, two-layer watertight closure and the presence of a sufficient soft tissue envelope in a healthy wound bed are requirements for grafting success.[57]

Distraction Osteogenesis

Transport-disc distraction has been used successfully in the reconstruction of large segmental defects, but it requires an intact soft tissue bed and periosteum to facilitate bone growth. Favorable settings include benign conditions not involving radiation and conditions not involving soft tissue defects.[57] Because there is no donor site, complications are limited to the surgical site; however, it is unclear whether this leads to improved outcomes with fewer overall infections or complications compared with free tissue transfer.[58]

Fixation

Trials in maxillofacial trauma have demonstrated that certain fixation plate combinations are less likely to result in postoperative complications. In reconstructive surgery, fixation techniques must also account for compromised blood flow and healing capabilities of the previously operated and irradiated tissue bed. Hardware infections can result from loosened screws (with the use of nonlocking plates), biofilm formation on the plate surface, osseous mobility, plate fracture, or plate exposure.[36] Reconstruction plates themselves are not associated with increased risk of infection, even in irradiated bone.[59] The current trend toward using 2-mm miniplates instead of or as adjuncts to reconstruction plates also has not been associated with increased complication rates.[36]

Biomaterials

Prefabricated and custom implants avoid donor site complications entirely and can be manipulated to replicate the normal contour of the defect site. These implants may be composed of materials such as natural or synthetic polymers, bioactive ceramics (e.g., hydroxyapatite), metals, or other scaffolds.[60] A review of these materials has found that outcome differences between these could be attributed more often to the size and location of the defect than to the properties of the implants themselves.[61] In particular, colonization of implants near mucosal surfaces should be avoided to reduce osteomyelitis or chronic infections requiring implant removal.[60,62] Recombinant human bone morphogenic proteins also have been reported with some success in the reconstruction of segmental defects of the mandible,[63] and although determination of efficacy and outcomes is ongoing, there does not appear to be an increased risk of infection with their use.

Dental Implants

Dental implants are used in areas of bone reconstruction for replacement of teeth and masticatory function. In patients who undergo reconstruction with osteoseptocutaneous flaps, thick subcutaneous tissue might not function as well as native keratinized gingiva, leading to increased mucositis and poor prosthesis hygiene.[64] Implants placed within the transplanted fibula free flap, however, have been shown to have similar complication rates compared with native mandibles or maxillae.[65] Palatal mucosal grafts and double-barreled fibulae have been reported as helpful in the optimization of dental implant outcomes.[66] Implant failures caused by infection have not been reported with significant difference in nonvascularized bone grafts versus free flaps.[67] Implant loss caused by periimplantitis is greater in patients who have undergone radiation therapy;[68,69] therefore, a waiting period (6 to 12 months)[70,71] has been recommended to allow the implanted bone to revascularize. To that end, hyperbaric oxygen (HBO) therapy has not been found to reduce implant failure or decrease infection rates.[72]

Computer-Assisted Design

Comparison of conventional fibular free flap reconstruction versus computer-aided design using surgical cutting guides has shown similar rates of postoperative infection and flap failure in a retrospective review of 68 patients.[73] A recent systematic review of 33 cases validates the potential of virtual surgical planning in improving oncologic reconstruction outcomes.[74] Another review of virtually planned iliac crest vascularized grafts found a statistically significant reduction in donor defect size and ischemia time compared with conventional surgery.[75] Operating time might be reduced[76] because of better presurgical planning, but it is unclear whether this modality can reduce infection or other complication rates. As research expands in this domain, the benefits of improved intraoperative efficiency may be realized for free vascularized flaps.

Infectious Complications

One of the primary goals for reconstruction of maxillofacial defects is optimization of the wound to prevent infectious complications. Dead space from the extirpation of the muscles of mastication, salivary glands, buccal fat, and other structures is complicated by constant motion of the remaining facial musculature: deglutition, mastication, and the cough reflex.[21] Poorly drained dead spaces can develop seromas or hematomas that lead to infection.[38] In turn, infection may spread and compromise the flap pedicle vasculature. Early identification and aggressive debridement, antibiotic therapy, and watertight closure are required,[77] especially in anticipation of contamination with upper aerodigestive tract flora. The infectious source should be controlled surgically, and the patient should be treated with appropriate antibiotic therapy, because spread can lead to thrombosis of the vascular pedicle and complete flap loss.[38,39,78-80]

Superficial infections (Table 27-1) have not been shown to alter morbidity after reconstructive surgery.[5] In an attempt to identify patients at risk for deep-incisional infections, one study has reported success in culturing wound drainage every other day after surgery, with a statistically significant, decreased incidence of deep infection after the third postoperative day of no culture growth.[81] Salivary fistulas occur infrequently (<5%); most fistulas will heal with secondary intention and only rarely pose a risk to anastomotic patency.[78]

Passive drains are not recommended, as wounds will contain persistent dead spaces, which contain inoculum for bacteria. The importance of proper drainage to prevent dead space and fluid accumulation in the head and neck reconstruction patient is paramount. Although some consideration has been given to the potential for active drains to compromise the patency of the vascular pedicle, they are generally preferred over passive drains in both free and pedicled flap anastomoses.[82] Of note, based on the guidelines published by the American Society of Health System Pharmacists, there are no data to support the continuation of antibiotics for the duration of indwelling drain placement.[83]

Microbes

The majority of infectious species in oncologic head and neck surgery are gram-negative aerobes and anaerobes,

TABLE 27-1	Criteria for Defining Surgical Site Infections in Head and Neck Reconstruction	
Classification	Historical Findings	Physical Findings
Superficial incisional SSI	Infection occurs within 30 days after operation and extends to skin or subcutaneous tissue only	Purulent drainage, pain, swelling, redness, heat, or growth of organisms in tissue culture
Deep incisional SSI	Infection occurs within 30 days after operation, or 1 year if related to an implanted material, and involves deeper soft tissues (e.g., fascia, muscle)	Purulent drainage, fever, pain, growth of organisms in tissue culture, or radiologic evidence of abscess
Organ or space SSI	Infection occurs within 30 days after the operation, or 1 year if related to an implanted material, and involves spaces manipulated during surgery but outside the area of incision	Purulent drainage, fever, pain, growth of organisms in tissue culture, or radiologic evidence of abscess

SSI, Surgical site infection.

Adapted from Mangram AJ, Horan TC, Pearson ML, et al. Guideline for prevention of surgical site infection, 1999. Hospital Infection Control Practices Advisory Committee. *Infect Control Hosp Epidemiol.* 1999;20(4):250-278.

especially those that produce β-lactamases. Nosocomial pathogens are also frequent causes of SSI; *Pseudomonas aeruginosa* is a predominant species and frequently resistant to standard perioperatively administered antibiotics.[84] Methicillin-resistant *Staphylococcus aureus* (MRSA), *Klebsiella pneumoniae,* and other enteric bacteria are other common nosocomial sources. However, the rate and causative organism of infections is not necessarily correlated to the number or type of bacterial contaminants in the surgical field.[7] In one report of more than 500 cultured free flap cases, existing skin or oral flora introduced to the wound during surgery were found to cause early wound infections, whereas late-onset infections included other bacteria acquired secondarily.[11] In this study, the majority of both donor and recipient site infections occurred more than 1 week postoperatively, leading to a recommendation for effective patient monitoring, follow-up, and perioperative antibiotic dosing as described in the following section. The tracheostomy site has been reported as a significant infectious risk in this regard, likely secondary to colonization with respiratory secretions.[6,29] Owing to multiple potential sources of contamination, wounds are often polymicrobial and may culture positive for fungi, especially *Candida albicans.*[14]

Hospital-Acquired Conditions and Remote Infections

Hospital-acquired infections are the most commonly acquired conditions described in patients with head and neck cancer and are likely prevalent to the same degree in patients with other diagnoses who have undergone reconstruction. In a nationwide cross-sectional sample, vascular catheter– and central line–associated infections accounted for more than 80% of such infected patients. Overall, the incidence of nosocomial infections was described as very low (<1%) and associated with more fragile patients, major surgical procedures, or urgent or emergent admissions.[85]

In another study of 225 patients, nonwound infections accounted for 10% of the patient population, with the most common causes being pneumonias or urinary tract infections. These patients had a statistically significant prolonged hospital stay by at least 3 days.[86] Atelectasis in the lungs should be minimized with the understanding that head and neck surgery often impairs the natural mechanisms of mucus clearance from the airways. Another retrospective study of oropharyngeal cancer removal with concomitant free flap reconstruction found that these remote infections are significantly more likely to occur in the setting of existing SSI.[21] The relationship between infection at either the wound or remote site may be related to the systemically compromised host, and demonstrates the importance of early detection and prompt treatment of either infectious site. In fact, a large retrospective review of general head and neck surgical patients found that the first two postoperative days are most important for the surveillance of cardiac and respiratory complications, and that high-risk patients may benefit from more intensive care during this period.[87]

Prevention

Prophylaxis

Prophylaxis is recommended for all clean-contaminated reconstructive surgeries of the head and neck,[88] although there is little consensus regarding the type of antibiotic prophylaxis in the literature (Table 27-2).[5] Antibiotic regimens are generally directed toward bacteriologic flora found along the mucosal lining of the upper aerodigestive tract. Importantly, coverage for *Pseudomonas* species, oral flora, and MRSA has been recommended for both early and late wound infections.[11] In tumor reconstruction, duration of antibiotic therapy beyond 24 hours has not been found clinically useful in reducing wound infections;[11,77,89,90]

TABLE 27-2 **Recommendations for Surgical Antimicrobial Prophylaxis**

Procedure Type	Recommended Agents	Alternative Agents	Strength of Evidence*
Clean	None	None	B
Clean with prosthesis	Cefazolin, cefuroxime	Clindamycin	C
Clean-contaminated (oncologic)	Cefazolin plus metronidazole, cefuroxime plus metronidazole, ampicillin-sulbactam	Clindamycin	A
Clean-contaminated (nononcologic)	Cefazolin plus metronidazole, cefuroxime with metronidazole, ampicillin-sulbactam	Clindamycin	B

*Strength of evidence involves randomized controlled trials or well-conducted cohort trials (A), case control studies or conflicting but generally positive studies (B), or expert opinion (C). Based on the comprehensive guideline, these recommendations would cover prophylaxis for surgery at donor sites for free vascularized or pedicled flaps commonly used in reconstruction.
Adapted from Bratzler DW, Dellinger EP, Olsen KM, et al. Clinical practice guidelines for antimicrobial prophylaxis in surgery. *Am J Health Syst Pharm.* 2013;70:195-283.

in fact, it might actually increase the rate of opportunistic infections.[3] Empiric therapies are used in cases of active infection. Institutional practice may deviate from these evidence-based recommendations because of the tremendous costs of failure[91] and poor outcomes, especially in the setting of postoperative infection.

Methicillin-Resistant *Staphylococcus aureus*

In a trial screening for MRSA before free flap reconstruction of the head and neck, only those who had previous MRSA infection, had a preexisting wound, or were from high-risk environments benefited from screening. Although some investigators do not recommend routine screening,[92] standard contact precautions and limited contact with multiple health care workers play an important role in limiting nosocomial exposure. Others advocate routine screening and decolonization of all surgical patients, citing successes in reduced SSI in general surgery and orthopedic procedures.[11] Most MRSA infections are acquired from the hospital environment, but prolonged courses of antibiotics are not an indication for MRSA prevention; instead, a standard course of perioperative and less than 1 day of postoperative antibiotics is recommended.[49] Nasal mupirocin has been reported to reduce the risk of MRSA infection and has been recommended for use in prolonged surgical cases in high-risk patients (e.g., poor nutritional status, prolonged antibiotic courses, ongoing steroid use). Case-by-case selection should be used to reduce the incidence of mupirocin-resistant MRSA.[93] Prolonged use (>24 or 48 hours) of systemic antibiotics is a prominent risk factor for resistant infections,[3] including MRSA.

Topical Antibiotics

Topical antimicrobials have been proposed as an adjunct in the prevention of SSIs, although the data in favor are not definitive. One randomized controlled trial evaluating 2% mupirocin ointment applied intranasally with 2% chlorhexidine gluconate showers for 5 days preceding surgery showed a strong but statistically insignificant trend toward benefit (seven patients needed to treat to prevent infection).[13] This regimen may be useful in patients who are at high risk for infection.[13] Oral cavity rinses are a mainstay in the decontamination before reconstructive surgery involving the oral mucosa. Most commonly, solutions containing chlorhexidine-gluconate are used in 0.12, 0.2, and 1% concentrations. These solutions have an antiseptic effect that lasts longer than povidone-iodine solutions, especially against anaerobes and with some effectiveness against aerobes. A randomized prospective trial comparing saline, iodine, chlorhexidine, and cetrimide found that mechanical cleansing with cetrimide or 1% chlorhexidine solution resulted in a statistically significant decrease in bacterial load.[94] Clindamycin has also been proposed for oral cavity rinses and for intraoperative irrigation of the neck and surgical sites with beneficial results.[95]

Nutrition

Extensive reconstruction often follows ablation for conditions predisposing patients to malnutrition through tumor-induced cachexia, excessive alcohol consumption, or poor dietary habits. Additionally, nutritional status and postoperative dysphagia can negatively affect surgical outcomes after head and neck surgery.[96] Preoperative hypoalbuminemia (<3.5 g/dL) has been considered as a prognostic marker for nutritional and inflammatory status and as a risk factor for SSI.[29,97] This has been corroborated in the gastrointestinal surgery literature, and is thought to be due to impairment of the immune system, of antibiotic penetration, and of wound edema.[98] Immunonutrition has been proposed as a method to reduce infectious complications in the postoperative period.[99] For example, enteral and parenteral feeds supplemented with arginine, which serves in the formation of nitric oxide, are thought to promote immune function and reduce infection.[100] A recent multicenter, prospective, randomized, double-blinded study found that immunonutrition has significant benefit when administered preoperatively, and postoperatively only when administered at greater than 75% of goal feeds. Near the goal feeding volume, systemic infections, SSIs (at the primary site, neck wound, and donor sites), and length of stay were significantly reduced.[101] A systematic review of arginine-enriched formulas found similar reductions in length of hospital stay even when only postoperative enteral immunonutrition was used.[100] It is less clear whether immunonutrition, also called *pharmaconutrition,* provides more or less benefit to malnourished versus well-nourished patients. Although there is significant clinical evidence of benefits in both head and neck reconstruction and other surgical specialties, improved clinical outcomes are thought to depend more on dosing of individual nutrients rather than standard formulations of immunonutrients.[102] Preoperative evaluation of nutritional status should help guide preoperative nutrition, perioperative adherence to feeding goals, and postoperative supplementation with immunonutrition when possible.[103]

Hyperbaric Oxygen

Postoperative infection complications in irradiated patients should be managed aggressively, regardless of HBO therapy, to prevent fistula formation or vessel rupture. Findings from the literature are equivocal regarding the role of preoperative or postoperative HBO therapy in reducing such complications, and it is the authors' opinion that HBO need not be routinely recommended in the treatment of ORN.[32] In fact, one study found a paradoxical increase in postoperative infections in patients who underwent HBO therapy,[104] whereas another randomized, double-blinded, and placebo-controlled multicenter trial found no benefit in cases of reconstruction for mandibular ORN.[105] There is some evidence for potential benefit in head and neck reconstruction,[106] but appropriate patient selection and therapeutic timing have yet to be defined. It is recommended that referral for HBO therapy should be considered in selected situations, such as in compromised recipient sites or large composite grafts or to aid in the survival of compromised or salvaged flaps.[107]

A recent study indicated 14 approved indications for HBO therapy. However, more studies are needed to evaluate the effectiveness of HBO in other types of infection, including SSIs.[108]

Summary

Despite the lack of high-level evidence from clinical trials regarding risk factors predisposing patients to SSI, it seems prudent to assess patients' risk preoperatively based on a general state of health and preexisting comorbidities. Previous history of surgery, radiation, or chemotherapy; poor nutritional status; length and complexity of reconstruction; and immune status may be useful indicators for closer patient observation. Reconstruction involving mucosal surfaces of the oral or nasal cavities, pharynx, or larynx, should be covered for gram-positive and anaerobic microbes both perioperatively and postoperatively for 24 hours. Topical antibiotic rinses in the oral cavity may also be useful in reducing infectious risk.

References

1. Smith GI, O'Brien CJ, Choy ET, et al. Clinical outcome and technical aspects of 263 radial forearm free flaps used in reconstruction of the oral cavity. *Br J Oral Maxillofac Surg.* 2005;43:199-204.
2. Cloke DJ, Green JE, Khan AL, et al. Factors influencing the development of wound infection following free-flap reconstruction for intra-oral cancer. *Br J Plast Surg.* 2004;57:556-560.
3. Lotfi CJ, de Cavalcanti RC, Costa e Silva AM, et al. Risk factors for surgical-site infections in head and neck cancer surgery. *Otolaryngol Head Neck Surg.* 2008;138:74-80.
4. Pecorari G, Riva G, Albera A, et al. Post-operative infections in head and neck cancer surgery: risk factors for different infection sites. *J Clin Med.* 2022;11(17):4969.
5. Penel N, Fournier C, Roussel-Delvallez M, et al. Prognostic significance of wound infections following major head and neck cancer surgery: an open non-comparative prospective study. *Support Care Cancer.* 2004;12:634-639.
6. Chaukar DA, Deshmukh AD, Majeed T, et al. Factors affecting wound complications in head and neck surgery: a prospective study. *Indian J Med Paediatr Oncol.* 2013;34:247-251.
7. Mazurek MJ, Rysz M, Jaworowski J, et al. Contamination of the surgical field in head and neck oncologic surgery. *Head Neck.* 2014;36:1408-1412.
8. Stabenau K, Akakpo K, Richmon J, et al. Postoperative wound infections in head and neck surgery: the current state of antiseptic and antibiotic practices. *Oral Oncol.* 2021;118:105361.
9. Penel N, Fournier C, Lefebvre D, et al. Multivariate analysis of risk factors for wound infection in head and neck squamous cell carcinoma surgery with opening of mucosa: study of 260 surgical procedures. *Oral Oncol Extra.* 2005;41:35-44.
10. Penel N, Fournier C, Lefebvre D, et al. Previous chemotherapy as a predictor of wound infections in nonmajor head and neck surgery: results of a prospective study. *Head Neck.* 2004;26:513-517.
11. Durand ML, Yarlagadda BB, Rich DL, et al. The time course and microbiology of surgical site infections after head and neck free flap surgery. *Laryngoscope.* 2014;125:1084-1089.
12. Huberman BA. Risks of wound infection in patients with head and neck cancer. *J Oral Maxillofac Surg.* 1990;48:1240-1241.
13. Shuman AG, Shuman EK, Hauff SJ, et al. Preoperative topical antimicrobial decolonization in head and neck surgery. *Laryngoscope.* 2012;122:2454-2460.
14. Ma CY, Ji T, Ow A, et al. Surgical site infection in elderly oral cancer patients: is the evaluation of comorbid conditions helpful in the identification of high-risk ones? *J Oral Maxillofac Surg.* 2012;70:2445-2452.
15. Yang R, Lubek JE, Dyalram D, et al. Head and neck cancer surgery in an elderly patient population: a retrospective review. *Int J Oral Maxillofac Surg.* 2014;43:1413-1417.
16. Frederick JW, Sweeny L, Carroll WR, et al. Outcomes in head and neck reconstruction by surgical site and donor site. *Laryngoscope.* 2013;123:1612-1617.
17. Shestak KC, Jones NF, Wu W, et al. Effect of advanced age and medical disease on the outcome of microvascular reconstruction for head and neck defects. *Head Neck.* 1992;14:14-18.
18. Weaver TS, Wester JL, Gleysteen JP, et al. Surgical outcomes in the elderly patient after osteocutaneous free flap transfer. *Laryngoscope.* 2014;124:2484-2488.
19. Wester JL, Lindau RH, Wax MK. Efficacy of free flap reconstruction of the head and neck in patients 90 years and older. *JAMA Otolaryngol Head Neck Surg.* 2013;139:49-53.
20. Ferrari S, Copelli C, Bianchi B, et al. Free flaps in elderly patients: outcomes and complications in head and neck reconstruction after oncological resection. *J Craniomaxillofac Surg.* 2013;41:167-171.
21. Karakida K, Aoki T, Ota Y, et al. Analysis of risk factors for surgical-site infections in 276 oral cancer surgeries with microvascular free-flap reconstructions at a single university hospital. *J Infect Chemother.* 2010;16:334-339.
22. Bozikov K, Arnez ZM. Factors predicting free flap complications in head and neck reconstruction. *J Plast Reconstr Aesthet Surg.* 2006;59:737-742.
23. Gugliotta Y, Rubattino S, Fasolis M. Postoperative infections associated with microvascular free flaps in head and neck reconstruction: Analysis of risk factors and results with a standardized prophylaxis protocol. *J Plast Reconstr Aesthet Surg.* 2023;87:61-68.
24. Liu SA, Wong YK, Poon CK, et al. Risk factors for wound infection after surgery in primary oral cavity cancer patients. *Laryngoscope.* 2007;117:166-171.
25. Ogihara H, Takeuchi K, Majima Y. Risk factors of postoperative infection in head and neck surgery. *Auris Nasus Larynx.* 2009;36:457-460.
26. Rossmiller SR, Cannady SB, Ghanem TA, et al. Transfusion criteria in free flap surgery. *Otolaryngol Head Neck Surg.* 2010;142:359-364.
27. Danan D, Smolkin ME, Varhegyi NE, et al. Impact of blood transfusions on patients with head and neck cancer undergoing free tissue transfer. *Laryngoscope.* 2015;125:86-91.
28. Perisanidis C, Dettke M, Papadogeorgakis N, et al. Transfusion of allogenic leukocyte-depleted packed red blood cells is associated

with postoperative morbidity in patients undergoing oral and oropharyngeal cancer surgery. *Oral Oncol.* 2012;48:372-378.

29. Lee DH, Kim SY, Nam SY, et al. Risk factors of surgical site infection in patients undergoing major oncological surgery for head and neck cancer. *Oral Oncol.* 2011;47:528-531.

30. Pohlenz P, Blessmann M, Heiland M, et al. Postoperative complications in 202 cases of microvascular head and neck reconstruction. *J Craniomaxillofac Surg.* 2007;35:311-315.

31. Sakakibara A, Hashikawa K, Yokoo S, et al. Risk factors and surgical refinements of postresective mandibular reconstruction: a retrospective study. *Plast Surg Int.* 2014;2014:893746.

32. Hirsch DL, Bell RB, Dierks EJ, et al. Analysis of microvascular free flaps for reconstruction of advanced mandibular osteoradionecrosis: a retrospective cohort study. *J Oral Maxillofac Surg.* 2008;66:2545-2556.

33. Arce K, Bell RB, Potter JK, et al. Vascularized free tissue transfer for reconstruction of ablative defects in oral and oropharyngeal cancer patients undergoing salvage surgery following concomitant chemoradiation. *Int J Oral Maxillofac Surg.* 2012;41:733-738.

34. Mücke T, Rau A, Weitz J, et al. Influence of irradiation and oncologic surgery on head and neck microsurgical reconstructions. *Oral Oncol.* 2012;48:367-371.

35. Lee S, Thiele C. Factors associated with free flap complications after head and neck reconstruction and the molecular basis of fibrotic tissue rearrangement in preirradiated soft tissue. *J Oral Maxillofac Surg.* 2010;68:2169-2178.

36. Shaw RJ, Kanatas AN, Lowe D, et al. Comparison of miniplates and reconstruction plates in mandibular reconstruction. *Head Neck.* 2004;26:456-463.

37. Zavattero E, Fasolis M, Garzino-Demo P, et al. Evaluation of plate-related complications and efficacy in fibula free flap mandibular reconstruction. *J Craniofac Surg.* 2014;25:397-399.

38. Wong CH, Wei FC. Microsurgical free flap in head and neck reconstruction. *Head Neck.* 2010;32:1236-1245.

39. Genden EM, Rinaldo A, Suárez C, et al. Complications of free flap transfers for head and neck reconstruction following cancer resection. *Oral Oncol.* 2004;40:979-984.

40. Decesare GE, Deleyiannis FW, Losee JE. Reconstruction of osteomyelitis defects of the craniofacial skeleton. *Semin Plast Surg.* 2009;23:119-131.

41. Thakker JS, Fernandes R. Evaluation of reconstructive techniques for anterior and middle skull base defects following tumor ablation. *J Oral Maxillofac Surg.* 2014;72:198-204.

42. Bell RB, Gregoire C. Reconstruction of mandibular continuity defects using recombinant human bone morphogenetic protein 2: a note of caution in an atmosphere of exuberance. *J Oral Maxillofac Surg.* 2009;67:2673-2678.

43. Chen SH, Chen HC, Horng SY, et al. Reconstruction for osteoradionecrosis of the mandible: superiority of free iliac bone flap to fibula flap in postoperative infection and healing. *Ann Plast Surg.* 2014;73(suppl 1):S18-S26.

44. Mücke T, Loeffelbein DJ, Kolk A, et al. Comparison of outcome of microvascular bony head and neck reconstructions using the fibular free flap and the iliac crest flap. *Br J Oral Maxillofac Surg.* 2013;51:514-519.

45. Momoh AO, Yu P, Skoracki RJ, et al. A prospective cohort study of fibula free flap donor-site morbidity in 157 consecutive patients. *Plast Reconstr Surg.* 2011;128:714-720.

46. Ho MW, Rogers SN, Brown JS, et al. Prospective evaluation of a negative pressure dressing system in the management of the fibula free flap donor site: a comparative analysis. *JAMA Otolaryngol Head Neck Surg.* 2013;139:1048-1053.

47. Wester JL, Pittman AL, Lindau RH, et al. AlloDerm with split-thickness skin graft for coverage of the forearm free flap donor site. *Otolaryngol Head Neck Surg.* 2014;150:47-52.

48. Hanna TC, McKenzie WS, Holmes JD. Full-thickness skin graft from the neck for coverage of the radial forearm free flap donor site. *J Oral Maxillofac Surg.* 2014;72:2054-2059.

49. Avery CME, Ameerally P, Castling B, et al. Infection of surgical wounds in the maxillofacial region and free flap donor sites with methicillin-resistant *Staphylococcus aureus. Br J Oral Maxillofac Surg.* 2006;44:217-221.

50. Mulvey CL, Pronovost PJ, Gourin CG. Hospital volume and failure to rescue after head and neck cancer surgery. *Otolaryngol Head Neck Surg.* 2015;152:783-789.

51. Chang DW, Langstein HN, Gupta A, et al. Reconstructive management of cranial base defects after tumor ablation. *Plast Reconstr Surg.* 2001;107:1346-1355; discussion 1356-1357.

52. Hanasono MM, Silva A, Skoracki RJ, et al. Skull base reconstruction: an updated approach. *Plast Reconstr Surg.* 2011;128:675-686.

53. van Gemert JTM, van Es RJJ, Van Cann EM, et al. Nonvascularized bone grafts for segmental reconstruction of the mandible: a reappraisal. *J Oral Maxillofac Surg.* 2009;67:1446-1452.

54. Baker A, McMahon J, Parmar S. Part I: Immediate reconstruction of continuity defects of the mandible after tumor surgery. *J Oral Maxillofac Surg.* 2001;59:1333-1339.

55. Carlson ER, Marx RE. Part II. Mandibular reconstruction using cancellous cellular bone grafts. *J Oral Maxillofac Surg.* 1996;54:889-897.

56. Schimmele SR. Part II: delayed reconstruction of continuity defects of the mandible after tumor surgery. *J Oral Maxillofac Surg.* 2001;59:1340-1344.

57. Hayden RE, Mullin DP, Patel AK. Reconstruction of the segmental mandibular defect: current state of the art. *Curr Opin Otolaryngol Head Neck Surg.* 2012;20(4):231-236.

58. Sacco AG, Chepeha DB. Current status of transport-disc-distraction osteogenesis for mandibular reconstruction. *Lancet Oncol.* 2007;8:323-330.

59. Boyd JB, Mulholland RS. Fixation of the vascularized bone graft in mandibular reconstruction. *Plast Reconstr Surg.* 1993;91:274-282.

60. Tevlin R, McArdle A, Atashroo D, et al. Biomaterials for craniofacial bone engineering. *J Dent Res.* 2014;93:1187-1195.

61. Neovius E, Engstrand T. Craniofacial reconstruction with bone and biomaterials: review over the last 11 years. *J Plast Reconstr Aesthet Surg.* 2010;63:1615-1623.

62. Engstrand T. Biomaterials and biologics in craniofacial reconstruction. *J Craniofac Surg.* 2012;23:239-242.

63. Herford AS. rhBMP-2 as an option for reconstructing mandibular continuity defects. *J Oral Maxillofac Surg.* 2009;67:2679-2684.

64. Fang W, Liu YP, Ma Q, Liu BL, Zhao Y. Long-Term Results of Mandibular Reconstruction of Continuity Defects with Fibula Free Flap and Implant-Borne Dental Rehabilitation. *Int J Oral Maxillofac Implants.* 2014 Dec 5. doi: 10.11607/jomi.3606. Epub ahead of print. PMID: 25506642.

65. Salinas TJ, Desa VP, Katnelson A, et al. Clinical evaluation of implants in radiated fibula flaps. *J Oral Maxillofac Surg.* 2010;68:524-529.

66. Chang YM, Wallace CG, Hsu YM, et al. Outcome of osseointegrated dental implants in double-barrel and vertically distracted fibula osteoseptocutaneous free flaps for segmental mandibular defect reconstruction. *Plast Reconstr Surg.* 2014;134:1033-1043.

67. Foster RD, Anthony JP, Sharma A, et al. Vascularized bone flaps versus nonvascularized bone grafts for mandibular reconstruction: an outcome analysis of primary bony union and endosseous implant success. *Head Neck.* 1999;21:66-71.

68. Granström G. Osseointegration in irradiated cancer patients: an analysis with respect to implant failures. *J Oral Maxillofac Surg.* 2005;63:579-585.

69. Ch'ng S, Skoracki RJ, Selber JC, Yu P, Martin JW, Hofstede TM, Chambers MS, Liu J, Hanasono MM. Osseointegrated implant-based dental rehabilitation in head and neck reconstruction patients. *Head Neck.* 2016 Apr;38 Suppl 1:E321-7. doi: 10.1002/hed.23993. Epub 2015 Jun 29. PMID: 25546139.

70. Teoh KH, Huryn JM, Patel S, et al. Implant prosthodontic rehabilitation of fibula free-flap reconstructed mandibles: a Memorial Sloan-Kettering Cancer Center review of prognostic factors and implant outcomes. *Int J Oral Maxillofac Implants.* 2005;20:738-746.

71. Cuesta-Gil M, Ochandiano Caicoya S, Riba-García F, et al. Oral rehabilitation with osseointegrated implants in oncologic patients. *J Oral Maxillofac Surg.* 2009;67:2485-2496.

72. Esposito M, Worthington HV. Interventions for replacing missing teeth: hyperbaric oxygen therapy for irradiated patients who require dental implants. *Cochrane Database Syst Rev.* 2013;(9):CD003603.

73. Seruya M, Fisher M, Rodriguez ED. Computer-assisted versus conventional free fibula flap technique for craniofacial reconstruction: an outcomes comparison. *Plast Reconstr Surg.* 2013;132:1219-1228.

74. Rodby KA, Turin S, Jacobs RJ, et al. Advances in oncologic head and neck reconstruction: systematic review and future considerations of virtual surgical planning and computer aided design/computer aided modeling. *J Plast Reconstr Aesthet Surg.* 2014;67:1171-1185.

75. Ayoub N, Ghassemi A, Rana M, et al. Evaluation of computer-assisted mandibular reconstruction with vascularized iliac crest bone graft compared to conventional surgery: a randomized prospective clinical trial. *Trials.* 2014;15:114.

76. Gil RS, Roig AM, Obispo CA, et al. Surgical planning and microvascular reconstruction of the mandible with a fibular flap using computer-aided design, rapid prototype modelling, and precontoured titanium reconstruction plates: a prospective study. *Br J Oral Maxillofac Surg.* 2015;53:49-53.

77. Coskun H, Erisen L, Basut O. Factors affecting wound infection rates in head and neck surgery. *Otolaryngol Head Neck Surg.* 2000;123:328-333.

78. Huang RY, Sercarz JA, Smith J, et al. Effect of salivary fistulas on free flap failure: a laboratory and clinical investigation. *Laryngoscope.* 2005;115:517-521.

79. Yoshimoto S, Kawabata K, Mitani H. Factors involved in free flap thrombosis after reconstructive surgery for head and neck cancer. *Auris Nasus Larynx.* 2010;37:212-216.

80. Chaine A, Pitak-Arnnop P, Hivelin M, et al. Postoperative complications of fibular free flaps in mandibular reconstruction: an analysis of 25 consecutive cases. *Oral Surg Oral Med Oral Pathol Oral Radiol Endod.* 2009;108:488-495.

81. Candau-Alvarez A, Linares-Sicilia MJ, Dean-Ferrer A, et al. Role of culture of postoperative drainage fluid in the prediction of infection of the surgical site after major oncological operations of the head and neck. *Br J Oral Maxillofac Surg.* 2015;53:200-203.

82. Barsaiyan G, Rogers SN. Active versus passive neck drainage in head and neck oncology surgery: completing the re-audit cycle: Re: Batstone MD, Lowe D, Shaw RJ, Brown JS, Vaughan ED, Rogers SN. Passive versus active drainage following neck dissection: a non-randomised prospective study. *Br J Oral Maxillofac Surg.* 2011;49:412-413.

83. Bratzler DW, Dellinger EP, Olsen KM, et al. Clinical practice guidelines for antimicrobial prophylaxis in surgery. *Am J Health Syst Pharm.* 2013;70:195-283.

84. Skitarelić N, Morović M, Manestar D. Antibiotic prophylaxis in clean-contaminated head and neck oncological surgery. *J Craniomaxillofac Surg.* 2007;35:15-20.

85. Kochhar A, Pronovost PJ, Gourin CG. Hospital-acquired conditions in head and neck cancer surgery. *Laryngoscope.* 2013;123:1660-1669.

86. Weber RS, Hankins P, Rosenbaum B, et al. Nonwound infections following head and neck oncologic surgery. *Laryngoscope.* 1993;103:22-27.

87. Buitelaar DR, Balm AJM, Antonini N, et al. Cardiovascular and respiratory complications after major head and neck surgery. *Head Neck.* 2006;28:595-602.

88. Kreutzer K, Storck K, Weitz J. Current evidence regarding prophylactic antibiotics in head and neck and maxillofacial surgery. *Biomed Res Int.* 2014;2014:879437.

89. Obeso S, Rodrigo JP, Sánchez R, et al. Antibiotic prophylaxis in otolaryngologic surgery. *Acta Otorrinolaringol Esp.* 2010;61:54-68.

90. Liu SA, Tung KC, Shiao JY, et al. Preliminary report of associated factors in wound infection after major head and neck neoplasm operations—does the duration of prophylactic antibiotic matter? *J Laryngol Otol.* 2008;122:403-408.

91. Penel N, Lefebvre JL, Cazin JL, et al. Additional direct medical costs associated with nosocomial infections after head and neck cancer surgery: a hospital-perspective analysis. *Int J Oral Maxillofac Surg.* 2008;37:135-139.

92. Supriya M, Shakeel M, Santangeli L, et al. Controlling MRSA in head and neck cancer patients: what works? *Otolaryngol Head Neck Surg.* 2009;140:224-227.

93. Miyake M, Ohbayashi Y, Iwasaki A, et al. Risk factors for methicillin-resistant *Staphylococcus aureus* (MRSA) and use of a nasal mupirocin ointment in oral cancer inpatients. *J Oral Maxillofac Surg.* 2007;65:2159-2163.

94. Kosutic D, Uglesic V, Perkovic D, et al. Preoperative antiseptics in clean/contaminated maxillofacial and oral surgery: prospective randomized study. *Int J Oral Maxillofac Surg.* 2009;38:160-165.

95. Grandis JR, Vickers RM, Rihs JD, et al. The efficacy of topical antibiotic prophylaxis for contaminated head and neck surgery. *Laryngoscope.* 1994;104:719-724.

96. Sadakane-Sakuramoto A, Hasegawa Y, Sugahara K, et al. Change in Nutritional Status and dysphagia after resection of head and neck cancer. *Nutrients.* 2021;13(7):2438.

97. Kamizono K, Sakuraba M, Nagamatsu S, et al. Statistical analysis of surgical site infection after head and neck reconstructive surgery. *Ann Surg Oncol.* 2014;21:1700-1705.

98. Hennessey DB, Burke JP, Ni-Dhonochu T, et al. Preoperative hypoalbuminemia is an independent risk factor for the development of surgical site infection following gastrointestinal surgery: a multi-institutional study. *Ann Surg.* 2010;252:325-329.

99. Snyderman CH, Kachman K, Molseed L, et al. Reduced postoperative infections with an immune-enhancing nutritional supplement. *Laryngoscope.* 1999;109:915-921.

100. Vidal-Casariego A, Calleja-Fernández A, Villar-Taibo R, et al. Efficacy of arginine-enriched enteral formulas in the reduction of surgical complications in head and neck cancer: a systematic review and meta-analysis. *Clin Nutr.* 2014;33:951-957.

101. Falewee MN, Schilf A, Boufflers E, et al. Reduced infections with perioperative immunonutrition in head and neck cancer: exploratory results of a multicenter, prospective, randomized, double-blind study. *Clin Nutr.* 2013;33:776-784.

102. Pierre JF, Heneghan AF, Lawson CM, et al. Pharmaconutrition review: physiological mechanisms. *J Parenter Enteral Nutr.* 2013;37:51S-65S.

103. de Luis DA, Culebras JM, Aller R, et al. Surgical infection and malnutrition. *Nutr Hosp.* 2014;30:509-513.

104. Nolen D, Cannady SB, Wax MK, et al. Comparison of complications in free flap reconstruction for osteoradionecrosis in patients with or without hyperbaric oxygen therapy. *Head Neck.* 2014;36:1701-1704.

105. Annane D, Depondt J, Aubert P, et al. Hyperbaric oxygen therapy for radionecrosis of the jaw: a randomized, placebo-controlled, double-blind trial from the ORN96 study group. *J Clin Oncol.* 2004;22:4893-4900.

106. Bennett MH, Feldmeier J, Hampson N, et al. Hyperbaric oxygen therapy for late radiation tissue injury. *Cochrane Database Syst Rev.* 2012;(5):CD005005.

107. Friedman HI, Friedman HIF, Fitzmaurice M, et al. An evidence-based appraisal of the use of hyperbaric oxygen on flaps and grafts. *Plast Reconstr Surg.* 2006;117:175S-190S; discussion 191S-192S.

108. Zhou D, Fu D, Yan L, et al. The role of hyperbaric oxygen therapy in the treatment of surgical site infections: a narrative review. *Medicina.* 2023;59(4):762.

28

Microbiologic Considerations With Dental and Craniofacial Implants

STUART E. LIEBLICH

The restoration of the structures with the use of implants has arguably been one of the defining advances in prosthetic replacement of body structures over the past 50 years. Once thought to be impossible to achieve, implants are placed routinely in dental and craniofacial practice with predictably excellent success rates. Much has been written about the ability of titanium to form a direct attachment to living bone, with Brånemark coining the term *osseointegration* to describe this bone–metal fusion.[1] Other materials such as hydroxyapatite, zirconia,[2] and various treatments of titanium surfaces have more recently emerged as potential ways to decrease the time needed to obtain osseointegration and to increase the success rates. Although the modifications of titanium surfaces do increase the success rates, materials such as zirconia have not shown advantages in clinical success other than in more closely approximating tooth color for dental implants.[3]

This chapter reviews the issues associated with the prevention and management of infections associated with surgical implant placement. The factors that are known to cause infection, the putative bacteria involved, and the means to control infection once it occurs are reviewed. Two types of implant infections—one affecting the apical region similar to a periapical lesion around teeth—are identified along with the means for treatment. The other is the vexing cause of the disease state of peri-implantitis, which is discussed including its management. Finally, as with any surgical procedure, the potential exists for serious and even life-threatening infections. The surgeon involved with implant placement must therefore appreciate these potential infections and be trained and experienced to deal with them appropriately.

Prophylaxis and Surgical Preparation

Implant placement for the restoration of teeth, for prosthetic ears and eyes, and to restore hearing are now considered a routine part of patient care. The benefits of implants and their ability to restore form and function for a patient have led to their widespread use in clinical practice.

However, as noted from the orthopedic literature, the dental implant also needs to survive in a potentially contaminated field.[4]

As with any foreign body, the amount of bacteria necessary to create an infection around an implant will be substantially less than in a clean surgical wound that does not involve any foreign body placement. For example, the placement of a suture reduces the number of bacteria necessary to create a wound infection by a factor of 1000. In addition, the placement of an intraoral endosseous dental implant is further complicated by the initial bacterial load present at the time of surgery, as well as the continued bombardment of the tissue to implant bond by bacteria throughout the lifespan of the fixture.[5]

Endosseous implants are also placed in extraoral sites for the restoration of craniofacial defects. Other types of implants are placed transcutaneously, perhaps in conjunction with free flap reconstructions into the oral cavity, thus having to resist infection by both skin and intraoral bacterium. The vast majority of implant cases are successful and without complications. However, the development of infection can lead to loss of the implant, as well as the surrounding bone, teeth, nerves, and extension into adjacent spaces. The practitioner placing implants needs to be acutely aware of these risks, practice appropriate technique to minimize the chances of infection, and be able to intervene rapidly if an infection should occur.

Previously many authors recommended the administration of prophylactic antibiotics in conjunction with implant surgery.[6,7] As with any type of prophylactic antibiotic administration, the most important dose for the patient is administered before the initiation of the surgical procedure. The decision to continue the antibiotics postoperatively has not been proven to be beneficial in well-controlled studies. Certain patient situations, such as complex grafting or pre-existing compromise of the immune system, may dictate an empiric decision to continue antibiotics for a 5- to 7-day course.

Gynther et al[8] studied the response of patients who received 1 g of penicillin preoperatively and every 8 hours thereafter for 10 days in comparison with a group that did not receive any antibiotics. They found no difference in the survival of implants in patients who did not receive any antibiotics preoperatively or postoperatively. They also reported no difference in the frequency of infections between the two groups. Despite this study, most other authors and protocols suggest the use of perioperative antibiotics. Verifying the use of antibiotics is the study by Dent et al,[9] who showed a failure rate of 2.6% with presurgical antibiotics and 4.0% without. Meta-analyses by Ati-Ali et al[10] and Sharaf et al[11] seem to present similar conclusions. Both reviews indicate that implant survival is improved with the use of a preoperative dose of antibiotics. The occurrence of postoperative infections is not clearly reduced with the use of antibiotics, but the survival rate of the implants is in these studies. A more recent multicenter double-blinded randomized clinical trial that was carried out by Momand et al[12] in 2021 did not show any differences in success rates of osseointegration, in either early (5 to 7 days) or late infections (up to 6 months) in groups receiving either placebo or amoxicillin preoperatively (single dose). Four different implant systems and various implant procedures looked at in this study also had no effect on outcomes. It should be noted that these patients did receive chlorhexidine rinses preoperatively or for an undefined time postsurgically.

Evidence supporting the continued use of antibiotics after surgery is not correlated with improved outcomes in most cases. However, comparative articles do discuss that implant procedures are highly heterogeneous because the sites may differ, grafting may be used, and host issues are difficult to control for (e.g., systemic disease, smoking). Therefore, the decision regarding postoperative antibiotic management also may be dictated by the patient's medical condition. Certain medical conditions, such as diabetes, may increase the risk of implant failures, although a recent study by Oates et al[13] showed no difference in implant stability after 1 year in patients with a normal hemoglobin A_{1C} in comparison with elevated levels. In their study of implants placed in the anterior mandible, the success rates with moderately elevated A_{1C} levels (6 to 8%) and those with levels greater than 8% were equivalent. They used only postoperative antibiotics for 7 days without a preoperative dose. No site-specific infections were noted. Other host factors, such as cigarette smoking,[14] have an increased risk of implant failures, but not necessarily because of infection.

The actual surgical procedure described by Brånemark and promulgated in the original protocols taught throughout the world used a full surgical patient draping technique. This originated through Dr. Brånemark's training as an orthopedic surgeon. Kraut[15] has written on this controversy as to whether a full surgical drape is necessary for working in a known contaminated field and did not show it significantly affected outcomes. Newer implant surgical protocols recommended by other implant companies do not specifically promote the use of full surgical draping. It is reported that the use of full surgical preparation may increase the "awareness" of the surgical team to maintain asepsis as much

as clinically possible with the understanding that the procedures are being performed in a contaminated field. However, surgically "clean" procedures using sterile instruments and gloves are acceptable as a minimum preparation.

There are two major classifications of endosseous implants placed: the endosseous fixture placed transorally and extraoral placement. Endosseous implants are typically placed intraorally into the maxilla, mandible, or zygoma. Occasionally, endosseous fixtures are placed extraorally to support prosthetic ears, eyes, or other facial structures. Transosseous implants, such as the small staple implant and Boskar transmandibular implant, were placed using a submental incision; they are rarely used at this time because of the successful outcomes of intraoral placement of endosseous implants. A suggested antibiotic regimen for implant placements is outlined in Box 28-1.

Chlorhexidine gluconate rinses (Peridex, PerioGard, etc.) are recommended for use immediately preoperatively and to be continued for 5 to 7 days postoperatively. With the use of chlorhexidine, the rate of complications caused by infection was reduced from 8.7 to 4.1%.[15] This will supplement the patient's use of saline rinses, because often their oral hygiene

---

• BOX 28-1 Antibiotic Administration for Implant Surgery

Intraoral Endosseous Implants Routine (antibiotics generally not indicated)
- Specific patient factors (diabetes, immunocompromised)
- Amoxicillin (2 g) or azithromycin (500 mg)

Intraoral Endosseous Implants (Entering Maxillary Sinus)
- Amoxicillin (2 g PO then 500 mg qid for 3 days) *or*
- Azithromycin (500 mg PO then 250 mg daily for 4 days)

Intraoral Implants With Extensive Local Grafting or Maxillary Sinus Grafting
- Amoxicillin with clavulanic acid (875 mg PO then 875 mg bid for 3 days)
- Clindamycin (600 mg PO then 300 mg PO tid for 3 days)

Transosseous Implants (With Skin and Intraoral Communication)
- Augmentin (875 mg PO then 875 mg bid for 3 days) *or*
- Penicillin V (2 g PO) and metronidazole (500 mg PO), then penicillin V (500 mg qid) and metronidazole (250 mg bid) for 3 days, *or*
- Azithromycin (500 mg PO then 250 mg PO daily for 4 days)

Extraoral Implants
- Cephalexin (1 g then 500 mg qid for 5 days) *or*
- Cephazolin (1 g IV) then cephalexin (500 mg qid) for 5 days, *or*
- Azithromycin (500 mg then 2500 mg bid for 5 days)

Note: All initial doses of antibiotics to be given preoperatively (ideally 1 hour before incision if oral route or just before incision if intravenous route).

IV, Intravenous; *PO,* by mouth.

regimen will be negatively affected because of the discomfort of the surgical site. There appears to be little downside to the use of these rinses in comparison with the potential risks of systemic antibiotics.

Before placing an implant, it is important to survey the surgical site clinically and radiographically to ascertain that no residual infection is present in the bone. Adjacent teeth should be evaluated for the presence of an occult periapical lesion, which could spread to and infect the implant.[16] This evaluation is critical because many patients now having implant procedures are partially dentate, in contrast to the fully edentulous patients in Brånemark's original treatment groups. Most early protocols recommend waiting at least 2 to 3 months following the removal of a tooth before inserting an implant. During that time, any residual infection in the bone should clear and form a soft tissue covering over the planned surgical site.

Infection adjacent to an implant site can potentially infect the implant as well. The surgical site needs to be clearly radiographed preoperatively to ascertain that the adjacent teeth are not endodontically involved. Ideally, any active endodontic lesions adjacent to the implant site are treated before endosseous implant placement.[17] Endodontically involved teeth typically exhibit a mixed flora type of infection. The most common of these organisms are *Propionibacterium acnes, Staphylococcus epidermidis, Streptococcus intermedius, Wolinella recta,* and *Porphyromonas* and *Prevotella* species.[18] These bacteria, when harbored in teeth or the periapical regions adjacent to an implant site, can contaminate the newly placed implant. The natural dentition also can be a source of bacteria that have been implicated in implant infections. Reducing plaque and overt bacterial contamination by presurgical hygiene visits should be considered.

The placement of an immediate implant into an extraction socket is no longer a controversial procedure. Many authors advocate waiting a period of months after the removal of a tooth to ensure that any residual infection has cleared and early bone healing has been initiated. Others recommend immediate placement if the extraction can be done atraumatically with good preservation of the local bony tissues and no preexisting infection is present. A final group proposes that even implants can be placed into infected teeth sockets. Novaes and Novaes[19] have published a protocol for infected sites that includes starting antibiotics 24 to 48 hours before the surgery, thorough debridement and irrigation of the socket, and continuation of the antibiotics for 10 days. Their results have been confirmed by others at this point via meta-analysis of smaller clinical and animal studies,[19] with a recommendation that antibiotics be used (although a protocol is not defined for the duration).

Patients with recalcitrant periodontal disease (defined as one not responding to conventional periodontal therapy and continuing to lose attachment around teeth) have not been shown to reduce implant survival if the teeth are extracted first.[20] In fact, two important periodontal pathogens, *Actinobacillus actinomycetemcomitans* and *Porphyromonas gingivalis,* are not found in the sites of implants of previous patients with periodontal disease who have had all of their teeth extracted.[21] However, the microbiology of the peri-implant region will differ in patients with periodontal disease who are still only partially edentulous with the persistence of organisms known to be periodontal pathogens around teeth.[22]

Overview of Implant Infections

Although the nonintegrated implant may exhibit a localized bacterial infection, it is often unclear whether the infection causes the failure to integrate or the infection is a result of the mobility of the implant and the presence of a connective tissue encapsulation. Reports as to the causes of failures of implants include factors such as increased load (especially during the healing phase), heat generated during the surgery, local contamination of the implant site, and host factors.[23] Because implant failures are not frequent, with 5-year success greater than 90% with most systems, it is difficult to control for all variables. Animal models may provide indications of the factors that actually lead to infection and eventual loss.

The microbiologic findings will differ significantly in the gingival tissues of healthy and failing implants. Unsuccessful implants with mobility, pain, and bleeding exhibit a large proportion of gram-negative anaerobic rods (*Bacteroides* species) and *Fusobacterium* species.[24] In contrast, healthy implant sites have predominately coccoid cells without the presence of spirochetes.[25] Other species identified in failing implants, including *A. actinomycetemcomitans, P. gingivalis,* and *Prevotella intermedia,* were detected by DNA probes.[26] The identification of the bacterial contamination of failing implants will therefore assist in the choice of antibiotic management. In testing the microbial sensitivity to antibiotics in failing implants, Sbordone et al[27] noted penicillin G and amoxicillin to have greater activity than even clindamycin, amoxicillin-clavulanate, and the combination of amoxicillin and metronidazole against the putative organisms isolated.

In addition to local bacterium surrounding an implant, the surfaces of contaminated implants are coated with a biofilm.[27] Biofilms develop on inert and living tissues, releasing antigens and reacting with the local tissues. Although the antibiotic treatment may temporarily reverse the symptoms, unless the surgical removal of the biofilm occurs, the symptoms will persist.[7]

The source of bacteria can come from the endogenous population of oral bacteria. The implant and its various components can harbor bacteria as well once inserted into the oral cavity. The space between the abutment and implant, as well as the internal aspect of the fixture, act as reservoirs for bacteria.[28]

Regarding hyperfunction as a cause of implant failure, Celletti et al[29] studied intentionally overloaded osseointegrated implants in a baboon model. Although they found failures of components and fractures of implants in some cases, the loss of integration or crestal bone loss with secondary infection did not occur.

The surface of an implant may predispose it to development of infection. Many authors report that the increased roughness may provide isolation of the bacteria from the systemic circulation to remove them. Polished metal cylinders required fortyfold more bacterial inoculum than for porous implants to create infection.[29] The concern with the use of hydroxyapatite implants is that they may be predisposed to bacterial contamination progressing to loss of osseointegration.[30] Although hydroxyapatite is reported to increase the success and speed of osseointegration, the potential for increased bacterial contamination has changed its use. Previous implants with hydroxyapatite on the gingival surface have been replaced with a polished titanium collar to reduce the risk of peri-implantitis (Figure 28-1). Controversy remains as to whether roughened implants are more susceptible to peri-implantitis (see later discussion). A systematic review of this topic by Jordana[32] indicates an increased incidence with rougher surface implants, whereas a consensus conference in 2021[32] did not implicate any surface with a higher incidence of progressive peri-implantitis.

Early Implant Infections

After implant placement, the raising of a subperiosteal flap with development of a hematoma can create a nidus for bacterial growth. Patients may have a vestibular fullness that creates difficulty with the seating of their prosthesis. If the patient has been taking antibiotics, the presence of a penicillinase-resistant bacterium, such as *Prevotella* species, should be suspected. The addition of metronidazole should be effective at eliminating the infection. The use of the provisional prosthesis may need to be delayed for 1 week. Early infections rarely require surgical drainage.

The transmission of a load to a submerged implant can lead to the loosening of the cover screw from the internal aspect of the implant. This usually creates an opening in the overlying mucosa, causing a localized superficial infection (Figure 28-2). A sinus tract also may be present. Reopening the incision and reseating the cover screw may resolve the local infection. In persistent cases of localized drainage, exposing the implant completely to the oral cavity by placing

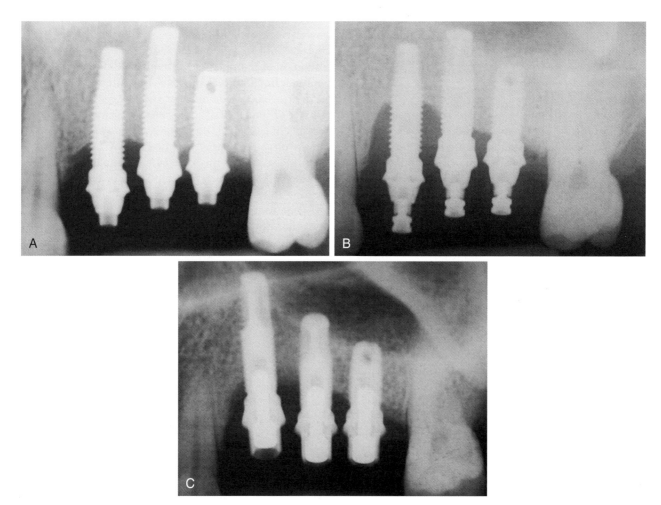

• **Figure 28-1** **A,** Bone level at final abutment placement. The anterior implant is a hydroxyapatite-coated implant. **B,** Bone level 4 months after abutment placement. Constant drainage from the anterior hydroxyapatite implant causing bone loss. Persistent drainage despite two surgical debridement procedures that included the placement of a local doxycycline delivery system. **C,** Anterior hydroxyapatite implant trephined out and replaced with a solid titanium fixture.

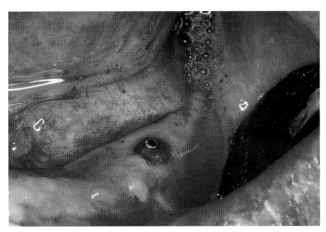

• **Figure 28-2** Local Infection Caused by Loosening of a Cover Screw from Forces Transmitted to it by an Overlying Removable Prosthesis. This infection will clear with reseating of the cover screw or alternatively placing a longer healing abutment to keep the site open and easier to clean. Antibiotics are generally not needed unless an adjacent space infection has occurred.

a longer healing abutment will resolve these localized infections. This maneuver is indicated only if the implant was solidly placed in bone at the initial surgery without the use of an associated graft.

Early implant failures can lead to the fixture being spontaneously exfoliated from the osteotomy site. The patient may acutely notice the surgical site being somewhat inflamed and painful, followed by immediate relief with the spontaneous loss of the implant. This type of implant failure is typically due to an acute infection that resolves with the loss of the implant. Further treatment with antibiotics is unnecessary if no other spaces are involved with the infection. A new implant, usually of a wider diameter, may be replaced after 4 to 8 weeks. Other signs of early failure include acute severe pain at the implant site. The placement of the fixture with mechanical retention and intimate contact to the native bone can create a compartment-type syndrome because of the effects of inflammation and infection. If a course of antibiotics (or supplemental antibiotics if the patient is already being treated) fails to resolve the pain, then consideration for early removal should be entertained, particularly for mandibular fixtures. Failure to address these issues promptly can lead to osteomyelitis of the mandible and extensive damage (discussed later).

Implants that compromise adjacent teeth can lead to development of an acute infection (Figure 28-3). Iatrogenic devitalization of an adjacent tooth to an implant site can create a periapical infection. This infection can then spread to involve adjacent implants in the region, leading to their loss as well. At least 3 mm of bone should separate the implant from a tooth to reduce this risk of local vascular compromise to an adjacent apex of a tooth. However, the surgeon needs to be aware that, because of the length of the implant and angulation of insertion, the apical end of the implant can impinge on adjacent structures even though an adequate space is present at the initial bone penetration site.

In addition, a "plaque front" has been shown to move laterally 2 mm to affect adjacent teeth[31] via an infrabony pocket. It seems likely that an implant within 2 mm of a periodontal pocket could also be adversely affected.

Apical Implantitis

Apical implantitis is a unique infection associated with the apical region of a dental implant (Figure 28-4). It has some parallels to an endodontic infection, because it localizes to the apical region of the implant and may exhibit symptoms of pain and fistula formation.[32] The spread of infection within the medullary bone has been shown to create pressure on the inferior alveolar nerve causing paresthesia and dysesthesia. In other cases, the finding is coincidentally noted as an asymptomatic radiolucency on a radiograph.

It is possible that the bone around the apical end of the newly placed implant can become compromised during the surgical procedure, permitting the build-up of heat. The lack of irrigation to the apical end of the drill can cause heat formation, which can be exacerbated if the drills become dull or excessive pressure is used. Gentle pressure and removing the bur every 15 to 20 seconds is recommended to clear any bone fragments from the drill flutes.[33] Compression of the bone and vascular compromise at the apex can also occur because of the biomechanics of achieving primary implant stabilization. This devitalized bone can then sequester, forming a nidus for bacterial contamination. Other potential causes and sources for the periapical implant infection to form are listed in Box 28-2.

Implants with apical infections that are removed and studied show extensive bacterial contamination, often in the apical vents or antirotational holes that are present in certain implant designs. The adjacent bone shows a histologic pattern consistent with localized suppurative osteomyelitis.[34] As expected from the extent of bone involvement, attempts at treating this type of infection solely with antibiotics have been unsuccessful.[18]

McAllister et al[35] described a surgical procedure to treat this type of infection. The procedure involves a thorough curettage of the apical region of all granulation tissue. This curettage should be completed with a titanium or plastic scaler to reduce the potential for damage to the implant. Resection of the exposed portion of the implant may be necessary if a large section is exposed and without bone coverage. Resection of the apical third may also remove the antirotational hole, which can continue to harbor bacteria and is mechanically difficult to debride thoroughly. Doxycycline powder can then be placed into the defect, left for 3 to 5 minutes, and then removed with irrigation. This will further debride and identify soft tissue remnants because of the cauterization effect of the acid environment it creates. The defect is filled with freeze-dried demineralized bone, autogenous bone, or alloplastic material (see Figure 28-4). A membrane can be placed over the defect, and the patient is prescribed antibiotics for a 10-day course. Balshi et al[36] reviewed three options for surgically approaching the apex

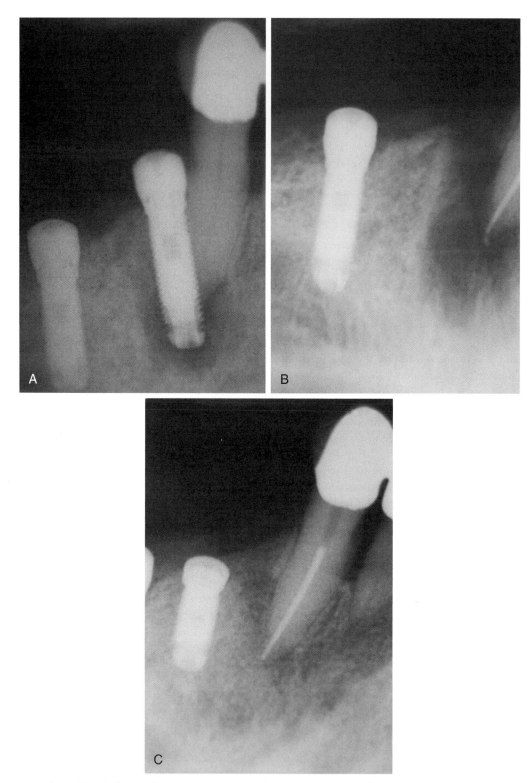

• **Figure 28-3** **A,** Fixture placement in close proximity to the apex of an adjacent tooth causing an iatrogenic infection of the tooth and implant. **B,** Subsequent infection required endodontic treatment of the tooth and removal of the grossly infected implant. **C,** After 3 months, resolution of the infection is demonstrated radiographically. Replacement of a new implant at an appropriate distance from the tooth facilitated successful completion of the case.

• **BOX 28-2** **Causes of Implant Periapical Lesion**

1. Contamination of the implant surface
2. Fenestration of the vestibular bone
3. Bone overheating during surgery
4. Excessive tightening of the implant with compression of the apical bone chips
5. Presence of preexisting bone pathology
6. Overloading of the implant
7. Poor quality of the bone site

Data from Piatelli A, Scarano A, Balleri P, et al. Clinical and histologic evaluation of an active "implant periapical lesion": a case report. *Int J Oral Maxillofac Implants*. 1998;13:713-716.

of infected mandibular implants: an intraoral transmandibular approach, a periosteal dissection, and an extraoral approach in select cases.

Peri-implantitis

The marginal tissues around implants have been of interest ever since osseointegrated implants were developed. The effect of plaque and bacterial contamination on the bone–implant junction was initially studied in the fully edentulous population. Adell et al[37] found that the presence of gingivitis around implants could occur with or without the presence of plaque, leading to the conclusion that the attachment and periodontal problems around implants are different from those of teeth. In contrast to teeth, the periodontal attachment to the implant abutment at the gingival level differs significantly. The collagen fibers from cementum are orientated in a perpendicular arrangement from the tooth, forming a direct attachment. Around implants, the collagen fibers are orientated parallel to the implant surface and without evidence of a direct attachment to the smooth titanium surface.[35] The term *peri-implantitis* is used to describe the diseased attachment state around implants.[36] The progression of peri-implantitis to loss of osseointegration is discussed as follows.

Peri-implantitis occurs when radiographic evidence of bone loss around the implant is found in conjunction with the clinical signs of localized infection. It is defined by bleeding and/or suppuration on probing along with radiographic evidence of bone loss. Biologic markers have identified that the bacteria associated with peri-implantitis are similar to those found in periodontal infections, originally leading to similar treatment recommendations.

Many authors report anecdotally that it is critical to have keratinized tissue around implants.[37] The theory is that since the attachment of soft tissues to the implant abutment is of a different nature than around natural teeth, the peri-implant area has a greater risk of breakdown. Indeed, the benefit to having immobile tissue around implants may be its ability to preserve the integrity of the connective tissue attachment at the gingival margin. However, the benefits of a keratinized border around the abutment in reducing the impact of peri-implantitis has only been shown around hydroxyapatite implants[38] and highly roughened surface titanium plasma-sprayed implants.[37]

Clinical classifications of peri-implant complications have been designated into various groups by authors.

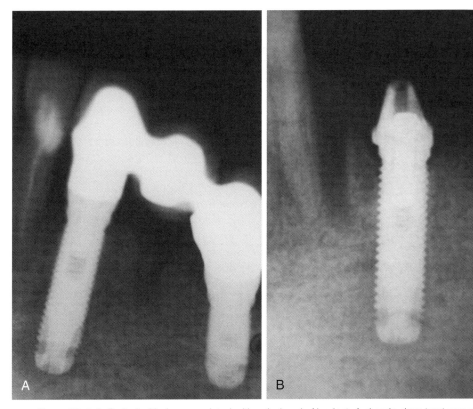

A

B

• **Figure 28-4** **A,** Periapical lesion associated with apical end of implant. A chronic sinus tract was noted in the mucobuccal fold. **B,** Treatment with surgical debridement, tetracycline powder, and extraction of the adjacent mobile, endodontically treated incisor.

Meffert used the terminology, "ailing, failing and failed" to describe implants in progressive stages of infection.[41] Ailing implants are defined as having bone loss with pocket formation. The failing implant has bone loss irrespective of therapy, bleeding on probing, and a purulent exudate. Failed implants have mobility, a dull sound on percussion, and peri-implant radiolucency. According to his classification system, implants that are ailing or failing may be able to be treated and maintained. Failed implants with frank mobility necessitate removal.

Peri-implantitis is defined as the pathologic changes confined to the surrounding hard and soft tissues adjacent to the implant and the contemporary diagnosis/terminology of this entity is outlined by Renvert. It is differentiated from peri-implant *mucositis,* which is a reversible inflammatory change in the soft tissue surrounding the implant. Peri-implant mucositis is analogous to gingivitis and is primarily an inflammatory disorder caused by plaque accumulation.[39,40] With conventional normal oral hygiene, the peri-implant mucositis will resolve with no permanent changes or bone loss.

Peri-implantitis is caused by the detrimental effects of anaerobic bacteria on the peri-implant tissue health. Support for this conclusion comes from various studies, including an experimental induction in humans[39] and development of an animal model of peri-implantitis.[41] The evidence for a bacterial cause is summarized in Box 28-3.

Peri-implantitis begins with bone loss at the coronal portion of the implant that becomes progressive and associated with a purulent exudate. The apical end of the implant maintains its osseointegration; therefore, the implant exhibits no mobility until the final stage of peri-implantitis is reached. The clinical diagnosis includes increased probing depths, patient reports of pain and spontaneous bleeding, and radiographic evidence of bone loss. Diagnostic markers such as interleukin-1B, proteases, glycosaminoglycan, and prostaglandin E$_2$ (PGE$_2$) levels may provide predictive

information of ongoing peri-implantitis that has not developed clinical manifestations.[42]

The microbiology of failing implants is associated with various species of bacteria. The typical periodontal pathogens (*P. gingivalis, P. intermedia,* and *A. actinomycetemcomitans*) are found in approximately half the cases of peri-implantitis. Other microorganisms such as *Staphylococcus* species, enteric bacteria, and *Candida* species are also found just as frequently around compromised implants.[43] These organisms are not typically associated with odontogenic periodontal disease states. Therefore, antimicrobial therapy is more responsive with tetracycline type of antibiotics such as minocycline. Peri-implantitis has an overall frequency of 5 to 10%. Rates of specific implant systems cannot be compared because of differences in reported diagnostic criteria.[36]

As peri-implantitis persists, additional attachment is lost. Bone levels will decrease and eventually can lead to the loss of integration. Periodontal probing is useful to determine whether bleeding on probing is present or if suppuration is found. Actual pocket depths are not as indicative of the disease, in contrast with teeth; however, increasing pocket depths over time are indications of the progression. Radiographic evidence of additional bone loss requires well-positioned parallel films with digital radiography and may provide a more sensitive indication of bone loss.

Certain types of implants may be more susceptible to peri-implantitis, based on the type of implant surface.[44] Hydroxyapatite-coated implants can harbor bacteria because of the surface roughness creating localized tissue reactions.[30] These reactions can persist and lead to loss of the implant. Wolinsky et al[48] reported that certain species of bacteria such as *Actinomyces viscosus, Fusobacterium* species, and *Peptostreptococcus prevotii* may preferentially adhere to hydroxyapatite, causing the increased propensity for peri-implantitis around these fixtures.[45]

The initial treatment of peri-implantitis is to confirm that all the components are seated on the implant fixture. Abutments with internal hexes can become offset and create a gap that traps plaque and bacteria, leading to a fistula. Loose components may also exhibit a localized tissue infection. After components are removed, the stability of the fixture is checked to ensure that the tissue response is not secondary to a failed implant.

Therapy for peri-implantitis can include subgingival debridement and removal of calculus. Calculus is not as adherent to titanium and is removed with graphite or plastic scalers to avoid damage to the implant surface. Cases of more extensive attachment loss will require open flap procedures and pocket reduction surgery. Doxycycline powder or minocycline chips can be placed into the defect has been shown to be effective as a topical means to suppress putative periodontal pathogens in the peri-implant defect.[46] Irrigation with subgingival chlorhexidine gluconate should be completed at the office, with the patient instructed on continuation of therapy at home. Antibiotic therapy is often instituted as well, although this has no proven benefit.

• BOX 28-3 Evidence for a Bacterial Cause of Peri-implantitis

1. Experimentally induced peri-implant mucositis: plaque accumulation leads to peri-implant mucositis.
2. Distinct differences in microflora of successful versus failing implants.
3. Successful implants experience no shifts in microflora over time.
4. Periodontal pathogens may be transmitted from residual teeth to implants.
5. Therapy that reduces peri-implant microflora improves symptoms.
6. Peri-implantitis can be induced by placing plaque-retentive ligatures in animals.
7. Edentulous implant patients with poor oral hygiene have more bone resorption than those with good hygiene.

Adapted from Mombelli A, Lang LP. The diagnosis and treatment of peri-implantitis. *Periodontol 2000.* 1998;17:63-76.

Some authors have recommended guided tissue regeneration procedures with membrane placement.[47] However, the placement of membrane into an area of infection often leads to complications of the membrane becoming secondarily infected and failure to restore bone height.[2] The use of autogenous bone blocks to treat the bone defects successfully has been described by Behneke et al.[50] Their protocol included debridement of soft tissues without touching the implant and air abrasion of the implant surface. Autogenous block grafts were harvested from either the retromolar or the symphysis region of the mandible. The blocks were stabilized against the implant with bone screws, and fibrin glue was used to retain bone chips to fill the residual defect. Their long-term successful treatment of 23 of 25 fixtures over a 6-month interval makes this one of the most successful protocols to be studied in a prospective fashion. However, there are no replication studies on this technique and it does not have a recommendation in current consensus management papers.

The propensity of rough-surfaced implants to retain bacteria and associated biofilm often requires special management to remove the coating. Implantoplasty with various air abrasion or direct mechanical smoothing of the surface has not been shown to improve outcomes or arrest the progression as reported by Koo et al.[51] Mechanical removal of the biofilm with aggressive instrument cleaning and use of titanium brushes is a recommended treatment modality.

An iatrogenic cause of peri-implantitis is the expression of cement hydraulically forced past the normal soft tissue barrier (Figure 28-5); this may be due to using an excessive amount of cement, as the restorative dentist may have more experience with tooth-supported restorations typically having a larger cement space. In contrast, the precision of implant reconstructions requires little cement. Wadwani et al[53] described this as a complication of cemented restorations and presented clinical techniques to reduce this occurrence. However, even a screw-retained implant prosthesis can develop peri-implantitis and studies such as de Brandeão have failed to show a difference in these two prosthetic modalities.

The prosthetic design of the implant restoration may also play a role in the presence of peri-implantitis. As noted in Figure 28-6 these are both screw-retained restorations but the open contacts between the two fixtures is creating a trap for bacteria. It also has been reported that overcontured, highly convex restorations and those with angles of emergence greater than 30 degrees may also predispose a site for peri-implantitis (Schwarz).

An analogous situation to peri-implantitis is associated with endosseous implants placed for craniofacial reconstruction (see Figure 28-6). Localized infections can form around the soft tissue surrounding the implants. The frequency of these infections is high, with 15 to 20% of patients experiencing an infection at some point.[49] Sebaceous crusting acts in a manner similar to calculus, causing a local tissue inflammation and perhaps creating a nidus for bacterial infection. Most of these infections are associated with *Staphylococcus aureus,* with additional reports implicating *Streptococcus* species and other gram-negative bacilli. As

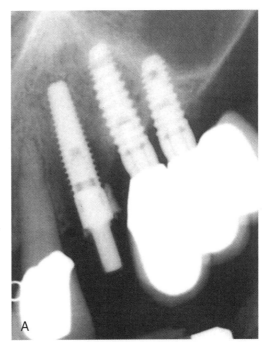

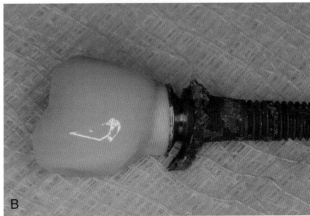

• **Figure 28-5 A,** Radiograph of implant with excessive cement. **B,** Fixture explanted because of chronic infection caused by excessive cement.

with intraoral implants, the development of an infection of the soft tissues does not always lead to osseointegration failure; however, the pain and erythema associated with the infection is substantially problematic.

There is a site-specific relationship to the success of craniofacial implants. In general, the endosseous fixtures placed in the mastoid and for ear reconstruction have a higher success rate than orbital implants.[50] The loss of orbital implants is related to a higher infection rate and exposure of the implant flange. The proximity of these implants to the nasal cavity and its native bacteria may account for the increased infection rate.

To improve the patient's ability to perform adequate hygiene, the dermal tissues are thinned as much as possible at the time of surgery. This also removes local skin appendages and reduces the mobility of the tissue around the implant that is critical to reduce local reactions.[51] Patients benefit from having a sufficiently long extension of the abutment and reduction of overhangs to facilitate hygiene.

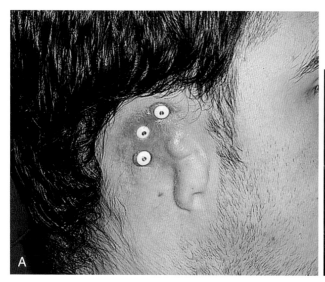
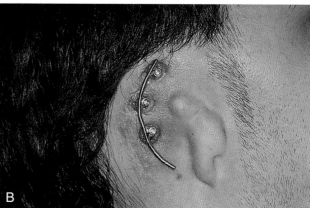

• **Figure 28-6 A,** Local tissue infection following external implants for an ear prosthesis. Cultures grew methicillin-resistant *Staphylococcus epidermidis,* demonstrating the need for culture and sensitivity testing. The overhanging plastic healing caps further impeded this patient's ability to perform adequate hygiene around the fixtures. **B,** Resolution of the infection with appropriate antibiotics, local cleansing, and placement of the final bar prosthesis that facilitated hygiene.

When managing the infections associated with craniofacial implants, attention is directed at improving hygiene with removal of all sebaceous crusting daily by the patient. Antimicrobial therapy is initiated on the basis of culture and sensitivity testing. Additional benefits of topical therapy with mupirocin (Bactroban) or oxytetracycline-hydrocortisone (Terra-Cortril) will help to resolve the infection. The placement of palatal tissue free grafts around the abutments of craniofacial implants has been suggested as a means to prevent the chronic infection (MP Powers, personal communication 1998). This tissue has a higher degree of keratinization and will reduce the mobility around the implant site.

The potential for yeast infections must be considered as well, especially under facial prostheses that create a warm, moist environment ideal for fungal growth. This consideration is supported by Abu-Serriah, who found yeasts associated with ear prosthesis implants but not with bone-anchored hearing aids in the same region.[49] Yeasts are not part of the normal microflora of skin and can be opportunistic with the removal of normal coagulase-negative staphylococci caused by antibiotic therapy. The most commonly isolated yeast is *Candida parapsilosis,* which is a known pathogen of endocarditis, ocular and dermal infections, arthritis, and peritonitis.[52]

A protocol for managing peri-implantitis is shown in Figure 28-7. The surgical treatment is a necessary adjunct to the need for home care and frequent office management.

Other Infections Associated With Implant Surgery

The reflection of a local flap and insertion of an implant can lead to severe infection in rare cases. The surgeon must be aware of the potential space involvement and urgently treat infections of the maxillofacial region should they occur. Because the implant is a persistent foreign body, it should be removed once an infection has spread from the local area adjacent to the fixture. The area around the implant should be explored, and necrotic bone should be removed. Specimens of bone and soft tissue are sent for culture and sensitivity testing.

Serious cases of infections have been reported when attempting to maintain a fixture in face of a spreading infection. Descending necrotizing fasciitis has been reported to be a consequence of implant surgery.[53] The cases in Figure 28-8 depict severe infections that developed into an osteomyelitis with pathologic fracture of the mandible. Of note in the author's (SEL) experience is that the development of osteomyelitis occurs in the anterior mandible. As expected, the blood flow to the distal aspects of the mandible is diminished, and the increased density of the bone leads to a more severe outcome. Aggressive treatment is indicated once the bone infection develops. Definitive treatment includes early removal of the implants and necrotic bone and stabilization of the pathologic fractures.

The placement of implants creates a site that is susceptible to the distant spread of osteomyelitis. Goldberg reports a case of *Klebsiella* osteomyelitis, which occurred 1 month after a severe urinary tract infection (MH Goldberg, personal communication 1998). Enteric rods such as these are not associated with failing implants.[25] The isolates from the bone in this case were consistent with the bacteria cultured from the urinary tract, with the same sensitivity profile. Therefore, the osteomyelitis was of a blood-borne spread. As again illustrated in this case, the infection did not resolve until the implants were removed, the necrotic bone was debrided, and the appropriate antibiotics were administered.

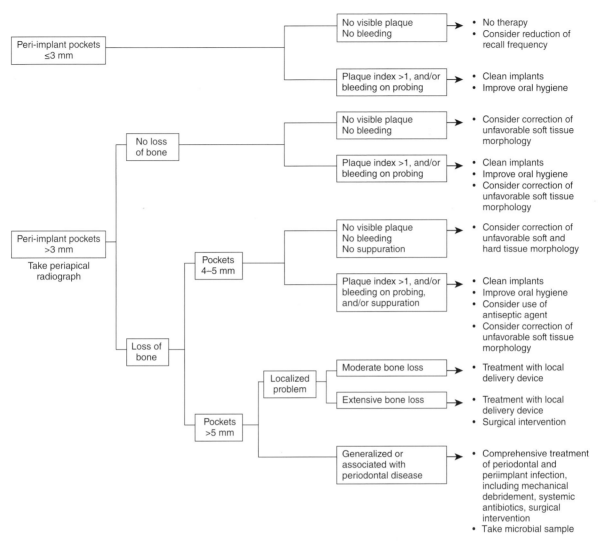

• **Figure 28-7** Protocol for Managing Peri-Implantitis. (From Mombelli A, Lang NP. The diagnosis and treatment of peri-implantitis. *Periodontol 2000*. 1998;17:71.)

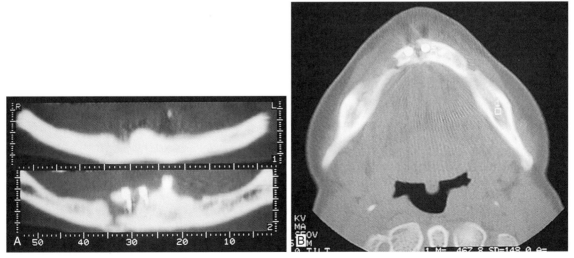

• **Figure 28-8** Examples of Sequestrum and Involucrum Formation as a Result of Infected Implants. Fixtures were left in place in spite of severe infection for months in an attempt to preserve the implants. Pathologic fracture and need for discontinuity bone grafting resulted. (Courtesy Dr. Morton H. Goldberg, Hartford, CT.)

References

1. Brånemark PI, Breine U, Adell R, et al. Intra-osseous anchorage of dental prosthesis. I: experimental studies. *Scand J Plast Reconstr Surg*. 1969;3:81-100.

2. Hurzler MB, Quinones CR, Schupback P, et al. Treatment of peri-implantitis using guided bone regeneration and bone grafts, alone or in combination, in beagle dogs. Part 2: histologic findings. *Int J Oral Maxillofac Implants*. 1997;12:168-175.

3. Manzano G, Herrero LR, Montero J. Comparison of clinical performance of zirconia implants and titanium implants in animal models: a systematic review. *Int J Oral Maxillofac Implants*. 2014;29:311-320.

4. Drake DR, Paul J, Keller JC. Primary bacterial colonization of implant surfaces. *Int J Oral Maxillfac Implants*. 1999;14:226-232.

5. Lee KH, Maiden MF, Tanner AC, et al. Microbiota of successful osseointegrated dental implants. *J Periodontol*. 1999;70:131-138.

6. Topazian RG. The basis of antibiotic prophylaxis. In: Worthington P, Brånemark PI, eds. *Advanced Osseointegration Surgery*. Chicago: Quintessence; 1992:57-66.

7. Trieger N. Antibiotics and anti-inflammatory agents in dental implantology. *Implant Dent*. 1999;8:343-346.

8. Gynther GW, Kondell PA, Moberg LE, et al. Dental implant installation without antibiotic prophylaxis. *Oral Surg Oral Med Oral Path Oral Radiol Endod*. 1998;85:509-511.

9. Dent CD, Olson JW, Farish SE, et al. The influence of preoperative antibiotics on success of endosseous implants up to and including stage II surgery: a study of 2,641 implants. *J Oral Maxillofac Surg*. 1997;55:19-24.

10. Ati-Ali J, Ata-Ali F, Ata-Ali F. Do antibiotics decrease implant failure and postoperative infections? A systematic review and meta-analysis. *Int J Oral Maxillofac Surg*. 2014;43:68-74.

11. Sharaf B, Jandali-Rifai M, Susarla SM, et al. Do perioperative antibiotics decrease implant failure? *J Oral Maxillofac Surg*. 2011;69:2345-2350.

12. Momand P, Becktor JP, Naimi-Akbar A, Tobin G, Götrick B. Effect of antibiotic prophylaxis in dental implant surgery: a multicentre placebocontrolled double-blinded randomized clinical trial. *Clin Implant Dent Relat Res*. 2022;24(1):116-124. Available at: https://doi.org/10.1111/cid.13068.

13. Oates TW, Galloway P, Alexander P, et al. The effects of elevated hemoglobin A1c in patients with type 2 diabetes mellitus on dental implants. *J Am Dent Assoc*. 2014;145:1218-1226.

14. Cavalcanti R, Oreglia F, Manfredonia MF, et al. The influence of smoking on the survival of dental implants: a 5-year pragmatic multicentre retrospective cohort study of 1727 patients. *Eur J Oral Implantol*. 2011;4:39-45.

15. Kraut RA. Clean operating conditions for the placement of intraoral implants. *J Oral Maxillofac Surg*. 1996;54:1337-1338.

16. Lambert PM, Morris HF, Ochi S. The influence of 0.12% chlorhexidine digluconate rinses on the incidence of infectious complications and implant success. *J Oral Maxillofac Surg*. 1997;55(12 suppl 5):25-30.

17. Takeshita F, Iyama S, Ayukawa Y, et al. Abscess formation around a hydroxyapatite-coated implant placed into the extraction socket with autogenous bone graft: a histological study using light microscopy, image processing, and confocal laser scanning microscopy. *J Periodontol*. 1997;68:299-305.

18. Sussman HI, Moss SS. Localized osteomyelitis secondary to endodontic-implant pathosis: a case report. *J Periodontol*. 1993;64:306-310.

19. Novaes AB, Novaes AB. Immediate implants placed into infected sites: a clinical report. *Int J Oral Maxillofac Implants*. 1995;10:609-613.

20. Palmer R. Evidence for survival of implants placed into infected sites is limited. *J Evid Based Dent Pract*. 2012;12(suppl 3):187-188.

21. Nevins M, Langer B. The successful us of osseointegrated implants for the treatment of the recalcitrant periodontal patient. *J Periodontol*. 1995;66:150-157.

22. Danser MM, van Winlelhoff AJ, van der Velden U. Periodontal bacteria colonizing oral mucous membranes in edentulous patients wearing dental implants. *J Periodontol*. 1997;68:209-216.

23. Becker W, Becker BE, Newman MG, et al. Clinical and microbiological findings that may contribute to dental implant failure. *Int J Oral Maxillofac Implants*. 1990;5:31-38.

24. Eckert SE, Meraw SJ, Cal E, et al. Analysis of incidence and associated factors with fractured implants: a retrospective study. *Int J Oral Maxillofac Implants*. 2000;15:662-667.

25. Augthun M, Conrads G. Microbial findings of deep peri-implant bone defects. *Int J Oral Maxillofac Implants*. 1997;12:106-112.

26. Mombelli A, van Oosten AC, Schurch E, et al. The microbiota associated with successful or failing osseointegrated titanium implants. *Oral Microbiol Immun*. 1987;2:145-151.

27. Sbordone L, Barone A, Ramaglia L, et al. Antimicrobial susceptibility of periodontopathic bacteria associated with failing implants. *J Periodontol*. 1995;66:69-74.

28. Costerton JW, Stewart PS, Greenberg EP. Bacterial biofilms: a common cause of persistent infections. *Science*. 1999;284:1318-1319.

29. Celletti R, Pameijer CH, Brachchetti G, et al. Evaluation of osseointegrated implants restored in non-axial functional occlusion with pre-angulated abutments. *J Periodontics Restorative Dent*. 1995;15:562-573.

30. Cordero J, Munuera L, Folgueira MD. The influence of the chemical composition and surface of the implant on infection. *Injury*. 1996;27:34-37.

31. Johnson BW. HA-coated dental implants: long-term consequences. *J Calif Dent Assoc*. 1992;20:33-34.

32. Jordana F, Susbielles L, Colat-Perro L. Periimplantitis and implant body roughness: a systematic review of literature. *Implant Dent*. 2018;27(6):672-681.

33. Schwarz F, Alcoforado G, Guerrero A, et al. Peri-implantitis: summary and consensus statements of group 3. The 6th EAO Consensus Conference 2021. *Clin Oral Implants Res*. 2021;32(suppl 21):245-253. Available at: https://doi.org/10.1111/clr.13827.

34. Waerhaug J. The infrabony pocket and its relationship to trauma from occlusion and subgingival plaque. *J Periodontol*. 1979;50:355-365.

35. McAllister B, Masters D, Meffert R. Treatment of implants demonstrating periapical radiolucencies. *Pract Periodontics Aesthet Dent*. 1992;4:37-41.

36. Balshi TJ, Pappas CE, Wolfinger GJ, et al. Management of an abscess around the apex of a mandibular root form implant: clinical report. *Implant Dent*. 1994;3:81-85.

37. Adell R, Lekholm U, Rocker B, et al. Marginal tissue reactions at osseointegrated titanium fixtures (I): a 3-year longitudinal prospective study. *Int J Oral Maxillofac Surg*. 1986;15:39-52.

38. Berglundh T, Lindhe J, Ericsson I, et al. The soft tissue barrier at implants and teeth. *Clin Oral Impl Res*. 1991;1:8-12.

39. Warrer K, Buser D, Lang NP, et al. Plaque-induced peri-implantitis in the presence or absence of keratinized mucosa: an experimental study in monkeys. *Clin Oral Implants Res*. 1995;6:131-138.

40. Hanisch O, Cortella CA, Boskovic MM, et al. Experimental breakdown around hydroxyapatite coated implants. *J Periodontol*. 1997;68:59-66.

41. Meffert RM. How to treat ailing and failing implants. *Implant Dent*. 1992;1:25-33.

42. Pontoriero R, Tonelli MP, Carnevale G, et al. Experimentally induced peri-mucositis: a clinical study in humans. *Clin Oral Implants Res*. 1994;5:254-259.

43. Renvert S, Persson GR, Pirih FQ, Camargo PM. Peri-implant health, peri-implant mucositis, and peri-implantitis: case definitions and diagnostic considerations. *J Clin Periodontol*. 2018;45(suppl 20):S278-S285. Available at: https://doi.org/10.1111/jcpe.12956.

44. Zitzmann NU, Berglundh T. Definition and prevalence of peri-implant disease. *J Clin Periodontol*. 2008;35:286-291.

45. Baron M, Haas R, Dortbudak O, et al. Experimentally induced peri-implantitis: a review of different treatment methods described in the literature. *Int J Oral Maxillofac Implants*. 2000;15:533-544.

46. Kao RT, Curtis DA, Murray PA. Diagnosis and management of peri-implant disease. *J Calif Dent Assoc*. 1997;25:872-880.

47. Salcetti JM, Moriarty JD, Cooper LF, et al. The clinical, microbial, and host response characteristics of the failing implant. *Int J Oral Maxillofac Implants*. 1997;12:32-42.

48. Wolinsky L, deCamargo P, Erard J, et al. A study of in vivo attachment of *Streptococcus sanguis* and *Actinomyces viscosus* to saliva treated titanium. *Int J Oral Maxillofac Implants*. 1989;4:27-31.

49. Jovanovic SA. Diagnosis and treatment of peri-implant disease. *Curr Opin Periodontol*. 1994;194-204.

50. Behneke A, Behneke N, d'Hoedt B. Treatment of peri-implantitis defects with autogenous bone grafts: six-month to 3-year results of a prospective study in 17 patients. *Int J Oral Maxillofac Implants*. 2000;15:125-138.

51. Koo K, Khoury F, Keeve P, et al. Implant surface decontamination by surgical treatment of periimplantitis: a literature review. *Implant Dent*. 2019;28(2):173-176.

52. Romeo E, Ghisolfi M, Murgolo N, et al. Therapy of peri-implantitis with respective surgery. *Clin Oral Implants Res*. 2005;16:9-18.

53. Wadwani C, Pineyro A, Zhang H, et al. Effect of implant abutment modification on the extrusion of excess cement at the crown-abutment margin. *Int J Oral Maxillofac Implants*. 2011;26:1241-1246.

29

Infections Associated With Aesthetic Facial Surgery

MOHAMMAD BANKI, CHARLES L. CASTIGLIONE, AND ELIE M. FERNEINI

Infections associated with facial aesthetic surgery are fortunately very rare; therefore, there are few published clinical reports. Reasons for a low infection rate include a lower risk of contamination of the surgical site, the generous blood supply of the head and neck, and patient selection factors (Figure 29-1). Facial aesthetic surgery sites are almost always rated as clean or clean/contaminated, and studies have shown very low associated infection rates.[1-7] Elective plastic surgery infection rates are lower than rates for other types of surgery. In general, patients undergoing elective surgery have a lower rate of postoperative infections than those undergoing emergent or semi-emergent surgery; the rate is even lower for aesthetic surgery.

Patients undergoing facial aesthetic surgery are generally concerned about their skin and overall facial appearance and as a result tend to use good skin care techniques. Facial skin is cleansed frequently and often exfoliated, and blemishes or acne are treated before surgery. Even for procedures involving intraoral and intranasal incisions, the risk of contamination is low. The use of facial or nasal implants may increase the risk of infection, but again the risk is relatively low.[1-3]

As with other types of surgery performed in the head and neck region, the abundant vascularity of the region lowers the risk of infections after facial aesthetic surgery. This allows for better healing and more resistance to infection. Grafted tissues are revascularized faster, and implants are integrated more quickly. Skin necrosis is less common; when it does occur, it will heal relatively quickly and with less risk of secondary infection.

Patient selection factors are most important. Facial aesthetic patients are usually healthy, even when older. Most surgeons performing aesthetic surgery will not operate on patients with significant comorbidities. Surgical site infections are greater in patients with obesity, diabetes mellitus, hypertension, and chronic obstructive pulmonary disease. Patients with significant cardiac or pulmonary disease are not candidates for such elective surgery. Diabetes mellitus and hypertension must be under control. Elevated blood pressure can lead to hematomas, which in turn can cause tissue necrosis and infection. Diabetes is associated with wound healing

issues and infection. Patients are also encouraged to lose weight before surgery. This will lower the risk of infection and tissue necrosis. Finally, smokers must stop smoking 3 weeks before surgery and maintain this cessation after surgery until the surgical site is well healed. Smoking is one of the greatest causes of wound healing problems. Because of these selection factors, the overall health of the patients having facial aesthetic surgery is better, thereby lowering the risk of infection.[1]

Prevention of wound infection is paramount for the facial aesthetic surgeon and for patients. Although patient selection is key, a careful execution of the surgical technique is also important. Appropriate skin washing and preparation are necessary, as well as attention to strict sterile technique. Meticulous surgical technique must be used to minimize tissue damage, avoid hematoma, and reduce wound tension, all of which can lead to tissue necrosis. Hematoma and necrotic skin provide a good medium for bacterial growth and can lead to both primary and secondary infections. Skin resurfacing techniques create large but superficial wounds that, with proper wound care, usually heal uneventfully. However, herpes simplex viral infections are of great concern, and prophylactic antiviral therapy is often given. The use of prophylactic antibiotics for facial aesthetic surgery is controversial, because most cases are clean or clean/contaminated. However, the consequences of infection after aesthetic surgery can be significant, including increased scarring and soft tissue distortion. This has prompted many surgeons to use at least a short course of prophylactic antibiotics. In cases involving bone or cartilage manipulation, or cases requiring the insertion of synthetic implants or nasal packing, antibiotic use is more common and they are used for a longer duration.[8]

If an infection is encountered after facial aesthetic surgery, treatment must be prompt and appropriately aggressive. Wound drainage, hematoma evacuation, and debridement of macroscopically necrotic tissue are necessary. Infected implants or foreign bodies must be removed. Culture and sensitivity testing should be done to help identify the infectious organism, and broad-spectrum antibiotic

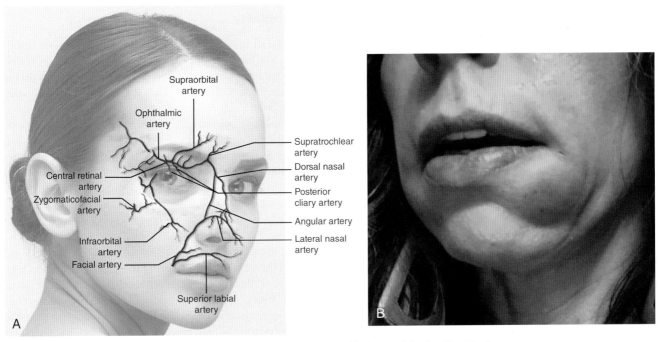

• **Figure 29-1 A,** Blood supply to the face. **B,** Early nodule after filler injection.

coverage to include methicillin-resistant *Staphylococcus aureus* (MRSA) should be started initially. Once the causative bacterium is determined, antibiotic therapy can be modified as indicated by culture and sensitivity. Frequent office follow-up is usually necessary. In some cases, consultation with an infectious disease specialist will be needed, particularly if the infection is not responding to routine therapeutic measures. MRSA has become a more common infectious agent, even for infections of the face. In cases of late developing and/or chronic infections, atypical *Mycobacterium* should be considered. These cases require frequent serial drainage and debridement initially, as well as coordinated treatment by an infectious disease specialist.[8-11]

As with any surgical infection or complication, frequent and careful evaluation by the clinician and the staff members is needed. The problem must be openly acknowledged, and a closely supervised treatment plan should be developed. Surgeons must be honest and empathetic with the patient, because these situations can be highly emotional. Patients often want the problem to "be fixed" quickly, but the surgeon must not rush to a quick solution and must use sound clinical judgment to treat the infection and the wound appropriately. Late revision surgery may be necessary and can be discussed as part of the overall treatment plan. If clinicians are truthful and supportive, patients are more satisfied and less likely to seek legal action.

Skin Resurfacing

The most commonly used skin resurfacing techniques are dermabrasion, chemical peel, and laser.[12] Many surgeons use antibacterial agents during the perioperative period to prevent infections despite lack of strong evidence to support

effectiveness of such a practice. The most common bacterial pathogens are *Staphylococcus* and *Streptococcus* species and *Pseudomonas aeruginosa*. Cephalexin (500 mg qid) or ciprofloxacin (500 mg bid) is used. In patients with a history of previous infections with MRSA, doxycycline (100 mg bid) or trimethoprim-sulfamethoxazole (160 mg/800 mg bid) may be prescribed. Patients undergoing skin resurfacing procedures may be given one of these antibacterial agents on the day preceding the procedure and maintained on the drug for 7 days after.[13]

Candida albicans is the most common fungal infection of the skin after skin resurfacing procedures. The use of a preventive antifungal regimen is indicated, especially when occlusive dressings are used, particularly when these dressings are applied for longer than 48 hours. These dressings promote healing by maintaining a moist environment that facilitates reepithelialization and reduces the discomfort associated with the procedure; however, this also creates a medium for fungal and bacterial growth. Fluconazole (100 mg daily) starting on the day preceding the procedure and continued for 7 days can be used as a preventive measure.[14,15]

Viral infections, particularly with herpes simplex virus, are the most feared infections after any skin ablative procedure because they may lead to significant scarring. All patients begin a preventive antiviral regimen. The risk of such infections is highest among individuals with a history of herpetic outbreaks and, in particular, when the procedure involves the perioral region where the virus is often dormant. Although the use of antiviral therapy does not always ensure suppression of such infections, the following agents have been proved effective: acyclovir (400 mg 5 times daily), valacyclovir (1000 mg bid), and famciclovir (500 mg bid). These agents should be started the day preceding the resurfacing procedure and continued from 7 to 14 days postoperatively.[16,17]

When an actual infection is noted as evidenced by increased pain, erythema, discharge, and even fever, it is imperative to treat the patient aggressively and concurrently for all three bacterial, fungal, and viral causes, because it is often difficult to determine the cause clinically. A consultation with an infectious disease specialist is indicated to prevent unsightly permanent scarring.[18-20]

Soft Tissue Fillers

Infection from soft tissue fillers is a rare event. It can manifest as single or multiple erythematous, fluctuant, and painful nodules. Treatment is usually with antibiotics against common skin flora. In fact, some authors have hypothesized that inflammatory nodules may be caused by a low-grade infection with bacteria (e.g., *Staphylococcus epidermidis* or *Propionibacterium acnes*) maintained around the soft tissue filler.[21,22] Abscess formation is usually more common in patients with human immunodeficiency virus (HIV) infection or facial lipoatrophy.[23]

Filler injections should not be performed if there is an adjacent site of infection (e.g., intraoral, mucosal, skin, or herpes labialis [for lip injection]). There are no evidence-based data to support the idea that fillers play a triggering role in recurrent herpes infection; therefore, there is no rationale in using an antiherpes prophylaxis regimen with every patient. However, patients with a history of developing a cold sore after a filler injection could benefit from it.[21,22]

Late infections also can occur, often as a tender, erythematous, warm nodule that may be fluctuant. The patient may develop systemic symptoms such as fever, chills, and malaise. Late manifestation raises suspicion for atypical bacteria, especially mycobacteria. Empiric antibiotic therapy should be started. In addition, tissue or aspirate should be sent for culture.[24] If the patient's condition does not improve after 48 hours, a punch biopsy should be performed to guide the tailored use of antibiotic therapy.[24] Some recent studies have shown that bacterial biofilms can be resistant to antibiotics and prevented by prophylactic antibiotics.[25,26]

Hypersensitivity reactions have been reported with various soft tissue fillers.[27] This is usually due to trace amounts of proteins present in the filler.[28] The surgeon must be able to differentiate between a hypersensitivity reaction and an infection. In fact, nodule formation is a common complication after the use of soft tissue fillers (see Figure 29-1, *B*). It is commonly categorized as inflammatory or noninflammatory. The timing of its occurrence is important for diagnosis: an inflammatory nodule can appear days to years after treatment; however, a noninflammatory nodule is usually seen immediately after implantation and is usually secondary to improper filler placement. Inflammatory nodules are more common with permanent fillers, such as silicone. These nodules can be secondary to infection or biofilm formation. Appropriate and prompt diagnosis is important in avoiding delay of treatment or long-term complications.[29,30]

Rhinoplasty

The overall incidence of infections associated with rhinoplasty has been reported at 3%. The use of prophylactic antibiotics has been advocated in nasal surgery, but there is no evidence to suggest that their use actually lowers the rate of infection.[31] The severity of such infections can range from minor incision site erythema to septicemia, toxic shock syndrome, necrotizing fasciitis, cavernous sinus thrombosis, or brain abscess. The use of antibiotics has been recommended when the host's immunity is compromised or suppressed, as well as with the use of alloplastic implants or when a hematoma is present. The use of nasal packing, especially beyond 24 hours, may also necessitate antibiotic coverage.[32-34]

Localized granulomas, cellulitis, or abscesses respond well to incision and drainage and the use of antibiotics. Septicemia, while rare, has been reported and can lead to circulatory failure, multiorgan system dysfunction, and disseminated intravascular coagulation. Intervention is directed at source control through surgery and supportive therapy with antibiotics, steroids, and fluid resuscitation.

The use of nasal packing after nasal surgery can lead to staphylococcal toxic shock syndrome (STSS). The incidence of STSS associated with rhinoplasty has been reported at 0.016%, and carries a mortality rate of approximately 11%. A patient with postnasal surgery fever, nausea, vomiting, diarrhea, hypotension, and an erythematous rash should quickly raise the suspicion of STSS. These nonspecific symptoms usually develop 3 to 5 days postoperatively. Susceptible individuals are the nasal carriers of *S. aureus* (18 to 50% of the healthy population). The syndrome is caused by the toxic shock syndrome toxin-1.[32,35,36] The use of antibiotics does not completely eliminate the risk of STSS in susceptible individuals. These patients are profoundly hypotensive and require intensive care with aggressive hemodynamic support, removal of any nasal packing, and immediate administration of intravenous broad-spectrum antibiotics while culture and Gram stain results are pending.[32,35,36] Because of the life-threatening nature of this infection, obtaining an infectious disease consultation is indicated.

Manipulation of the perpendicular plate of the ethmoid bone during septoplasty can lead to the traumatic fracture of the cribriform plate, causing cerebrospinal fluid leak and pneumocephalus.[37] This, in turn, can result in an ascending intracranial infection.[38] Meningitis, subdural empyema, cerebral abscess, and carotid cavernous fistula have all been reported to occur after rhinoplasty through this mechanism.[38-40]

Acute and chronic sinusitis could occur after a rhinoplasty procedure secondary to disruption of the osteomeatal complex. If medical management fails to address the problem, functional endoscopic sinus surgery may be required for definitive treatment.[41]

Postnasal surgery infections are often associated with the use of alloplastic implants. The most commonly used materials in such implants are silicone, expanded polytetrafluoroethylene

(Gore-Tex), and porous high-density polyethylene (Medpor). Nasal reconstruction presents a significant challenge in trying to achieve the dual goals of restoring an aesthetic nasal contour and nasal airway patency for respiratory function. Silicone rubber implants have been the most commonly used material worldwide. Silicone has had popularity, especially for the augmentation of the Asian nose. Silicone polymer implants, however, have a smooth surface and a lack of porosity, which precludes any soft tissue ingrowth. This property leads to infection through frank exposure or late infection by hematogenous bacterial seeding. Extrusion rates of 24 to 55% have been reported. Expanded polytetrafluoroethylene is a microporous woven polymer, and host tissue ingrowth is often limited by the small pore size (22 μm). These implants are usually well tolerated with a less than 2% risk of infection. Porous high-density polyethylene has larger internal pores (100 to 250 μm) that allow for soft tissue and bone ingrowth. This, in turn, provides an avenue for host immune response and leads to better resistance to exposure and infection. In general, regardless of the material used, all alloplastic implants used for nasal reconstruction are prone to infection if inoculation with a pathogen occurs. Minimal handling of these materials during surgery and the use of perioperative antibiotics may reduce the infection risk. In addition, soaking the implant in an antibiotic solution (bacitracin, 50,000 U in 1 L of normal saline) will reduce the incidence of implant-related infections.[42-44]

Facelift and Forehead Lift

Because of the rich vascularity of the face, postoperative rhytidectomy infection rates are extremely low and range from 0.1 to 1% (Figure 29-2). In fact, a retrospective review of 6166 consecutive facelifts found a 0.18% incidence of

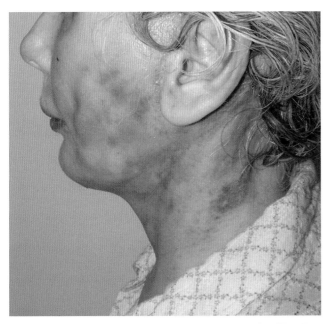

• **Figure 29-2** Unilateral Infected Hematoma 6 Days after Rhytidectomy. (Courtesy Dr. Michael Will.)

infections requiring hospitalization. The majority of these cases yielded cultures positive for *Staphylococcus* species.[45] A more recent review of 780 patients undergoing deepplane facelift found a 0.6% incidence of surgical site infection. Four of the five patients with an infection produced cultures that were positive for MRSA, and two of those patients required hospitalization.[46] A 2020 review of the TOPS database identified a 0.89% incidence of infection after facelift surgery.[47,48] There is little evidence that the use of antibiotics prevents or lowers an already low rate of infection, and yet most surgeons still debate their necessity. Among the surgeons using antibiotics, there is a significant difference in the type of antibiotics used. It appears that the more experienced surgeons tend to use antibiotics less frequently. The use of antibiotics by surgeons seems to be higher when operating on patients who are immunocompromised, such as those with diabetes, the ones receiving immunosuppressive therapy, and smokers. There is no evidence to support the use of postoperative antibiotics in facelift surgery. A 2002 survey, however, found that 52% ($n = 881/1704$) of respondents prescribe postoperative antibiotics after facelift surgery.[49] The signs and symptoms of infection can include the onset of localized tenderness especially with associated erythema and the presence of exudative discharge, swelling, and fever. Perioperative prophylactic antibiotics, if used, should be started between 30 and 120 minutes before the initial skin incision and discontinued within 48 hours of surgery. Principles of infection management should be applied when an infection is noted, including culture and sensitivity testing, incision and drainage or aspiration of any abscesses, removal of any infected sutures, and initiation of empiric antibiotic therapy until speciation and susceptibility studies are available. Proper wound care after a facelift with the use of half-strength hydrogen peroxide and application of a topical antibiotic ointment may reduce the infection rate. When the infection appears unremitting despite the listed measures, or is spreading, an infectious disease consultation is appropriate.[9]

The incidence of infections associated with MRSA is on the rise in all surgical fields, including in soft tissue and cosmetic surgery.[9] Recent hospitalization, recent use of antimicrobial therapy, history of MRSA colonization, diabetes, obesity, and smoking are some of the risk factors associated with soft tissue infections with MRSA after rhytidectomy. Early detection and treatment can tremendously reduce the morbidity associated with this resistant strain, because the infection can spread rapidly along the surgical dissection planes. Vancomycin, linezolid, daptomycin, tigecycline, trimethoprim-sulfamethoxazole, minocycline, clindamycin, fluoroquinolone, and rifampin are among the antibiotics used to combat MRSA infection.[9] Given its ever-evolving resistance profile, it is critical to determine the susceptibility of MRSA to these agents on a case-by-case basis.[50]

Although a search of the literature yields few if any evidence-based studies on infections associated with forehead lift, the surgical and medical management of such infections follows the general guidelines presented earlier for facelift.

Blepharoplasty

Infections after aesthetic eyelid surgery are uncommon and can range from mild wound dehiscence secondary to epidermal inclusion cysts and granulomas to significant periorbital cellulitis and abscess that can lead to blindness. The minor wound separations are readily amenable to local wound care and application of topical ophthalmic antibiotics. These wounds normally heal without any sequelae and rarely need further surgical revision. Patients with orbital cellulitis often exhibit sudden onset of periorbital erythema, swelling, and pain. Examination may also reveal conjunctival injection, chemosis, and restrictions in the range of motion in the affected eye. Although the most feared postoperative blepharoplasty complication is a retrobulbar hemorrhage that results in permanent loss of vision, there are rare reports of blindness secondary to postseptal orbital cellulitis also as a result of compartment syndrome phenomenon. In addition to intense erythema and pain, the globe appears tense, proptotic, and resistant to retropulsion. There is also the presence of concomitant ophthalmoplegia and relative afferent pupillary defect (Marcus Gunn pupil). This constitutes a surgical emergency requiring immediate orbital decompression, which most commonly is achieved through lateral canthotomy and cantholysis. Failure to do so will lead to the compression and occlusion of the central retinal artery and optic nerve vasculature with the resultant permanent blindness. An ophthalmologic consultation after performing the immediate sight-saving surgical decompression is indicated. Medical management is directed at reducing orbital content inflammation, edema, and optic neuritis with the use of intravenous acetazolamide, mannitol, and corticosteroids.[51-54]

Otoplasty

Similar to other structures of the head and neck, the ears are also highly vascular and therefore a low infection rate after otoplasty of approximately 2% has been reported (Figure 29-3). Infections are usually caused by normal flora of the skin and ear canal. The most common responsible microorganisms are *S. aureus, Escherichia coli,* and *Pseudomonas aeruginosa.* The initial presentation of an infection is usually on the third to fifth postoperative days, and it involves sudden onset of pain refractory to analgesic medications. Because hematomas are also painful, it is critical to examine the patient's ear to institute the proper management. Aural hematomas require evacuation followed by application of a pressure dressing to prevent fluid reaccumulation, whereas a cellulitic process or an abscess is treated by removing the sutures at the affected site to allow for drainage. Any purulent exudate is cultured, and empiric enteral antibiotic therapy is initiated. Appropriate antimicrobials for these infections are amoxicillin plus clavulanate (875 mg bid) or ciprofloxacin (750 mg bid). The choice of antibiotic may have to be modified after culture and sensitivity study results become available. A rapidly progressing infection may require intravenous antibiotics and an infectious disease consultation.[55,56]

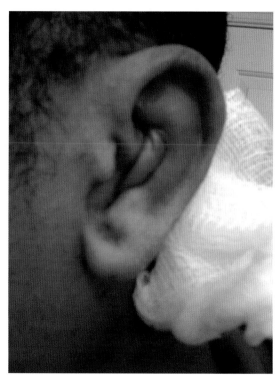

• **Figure 29-3** Perichondritis 7 Days after Otoplasty. (Courtesy Dr. Michael Will.)

Facial Implants

The use of alloplastic implantable materials to achieve improved facial contours has revolutionized the field of facial cosmetic surgery. These implants are used to augment different facial areas, including the chin, mandible, malar area, nose, ear, and orbit and periorbital areas. Most alloplastic facial implants are synthetic polymers. They may be solid polymers, such as polydimethylsiloxane and polymethylmethacrylate; porous polymers, such as high-density porous polyethylene and expanded polytetrafluoroethylene; or meshed polymers, such as polyethylene terephthalate. The ideal implant material is nonantigenic, durable, nontoxic, and resistant to infection.[57] Infection and extrusion of alloplastic implants are serious complications and fortunately are rare. However, infection can occur with any facial implantation procedure and is more common with intraoral approaches. Some studies have recommended soaking the implant in an antibiotic solution (bacitracin, 50,000 U in 1 L of normal saline), and using perioperative antibiotics to reduce the incidence of implant-related infections.[57,58] The use of prophylactic antibiotics, proper dissection, and implant fixation can reduce the rate of acute and late infection rates to 3%.[59] Commonly cultured organisms include staphylococcal and streptococcal species and anaerobes. Preoperative antibiotics (ideally 30 to 45 minutes before the initial incision) and postoperative antibiotics for 5 to 7 days are usually recommended to decrease the risk of infection. Antibiotics should be broad spectrum and have good gram-positive and anaerobic coverage. Infection usually requires implant removal; however, some facial implants with good vascular ingrowth (e.g., high-density porous polyethelene) may be salvageable with only an incision and drainage and antibiotics.

Infection rates vary depending on the type of facial implant and the site of implantation. The mean rates vary from 0 to 5.3%.[59] The highest rate of infection has been associated with nasal surgical mesh (5.3%) and the lowest with porous polyethylene in the malar area (0%).[59] When performing chin augmentation, the submental approach is favored over the transoral one to decrease the chance of infection. There are cases of late infection of these implants, even 10 years after placement; this is most likely due to seeding from a dental source.[60,61]

Hair Transplantation

Hair transplantation is generally safe and is the most common cosmetic surgery procedure performed in men.[62] An infection rate less than 0.1% associated with this procedure has been reported in the literature.[63] Although most of these infections are limited to pustular lesions that respond to antimicrobial therapy and local wound care, significant infections such as bacteremia and sepsis, septic pulmonary embolism, and *S. aureus* osteomyelitis of the calvarium have been reported.[64,65] A sudden onset of increased pain, erythema, and the presence of a purulent exudate or fever should raise the suspicion for a wound infection. Local measures such as incision and drainage, possible debridement, and obtaining a sample of any wound fluid for culture and sensitivity would be the first steps in the management of these infections. Broad-spectrum antimicrobials are then initiated and later adjusted to a narrower, species-specific coverage once the culture and sensitivity results become available.

Summary

Infections after facial aesthetic surgery are rare because the surgical site has less risk of contamination, the blood supply to the area is excellent, and patients tend to be healthier. Prevention of infection is paramount, and it requires good patient selection, proper patient preparation, and meticulous surgical technique. The use of prophylactic antibiotics is controversial, but they should be strongly considered for procedures involving bone or cartilage manipulation, implant or graft placement, or packing insertion. Skin resurfacing procedures may be associated with herpes simplex viral infections. Treatment of infection should be prompt and should include adequate drainage/debridement, foreign body removal, culture and sensitivity testing, initial broad-spectrum antibiotic therapy, and eventual tailored therapy based on culture and sensitivity results, and the use of an infectious disease consultant for complex cases. MRSA should be considered in cases of early infection. For late or chronic infections, atypical mycobacterial infections should be suspected. In all cases, frequent follow-up with the surgeon and the staff members is required, and sound surgical judgment and empathetic care are necessary.

References

1. Miotin LM, Jordan SW, Hanwright P, et al. The relationship between preoperative wound classification and postoperative infection: a multi-institutional analysis of 15,289 patients. *Arch Plast Surg.* 2013;40:522-529.
2. Andenaes K, Amland PF, Lingaas E, et al. A prospective, randomized surveillance study of postoperative wound infections after plastic surgery: a study of incidence and surveillance methods. *Plast Reconstr Surg.* 1995;96:948-956.
3. Gravante G, Caruso R, Araco A, et al. Infections after plastic procedures: incidences, etiologies, risk factors, and antibiotic prophylaxis. *Aesthetic Plast Surg.* 2008;32:243-251.
4. Kirkland KB, Briggs JP, Trivette SL, et al. The impact of surgical-site infections in the 1990s: attributable mortality, excess length of hospitalization, and extra costs. *Infect Control Hosp Epidemiol.* 1999;20:725-730.
5. Ortega G, Rhee DS, Papandria DJ, et al. An evaluation of surgical site infections by wound classification system using the ACS-NSQIP. *J Surg Res.* 2012;174:33-38.
6. Drapeau CM, D'Aniello C, Brafa A, et al. Surgical site infections in plastic surgery: an Italian multicenter study. *J Surg Res.* 2007; 143:393-397.
7. Sylaidis P, Wood S, Murray DS. Postoperative infection following clean facial surgery. *Ann Plast Surg.* 1997;39:342-346.
8. Hsu P, Bullocks J, Matthews M. Infection prophylaxis update. *Semin Plast Surg.* 2006;20:241-248.
9. Zoumaian RA, Rosenberg DB. Methicillin-resistant *Staphylococcus aureus*-positive surgical site infections in face-lift surgery. *Arch Facial Plast Surg.* 2008;10:116-123.
10. Centers for Disease Control and Prevention (CDC). *Mycobacterium chelonae* infections associated with face lifts. *MMWR Morb Mortal Wkly Rep.* 2004;53:192-194.
11. Mauriello JA, Atypical Mycobacterial Study Group. Atypical mycobacterial infection of the periocular region after periocular and facial surgery. *Ophthal Plast Reconstr Surg.* 2003;19:182-188.
12. Kim EK, Hovsepian RV, Mathew P, et al. Dermabrasion. *Clin Plast Surg.* 2011;38:391-395.
13. Manuskiatti WL, Fitzpatrick RE, Goldman MP, et al. Prophylactic antibiotics in patients undergoing laser resurfacing of the skin. *J Am Acad Dermatol.* 1999;40:77-84.
14. Alam M, Pantanowitz L, Harton AM, et al. A prospective trial of fungal colonization after laser resurfacing of the face: correlation between culture positivity and symptoms of pruritus. *Dermatol Surg.* 2003;29:255-260.
15. Setyadi HG, Jacobs AA, Markus RF. Infectious complications after nonablative fractional resurfacing treatment. *Dermatol Surg.* 2008;34:1595-1598.
16. Beeson WH, Rachel JD. Valacyclovir prophylaxis for herpes simplex virus infection or infection recurrence following laser skin resurfacing. *Dermatol Surg.* 2002;28:331-336.
17. Gilbert S. Improving the outcome of facial resurfacing–prevention of herpes simplex virus type 1 reactivation. *J Antimicrob Chemother.* 2001;47(suppl T1):29-34.
18. Halepas S, Lee KC, Higham ZL, Ferneini EM. A 20 year analysis of adverse events and litigation with light-based skin resurfacing procedures. *J Oral Maxillofac Surg.* 2020;78:619-628.
19. Halepas S, Muchemi A, Higham Z, Ferneini EM. The past decade in courts, what OMS should know about facial cosmetic surgery. *J Oral Maxillofac Surg.* 2021;79:1743-1749.
20. Agrawal N, Smith G, Heffelfinger R. Ablative skin resurfacing. *Facial Plast Surg.* 2014;30:55-61.

21. Christensen L. Normal and pathologic tissue reactions to soft tissue gel fillers. *Dermatol Surg.* 2007;33:S168-S175.

22. Christensen L, Breiting V, Janssen M, et al. Adverse reactions to injectable soft tissue permanent fillers. *Aesthetic Plast Surg.* 2005;29:34-48.

23. Kadouch JA, Kadouch DJ, Fortuin S, et al. Delayed-onset complications of facial soft tissue augmentation with permanent fillers in 85 patients. *Dermatol Surg.* 2013;39:1474-1485.

24. Sclafani AP, Fagien S. Treatment of injectable soft tissue filler complications. *Dermatol Surg.* 2009;35(suppl 2):1672-1680.

25. Halepas S, Peters S, Goldsmith J, Ferneini EM. Vascular compromise following soft tissue facial fillers: case report and review of current treatment protocols. *J Oral Maxillofac Surg.* 2020;78:440-445.

26. Aldhede M, Er O, Eickhardt S, et al. Bacterial biofilm formation and treatment in soft tissue fillers. *Pathog Dis.* 2014;70:339-346.

27. Ferneini EM, Banki M, Ferneini CM, et al. Hypersensitivity reaction to facial augmentation with a hyaluronic acid filler: case report and review of literature. *Am J Cosmet Surg.* 2013;30:231-234.

28. Ferneini EM, Boynton T, Almunajed H, et al. Review of facial fillers and injectable neurotoxins. *Am J Cosmet Surg.* 2013;30:53-60.

29. Beauvais D, Ferneini EM. Complications and litigation associated with injectable facial fillers: a cross-sectional study. *J Oral Maxillofac Surg.* 2020;78(1):133-140.

30. Ledon JA, Savas JA, Yang S, et al. Inflammatory nodules following soft tissue filler use: a review of causative agents, pathology and treatment options. *Am J Clin Dermatol.* 2013;14:401-411.

31. Ferneini EM, Halepas S, Sajdlowska J, Weyman D, Bandeff B, Grady J. Systemic antibiotic prophylaxis in rhinoplasty: meta-analysis with recommendations from the literature. *Conn Med.* 2019;83(10):489-497.

32. Jacobson JA, Kasworm EM. Toxic shock syndrome after nasal surgery: case reports and analysis of risk factors. *Arch Otolaryngol Head Neck Surg.* 1986;112:329-332.

33. Cabouli JL, Guerrissi JO, Mileto A, et al. Local infection following aesthetic rhinoplasty. *Ann Plast Surg.* 1986;17:306-309.

34. Rajan GP, Fergie N, Fischer U, et al. Antibiotic prophylaxis in septorhinoplasty? A prospective, randomized study. *Plast Reconstr Surg.* 2005;116:1995-1998.

35. Holt GR, Garner ET, McLarey D. Postoperative sequelae and complications of rhinoplasty. *Otolaryngol Clin North Am.* 1987;20:853-876.

36. Thumfart WT, Völklein C. Systemic and other complications. *Facial Plast Surg.* 1997;13:61-69.

37. Hallock GG, Trier WC. Cerebrospinal fluid rhinorrhea following rhinoplasty. *Plast Reconstr Surg.* 1983;71:109-113.

38. Lewin ML, Argamaso RV, Friedman S. Localized cerebritis following an esthetic rhinoplasty. *Plast Reconstr Surg.* 1979;64:720-723.

39. Pothula VB, Reddy KT, Nixon TE. Carotico-cavernous fistula following septorhinoplasty. *J Laryngol Otol.* 1999;113:844-846.

40. Guyuron B, Licotal L. Arteriovenous malformation following rhinoplasty. *Plast Reconstr Surg.* 1986;77:474-475.

41. Millman B, Smith R. The potential pitfalls of concurrent rhinoplasty and endoscopic sinus surgery. *Laryngoscope.* 2002;112:1193-1196.

42. Winkler AA, Soler ZM, Leong PL, et al. Complications associated with alloplastic implants in rhinoplasty. *Arch Facial Plast Surg.* 2012;14:437-441.

43. Loyo M, Ishii LE. Safety of alloplastic materials in rhinoplasty. *JAMA Facial Plast Surg.* 2013;15:162-163.

44. Peled ZM, Warren AG, Johnston P, et al. The use of alloplastic materials in rhinoplasty surgery: a meta-analysis. *Plast Reconstr Surg.* 2008;121:85e-92e.

45. LeRoy Jr JL, Rees TD, Nolan WB III. Infections requiring hospital readmission following face lift surgery: incidence, treatment, and sequelae. *Plast Reconstr Surg.* 1994;93(3):533-536.

46. Zoumalan RA, Rosenberg DB. Methicillin-resistant Staphylococcus aureus–positive surgical site infections in face-lift surgery. *Arch Facial Plast Surg.* 2008;10(2):116-123.

47. Chopan M, Samant S, Mast BA. Contemporary analysis of rhytidectomy using the Tracking Operations and Outcomes for Plastic Surgeons database with 13,346 patients. *Plast Reconstr Surg.* 2020;145(6):1402-1408.

48. Sinclair N, Coombs DM, Kwiecien G, Zins JE. How to prevent and treat complications in facelift surgery. Part 1: short-term complications. *Aesthet Surg J Open Forum.* 2021;3(1):ojab007. Available at: https://www.ncbi.nlm.nih.gov/pmc/articles/PMC8240741/.

49. Perrotti JA, Castor SA, Perez PC, Zins JE. Antibiotic use in aesthetic surgery: a national survey and literature review. *Plast Reconstr Surg.* 2002;109(5):1685-1693; discussion 1694.

50. Ferneini EM, Beauvais D, Castiglione C. Antibiotics in rhytidectomy surgery: evidence-based recommendations. *Conn Med.* 2018;82(5):271-275.

51. Lee EW, Holtebeck AC, Harrison AR. Infection rates in outpatient eyelid surgery. *Ophthal Plast Reconstr Surg.* 2009;25:109-110.

52. Whipple KM, Lim LH, Korn BS, et al. Blepharoplasty complications: prevention and management. *Clin Plast Surg.* 2013;40:213-224.

53. Klapper SR, Patrinely JR. Management of cosmetic eyelid surgery complications. *Semin Plast Surg.* 2007;21:80-93.

54. Carter SR, Stewart JM, Khan J, et al. Infection after blepharoplasty with and without carbon dioxide laser resurfacing. *Ophthalmology.* 2003;110:1430-1432.

55. Handler EB, Song T, Shih C. Complications of otoplasty. *Facial Plast Surg Clin North Am.* 2013;21:653-662.

56. Limandjaja GC, Breugem CC, Mink van der Molen AB, et al. Complications of otoplasty: a literature review. *J Plast Reconstr Aesthet Surg.* 2009;62:19-27.

57. Binder WJ, Moelleken B, Tobias G. Aesthetic facial implants. In: Papel ID, ed. *Facial Plastic and Reconstructive Surgery.* 4th ed. New York: Thieme Medical Publishing; 2016:276-298.

58. Yaremchuk MJ. Facial skeletal reconstruction using porous polyethylene implants. *Plast Reconstr Surg.* 2003;111:1818-1827.

59. Rubin JP, Yaremchick MJ. Complications and toxicities of implantable biomaterials used in facial reconstructive and aesthetic surgery: a comprehensive review of the literature. *Plast Reconstr Surg.* 1997;100:1336-1353.

60. Ferneini EM, Halepas S. Antibiotic prophylaxis in facial implant surgery: review of the current literature. *Conn Med.* 2018;82(10):593-597.

61. Terino EO. Complications of chin and malar augmentation. In: Peck G, ed. *Complications and Problems in Aesthetic Plastic Surgery.* New York: Gower Medical Publishers; 1992.

62. Vallis CP. Hair replacement surgery. In: McCarthy JG, ed. *Plastic Surgery.* 3rd ed. Philadelphia: WB Saunders; 1990.

63. Unger WP. Treatment for baldness. In: Aston SJ, Beasley RW, Thorne CHM, eds. *Grabb and Smith's Plastic Surgery.* 5th ed. Philadelphia: Lippincott-Raven; 1998.

64. Hirsch BE, Salibian MS, Arunabh R, et al. *Staphylococcus aureus* sepsis complicating hair transplant. *Infect Dis Clin Pract.* 2001;10:101-102.

65. Jones JW, Ignelzi RJ, Frank DH, et al. Osteomyelitis of the skull following scalp reduction and hair plug transplantation. *Ann Plast Surg.* 1980;5:480-482.

30

Tuberculosis and Mycobacterial Infections of the Head and Neck

ELIE M. FERNEINI, STEVEN HALEPAS, KEYUR Y. NAIK

Tuberculosis (TB) is one of the world's deadliest infectious diseases and disproportionately affects developing and underdeveloped countries. In the 1980s, the advent of the bacille Calmette-Guérin (BCG) vaccine promised a reduction in the spread of TB and initially a decrease in incidence was reported. However, multidrug-resistant TB and the rise of the human immunodeficiency virus (HIV) pandemic quickly saw a reversal in this trend. In 2021, 10.6 million people fell ill with TB worldwide, an increase of 4.5% from 2020.[1]

Pulmonary TB is the most common manifestation of a mycobacterial infection. However, in 2009, almost one fifth of all mycobacterial infections in the United States were extrapulmonary,[2] with infection of the head and neck being the most common form of extrapulmonary mycobacterial disease.[3,4] Extrapulmonary TB infections prove to be diagnostically challenging because of the frequently unique presentation. This is particularly true in the head and neck region.

This chapter discusses TB and nontuberculous mycobacterial infections of the head and neck, including cervical lymphadenitis, mycobacterial otic infections, mycobacterial ocular infections, and laryngeal, nasal, pharyngeal, salivary gland, and oral cavity TB.

Cervical Lymphadenitis

Mycobacterial infection involving the cervical lymph nodes is the most common extrapulmonary manifestation of TB.[5] Patients can exhibit an isolated affected node or a collection of involved nodes. The skin overlying the lesion can appear erythremic and may be tender to palpation.[6] While the presentations frequently overlap, it is important to differentiate between a tuberculous and nontuberculous lymphadenitis as the clinical course and treatment are different (Table 30-1).

Tuberculous Lymphadenitis

Tuberculous lymphadenitis is thought to be a result of lymphohematogenous dissemination of *Mycobacterium tuberculosis* (MTB) after initial pulmonary exposure. As the incidence of MTB infections in childhood has decreased, the peak age of patients with MTB lymphadenitis has shifted to 30 to 40 years. Although pulmonary MTB is more common in males and older patients, MTB lymphadenitis is more common in females and in patients from areas with endemic MTB. Adult patients generally exhibit slowly enlarging, painless lymph nodes that most often involve the cervical and supraclavicular nodes. Chest radiographs will generally appear normal, and any abnormalities usually represent healed MTB infections, suggesting that in adults MTB lymphadenitis is a consequence of reactivation of latent infection.[7] This is in sharp contrast to children and immunocompromised adults, who typically show a rapid progression from initial exposure and infection to involvement of the cervical lymph nodes.[8] Therefore, radiographs in these populations will generally show evidence of active MTB infection. Classic constitutional symptoms of fever, chills, night sweats, anorexia, weight loss, and hemoptysis are generally absent, but may be present in immunocompromised patients.[9]

Mantoux purified protein derivative (PPD) skin test will be positive in up to 96% of immunocompetent patients with MTB lymphadenitis. For definitive diagnosis, acid-fast bacilli must be identified by culture, in a polymerase chain reaction (PCR) smear of biopsy, or in fine-needle aspirate. Biopsy has traditionally been used to aid in diagnosis through visualization of granulomatous inflammation and it is still recommended in cases involving multiple nodes (Figure 30-1).[8] However, fine-needle aspiration is less invasive and has comparable sensitivity for diagnosis by culture of acid-fast bacteria.[10] Molecular techniques such as PCR have shown up to 100% sensitivity with 96% specificity,[11] with a more rapid turnaround time than conventional methods and the potential to allow speciation of mycobacterial strains.[12]

The treatment of MTB lymphadenitis involves a 6-month course of antibiotics.[13] A 2-month, four-drug regimen with isoniazid, rifampin, pyrazinamide, and ethambutol should be followed with an additional 4 months of isoniazid and

Characteristic	Tuberculous	Nontuberculous
Age	Adults (30-40 y)	Children (1-5 y), immunocompromised adults
Involved nodes	Posterior cervical, supraclavicular, unilateral or bilateral	Submandibular, submental Unilateral
Classic symptoms	Usually absent	Absent
History of tuberculosis exposure	Common in children, uncommon in adults	Uncommon
Tuberculin skin test	Usually positive	Usually negative
Radiograph findings	Abnormal in children, normal in adults	Usually normal
Primary treatment	Antimicrobial therapy	Surgical excision

TABLE 30-1 Common Features of Tuberculous and Nontuberculous Cervical Lymphadenitis

• BOX 30-1 Nontuberculous Mycobacterial Head and Neck Pathogens

- *Mycobacterium avium*
- *Mycobacterium bohemicum*
- *Mycobacterium chelonae*
- *Mycobacterium fortuitum*
- *Mycobacterium genavense*
- *Mycobacterium haemophilum*
- *Mycobacterium kansasii*
- *Mycobacterium malmoense*
- *Mycobacterium marinum*
- *Mycobacterium scrofulaceum*
- *Mycobacterium szulgai*

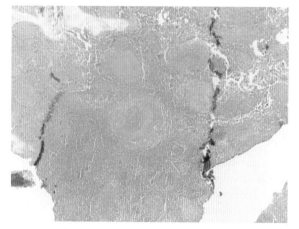

• **Figure 30-1** Granulomatous Reaction of Tuberculosis in Cervical Lymph Node. (From Durucan G, Baglam T, Karatas E, Oz A. Simultaneous mycobacterial infection of tonsil and cervical lymph node: evidence to portal of entry. *Int J Pediatr Otorhinolaryngol Extra.* 2010; 5[3]:97-98.)

rifampin. A relatively common side-effect of therapy is a paradoxical upgrading reaction (PUR) involving new or enlarged nodes in patients after at least 10 days of treatment.[14] Symptoms are thought to be a result of a robust immune response to MTB after the release of mycobacterial antigens from antibiotic treatment. PUR may be exacerbated in HIV-positive patients who also initiate antiretroviral treatment. If PUR or treatment failure occurs, surgical excision is recommended.[15]

In pregnant patients, medical therapy should be delayed, and involved cervical nodes should be excised during the

second or third trimesters.[16] Any fluctuant abscesses should be frequently aspirated during pregnancy. After delivery, a full course of antimicrobial drugs should be administered.

Nontuberculous Lymphadenitis

Nontuberculous mycobacterial (NTM) lymphadenitis is likely acquired through the oral mucosa by contaminated water or soil. The *Mycobacterium avium* complex accounts for 80% of infections, with the other 20% being caused by *M. kansasii, M. haemophilum, M. szulgai, M. malmoense,* and *M. genavense* (Box 30-1).[17] NTM lymphadenitis is generally a disease of children between 1 and 5 years of age and immunocompromised adults. Patients exhibit nontender, unilateral inflammation of the submandibular, anterior cervical, or submental lymph nodes. The overlying skin may appear thin, shiny, and erythematous and may suppurate and form a draining sinus tract.[18]

Unlike MTB, systemic symptoms are absent, chest radiographs almost always appear normal, and a PPD skin test result is generally negative. Therefore, diagnosis requires a high degree of clinical suspicion. Positive identification of the bacteria is necessary to confirm the infection as with MTB lymphadenitis. In addition, fluid from draining wounds should be collected and evaluated for acid-fast bacteria.[19]

Treatment for NTM lymphadenitis involves three options: surgical excision, medical management, and observation. Unlike MTB for which a medical therapy is the first line of treatment, surgical excision has been the preferred treatment in NTB because of the reduced healing time, complete cure rate, and better cosmetic outcome. Direct comparison of surgical excision to antimicrobial therapy has shown a 96% versus a 66% cure rate. For patients in whom complete excision is not an option because of anatomic considerations (e.g., facial nerve involvement) or recurrent disease, a 3- to 6-month therapy regimen with clarithromycin or azithromycin combined with ethambutol or rifampin can be beneficial. Many cases of NTM lymphadenitis will resolve without intervention within 6 to 12 months with scarring of the overlying skin.[20] Therefore, treatment should account for the risks associated with surgery compared with the prolonged course of treatment with antimicrobial drugs and cosmetic outcomes of observation.

Mycobacterial Otic Infections

Mycobacterial otic infections may be of MTB or NTM origin. Otic mycobacterial infection is not common and accounts for only 0.04% of all otitis media infections.[21] MTB otitis media can result from hematogenous dissemination or local spread after pulmonary infection. In contrast, NTM otitis develops from a preexisting middle ear disease with a perforation of the tympanic membrane (Figure 30-2). In both cases, patients exhibit otorrhea and granulation tissue in the external and middle ear and mastoid cavity. MTB otic infections can have significant sequelae including facial palsy, abscess formation, or bone necrosis in up to 16 to 40% of those infected.[22]

Children infected with MTB will frequently have abnormal chest radiographs, but adults with MTB or patients with NTM infections will have normal radiographs. A PPD skin test result is positive in 88% of MTB cases and negative in NTM cases.[23] Identification of acid-fast bacilli from external ear canal cultures has been reported to be positive in 5 to 35% of cases, and confirmation by staining or culture can be hampered by secondary bacterial infection.[24]

Treatment for MTB otic infections includes 6 months of systemic chemotherapy, with otorrhea and granulation formation reported to resolve within 2 months.[25] After completion of therapy, surgery may be indicated to improve hearing or treat facial paralysis. In contrast, for treatment of NTM otic infection, surgery remains the primary modality of treatment.

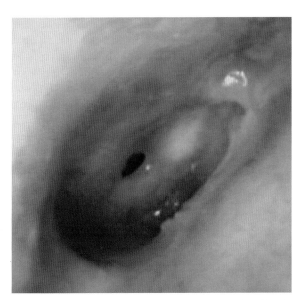

• **Figure 30-2** The Tympanic Membrane Showing a Small Perforation with Copious, Serous Otorrhea Caused by *Mycobacterium abscessus*. (From Sugimoto H, Ito M, Hatano M, et al. A case of chronic otitis media caused by *Mycobacterium abscessus*. *Auris Nasus Larynx*. 2010;37:636-639.)

Removal of tympanostomy tubes, surgical removal of the granulation tissue, and chemotherapy are recommended.

Mycobacterial Ocular Infections

Ocular infections are common in disseminated, head and neck MTB infection and occur with an incidence of 1 to 2% in immunocompetent individuals.[26] Up to 60% of ocular MTB cases were in patients with HIV.[27] Most patients are asymptomatic, but 27% have visual impairment.[28] The most common ocular manifestation is choroiditis, affecting the iris, ciliary body, or choroids. Choroiditis can manifest as a choroidal tuberculoma and appears as multiple disseminated nodules or a single nodule on ocular examination.[29] In children, the surrounding structures of the orbit may be involved, such as lacrimal ducts or sinuses. Painful swelling of the eyelids, epiphora, diminished vision, photophobia, redness, and scleritis are also signs of orbital MTB infection. Other ocular involvement includes retinitis, vitritis, scleritis, and conjunctivitis. Because isolation of bacteria from the orbit is difficult, diagnosis often relies on the presence of bacteria in other sites along with the ocular findings. Treatment relies on systemic antituberculosis therapy. It bears mentioning that some certain ocular diseases are secondary to infection with MTB. These diseases manifest as an allergic reaction (phlyctenular keratoconjunctivitis) or immune-mediated hypersensitivity (tuberculous keratitis) to tuberculous antigens. Treatment of these secondary infections includes the use of topical corticosteroids in addition to antimicrobial therapy.

NTM ocular infections are most commonly caused by *Mycobacterium fortuitum* and *Mycobacterium chelonae*. The most common diagnoses were keratitis, scleral buckle infections, and socket or implant infections.[30] Infection occurs after corneal trauma by contact lens, ocular surgery, or foreign-body injury. Clinical presentation is indistinguishable from fungal infection, and includes cracked windshield appearance, ring infiltrate, satellite lesions, and infectious crystalline keratopathy.[31] Corneal scraping or biopsy is required to obtain sufficient material for positive identification of NTM. Because most first-line drugs used against MTB have no activity against *M. fortuitum* and *M. chelonae*, susceptibility screening is suggested. Reports suggest that clarithromycin is effective in 93%, amikacin is effective in 81%, and moxifloxacin is effective in 21% of cases.[32] Despite these excellent in vitro susceptibility profiles, treatment outcomes still remain generally poor and illustrate the need to recognize and treat ocular NTB infection early.

Laryngeal Tuberculosis

Laryngeal TB is rare form of extrapulmonary TB.[33] The spread of infection is direct from a bronchus or hematogenous spread. The most common symptom associated with laryngeal TB is hoarseness that may be accompanied by odynophagia, dysphagia, cough, otalgia, and stridor. Tuberculous lesions are ulcerofungative, ulcerative, nonspecific inflammations or polypoid masses. These lesions are seen most frequently in the anterior or posterior glottis, but have been seen throughout the larynx and may be difficult to distinguish from cancerous lesions. To differentiate malignant lesions from those caused by TB, biopsy and histopathologic examination is required. Because laryngeal MTB occurs in association with pulmonary MTB, a chest radiograph normally shows abnormalities and PPD skin test result is positive. Although sputum cultures are useful in the diagnosis of active pulmonary TB, sputum microscopy is positive in only approximately 20% of patients with laryngeal TB.[34] Once the diagnosis is made, treatment with a standard antituberculin regimen results in a quick clinical response.[35]

Nasal Tuberculosis

Primary nasal TB can be caused by inhalation of MTB particles or from digital inoculation. Patients complain of nonspecific symptoms, particularly nasal obstruction due to a buildup of mucus or postnasal drip. Physical examination may reveal pale nasal mucosa with nodules, more frequently on the nasal septum than on the lateral walls.[36] Confirmation of the diagnosis must include biopsy and culture to rule out other acid-fast bacilli such as *Mycobacterium laprae*.[37] Nasal secretions and swab specimens are low yield and should not be used to rule out MTB infection.[38] Although nasal TB is rare, treatment with standard antituberculin therapy has shown improvement of symptoms in case reports.[39]

Pharyngeal Tuberculosis

MTB infections rarely affect the oropharynx or nasopharynx. MTB infections of the pharynx are more frequently primary infections with no involvement of the lungs seen on radiograph.[40] Clinical presentations of nasopharyngeal TB are varied, and case reports range from patients with no symptoms to patients with epistaxis, chronic cough, postnasal drip, and nasal obstruction.[41] Adenoid hypertrophy and cervical lymphadenopathy commonly accompany pharyngeal MTB infections.[42] Patients respond rapidly to treatment with standard antituberculin drug regimens.

Salivary Gland Tuberculosis

Salivary gland MTB infection is extremely rare and when present is more commonly found in the parotid gland than in the submandibular or sublingual glands. Infection of the salivary glands is thought to follow a preceding tooth or tonsil infection that spreads through the lymphatics or by retrograde migration through Stensen's duct. The course of infection proceeds as a slow-growing, firm, nodular mass, and weeks to months may pass before a patient seeks medical attention. Patients are generally healthy with no evidence of MTB systemic disease, and masses are difficult to distinguish from salivary gland neoplasms, making diagnosis a challenge.[43] Confirmation of suspected cases requires fine-needle aspiration and positive PCR identification.[43,44] Incisional biopsy should be avoided because it can lead to a chronic fistula.[41] Treatment with standard antituberculosis therapy has been successful when given for up to 12 months. In cases of treatment failure, ablative surgery of the affected gland should be performed.[45]

Oral Cavity Tuberculosis

Infection of the oral mucosa by MTB represents less than 1% of the extrapulmonary MTB infections, with secondary infections occurring more frequently than primary infections.[46] Despite the high levels of MTB in the oral cavity during a pulmonary infection, the paucity of lesions in the oral cavity suggests a protective effect of saliva among other barriers in the oral cavity, such as thick epithelial covering.[47] Injury to the mucosa through poor dental hygiene, local trauma, or irritation can lead to self-inoculation through sputum. Lesions occur most commonly on the tongue; they may also be found on the palate, lips, buccal mucosa, gingiva, palatine tonsil, and floor of the mouth. These lesions appear in many forms as ulcers, nodules, tuberculomas, or periapical granulomas, and they are commonly painful.[48] Cases should be confirmed by histopathologic examination to differentiate from carcinoma and treated with a standard TB regimen as discussed previously.[49] The majority of cases are secondary to pulmonary infection; therefore, a case of oral MTB should lead the clinician to evaluate the patient for underlying systemic infection.

Summary

Mycobacterial infections is an increasingly significant global health problem. Multidrug-resistant mycobacteria and the spread of HIV have both led to an increasing incidence of disease particularly in the developing and underdeveloped world. These infections can be divided into two categories: *M. tuberculosis* and nontuberculous mycobacterial infections. MTB is a systemic infection that typically originates as a pulmonary infection and then spreads to regions of the head and neck, including the cervical lymph nodes and the ocular, otic, laryngeal, pharyngeal, and oral spaces. MTB infection is treated medically with multiple agents, although resistance has become an increasing problem and has worsened the burden of disease worldwide. In contrast, NTM lymphadenitis can establish infection in the cervical lymph nodes and ocular and aural spaces but cannot be managed with medications used for MTB. These infections can require surgical intervention; therefore, it is imperative that the distinction between mycobacterial infections be made quickly to allow proper control and management of disease.

References

1. World Health Organization. *Global Tuberculosis Report 2022.* Geneva: World Health Organization; 2022.

2. Peto HM, Pratt RH, Harrington TA, LoBue PA, Armstrong LR. Epidemiology of extrapulmonary tuberculosis in the United States, 1993-2006. *Clin Infect Dis.* 2009;49:1350-1357.

3. Al-Serhani AM. Mycobacterial infection of the head and neck: presentation and diagnosis. *Laryngoscope.* 2001;111(11 Pt 1):2012-2016.

4. Mandpe A, Lee K. Tuberculous infections of the head and neck. *Curr Opin Otolaryngol Head Neck Surg.* 1998;l6:190.

5. Dabrowski MT, Keith AO. Three cases of mycobacterial cervical lymphadenitis. *J Laryngol Otol.* 1994;108:514-515.

6. Rahal A, Abela A, Arcand PH, et al. Nontuberculous mycobacterial adenitis of the head and neck in children: experience from a tertiary care pediatric center. *Laryngoscope.* 2001;111:1791-1796.

7. Shriner KA, Mathisen GE, Goetz MB. Comparison of mycobacterial lymphadenitis among persons infected with human immunodeficiency virus and seronegative controls. *Clin Infect Dis.* 1992;15:601-605.

8. Blaikley JF, Khalid S, Ormerod LP. Management of peripheral lymph node tuberculosis in routine practice: an unselected 10-year cohort. *Int J Tuberc Lung Dis.* 2011;15:375-378.

9. Handa U, Mundi I, Mohan S. Nodal tuberculosis revisited: a review. *J Infect Dev Ctries.* 2012;6:6-12.

10. Knox J, Wong JSJ, Trevan PG, Karunajeewa H. Diagnosis of tuberculous lymphadenitis using fine needle aspiration biopsy. *Intern Med J.* 2012;42:1029-1036.

11. Kim DW, Jung JS, Ha TK, Park K. Individual and combined diagnostic accuracy of ultrasound diagnosis, ultrasound-guided fine-needle aspiration and polymerase chain reaction in identifying tuberculous lymph nodes in the neck. *Ultrasound Med Biol.* 2013;39:2308-2314.

12. Park DY, Kim JY, Choi KU, et al. Comparison of polymerase chain reaction with histopathologic features for diagnosis of tuberculosis in formalin-fixed, paraffin-embedded histologic specimens. *Arch Pathol Lab Med.* 2003;127:326-330.

13. American Thoracic Society, Centers for Disease Control and Prevention, Infectious Diseases Society of America. In: *Control CFD: Treatment of Tuberculosis.* New York: ATS, CDC, IDSA; 2003:1-77. Available at: https://www.cdc.gov/mmwr/preview/mmwrhtml/rr5211a1.htm

14. Hawkey CR, Yap T, Pereira J, et al. Characterization and management of paradoxical upgrading reactions in HIV-uninfected patients with lymph node tuberculosis. *Clin Infect Dis.* 2005;40:1368-1371.

15. Munck K, Mandpe AH. Mycobacterial infections of the head and neck. *Otolaryngol Clin North Am.* 2003;36:569-576.

16. Lindeboom JA, Kuijper EJ, Bruijnsteijn van Coppenraet ES, Lindeboom R, Prins JM. Surgical excision versus antibiotic treatment for nontuberculous mycobacterial cervicofacial lymphadenitis in children: a multicenter, randomized, controlled trial. *Clin Infect Dis.* 2007;44:1057-1064.

17. Perlman DC, D'Amico R, Salomon N. Mycobacterial infections of the head and neck. *Curr Infect Dis Rep.* 2001;3:233-241.

18. Hatzenbuehler LA, Starke JR. Common presentations of nontuberculous mycobacterial infections. *Pediatr Infect Dis J.* 2014;33:89-91.

19. Amir J. Non-tuberculous mycobacterial lymphadenitis in children: diagnosis and management. *Isr Med Assoc J.* 2010;12:49-52.

20. Zeharia A, Eidlitz-Markus T, Haimi-Cohen Y, Samra Z, Kaufman L, Amir J. Management of nontuberculous mycobacteria-induced cervical lymphadenitis with observation alone. *Pediatr Infect Dis J.* 2008;27:920-922.

21. Jeanes AL, Friedmann I. Tuberculosis of the middle ear. *Tubercle.* 1960;41:109-116.

22. Skolnik PR, Nadol Jr JB, Baker AS. Tuberculosis of the middle ear: review of the literature with an instructive case report. *Rev Infect Dis.* 1986;8:403-410.

23. Greenfield BJ, Selesnick SH, Fisher L, Ward RF, Kimmelman CP, Harrison WG. Aural tuberculosis. *Am J Otol.* 1995;16:175-182.

24. Odetoyinbo O. Early diagnosis of tuberculous otitis media. *J Laryngol Otol.* 1988;102:133-135.

25. Singh B. Role of surgery in tuberculous mastoiditis. *J Laryngol Otol.* 1991;105:907-915.

26. Thompson MJ, Albert DM. Ocular tuberculosis. *Arch Ophthalmol.* 2005;123:844-849.

27. Babu RB, Sudharshan S, Kumaraswamy N, Therese L, Biswas J. Ocular tuberculosis in acquired immunodeficiency syndrome. *Am J Ophthalmol.* 2006;142:413-418.

28. Bouza E, Merino P, Muñoz P, Sanchez-Carrillo C, Yáñez J, Cortás C. Ocular tuberculosis: a prospective study in a general hospital. *Medicine (Baltimore).* 1997;76:53-61.

29. Lazarus AA, Thilagar B. Tuberculosis of pericardium, larynx, and other uncommon sites. *Dis Mon.* 2007;53:46-54.

30. Girgis DO, Karp CL, Miller D. Ocular infections caused by non-tuberculous mycobacteria: update on epidemiology and management. *Clin Experiment Ophthalmol.* 2012;40:467-475.

31. Garg P. Fungal, mycobacterial, and *Nocardia* infections and the eye: an update. *Eye (Lond).* 2012;26:245-251.

32. Lalitha P, Rathinam SR, Srinivasan M. Ocular infections due to non-tuberculous mycobacteria. *Indian J Med Microbiol.* 2004;22:231-237.

33. Shin JE, Nam SY, You SJ, Kim SY. Changing trends in clinical manifestations of laryngeal tuberculosis. *Laryngoscope.* 2000;110:1950-1953.

34. Nishiike S, Irifune M, Doi K, Sawada T, Kubo T. Laryngeal tuberculosis: a report of 15 cases. *Ann Otol Rhinol Laryngol.* 2002;111:916-918.

35. Soda A, Rubio H, Salazar M, Ganem J, Berlanga D, Sanchez A. Tuberculosis of the larynx: clinical aspects in 19 patients. *Laryngoscope.* 1989;99:1147-1150.

36. Masterson L, Srouji I, Kent R, Bath AP. Nasal tuberculosis: an update of current clinical and laboratory investigation. *J Laryngol Otol.* 2011;125:210-213.

37. Williams RG, Douglas-Jones T. *Mycobacterium* marches back. *J Laryngol Otol.* 1995;109:5-13.

38. Goguen LA, Karmody CS. Nasal tuberculosis. *Otolaryngol Head Neck Surg.* 1995;113:131-135.

39. Kim YM, Kim AY, Park YH, Kim DH, Rha KS. Eight cases of nasal tuberculosis. *Otolaryngol Head Neck Surg.* 2007;137:500-504.

40. Srirompotong S, Yimtae K, Jintakanon D. Nasopharyngeal tuberculosis: manifestations between 1991 and 2000. *Otolaryngol Head Neck Surg.* 2004;131:762-764.

41. Güneri EA, Ikiz AO, Atabey N, Izci O, Sütay S. Polymerase chain reaction in the diagnosis of parotid gland tuberculosis. *J Laryngol Otol.* 1998;112:494-496.

42. Patil C, Patel RK, Deshmukh P, Biswas J, John B. Primary tuberculosis of nasopharynx (adenoid): a rare presentation. *Asian Pac J Trop Med.* 2013;6:246-248.

43. Tse GM, Ma TFK, Chan ABW, et al. Tuberculosis of the nasopharynx: a rare entity revisited. *Laryngoscope.* 2003;113:737-740.

44. Kim YH, Jeong WJ, Jung KY, et al. Diagnosis of major salivary gland tuberculosis: experience of eight cases and review of the literature. *Acta Otolaryngol.* 2005;125:1318-1322.

45. Tauro LF, George C, Kamath A, Swethadri GK, Gatty R. Primary tuberculosis of submandibular salivary gland. *J Glob Infect Dis.* 2011;3:82-85.

46. Saunders NC, Albert DM. Tuberculous mastoiditis: when is surgery indicated? *Int J Pediatr Otorhinolaryngol.* 2002;65:59-63.

47. Haddad NM, Zaytoun GM, Hadi U. Tuberculosis of the soft palate: an unusual presentation of oral tuberculosis. *Otolaryngol Head Neck Surg.* 1987;97:91-92.

48. Prada JL, Kindelan JM, Villanueva JL, et al. Tuberculosis of the tongue in two immunocompetent patients. *Clin Infect Dis.* 1994;19:200-202.

49. Dixit R, Sharma S, Nuwal P. Tuberculosis of oral cavity. *Indian J Tuberc.* 2008;55:51-53.

31

Anesthetic Considerations in Head, Neck, and Orofacial Infections

WILLIAM CHUNG

Infections involving the deep fascial spaces of the oropharynx and head and neck regions present a multitude of challenges for the treating surgeon and anesthetist, none more concerning or ominous than airway obstruction or complete loss of the airway. Infections in the maxillofacial region have the potential to complicate treatment because of its ability to cause trismus and edema with resultant pathologic changes to normal anatomic structures such as displacement of the tongue or airway deviation that results in a true emergent medical crisis. This chapter will discuss anesthetic considerations in the management of the airway of a patient with a head and neck infection.

Anatomy of the Airway

Head and neck infections pose numerous challenges to their successful management and treatment. Several infections such as those located in the masseteric, infratemporal, pterygomandibular, or lateral pharyngeal spaces are bordered by the masticatory muscles and thus can result in trismus. Other infections involving the lateral pharyngeal or retropharyngeal spaces lie directly adjacent to the airway. Also complicating the situation is that cleavage planes exist within the base of the tongue that allow submandibular and sublingual infections to pass posteriorly toward the epiglottis.[1] These factors contribute to the imminent danger that deep fascial space infections pose. The surgeon should not underestimate the morbidity or mortality associated with this group of infections because they can spread rapidly to adjacent areas and in severe cases could result in aspiration of infected material and cause bronchopneumonia.[2-4]

Evaluation of the Patient

Time is of the essence when evaluating a patient with a presumed head and neck infection. The surgeon should perform the initial survey expeditiously and forego obtaining a thorough medical history if the patient is in imminent danger of experiencing respiratory distress or loss of an airway. An experienced clinician will be aware of less obvious signs and symptoms consistent with pending hypoxia, such as agitation or irritability, which in turn can develop into an altered level of consciousness. If complete obstruction of the airway occurs and the brain is deprived of oxygen, permanent damage can occur in as few as 4 to 6 minutes.[5] An evaluation of an infected patient's ventilatory effort and oxygenation level is standard, and use of a pulse oximeter facilitates this objective. A slow declining trend in the patient's oxygen saturation level may indicate a need for establishing a more definitive and protected airway.

History

Predicting the difficulty in mask ventilation or intubation of a patient particularly in the setting of a head and neck infection is not an exact science. Thus, identifying any factors that improve the ability to predict difficult ventilation or intubation is critical before administering any anesthetic or analgesic medications. Accurate answers to questions such as the time, onset, progression of, and severity of symptoms, and what therapies, if any, have already been implemented must be obtained. The report of dysphagia in the setting of an infection is not uncommon because of lingual and pharyngeal edema and involvement of the masticatory muscles. A complaint of dysphagia and dyspnea or an inability to handle oral secretions likely indicate upper airway edema or narrowing, respectively, making further investigation all-important. A muffled voice is a sign of a narrowed upper airway, whereas a hoarse voice may be consistent with an infection that has reached the glottis. Determining a history of other conditions that can have an impact on both the surgery and anesthesia for a patient with a head and neck infection include a history of stridor, obstructive sleep apnea,[6-8] cervical disorders, or systemic diseases such as diabetes or arthritis, particularly involvement of the temporomandibular joints.

Physical Examination

A detailed examination of an infected patient must determine the presence of any of the following findings: limited interincisal opening, a swollen or displaced tongue, decreased airway space, swelling of the pharynx, and the presence of either congenital or acquired deformities of the hard and soft tissues in the maxillofacial region. Also, of importance is determining any difficulty in extension or flexion of the neck, which may indicate involvement of deep fascial spaces.

The presence of trismus, or limited interincisal opening, should elevate the surgeon's level of concern because of impeding access to, and visualization of, structures in the oropharynx in the event direct laryngoscopy is required[9-11] (Figure 31-1). An opening that is less than 20 mm may make direct laryngoscopy for intubation challenging, particularly for an inexperienced anesthetist. However, the degree of trismus may partially improve if the limited opening was a result of pain and inflammation. The progression of edema may cause distortion or displacement of critical structures such as the tongue or floor of mouth, submandibular and sublingual spaces, or the thyroid cartilage or trachea more inferiorly (Figure 31-2). When edema involves the pharynx and supraglottic areas, the patient will not tolerate being placed in a semisupine or supine position and will sit upright with extension of the head forward and flexion of the neck, which is described as the "sniffing" position (Figure 31-3). All of these changes can have an adverse impact on the ability to reduce the risk of respiratory distress or protect the airway.

Assessment of the Airway and Risk for Compromise

Methods used to predict the success of laryngoscopy and intubation require simplicity and reproducibility.[12-14] One such method is the Mallampati score, an assessment of the airway based on the ability of the surgeon to visualize the uvula and faucial pillars with the patient sitting upright, mouth wide open, and tongue maximally protruded. The higher score corresponds to a more difficult intubation as well as a higher incidence of sleep apnea.[15] Another assessment tool is the

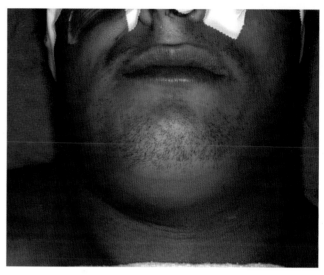

• **Figure 31-2** Fascial Space Infection Involving Both Submental and Submandibular Spaces. Note erythema and edema from abscessed right mandibular molar and bicuspid teeth. (Courtesy of Dr. William Chung, Indianapolis, IN)

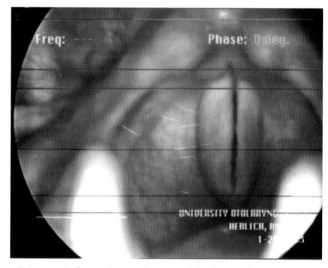

• **Figure 31-3** Supraglottic Edema Involving Vocal Cords. (Courtesy Dr. Andrew Herlich, University of Pittsburgh, Pittsburgh, PA).

thyromental distance, which is the distance from the prominence of the thyroid cartilage to the menton with complete head extension. A thyromental distance less than 6.5 cm (three fingerbreadths) serves as an indicator for difficult mask ventilation, laryngoscopy, supraglottic airway placement, or endotracheal intubation.[16] In another study, Karkouti et al.[17] recommended evaluating the following variables: mouth opening, chin protrusion, and atlanto-occipital extension. Their study produced a highly reliable and predictive model to determine difficult intubation, with an 86.8% sensitivity and 96.0% specificity.

Potential challenges with delivering positive pressure ventilation also must be considered when assessing airway management in head and neck infections.[18] Atypical anatomy or edema can distort and displace critical structures such as the tongue and pharynx complicating what otherwise

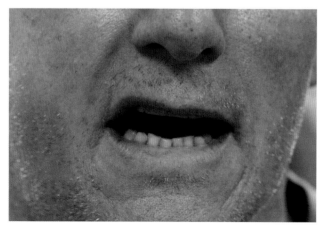

• **Figure 31-1** Trismus Resulting from an Infection Involving the Pterygomandibular and Lateral Pharyngeal Spaces.

would be a routine task such as bag-mask ventilation. Each method has its own limitations, but performed correctly, they can assist in predicting a difficult intubation, particularly in the setting of a head and neck infection.

Diagnostic Tests

Unless a concern exists for the progression of respiratory distress or airway obstruction, completion of diagnostic imaging should not be delayed. Advanced imaging, specifically computed tomography (CT), has become the standard of care in the overall assessment of head and neck infections.[19] Use of intravenous contrast dye further improves the accuracy of the study by enhancing phlegmonous tissues and can delineate any abscesses or necrotic areas.[20] Additional diagnostic modalities such as video laryngoscopy and fiberoptic examination enable the surgeon to directly visualize the airway and adjacent structures, augmenting the information provided by any obtained imaging.

Categorization of Urgency for Treatment

A system to stratify patients into specific categories discerning the urgency for treatment was created by Brown and Sataloff.[21] The categories included:
1. Occult impending respiratory distress
2. Obvious respiratory distress
3. Total or nearly total airway obstruction.

Occult impending respiratory distress refers to a patient's risk of experiencing airway difficulty after medication or manipulation. Muscular relaxation may result from the administration of certain medications that may impair the patient's compensatory respiratory mechanisms and compromise the airway. Categorization in the *obvious respiratory distress* occurs if an infected patient experiences stridor, labored breathing, intercostal retractions, and tracheal tug, which can eventually produce fatigue, adversely affecting the patient's ventilatory effort and potentially resulting in insufficient oxygenation. *Total or near-total airway obstruction* involves a patient experiencing hypoxia, hypercarbia, and delirium. Patients who fall into this category emergently require an established and protected airway.

Corticosteroids

Inflammation associated with an infection has the potential to spread beyond the borders of the infection, which can potentially lead to a series of deleterious effects such as swelling and distortion of airway-related structures and eventual airway obstruction. Administration of corticosteroids can prevent or reduce the inflammatory process that occurs within tissues and avoid tissue damage, exerting various effects such as suppression of capillary dilation and permeability, leukocyte migration, and phagocytosis. Corticosteroid therapy does not come without its potential risks, but short-term use was determined to have minimal risks.[22] Additionally, corticosteroids have been used in the

treatment of inflamed structures of both the oropharynx and airway such as the epiglottis, larynx, and trachea.[22,23] However, a paucity of studies exists to support the use of steroids in the setting of head and neck infections,[24] and multiple studies refute the clinical benefits of corticosteroid administration for the treatment of infections, as well as reducing postextubation airway edema.[25-27] Thus, administration of corticosteroids for the treatment of head and neck infections is not routinely recommended.

Anesthesia

Purulence that is produced from an infection lowers the pH of infected tissue compared to its surroundings. The pH of pus ranges between 5 and 6, and the excess hydrogen ions that exist within infected tissue causes more of the local anesthetic molecules to change into its ionized, or cationic, form. However, it is the nonionized, or base, form of the local anesthetic molecule that rapidly diffuses through cell membranes to reach neural tissue to produce its intended effect. Thus, the inflammatory process and developing infection make attaining a sufficient or clinically effective level of local anesthesia challenging.

Sedation and Analgesia

When sufficient anesthesia is unsuccessful with local anesthesia alone, the patient will require additional medications to proceed with an incision and drainage of the infection. Proper patient selection is paramount when conscious sedation and analgesia is considered. Factors such as limited oral opening, deviation and distortion of upper airway structures, narrowing of the airway, and the proposed location of the surgical incision and drainage must be taken into account. Although administering sedation and analgesia may increase the patient's ability to tolerate the proposed surgical procedure, oversedation of the patient may result in depression of the hypoxic or hypercapnic respiratory drive, obtund any protective airway reflexes, or cause airway obstruction. Upper airway obstruction from moderate sedation occurs from decreased muscle tone of the pharyngeal muscles, which results in obstruction of air movement despite performing mask ventilation. Partial obstruction at this level will produce sounds similar to snoring from the turbulent airflow. Complete obstruction can lead to apnea and is characterized by no air movement and an absence of respiratory sounds. Apnea is a true medical emergency that can result in hypoxemia, hypercarbia, negative pressure pulmonary edema, and cardiac arrest.

Proper identification of involved fascial space(s) is essential when sedation and analgesia is considered. Sublingual or lateral pharyngeal space involvement requires a higher level of attention because of its proximity to the airway when administering conscious sedation and analgesia. The patient's level of consciousness must be determined before the administration of any sedative or analgesic medications to avoid oversedation and the potential for a loss of the airway. The presence and severity of trismus directly affects the decision to use sedation and analgesia medications. Titration of these medications may facilitate opening of the oral cavity with a ratchet-type mouth prop to enable visualization of critical areas such as the floor of mouth and pharynx. If sedation and analgesia does not improve mouth opening, further administration of these medications should be discontinued to prevent the patient from becoming oversedated and the surgeon potentially losing control of the airway. An option at this juncture is to perform an awake intubation (discussed later in this chapter), which is assisted by topicalization of the oropharynx and/or decreasing the gag reflex. Sedating the patient and anesthetizing the airway may allow visualization of the glottis to more accurately determine the feasibility of endotracheal intubation.

Pain and anxiety reduce gastric pH and delay gastric emptying time, so determining an accurate fasting status is paramount to prevent aspiration from either gastric contents or from rupture of abscess contents. In a nonemergent scenario, the patient should fast from solid foods for 8 hours and fast from clear liquids for a minimum of 2 hours. If an infection does not pose an imminent threat to the airway and an appropriate fasting period has not been achieved, the surgeon may consider delaying the procedure or further administration of anesthetic medications until such time has been determined.

Sedation and analgesia are considered in the surgical management of orofacial infections when effective local anesthesia is unattainable and is typically produced by administration of benzodiazepines and opioids. Benzodiazepines produce sedation, anxiolysis, and amnesia, and opioids provide analgesia. These medications must be titrated slowly to avoid oversedation and respiratory depression, but reversal agents exist for both groups of medications.[28,29] The potential for respiratory depression from these medications require administration of supplemental oxygen and continuous monitoring of the patient's oxygen saturation, carbon dioxide levels, and vital signs during and after the procedure.

Ketamine and Dexmedetomidine

Ketamine is an anesthetic agent that possesses multiple characteristics that make its administration advantageous in the setting of head and neck infections. Ketamine induces a state of "dissociative anethesia," or a trance-like state while also providing analgesia, sedation, and amnesia.[30] Additional clinical advantages of ketamine include maintenance of airway reflexes, ventilatory drive, and functional residual capacity, moderate bronchodilation, and a slow anesthetic emergence. When used as an adjunct agent in combination with benzodiazepines or propofol, ketamine can be administered in smaller subanesthetic doses, shortening the recovery period, yet still providing effective analgesia.

Another anesthetic agent that produces analgesia and sedation without respiratory depression is dexmedetomidine. This α_2-selective adrenoceptor agonist reduces anesthetic and opioid requirements and makes its use advantageous in patients who have an orofacial infection that also may be at risk for a compromised airway. Dexmedetomidine is administered intravenously by a bolus followed by continuous infusion. It is also administered intranasally in pediatric patients as an alternative to midazolam.[31] However, the intranasal administration of dexmedetomidine carries the potential for developing hypotension or bradycardia and a longer recovery time, which makes this route more challenging if a concern for a compromised airway exists.

General Anesthesia

General anesthesia may be inevitable if all previous methods of anesthesia fail to provide adequate anesthesia for a patient during surgical intervention for an infection. Endotracheal intubation also may be necessary if trismus cannot be overcome with sedation and analgesia and a risk for loss of the airway becomes more evident. The obvious advantage of endotracheal intubation is that it provides a secured and established airway in the setting of pending airway obstruction and may also protect the patient from aspiration if the abscess cavity is traumatized with resultant rupture of the contents.

Although surgical access to structures in the oropharynx is improved with nasotracheal intubation, orotracheal intubation is the preferred method for an orofacial or head and neck infection, particularly if a concern exists for loss of an airway. Orotracheal intubation is faster and can be simpler than nasotracheal intubation, and nasotracheal intubation may be more challenging, particularly in the setting of a difficult airway from an orofacial infection, if the anesthetist is less experienced with nasal intubations. Lastly, multiple failed attempts at nasotracheal intubation may increase the risk of complications such as epistaxis, mucosal laceration, increased airway edema, false passage of the endotracheal tube, or iatrogenic rupture of abscess contents into the trachea and potential aspiration.

The nasotracheal route is often preferred during an awake intubation, and an endotracheal tube can be left in place for a longer period because of better patient tolerance of the tube in the nasal cavity versus the oral cavity and less risk of accidental extubation. If the nasal route is planned, intubating the naris opposite the side of the infection may avoid or minimize trauma to structures affected by the infection. However, nasal intubation is contraindicated in the setting of a lateral pharyngeal or retropharyngeal space infection because of the increased risk of abscess rupture and subsequent aspiration.

If airway edema progresses and obstruction is becoming more apparent, determining the anatomic level of the obstruction is paramount before ventilatory efforts become compromised. If the obstruction is located in the upper airway, placement of either an oropharyngeal or nasopharyngeal airway, depending on the location of the infection, will possibly prevent inadvertent rupture of the abscess during further manipulation of the oral cavity to establish an open airway. When delivering positive pressure ventilation, a self-inflating resuscitation bag may be used, which has the advantage of not requiring a compressed gas source for proper function. This type of resuscitation bag also contains an exhalation valve to prevent rebreathing. If ventilatory efforts improve, the decision can be made to proceed with intubation; if ventilatory efforts continue to be difficult, use of additional airway adjuncts or a surgical airway will need to be considered.

If establishing a secured airway on an emergent basis does not appear imminent, a more controlled induction of anesthesia is accomplished by administering a volatile inhalational agent through a mask. Although intravenous medications can be titrated to achieve a desired depth of anesthesia during induction, these medications can also cause respiratory depression that can contribute to airway obstruction. Inhalational agents allow spontaneous ventilation, which facilitates maintenance of a patent airway even as the depth of anesthesia increases.

Several favorable clinical characteristics of an inhalational anesthetic agent include high potency; low solubility in blood and tissues, which allows for rapid recovery; and not irritating to the airway. Desflurane, sevoflurane, and isoflurane are several more commonly used agents for induction or maintenance anesthesia, but sevoflurane has a low blood-gas partition coefficient, allowing it to be titrated faster to achieve the intended depth of anesthesia.[32]

Patient comfort and cooperation is paramount for patient safety during an awake intubation. Providing the patient with an explanation of the process allows the patient to anticipate the subsequent steps of the awake intubation. Providing sedation during an awake intubation assists in decreasing patient anxiety while minimizing undesirable changes in the patient's hemodynamic stability, and oversedation must be avoided, which can produce oxygen desaturation and impede maintaining a secure airway. Supplemental oxygen delivery with appropriate anesthesia monitoring throughout the entire process is compulsory to avoid hypoxia, and agitation or combativeness during the intubation may not be the product of discomfort and anxiety, but rather may be the result of hypoxia. Any patient undergoing endotracheal intubation requires preoxygenation with 100% oxygen for 3 minutes to reduce the chance of hypoxia[33] while also maintaining oxygen saturation over 80% in a 70-kg adult for approximately 8 minutes or for 2½ minutes in a healthy child. Oxygen saturation and capnographic monitoring can be facilitated by attaching a nasopharyngeal airway to an endotracheal tube adaptor that is subsequently connected to the anesthesia circuit.[34]

Reducing both airway reactivity during manipulation and the gag reflex will increase patient compliance and safety during an awake fiberoptic intubation, and application of topical anesthetics or nerve blocks accomplish this goal.[35,36] Topicalization of the pharynx can be achieved with viscous lidocaine by either a swish and swallow technique or direct application onto the pharyngeal tissues with the viscous lidocaine that has been placed on the end of a tongue depressor.

Topical anesthesia of the pharynx also can be achieved with nebulized lidocaine administered by a mouthpiece or facemask. Anesthetizing other airway-related structures to reduce the gag reflex may further improve patient tolerance and safety during an awake fiberoptic intubation. The base of tongue, vallecula, and epiglottis can be anesthetized with a superior laryngeal nerve block, which is accomplished by administration of 1 to 2 mL of 2% lidocaine just lateral to the midline above the thyroid notch into the thyroid membrane. A glossopharyngeal nerve block anesthetizes the posterior third of the tongue, vallecula, anterior epiglottis, tonsillar pillars, and pharynx after depositing 1 to 2 mL of lidocaine into the inferior aspect of the anterior tonsillar pillars. Additionally, anesthesia of the larynx can be performed by transtracheal administration of 4 mL of 4% lidocaine through the cricothyroid membrane. The anesthetic must only be administered after a positive aspiration of air is confirmed. Attention must be given to avoid administering any nerve block if the transcutaneous injection runs the risk of traversing the abscess cavity, causing spread of the infection or possible rupture and spillage of the contents.

Performing a successful nasal intubation can be augmented by use of various adjuncts, such as a *video laryngoscope, fiberoptic laryngoscope,* or *lighted stylet.* Furthermore, a specific technique has been described to assist in nasal intubation where structures may be misaligned, making passage of the endotracheal tube more challenging.[37,38] When repeated attempts to establish nasotracheal intubation have failed, the endotracheal tube does not need to be completely removed to continue oxygenating the patient. Rather, oxygen still can be delivered through the endotracheal tube by holding the patient's mouth and nares closed while keeping the airway in an open position and oxygen is delivered with positive pressure ventilation by bag-mask ventilation.

A *video laryngoscope* is now routinely available in most operating rooms. Video laryngoscopy provides a rapid and clear indirect view of the glottis, and when the anesthetist is familiar with and experienced with its use, a nasal intubation can be easier and more predictable, particularly when trismus or a narrowed airway is present. If the anesthetist is inexperienced or unfamiliar with the use of a video laryngoscope, then this modality does not guarantee a faster or safer intubation. Use of a *fiberoptic laryngoscope* is considered the standard of care when an awake nasotracheal intubation is required. A fiberoptic scope is flexible, so the tip can be purposefully directed by the anesthetist through the fiberoptic cable. This specific functionality is particularly valuable, especially if the nasoendotracheal tube must navigate through edematous, distorted tissues in the acute setting of a head and neck infection.[39] Finally, a *lighted stylet* provides transillumination of the external neck by providing a light source at the tip of the endotracheal tube, assisting the anesthetist to locate the tip of the tube. The American Society of Anesthesiologists recognizes the use of a lighted stylet in management of a difficult airway.[40,41] The lighted stylet may avert the anesthetist from having to perform a blind nasal intubation for a head and neck infection.

Gastric regurgitation and insufflation during anesthesia induction and positive pressure ventilation is minimized by use of the Sellick maneuver, which requires downward pressure on the cricoid cartilage that results in temporary esophageal closure between the cricoid cartilage and cervical vertebrae. The effectiveness of the Sellick maneuver depends on the amount of pressure applied to the cricoid cartilage.[42,43] Although this maneuver is the standard of care for preventing aspiration of gastric contents in obtunded patients, it does not prevent aspiration from ruptured material within an abscess.

Supraglottic Airway

The laryngeal mask airway (LMA) enables potential ventilation when the patient cannot not be ventilated with a facemask or endotracheal intubation has failed. Although an LMA can be inserted blindly, it does not protect against pulmonary aspiration because the seal the LMA creates is located in the hypopharynx and supraglottis.[44] By nature of its design, the patient's glottis can be directly visualized by placing a fiberoptic endoscope through the tube of the LMA. A more definitive airway can be placed after the LMA is secured and the patient is appropriately ventilated. An endotracheal tube without a balloon can be placed through an LMA with the assistance of a tube exchanger inserted in the endotracheal tube.[45,46] A no. 6 endotracheal tube can be passed through a no. 3 LMA, and a no. 5 endotracheal tube can be passed through a no. 4 LMA.

Surgical Airway

When an infection progresses and begins to cause airway obstruction and efforts to ventilate the patient are compromised, an emergent need arises to establish a secured and protected airway. The patient must be sedated to allow for laryngoscopy to place an endotracheal tube. If endotracheal intubation fails, a surgical airway via a cricothyrotomy or a tracheotomy can be performed[47,48] before oxygen deprivation causes irreversible organ damage. However, a surgical airway is not without inherent risks.[49]

If a surgical airway must be performed emergently and time has not permitted adequate sedation and analgesia, the patient's lack of sedation will have preserved intact airway reflexes to facilitate placement of a cuffed endotracheal or tracheotomy tube to protect the lower airway. Complications related to performing a tracheotomy include bleeding, displacement of the tracheotomy tube, creation of a false passage to the trachea while inserting the tracheotomy tube, or causing either a pneumothorax or pneumomediastinum positive pressure ventilation through the false passage. Other complications include formation of a cutaneous fistula from the trachea or tracheal stenosis at the site of tracheotomy after decannulation.[50] Most patients will not experience symptoms of tracheal stenosis unless a significant portion of the trachea becomes obstructed.

Pulmonary Aspiration

Administering sedation and analgesia can impair a patient's protective airway reflexes, so decreasing the amount of sedation, particularly in patients who are at risk for aspiration or impaired gastric emptying, may lower this risk. To further avoid or minimize the risk of aspiration, a Yankauer suction tip on high-volume suction must be readily available to evacuate any purulence and secretions, especially during anesthesia induction. Patient positioning may also assist in avoiding complications related to aspiration of ruptured contents of an abscess. Placing the patient in a Trendelenburg position during induction may prevent pus from entering the trachea.

There is a paucity of reports regarding the incidence of aspiration from a ruptured infection of the head and neck region, so the true incidence of such an event is unknown. One particular study documented mediastinal or endothoracic spread from deep space abscesses of odontogenic origin.[51] Furthermore, no statistics exist for the mortality rate from aspiration of an orofacial infection. However, a 70% mortality rate has been documented from aspiration of any source.[52,53] The organisms most commonly isolated from the pulmonary aspirate were bacteria routinely cultured in oropharyngeal infections: *Fusobacterium nucleatum, Bacteroides melaninogenicus, Bacteroides oralis,* and *Peptostreptococcus* and *Peptococcus* species.[54] The antibiotic of choice in those who are not allergic is clindamycin. It is not inconceivable that an infection related to aspiration pneumonia can be prolonged. Thus, a transtracheal aspirate should be obtained to reculture the aspirate to determine any changes in its flora.[55]

Extubation Post Infection

The potential for severe complications during both intubation and extubation of a patient exist,[56] and the anatomic changes and airway-related complexities associated with a head and neck infection demands a greater understanding of the criteria for both processes. Several clinical criteria exist to determine the safety for extubation after treatment of a head and neck infection. Physical examination of the masticatory muscles and perioral structures can determine any improvement in the ease and amount of mouth opening after the procedure. Improvement in the patient's trismus enables the surgeon to inspect the floor of mouth and oropharynx. The surgeon can gauge improvement in the resolution of airway edema around the glottis and upper airway by determining if the patient can breathe around the endotracheal tube after deflating the tube cuff as well as using a fiberoptic laryngoscope. Finally, advanced imaging allows for evaluating the presence of postoperative airway edema and confirmation of surgical drainage of the abscess.

If reintubation appears imminent, the use of an endotracheal tube changer to facilitate this process has been described in the American Society of Anesthesiologists Task Force on Management of the Difficult Airway.[40] The tube changer is inserted just below the tip of the endotracheal tube above the carina, and it is designed such that jet ventilation can be delivered through it. The tube changer is typically removed within 1 hour of extubation[57] but can be left in place for several hours if reintubation may be anticipated. Furthermore, a fiberoptic laryngoscope can function in a role similar to that of a tube changer when reintubation becomes necessary.

Conclusion

As in any clinical scenario in which airway obstruction is a possibility, securing the airway in the setting of a head and neck infection in the safest manner possible is paramount to avoid respiratory compromise and loss of the airway. Patient comfort and cooperation are essential for successful management of the infection, and sedation and analgesia are often administered to provide the level of required anesthesia for a patient to tolerate a procedure that local anesthesia alone cannot sufficiently provide. Several adjuncts such as video and fiberoptic laryngoscopes exist to assist with endotracheal intubation in the setting of a narrowed or distorted airway, and oxygenation with appropriate anesthesia monitoring is compulsory to avoid hypoxia. A surgical airway should be considered a last resort if ventilation can be effectively performed through an established secured supraglottic device or endotracheal tube.

References

1. Grodinsky M. Ludwig's angina: an anatomical and clinical study with review of literature. *Surgery*. 1939;5:678.
2. Jevon P, Abdelrahman A, Pigadas N. Management of odontogenic infections and sepsis: an update. *Br Dent J*. 2020;229(6):363-370.
3. Rautaporras N, Furuholm J, Uittamo J, et al. Deep odontogenic infections: identifying risk factors for nosocomial pneumonia. *Clin Oral Investig*. 2021;25(4):1925-1932.
4. Saifeldeen K, Evans R. Ludwig's angina. *Emerg Med J*. 2004; 21:242-243.
5. Bernat JL. Coma, vegetative state, and brain death. In: Goldman L, Shafer AI, eds. *Cecil Medicine*. 24th ed. Philadelphia: Saunders-Elsevier; 2011.
6. Young T, Palta M, Dempsey J, et al. The occurrence of sleep-disordered breathing among middle-aged adults. *N Engl J Med*. 1993;328(17):1230-1235.
7. Turner K, VanDenkerkhof E, Lam M, et al. Perioperative care of patients with obstructive sleep apnea: a survey of Canadian anesthesiologists. *Can J Anaesth*. 2006;53(3):299-304.
8. Gross JB, Bachenberg KL, Benumof JL, et al. Practice guidelines for the perioperative management of patients with obstructive sleep apnea: a report by the American Society of Anesthesiologists Task Force on Perioperative Management of Patients with Obstructive Sleep Apnea. *Anesthesiology*. 2006;104:1081-1093.
9. Ovassapian A. Management of the difficult airway. In: Ovassapian A, ed. *Fiberoptic Endoscopy and the Difficult Airway*. 2nd ed. Philadelphia: Lippincott-Raven; 1996.
10. Mallampati SR, Gatt SP, Gugino LD, et al. A clinical sign to predict difficult tracheal intubation: a prospective study. *Can Anaesth Soc J*. 1985;32:429.
11. Wilson ME, Speigelhlter D, Roberson JA, et al. Predicting difficult intubation. *Br J Anaesth*. 1988;61:211.
12. Shiga T, Wajima Z, Inoue T, et al. Predicting difficult intubation in apparently normal patients: a meta-analysis of bedside screening test performance. *Anesthesiology*. 2005;103:429-437.
13. Eberhart LH, Arndt C, Aust HJ, et al. A simplified risk score to predict difficult intubation: development and prospective evaluation in 3763 patients. *Eur J Anaesthesiol*. 2010;27:935-940.
14. Frova G, Sorbello M. Algorithms for difficult airway management: a review. *Minerva Anestesiol*. 2009;5:201-209.
15. Nuckton TJ, Glidden DV, Browner WS, et al. Physical examination: Mallampati score as an independent predictor of obstructive sleep apnea. *Sleep*. 2006;29(7):903-908.
16. Ambesh SP, Singh N, Rao PB, et al. A combination of the modified Mallampati score, thyromental distance, anatomical abnormality, and cervical mobility (M-TAC) predicts difficult laryngoscopy better than Mallampati classification. *Acta Anaesthesiol Taiwan*. 2013;51:58-62.
17. Karkouti K, Keith Rose D, Wiggleworth D, et al. Predicting difficult intubation: a multivariate analysis. *Can J Anaesth*. 2000; 47:730.
18. El-Orbany M, Woehlck HJ. Difficult mask ventilation. *Anesh Analg*. 2009;109:1870-1880.
19. Cunqueiro A, Gomes W, Lee P, Dym RJ. CT of the neck: image analysis and reporting in the emergency setting. *Radiographics*. 2019;39(6):1760-1781. Available at: https://doi.org/10.1148/rg.2019190012.
20. Gonzalez-Beicos A, Nunez D. Imaging of acute head and neck infections. *Radiol Clin North Am*. 2012;50:73-83.
21. Brown AC, Sataloff RT. Special anesthetic techniques in head and neck surgery. *Otolaryngol Clin North Am*. 1981;14:587.
22. Shah RK, Stocks C. Epiglottitis in the United States: national trends, variances, prognosis, and management. *Laryngoscope*. 2010;120(6):1256-1262.
23. Ozbek C, Aygenc E, Tuna EU, et al. Use of steroids in the treatment of peritonsillar abscess. *J Laryngol Otol*. 2004;118:439-442.
24. Barret A. Dexamethasone as an adjunct in oropharyngeal obstruction in a patient with leukemia. *Oral Surg Oral Med Oral Pathol*. 1990;70:741.
25. Darmon JY, Rauss A, Dreyfuss D, et al. Evaluation of risk factors for laryngeal edema after tracheal extubation in adults and its prevalence by dexamethasone: a placebo-controlled, double-blind, multicenter study. *Anesthesiology*. 1992;77:245-251.
26. Anene O, Meert KL, Uy H, et al. Dexamethasone for the prevention of postextubation airway obstruction: a prospective randomized, double-blind, placebo-controlled trial. *Crit Care Med*. 1996;24:1666.
27. Ho LI, Harn HJ, Lien TC, et al. Postextubation laryngeal edema in adults: risk factor evaluation and prevention by hydrocortisone. *Intensive Care Med*. 1996;22:933.
28. Blouin RT, Conrad PF, Perrault S, et al. The effect of flumazenil on midazolam-induced depression of the ventilatory response to hypoxia during isohypercarbia. *Anesthesiology*. 1993;78:635.
29. Gross JB, Weller RS, Conrad P. Flumazenil antagonism of midazolam-induced ventilatory drive during sedation with midazolam and alfentanil. *Anesthesiology*. 1996;78:635.
30. Gitlin J, Chamadia S, Locascio J, et al. Dissociative and analgesic properties of ketamine are independent. *Anesthesiology*. 2020; 133:1021-1028.
31. Sun Y, Huang Y, Jiang H. Is dexmedetomidine superior to midazolam as a premedication in children? A meta-analysis of randomized controlled trials. *Pediatr Anesth*. 2014;24:863-874.

32. Brioni J, Varughese S, Ahmed R, Bein B. A clinical review of inhalational anesthesia with sevoflurane: from early research to emerging topics. *J Anesth.* 2017;31:764-778.

33. Berthound M, Read D, Norman J. Preoxygenation—how long? *Anesthesia.* 1983;38:96-102.

34. Roelofse J, Joubert JJ, Payne KA. The Loumanen oral airway and endotracheal tube holder as an aid to pediatric fiberoptic endoscopy. *J Oral Maxillofac Surg.* 1990;48:533-534.

35. Kostyk P, Francois K, Salik I. Airway anesthesia for awake tracheal intubation: a review of the literature. *Cureus.* 2021;13(7):e16315.

36. Sitzman BT, Rich GF, Rockwell JJ, et al. Local anesthesia administration for awake direct laryngoscopy. *Anesthesiology.* 1997;86:34-40.

37. Ackerman WE, Phero JC. An aid to nasotracheal intubation. *J Oral Maxillofac Surg.* 1989;47:1341.

38. Gorback MS. Inflation of the endotracheal tube cuff as an aid to blind nasal endotracheal intubation. *Anesth Analg.* 1987; 66:916-917.

39. Stella JP, Kageler W, Epker BN. Fiberoptic endotracheal intubation in oral and maxillofacial surgery. *J Oral Maxillofac Surg.* 1986;44:923-925.

40. The American Society of Anesthesiologists Task Force on Management of the Difficult Airway. Practice guidelines for management of the difficult airway. *Anesthesiology.* 1993;78:597-602.

41. Davis L, Cook-Sather SD, Shreiner MS. Lighted stylet tracheal intubation; a review. *Anesth Analg.* 2000;90:745-756.

42. Ovassapian A, Salem M. Sellick's maneuver: to do or not do. *Anesth Analg.* 2009;109(5):1360-1362.

43. Moied AS, Jyotishka P. Cricoid pressure: a misnomer in pediatric anaesthesia. *J Emerg Trauma Shock.* 2010;3(1):96-97.

44. Benumof JL. Laryngeal mask airway and the ASA difficult airway algorithm. *Anesthesiology.* 1996;84:686-699.

45. Heath ML, Allagain J. Intubation through the laryngeal mask: a technique for unexpected difficult intubation. *Anaesthesia.* 1991;46:545-548.

46. Silk JM, Hill HM, Calder I. Difficult intubation and the laryngeal mask. *Eur J Anaesthesiol.* 1991;4(suppl):47-51.

47. Demas PN, Sotereanos GC. The use of tracheotomy in oral and maxillofacial surgery. *J Oral Maxillofac Surg.* 1988;43:483.

48. Feinberg SE, Peterson LJ. Use of cricothyroidostomy in oral and maxillofacial surgery. *J Oral Maxillofac Surg.* 1987;45:873.

49. Zasso F, You-Ten K, Ryu M, et al. Complications of cricothyrotomy and tracheotomy in emergency surgical airway management: a systematic review. *Br J Anaesth.* 2020;125:213-214.

50. Wright C, Li S, Geller A, et al. Postintubation tracheal stenosis: management and results 1993-2017. *Ann Thorac Surg.* 2019; 108:1471-1477.

51. Toews A, de la Roche AG. Oropharyngeal sepsis with endothoracic spread. *Can J Surg.* 1980;23:265.

52. LeFrock J, Clark T, Davies B, et al. Aspiration pneumonia: a ten-year review. *Am Surg.* 1979;45:305-313.

53. Lanspa MJ, Jones BE, Brown SM, Dean NC. Mortality, morbidity, and disease severity of patients with aspiration pneumonia. *J Hosp Med.* 2013;8:83-90.

54. Gorbach SL, Barlett JG. Anaerobic infections. *N Engl J Med.* 1974;290:1237.

55. Marik PE. Aspiration pneumonitis and aspiration pneumonia. *N Engl J Med.* 2001;344:665-671.

56. Caplan RA, Posner KL, Ward RJ, et al. Adverse respiratory events in anesthesia: a closed claim analysis. *Anesthesiology.* 1990;72:828.

57. Miller J, Lovino W, Fine J, et al. High-frequency jet ventilation in oral and maxillofacial surgery. *J Oral Maxillofac Surg.* 1982;40:790.

32

Perioperative Infection Control

KAYLIE CATLIN, CHAD DAMMLING, SHELLY ABRAMOWICZ, AND BRIAN KINARD

Health Care–Associated Infections

The prevention of health care–associated infections (HCAIs) has been a goal of regulatory organizations for over a decade. As of 2008, it was estimated that 5 to 10% of hospitalized patients (nearly 2 million patients) develop an HCAI, leading to approximately 100,000 deaths and 4.5 to 6.5 billion dollars in extra health care costs per year.[1] In response to these alarming statistics, the Society for Healthcare Epidemiology of America and the Infectious Diseases Society of America Standards and Practice Guidelines Committee appointed a task force dedicated to publishing concise recommendations for the prevention of common HCAIs in acute care hospitals. The first iteration of this compendium was published in 2008, and updates were published in 2014 and 2022.[1-3] The 2008 compendium addressed four device- and procedure-associated HCAIs: central line–associated bloodstream infections (CLABSIs), ventilator-associated pneumonia (VAP), catheter-associated urinary tract infections (CAUTIs), and surgical site infections (SSIs). Two organism-specific categories were also addressed because of an increasing incidence and high morbidity: methicillin-resistant *Staphylococcus aureus* (MRSA) infection and *Clostridium* (now *Clostridioides*) *difficile* infection (CDI). A revised 2014 compendium added an additional category of targeted improvement in hand hygiene.[2] All hospitalized patients are at risk for development of an HCAI, and it is the responsibility of the surgeon to screen patients appropriately and implement approved preventive practices. This chapter will highlight updated recommendations targeted to reduce the incidence of HCAIs, with a special focus on the prevention of perioperative infections and SSIs.

Central Line–Associated Bloodstream Infection

The compendium of strategies to prevent HCAIs in acute care hospitals offered several recommendations for the prevention of CLABSI before, during, and after central line insertion. The compendium endorses completion of an educational program for all health care providers involved in the placement of central venous catheters (CVCs), as well as

periodic retraining and competency assessments. At the time of insertion, skin preparation should be performed with an alcohol-chlorhexidine solution.[2] The 2022 compendium established the subclavian vein as the preferred site of access for CVCs in intensive care unit (ICU) patients, and recommended that ultrasound guidance is standard practice for catheter insertion.[3] The femoral vein should be avoided for central line placement, especially in obese patients because of presence of groin bacteria and difficulty in cleaning. ICU patients over the age of 2 months should be bathed daily with a chlorhexidine preparation, and in patients over 2 months of age, the use of chlorhexidine-containing dressings is now considered an essential practice.[3] The use of antiseptic- or antimicrobial-impregnated CVCs is considered an additional approach that may be used for patient populations or hospital units with CLABSI rates above institutional goals. However, the compendium recommends against the use of antimicrobial prophylaxis for short-term or tunneled catheter insertion or while catheters are in situ.[3]

Ventilator-Associated Pneumonia

To decrease the risk of VAP, the compendium recommends avoiding intubation whenever possible in favor of noninvasive positive pressure ventilation. In intubated patients, sedation should be minimized (or weaned when possible) and spontaneous breathing trials with assessment for extubation should be completed daily. Interventions that decrease secretion pooling superior to the endotracheal tube cuff are especially important in patients who require intubation for 48 to 72 hours. Head of bed elevation to 30 to 45 degrees is recommended, although with lower quality of evidence rating.[1,2] Other strategies to reduce the risk of VAP include selective decontamination of the oropharynx, performance of oral care with chlorhexidine, and provision of mechanical toothbrushing.

Catheter-Associated Urinary Tract Infection

To reduce the incidence of CAUTIs, urinary catheters should be inserted only when necessary and removed as soon as possible. Other methods of bladder management should be considered, including the use of bladder scanners and intermittent catheterization. Other recommendations for the prevention of CAUTIs include the use of small catheters to reduce urethral trauma, placement of catheters only by trained, dedicated personnel, use of sterile technique during catheter placement, and proper securing of catheters after insertion to prevent movement.[1,2]

Surgical Site Infection

The compendium recommends the following basic practices for the prevention of SSI. Antibiotic prophylaxis should be administered in accordance with evidence-based standards and guidelines. Hair should not be removed at the surgical site unless it interferes with the procedure; when it is removed, clippers are preferred to razors. Blood glucose should be controlled, especially in cardiac patients. Core temperature of 35.5°C (95.9°F) should be maintained perioperatively. Tissue oxygenation should be maximized by the administration of supplemental oxygen during and immediately after surgery. Alcohol-containing preparatory solutions should be used to prepare the skin whenever possible. Hospitals should perform routine surveillance for SSI and use automated data whenever possible.[1,2] Each of these strategies will be discussed in detail with evidentiary support later in this chapter.

Hand Hygiene

Generally, hand hygiene should be performed with an alcohol-based rub or, alternatively, an antimicrobial or nonantimicrobial soap when hands are visibly soiled. Hospitals are instructed to monitor compliance with hand hygiene and implement multimodal strategies for adherence. Situations that require specific approaches to hand hygiene include outbreaks of norovirus or of *C. difficile*. In addition to contact precautions, hands should be washed with soap and water after caring for each patient with known or suspected infection of norovirus or *C. difficile*.[2]

Methicillin-Resistant *Staphylococcus aureus*

The compendium recommends that hospitals conduct MRSA risk assessments and implement an active surveillance testing (AST) program to control and prevent MRSA. If health care providers are linked epidemiologically to a cluster of MRSA infections, they are advised to be screened for MRSA infection or colonization. As part of the AST, MRSA-colonized patients should receive targeted decolonization therapy, and all ICU patients should be treated with universal MRSA decolonization. The compendium also advised the use of gowns and gloves when treating all ICU patients, though this intervention was noted to have lower quality of evidentiary support.[1,2]

Clostridioides difficile Infection

In 2011, *C. difficile* was responsible for an estimated 453,000 infections nationally, as well as 29,300 deaths.[4]

Most strategies mentioned in the compendium to address CDI were thought to be of low or moderate evidentiary support. Basic strategies to reduce CDI include judicious antimicrobial prescribing practices, use of contact precautions for infected patients, and adequate cleaning and disinfection of equipment and environment (with Environmental Protection Agency–approved sporicidal disinfectant or diluted sodium hypochlorite). There is moderate-quality evidence to support placing patients who have diarrhea under contact precautions while *C. difficile* testing is pending. It may be beneficial to extend the duration of contact precautions for patients with known CDI until hospital discharge, regardless of symptoms. As mentioned previously, during outbreaks of CDI, hand hygiene should be completed with soap and water whenever exiting the room of a patient with a CDI.[1,2]

Outcomes Assessment

Since the publication of the initial Compendium in 2008, the Centers for Disease Control and Prevention (CDC) began conducting surveys to assess the prevalence of HCAIs. In 2011, a multistate point prevalence survey including 11,282 patients at 183 hospitals showed that 4% of hospitalized patients had an HCAI.[5] In 2015, the survey was repeated across 10 states and 199 hospitals, many of which had participated in the 2011 survey, to evaluate changes in the incidence of HCAIs as a result of broad reporting requirements and targeted prevention efforts.[6] Of the 12,299 patients surveyed, researchers identified 427 HCAIs in 394 patients (3.2%). Of these, the most common type was pneumonia (25.7%), followed by gastrointestinal infections (21.3%, predominantly CDI), and SSIs (16.2%). Patient age older than 40, larger hospital size, length of stay, and the presence of a ventilator or central catheter were independently associated with HCAIs. Of the 69 SSIs identified in the 2015 survey, 16% were attributed to "other" operative procedures, followed by colon surgeries (10%), hip replacements (10%), and spinal fusions (7%).[6] The most frequently identified organisms implicated overall in HCAIs were *C. difficile, S. aureus,* and *Escherichia coli.* Using data from the National Inpatient Sample stratified by patient age and length of stay, the survey results can be extrapolated to estimate a disease burden of 633,300 patients with an HCAI (95% confidence interval [CI] [216,000; 1,912,700]) and 687,200 total HCAIs (95% CI [181,400; 2,691,200]) in U.S. hospitals in 2015.[6]

When comparing the 2015 survey and its predecessor, researchers found that fewer patients had HCAIs in 2015 (3.2%; 95% CI [2.9 to 3.5]) than in 2011 (4.0%; 95% CI [3.7 to 4.4]). When adjusted for multiple confounding factors, hospitalized patients in the 2015 survey were 16% less likely to have an HCAI than patients in the 2011 survey (risk ratio [RR] 0.84; 95% CI [0.74 to 0.95]). Most of this reduction was due to significant decreases in the rate of CAUTIs ($P = .005$) and SSIs ($P < .001$).[6] However, there was no significant difference in the prevalence of pneumonia and CDI, nor a difference in the outcome of patients hospitalized with HCAIs (i.e., mortality). These results demonstrate a partial success of evidence-based interventions in reducing national rates of HAIs, particularly CAUTIs and SSIs. However, more effort is needed to decrease overall disease burden and reduce mortality among patients with HAIs.[6]

Focus on Surgical Site Infections

As noted previously, SSIs still account for a significant proportion of HCAIs (16.2%).[6] SSIs are categorized as either superficial incisional, deep incisional, or organ/space.[7,8] Superficial incisional SSIs involve only the skin or subcutaneous tissue, not including suture abscesses. A deep incisional SSI involves the deep soft tissue such as the fascia and muscle. An organ/space SSI involves any organ or space that was accessed during surgery.[8] In all cases, an SSI is defined as occurring within 30 days of surgery unless an implant was placed; in these cases, it is defined as occurring within 1 year of surgery.[7] The microbes most likely to be responsible for SSIs are those endogenous flora that are present on the skin, mucosa, or viscera contiguous with the operative site.[8] Logically, the likelihood of developing an SSI depends on the location, nature, and cleanliness of the surgical site. The CDC defines wound class risk in four categories: clean, clean-contaminated, contaminated, and dirty.[8] In lower wound classes, the organisms responsible for SSI are most likely derived from the skin or external environment. With increasing wound class, these microbes are more likely derived from internal body linings, such as the gastrointestinal and genitourinary tracts. Higher wound class is directly correlated to risk of SSI.[8]

Table 32-1 summarizes the wound classification system, with examples of wound classification in routine head and neck surgical procedures.[8,9]

There are numerous patient, operative, and microbial factors that may contribute to the development of SSI. The National Nosocomial Infection Surveillance (NNIS) system has been developed to predict risk of SSI based on 3 factors.

These include (1) American Society of Anesthesiologists (ASA) preoperative score greater than 3, (2) wound classification of contaminated or dirty, and (3) an operation length greater than the 75th percentile for expected procedure time. A higher NNIS score is correlated to greater risk of SSI.[8] Specific patient risk factors that will be discussed include hyperglycemia, smoking habits, malnutrition, age, obesity, coexisting infections, prolonged hospitalization, altered immune response, and perioperative transfusions.[7,8] Perioperative factors that may influence the risk of SSI include administration of prophylactic antibiotics, skin care, operating room environment, temperature, glucose control, wound treatment, and oxygenation.[8] These risk factors are illustrated in the following table and will be discussed in detail later in this text.

Patient Risk Factors	Operative Risk Factors
Age	Preoperative skin preparation
Nutritional status	Duration of operation
Hyperglycemia/diabetes	Antimicrobial prophylaxis
Smoking	Perioperative oxygenation
Obesity	Inadequate sterilization of instruments
Coexisting infections	Surgical technique
Altered immune response	Operating room environment
Prolonged hospitalization	Topical antibiotics/antiseptics

Patient Risk Factors

Age

Age has been described as a risk factor associated with the development of SSI.[8,10] Several variables have been proposed to explain the relationship between age and risk of SSI, including increased prevalence of comorbid conditions, higher severity of acute illness, poor nutritional status, and immune dysfunction.[11] A cohort study conducted by Kaye et al.[11] included 144,485 consecutive surgical

---

TABLE 32-1	Centers for Disease Control and Prevention Wound Classification System and Surgical Site Infection Risk

Class	Type	Descriptor	Infection Risk
1	Clean	An uninfected operative wound in which no inflammation is encountered and the respiratory, alimentary, or genitourinary tract is not entered (e.g., parotidectomy, lymph node excision).	<2%
2	Clean-contaminated	An operative wound in which the respiratory, alimentary, or genitourinary tracts are entered under controlled conditions and without unusual contamination (e.g., orthognathic surgery, cleft lip and palate surgery, cyst enucleation).	<10%
3	Contaminated	Open, fresh, accidental wounds. In addition, operations with major breaks in sterile technique and incisions in which acute, nonpurulent inflammation is encountered (e.g., mandibular fractures, chronic open wounds).	Approximately 20%
4	Dirty-infected	Old traumatic wounds with retained devitalized tissue and those that involve existing clinical infection (e.g., odontogenic abscesses).	Approximately 40%

Adapted from Dammling C, Abramowicz S, Kinard B. Current concepts in prophylactic antibiotics in oral and maxillofacial surgery. *Oral Maxillofac Surg Clin North Am.* 2022;34(1):157-167. https://doi.org/10.1016/j.coms.2021.08.015.[9]

patients at 11 hospitals between 1991 and 2002. After adjusting for confounding variables (ASA score, wound class, operative duration, type of operative procedure, and type of hospital), increasing age was found to be an independent risk factor for the development of SSI ($P = .002$), with risk of SSI increasing by 1.1% per year between ages 17 and 65. Interestingly, risk of SSI decreased by 1.2% for each additional year beyond age 65. The authors proposed this finding may relate to surgical selection bias, as healthier elderly patients are more likely to undergo surgery than their more frail peers.[10,11]

Although unmodifiable, it is important to recognize that elderly patients who develop SSI have higher mortality rates, prolonged hospitalizations, and increased hospital costs compared to younger patients with SSIs.[10] Thus, rigorous adherence to interventions for the prevention of SSIs should be employed in elderly patients. Consideration of age as a risk factor for the development of SSI is also an important component of any risk-benefit discussion.

Hyperglycemia

Hyperglycemia is common in both diabetic and nondiabetic patients in the postoperative period as a result of surgical stress. The effects of hyperglycemia on the immune response are well known—decreased white blood cell counts, impaired chemotaxis and phagocytosis, and decreased complement binding to the surface of bacteria, resulting in poor wound healing and increased risk of infection. Various studies have demonstrated increased morbidity and mortality in critically ill patients with hyperglycemia, even in nondiabetic patients.[12,13] Van den Berghe et al performed a landmark prospective, randomized controlled trial involving 1548 surgical ICU patients on mechanical ventilation.[13] The authors found that intensive insulin therapy administered by infusion with maintenance of blood glucose between 80 and 110 mg/dL reduced mortality from 8.0 to 4.6%. The most significant mortality reduction involved multisystem organ failure related to sepsis. Intensive insulin therapy also reduced in-hospital bloodstream infections in the study population by 46%.[13] These data prompted several additional studies to evaluate the role of strict glucose control in preventing SSI. Most studies demonstrating the role of hyperglycemia as a risk factor for SSI have been completed in cardiac surgery patients,[14] although other surgical populations (colorectal, spinal, pancreatic, vascular, and breast surgery) have been studied as well.[14,15]

Both the CDC and the World Health Organization (WHO) recommend perioperative blood glucose control less than 200 mg/dL.[16,17] However, controversy remains regarding the timing of insulin therapy, ideal target glucose ranges, and the optimal delivery method. In their 2016 report on recommendations for prevention of SSI, the WHO conducted a systematic review of 15 RCTs to establish an optimal glycemic management protocol. Overall, an intensive protocol with target blood glucose concentrations less than 150 mg/dL was significantly associated with reduced risk of developing an SSI (odds ratio [OR] 0.43; 95% CI [0.29, 0.64]). However, no difference was identified between studies using an upper limit glucose range of 100 to 150 mg/dL versus a stricter target of less than 110 mg/dL.[17] A target blood glucose range less than 150 mg/dL in the perioperative period likely decreases the risk of SSI without concomitantly elevating the risk of severe hypoglycemia.

Other studies have attempted to elucidate if glycosylated hemoglobin (HbA1c), which measures average blood glucose levels over 3 months, is independently related to postoperative wound complications. Traditionally, glycemic management recommendations describe a target HbA1c less than 7.0%.[8] However, recent studies suggest that when similar ranges of perioperative blood glucose are achieved, preoperative HbA1c is not an independent risk factor for development of SSI.[18] Blankush et al.[19] reviewed 2200 charts of patients with preoperative HbA1c undergoing elective procedures across all surgical specialties from 2010 to 2014. They followed patients for 30 days to determine the incidence of postoperative infection. When comparing patients with HbA1c less than 6.5% and patients with HbA1c of 6.5% or greater, the authors found that HbA1c was not an independent risk factor for development of postoperative infection except in select patient subgroups (age ≥81 or dirty wounds).[19] The CDC does not currently state recommendations for target preoperative HbA1c to reduce risk of SSI.[16]

Nutritional Status

Malnutrition and chronic hypoalbuminemia are associated with poor surgical outcomes, including delayed wound healing, higher risk of infection, impaired cardiac and respiratory function, poor quality of life, and higher readmission and mortality rates.[8,10,20,21] Various screening tools have been developed to detect malnutrition in the preoperative period, including the Subjective Global Assessment, the patient-generated Subjective Global Assessment, and the Malnutrition Universal Screening Tool.[22] The Duke University Pre-Operative Nutrition Score, which has adopted questions from the Malnutrition Universal Screening Tool, identifies patients who are at risk for surgical complications based on nutritional status. This assessment tool is shown in Figure 32-1. It is recommended that any patients with "Yes" screening answers or preoperative albumin less than 3.0 be referred to a dietitian for formal nutritional assessment and optimization before surgery.[21]

Preoperative assessment of nutritional status is especially important in patients undergoing head and neck surgery, which can severely compromise oral intake.[9] Son et al.[23] conducted a retrospective study of 369 patients undergoing head and neck cancer surgery; 104 (28.2%) patients developed an SSI postoperatively. The authors found that patients with low preoperative serum albumin levels (<3.3 g/L) had a threefold increased risk of developing an SSI. Weight loss at diagnosis greater than 5% was also independently predictive of SSI.[23] For patients with high

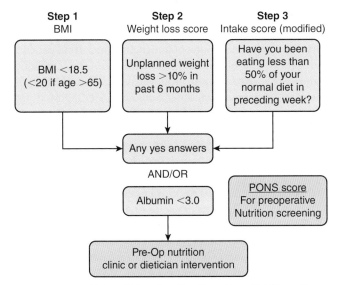

| Step 1 | Step 2 | Step 3 |
| BMI | Weight loss score | Intake score (modified) |

BMI <18.5 (<20 if age >65)

Unplanned weight loss >10% in past 6 months

Have you been eating less than 50% of your normal diet in preceding week?

Any yes answers

AND/OR

Albumin <3.0

PONS score For preoperative Nutrition screening

Pre-Op nutrition clinic or dietician intervention

- **Figure 32-1** Duke University Pre-Operative Nutrition Score (PONS). This validated tool assesses preoperative malnutrition risk. Any patients who score 1 or more should be referred to a dietitian for evaluation and optimization of nutrition status before undergoing surgery. *BMI,* Body mass index. (Obtained from: Wischmeyer PE, Carli F, Evans DC, et al. American Society for Enhanced Recovery and Perioperative Quality Initiative joint consensus statement on nutrition screening and therapy within a surgical enhanced recovery pathway. *Anesth Analg.* 2018; 126[6]:1883. DOI:10.1213/ANE.0000000000002743.[21])

nutritional risk, enteral supplementation starting 7 to 14 days before surgery with high-carbohydrate, high-protein formulas has been shown to considerably reduce postoperative complications.[20,21]

Optimizing nutrition in the postoperative period is also critical to reduce the risk of developing an HCAI. Lee et al.[24] followed 337 patients undergoing clean-contaminated surgery for oropharyngeal squamous cell carcinoma. Perioperative measurements of serum albumin, glucose, and hemoglobin levels were examined to determine if they were associated with development of an SSI. SSI was detected in 88 (26.1%) patients. After conducting multiple regression analyses, the authors found that only low serum albumin (<2.5 g/dL) in the postoperative period was independently associated with risk of developing an SSI ($P = .003$). Additionally, duration of hospitalization was negatively correlated to postoperative albumin, indicating that patients with longer hospital stays were more likely to have poor nutritional status.[24] Other studies have concluded that initiating enteral feeding within 36 hours of hospitalization has been shown to decrease risk of developing a nosocomial infection by half in critically ill and injured patients.[25] Postoperative supplementation should target an energy intake of 30 to 35 kcal/kg body weight per day and should be rich in glucose and amino acids to promote wound healing. Close attention to nutrition and early initiation of enteral feeding can reduce overall health care costs and duration of hospitalization and improve patient outcomes.[20]

Obesity

Obesity is a recognized risk factor for perioperative development of HCAIs, including SSI. Increased risk of SSI may be attributed to both systemic and local factors related to obesity. Excessive adiposity at the surgical site likely contributes to longer duration of the procedure and increased tissue trauma from retraction. Obesity also is linked to immune dysregulation, which can impair host defense mechanisms and increase vulnerability to wound complications and infection. Waisbren et al.[26] conducted a prospective study including 591 patients aged 18 to 64 years undergoing elective surgery from September 2008 to February 2009. BMI and percent body fat (% BF) were calculated for each patient, and surgical outcomes were recorded up to 30 days postoperatively. The prevalence of SSI in obese patients was 5.0% for nonobese patients and 15.2% for obese patients ($P < .0001$). Overall, obesity (defined by >25% BF in men and >31% BF in women) was associated with a five-fold increased risk for developing an SSI. In contrast, BMI-defined obesity was not found to be significantly related to development of SSI, likely because it does not take into account overall body composition and may inaccurately reflect body fat content.[26]

Progressive obesity has also been linked to higher rates of SSIs in patients undergoing colorectal and orthopedic surgery, as well as women undergoing cesarean sections.[27-29] Unfortunately, there is limited research to support preoperative weight loss interventions as a strategy to reduce postoperative complications. A meta-analysis of 16 studies conducted between 1995 and 2016 and including 6060 patients undergoing elective surgery (predominantly bariatric surgery) attempted to evaluate the effect of preoperative weight loss interventions on postoperative complications. The authors' primary outcome, all-cause in-hospital mortality, was not significantly different between the intervention and control groups. The use of preoperative weight loss programs also did not significantly reduce duration of operation or incidence of postoperative infection.[30] Clearly, obesity is a significant risk factor for development of postoperative wound complications, but more research is needed to understand the role of weight loss interventions in preoperative optimization.

Smoking

Cigarette smoking is well-known to cause vascular constriction, decreased tissue perfusion, and attenuation of the inflammatory healing response, thus delaying wound healing and increasing susceptibility to SSI. Numerous studies have demonstrated that smoking increases the risk of developing an SSI by at least twofold.[8] Sørenson conducted a systematic review and meta-analysis of 140 cohort studies involving 479,150 patients undergoing a wide variety of surgical procedures. Pooled adjusted odds ratios demonstrated that smoking was significantly associated with wound necrosis (OR 3.6, 95% CI [2.62, 4.93]), healing delay and dehiscence, (OR 2.07; 95% CI [1.53, 2.81]), SSI (OR 1.79;

95% CI [1.57, 2.04]), wound complications (OR 2.27; 95% CI [1.82, 2.84]), hernia formation (OR 2.07; 95% CI [1.23, 3.47]), and lack of fistula or bone healing (OR 2.44; 95% CI [1.66, 3.58]). The review also sought to quantify the risk of wound complications associated with former smokers (when defined, cessation period ranged from 2 to 52 weeks before surgery, median 4 weeks) compared with current or never smokers. Sørenson found that former smokers had significantly more wound complications than never smokers (adjusted OR 1.31; 95% CI [1.10, 1.56]) but fewer wound complications when compared with current smokers (adjusted OR 0.28; 95% CI [0.12, 0.72]).[31] Another meta-analysis by Mills et al.[32] evaluated the effect of preoperative smoking cessation on postoperative complications. The authors pooled six randomized controlled trials that evaluated the influence of smoking interventions on postoperative complications. They found that implementation of a preoperative smoking cessation program reduced risk of postoperative complications by 41% (95% CI [15, 59%]). Furthermore, each additional week of cessation increased the magnitude of effect by 19%, with trials of at least 4 weeks' duration having a significantly larger treatment effect than shorter trials.[32] These data support guidelines that recommend smoking cessation 30 days before surgery.[8]

Operative Risk Factors

Prophylactic Antibiotics

Antibiotic prophylaxis is defined as the administration of antibiotics before contamination by surgical incision has occurred and is given with the intention of preventing SSI resulting from transient bacteremia from physiologic flora.[8,9] A review of meta-analyses published between 1990 and 2006 on the subject, including 256 clinical trials of 43,809 patients undergoing 21 different types of surgery, concluded that antibiotic prophylaxis is effective in preventing wound infection.[33] This meta-analysis also found that the efficacy of prophylactic antibiotics was not correlated to surgical wound classification, indicating that it is likely beneficial regardless of the type of surgery to be performed. The study supported the use of antibiotic prophylaxis, but did not take into account some of the adverse consequences associated with antibiotic prophylaxis, including possible patient side effects, the effect of antibiotic use on microbial resistance, and cost.[33]

Effective antibiotic prophylaxis must account for proper timing of administration as well as proper antibiotic selection and dose. The Centers for Medicare and Medicaid Services Surgical Care Improvement Project (SCIP) has established a 60-minute window during which antibiotic prophylaxis should be administered before surgery start, whereby the objective is to have a bactericidal concentration of the antibiotic in the serum and tissues at the time of first incision.[16] Recently, studies have been conducted to evaluate whether a shorter interval (i.e., 30 minutes) from infusion to incision is recommended. The TAPAS study was an observational cohort study conducted between March 2010 to 2012 at a tertiary care center in Amsterdam, the Netherlands. Of the 3001 eligible patients, 1550 patients received antibiotic prophylaxis within 30 minutes before incision and 1062 patients between 30 and 60 minutes before incision. The remaining patients received antibiotic prophylaxis outside of the recommended 60-minute window. Subjects were followed for 30 days postoperatively (or 1 year in the case of implantation of a foreign body), during which 161 (5.4%) SSIs were diagnosed, of which 95 (59%) were superficial and 66 (41%) were deep. Researchers found that there was no conclusive evidence of a difference in SSI risk when antibiotic prophylaxis was administered 0 to 30 minutes or 30 to 60 minutes before incision (OR 0.82, 95% CI [0.57, 1.19]).[34]

Redosing of antibiotics should occur if the length of surgery extends beyond the half-life of the antibiotic being used, with consideration of creatinine clearance in patients who need renal dosing. Some authors recommend that an additional dose should be provided if the procedure is 1 to 2 times the half-life of the antibiotic or when there has been substantial blood loss.[35] In clean and clean-contaminated procedures, antibiotics should be discontinued once the surgical incision has been closed.[15,16]

In addition to appropriate timing of administration, antimicrobial prophylaxis should be directed toward the microbial flora most likely implicated in an SSI depending on the site and nature of the procedure performed. In the National Healthcare Safety Network surveillance report on 21,100 isolates from 2009 to 2010, the most frequently identified pathogen in all SSIs was *Staphylococcus aureus*, followed by coagulase-negative staphylococci, *E. coli, Enterococcus faecalis,* and *Pseudomonas aeruginosa.*[7,8] For head and neck surgeries specifically, contact with flora of the skin and upper aerodigestive tract contribute to polymicrobial SSIs. In oropharyngeal secretions, anaerobic colonizers are commonly encountered, including *Peptostreptococcus* and *Fusobacterium*. Additionally, *Staphylococcus aureus, Staphylococcus epidermidis,* and *Streptococcus* species are frequently isolated from the skin.[36] Cefazolin is the most frequently selected preoperative antibiotic because it has proven efficacy against skin flora. Clindamycin is a common alternative in patients allergic to penicillin or cephalosporins, although it may be inferior to cefazolin in the prevention of SSI in head and neck surgeries.[9,15,36] Judicious use of antimicrobial prophylaxis should be specific to the pathogens at the surgical site and administered for the shortest amount of time possible to reduce adverse effects, excess cost, and the risk of antibiotic resistance.[9,37] Specific antibiotic prophylaxis recommendations for various oral and maxillofacial procedures may be found later in this chapter.

Review: Antimicrobial Prophylaxis in Specific Surgical Populations

Third Molars

The role of antibiotics in preventing complications associated with third molar surgery has been a topic of review for several decades. The two major inflammatory complications associated with third molar surgery are alveolar osteitis and SSI.[37] Alveolar osteitis (AO), although not directly representative of a bacterial infection, is an inflammatory complication with a reported frequency of 25 to 30% in mandibular third molar extraction.[38] The incidence of AO increases with longer operative time, increased tissue trauma, and presence of preexisting microbial contamination.[39,40] The estimated frequency of SSI after third molar surgery has been estimated as 1 to 6%, with higher rates corresponding with greater degrees of impaction.[41,42] Despite their low incidence rate, postoperative AO and SSI are associated with significant pain and functional impairment, increased overall health care costs, and in severe cases, hospitalization and possible airway compromise.[40] However, given their relative infrequency, any evidence supporting the use of antimicrobial prophylaxis to prevent postoperative inflammatory complications in patients undergoing third molar removal should be weighed against the risk of adverse effects at a patient (6 to 7%) and population level.[37]

Ren and Malmstrom performed a thorough meta-analysis of 20 randomized controlled clinical trials evaluating antibiotic use in third molar extractions published between 1974 and 2007.[40] The primary outcomes evaluated were AO and SSI; 16 studies involving 2932 patients reported AO as an outcome. AO occurred in 14.4% of patients who did not receive preoperative systemic antibiotics and in 6.2% of patients who did receive preoperative systemic antibiotics (OR 2.175). The authors also evaluated 12 studies involving 2396 patients that were included in the final analysis with SSI as the primary outcome. SSI occurred in 4% of patients who did receive antibiotic prophylaxis and in 6.1% of patients who did not receive antibiotics (OR 1.794). The number needed to treat (NNT) was 25, indicating that on average 25 patients would need to be treated with systemic antibiotics to prevent one case of postoperative wound infection.

Ren and Malstrom also completed subgroup analyses to elucidate a preferred antibiotic type and dosing regimen aimed at preventing postoperative complications. According to the analysis, preoperative systemic antibiotics (parenteral or enteral), given as a single dose or as a first dose in a multiday regimen, resulted in a significant reduction in the incidence of AO, with an NNT of 13. The effect of preoperative dosing only was less predictable in reducing development of SSI. In contrast, exclusive use of postoperative antibiotics, which were administered after surgery was completed, did not significantly reduce the incidence of postoperative complications, implying that adequate tissue concentrations of the antibiotic must be present before first incision to have a beneficial effect. Several studies included in the meta-analysis compared the rate of postoperative complications in patients treated with a broad-spectrum antibiotic (penicillin) versus an antianaerobic agent only (metronidazole). In their final analysis, the authors found that both penicillin and metronidazole were effective in reducing AO, but metronidazole was not as effective as

penicillin in prevention of SSI.[40] In conclusion, the authors recommend preoperative dosing with a single dose of penicillin or its derivative 30 to 90 minutes before surgery as the most cost-effective strategy for third molar extractions. For patients with known risk factors for postoperative complications, there is moderate evidence to support 3 to 5 days of treatment after the procedure to prevent postoperative SSI and AO.[40]

A 2021 Cochrane review also attempted to establish clear guidelines regarding the administration of antibiotic prophylaxis for dental extractions. The authors identified 23 trials involving 3206 participants; the majority of studies exclusively pertained to postoperative complications after third molar extractions. Compared to a placebo, antibiotic prophylaxis reduced the risk of SSI by 66% (RR 0.34; 95% CI [0.19, 0.64]; 1728 participants; 12 studies; low-certainty evidence), with an NNT of 19. They also found that antibiotic prophylaxis reduced the risk of AO by 34% (RR 0.66; 95% CI [0.45, 0.97]; 1882 participants; 13 studies; low-certainty evidence), with an NNT of 46. Unlike Ren and Malmstrom, the authors found no evidence to support that timing of antibiotic administration (preoperative, postoperative, or both) was a significant variable. Given this evidence, the authors supported use of antibiotic prophylaxis before extraction of impacted third molars on the basis of each patient's clinical condition (i.e., immune status, comorbidities, age) and the level of surgical complexity.[43]

Many of the trials evaluating the relationship between antibiotic prophylaxis and postoperative wound complications have taken place in settings substantially different from the standard U.S. oral surgery ambulatory model, as well as with nonstandard dosing strategies and antibiotic regimens, which limits the generalizability of their results.[44] Halpern and Dodson conducted a well-designed randomized controlled trial of 118 subjects undergoing removal of at least one impacted third molar with ambulatory anesthesia. The authors found that the administration of a single dose of preoperative intravenous antibiotics (penicillin or clindamycin in allergic patients) significantly reduced the incidence of postoperative SSI in the treatment group (0%) compared to the placebo group (8.5%), $P = .03$, NNT = 12.[45] No cases of AO were diagnosed. All SSI were associated with the removal of partial bony or full bony impacted mandibular third molars. This study provides good evidence that in a typical ambulatory surgical setting, single-dose intravenous antibiotic prophylaxis administered 60 minutes before first incision can effectively reduce SSI rate among patients undergoing extraction of multiple third molars.[44,45]

There is new evidence supporting the role of antibiotic prophylaxis in controlling postoperative pain after third molar extractions. Yanine et al.[46] conducted a randomized, double-blind controlled trial of 154 patients, half of which received 2 g of amoxicillin 1 hour before surgery and half of which received placebo. In total, 4.5% of patients experienced postoperative infections. The authors found that antibiotic prophylaxis did not prevent postoperative AO or SSI (RR = 0.44; 95% CI [0.08, 1.99], $P = .41$, NNT = 26).

However, antibiotic prophylaxis was associated with a reduced need for rescue analgesia (RR = .49; 95% CI [0.32, 0.75], $P < .05$, NNT = 3).[46] The results from a randomized controlled trial of 59 young patients (ages 15 to 19) undergoing third molar surgery also determined that postoperative pain and analgesic intake was lower in patients who received 2 g amoxicillin 1 hour before third molar surgery.[47]

Researchers have also investigated the use of antiseptic rinses to prevent postoperative inflammatory complications in third molar surgery. Current data suggests that postoperative chlorhexidine rinses have a significant and clinically relevant effect on the prevention of AO after surgical removal of mandibular third molars.[48] This claim is supported by a 2022 Cochrane review that compared the use of antiseptic rinses and intrasocket gel placement with placebo. The authors evaluated 39 trials involving 6219 patients. They concluded that rinsing before and after tooth extraction with chlorhexidine 0.12% or 0.2% strength, as well as placement of 0.2% chlorhexidine gel in the extraction socket, are beneficial at reducing the incidence of AO.[49] A meta-analysis by Caso et al. also provided strong evidence that the combined use of chlorhexidine rinse preoperatively and for several days postoperatively produced a significant reduction in the rate of AO.[50] In summary, postoperative chlorhexidine rinses seem to decrease the risk of AO after third molar extraction, but further study is necessary to determine an ideal protocol.

Orthognathic Surgery

Orthognathic surgery is classified as a clean-contaminated procedure, because it involves making an incision through the oral mucosa. Without any prophylactic antibiotics, the rate of SSI ranges from 10 to 25%.[9] Surgical variables that may increase risk of SSI include operation on the mandible, which is less vascular and more susceptible to pooling of food and saliva at the incision compared to the maxilla, and operation on both jaws.[37,51,52] A dose of preoperative antibiotics (typically cefazolin) has been shown to reduce SSI and is indicated within 60 minutes before first incision.[9,53] Some investigators have advocated for extended regimens of antibiotic prophylaxis after surgery, although the data to support this are mixed. Chow et al.[52] conducted a retrospective study of 2910 orthognathic procedures over a 15-year period. The overall postoperative infection rate was 7.4%. The authors found that patients who had received only one preoperative antibiotic dose had a significantly higher rate of infection (17.3%) than those who received both preoperative and postoperative antibiotics (5.1%). The duration of postoperative antibiotics ranged from 2 to 14 days. Interestingly, the duration of postoperative antibiotics (beyond 2 days) as well as the type of antibiotic given did not significantly affect the infection rate.[52] Danda and Ravi performed a meta-analysis to determine the role of postoperative antibiotics in orthognathic surgery. In total, they reviewed 532 patients in eight clinical trials. Patients were grouped according to duration of postoperative antibiotics: short-term (<24 hours) or extended-term (>24 hours). SSI occurred in 30 of 268 patients in the short-term prophylaxis group (11.2%) and in 10 of 264 patients in the extended-term group (3.8%), $P < .01$. Like Chow, the authors found that the most profound effect on reduction of SSI was observed at 2 days of postoperative antibiotic use (OR, 8.2; 95% CI [0.39 to 169.89]), but they did not find evidence that the duration of extended antibiotic administration beyond 2 days had a significant effect on the incidence of SSI.[54] Davis et al.[51] conducted a prospective, double-blind randomized controlled trial involving 171 patients undergoing orthognathic surgery to evaluate if 3 days of postoperative antibiotics was superior to 1 day of antibiotics in preventing SSI. All patients received 1 day of intravenous antibiotics immediately postoperatively. Patients were subsequently randomized to receive 2 days of either additional antibiotics or placebo. The authors found that groups receiving 3 days of postoperative antibiotics (cefazolin and cephalexin) had a lower incidence of SSI (7.0%) compared with the group receiving a placebo (17.6%, $P = .04$).[51]

Currently, there is no general consensus regarding the preferred duration for antimicrobial prophylaxis after orthognathic surgery, but weak evidence suggests that implementation of extended postoperative antibiotic regimens may be superior to perioperative antibiotic prophylaxis only in reducing incidence of SSI. A consideration of individual patient risk factors for developing infection (i.e., performance of adjunctive procedures, immunocompromised patients, higher surgical complexity/duration) should be balanced with the risk of adverse effects when deciding appropriate duration of antimicrobial prophylaxis.

Facial Fractures

Maxillofacial fractures are fractures of the bony facial skeleton, including the maxilla, mandible, zygoma, nasal bones, orbits, and the frontal sinus. Long-term sequelae of facial fractures include cosmetic deformities, occlusal disharmony, limited mouth opening, and neurosensory disturbances. Patients with facial fractures may undergo one of three treatment modalities: observation, closed reduction, and open reduction with or without internal fixation.

Postoperative SSI after open reduction and internal fixation of maxillofacial fractures ranges from 0 to 30%, with a mean of 12%.[55] Risk factors for postoperative SSI include site of fracture (i.e., mandibular symphysis, angle, or body),[56] open fracture (i.e., disruption of the oral mucosa, gingiva, or tooth socket),[56] preoperative infection, more than 72 hours delay between fracture and operative repair, and patient comorbidities.[55] Numerous investigators have explored the role of antibiotic prophylaxis in preventing SSI after maxillofacial trauma.

Antibiotic prophylaxis can be administered preoperatively (from time of injury until 2 hours before surgical intervention), perioperatively (within 60 minutes of first incision and concluding <24 hours after surgery), or postoperatively.[55] Multiple studies have supported the efficacy of perioperative antibiotics in preventing SSI for patients with maxillofacial trauma involving the dentate region of the mandible, exposed to the oral cavity, and undergoing open repair.[57] Antibiotic prophylaxis is unlikely to benefit patients with nonoperative fractures of the maxilla, zygoma, or nondentate region of the mandible, as the rate of SSI is exceedingly low in this group.[56] There is also little evidence to support a role for postoperative antibiotic prophylaxis more than 24 hours after operative intervention regardless of the injury pattern, mechanism, or treatment.[58]

Studies regarding the usage of antibiotic prophylaxis to reduce SSI in patients with craniomaxillofacial trauma can be summarized in the following recommendations, derived from guidelines at a large Level 1 trauma center. Overall, the evidence supports the use of a single dose of perioperative antibiotics in all facial thirds in patients undergoing open surgical repair.[59] Preoperative antibiotics should be reserved for patients with open mandible fractures (i.e., mucosal, gingival, or tooth socket disruption) or fractures of the dentate segment of the mandible for 7 days or until the time of operative repair.[59,60] Postoperative antibiotic regimens more than 24 hours after surgical repair are not beneficial except in specific cases of penetrating trauma or host immune compromise. Nonoperative fractures that do not fall into any of the other above categories do not require antibiotic prophylaxis.[60] In the setting of maxillofacial fractures, antibiotic prophylaxis should be specific to oral and respiratory flora, and provide appropriate gram-positive cocci, gram-negative bacteria, and anaerobic coverage. The first-line antibiotic is typically ampicillin-sulbactam, administered intravenously for adult patients at a dose of 3 g every 6 hours, and for pediatric patients at a dose of 300 mg/kg/day, with a maximum dose of 12 g/day. For penicillin-allergic patients, the alternative is clindamycin administered intravenously at a dose of 20-40 mg/kg/day and a maximum daily dose of 2.7 g/day.[60] Transition to an oral agent is appropriate for patients being discharged. Figure 32-2 presents an algorithm for determining the use of antibiotic prophylaxis in facial trauma at a Level 1 trauma center.[59,60]

Dental Implants and Bone Grafting

Dental implants and bone grafting are standard ambulatory procedures performed by most oral and maxillofacial surgeons intended for the rehabilitation of fully or partially edentulous jaws. Dental implant success rates are overall high (95 to 99%), but failures are associated with surgical trauma, lack of primary stability, and infection.[37] Infections around foreign bodies such as implants or grafting materials are particularly difficult to treat because of biofilm formation and often require removal of the prosthesis. A variety of prophylactic antibiotic regimens have been suggested to reduce the risk of SSI when performing dental implant and bone grafting procedures.

A 2013 Cochrane review analyzed six randomized controlled trials with 1162 participants. All of the trials compared various regimens of prophylactic amoxicillin versus placebo in patients undergoing dental implant place-

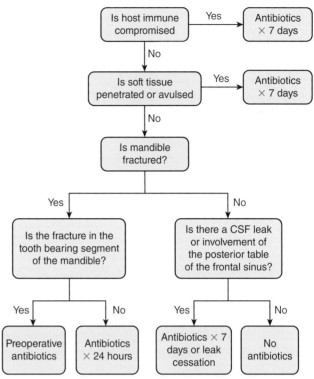

• **Figure 32-2** Algorithm for Antibiotic Prophylaxis in Facial Trauma. Preoperative antibiotics for 7 days or until the time of fracture repair is recommended in patients with open fractures involving dentate segments of the mandible. A single dose of perioperative antibiotics is recommended in all patients with operative facial fractures undergoing surgical repair. Otherwise, extended courses of antibiotics (>24 hours) are indicated only for facial fractures in patients with immune compromise, penetrating soft tissue injuries, or cerebrospinal fluid (CSF) leaks. (From Michel JC, Amin D, Gelbard RB, Abramowicz S. An evidence-based approach to antibiotic use in maxillofacial trauma. *Oral Surg Oral Med Oral Pathol Oral Radiol.* 2022;134[2]:151-158. https://doi.org/10.1016/j.oooo.2021.12.135.)

ment. A meta-analysis of the six trials demonstrated a significantly lower number of implant failures in the group receiving antibiotics (RR 0.33; 95% CI [0.16, 0.67], P = .002). The NNT was calculated as 25, based on an implant failure rate estimated as 6% in the control group. Interestingly, there was no statistically significant difference in infection rate between the antibiotic and placebo groups (RR 0.69; 95% CI [0.36, 1.35]). The authors recommended administration of 2 g amoxicillin 1 hour preoperatively to reduce implant failure rate.[61] Further research from the Dental Implant Clinical Research Group also supported the use of antibiotic prophylaxis for dental implant surgery. Data for the placement of 2973 implants were correlated with failure from initial osseointegration to prosthesis loading and 36 months postoperatively.[62] Antibiotic prophylaxis was associated with a reduced risk of implant failure (4.6%) compared to no antibiotic use (10%) at all stages of healing. Other studies have contradicted these findings, suggesting that antibiotic prophylaxis may not be beneficial in specific clinical scenarios. Randomized controlled trials completed by both Anitua et al[63] and Tan et al[64] found no difference in the implant complications rates when comparing antibiotic prophylaxis with amoxicillin versus placebo in patients undergoing uncomplicated single implant placement. However, these studies had relatively short follow-up periods (3 and 2 months, respectively).

Resnik and Misch[65] published a classification system and protocol to guide practitioners in prescribing an appropriate antibiotic prophylaxis regimen for patients undergoing dental implant procedures based on a range of procedural, local, and systemic factors. The authors identified several risk factors for peri-implant infection, including patient immune status, smoking, comorbidities, and malnutrition. Local host factors that were described as risk factors for implant failure included periodontal disease, type of grafting material, existing tissue inflammation, presence of odontogenic infections, incision design, surgical technique, poor oral hygiene, and increased duration of surgery. The Misch International Implant Institute prophylaxis protocol classifies implant procedures into four types based on complexity and presence of risk factors. For type 1 procedures (e.g., single tooth implants, second-stage surgeries), Resnik and Misch recommend postoperative antiseptic rinse with chlorhexidine only and no administration of systemic antibiotics. For type 2 procedures (e.g., socket grafting, multiple implant placement, immediate implant placement), the authors recommend a preoperative loading dose of antibiotics 1 hour before surgery, followed by a single postoperative dose 6 hours later and postoperative chlorhexidine rinse for 2 weeks. For type 3 procedures (e.g., multiple immediate implants, membrane bone grafting, extensive soft tissue reflection), it is advisable to administer preoperative followed by 3 days of postoperative systemic antibiotics in addition to a chlorhexidine rinse. Finally, for type 4 procedures (full-arch implants, sinus procedures, and autogenous bone grafts, particularly in medically compromised patients), antibiotics should be continued for 5 days postoperatively. The authors recommend amoxicillin as first-line because of its high bioavailability, low toxicity, and broad coverage of oral bacteria. Alternatively, amoxicillin-clavulanic acid may be used in patients undergoing sinus augmentation because of the high incidence of β-lactamase producing bacteria involved in sinus infections.[65]

Skin Care

Hair Removal

Previously, it was thought that preoperative hair removal would reduce bacterial load and result in a decreased incidence of SSI. An updated Cochrane review by Tanner et al in 2021 examined 19 randomized and 6 quasi-randomized trials involving 8919 total study participants. The authors found that there was no significant difference in risk of SSI when no hair removal was compared with hair removal using clippers, and there was an increased risk of SSI in participants who had hair removal with a razor compared with no hair removal.[66] Based on this evidence, the authors recommend that if hair at the surgical site must be removed for operative reasons, using clippers rather than a razor is the preferred method. If hair is to be removed, most studies agree that it should be removed immediately before surgery.[8,15]

Skin Preparation (Patient)

Appropriate skin disinfection before surgery is an important step in reducing bacterial colonization and preventing SSIs. Established guidelines address appropriate skin hygiene for both the immediate preoperative period and the day before surgery. Currently, the CDC advises patients to bathe or shower with soap or an antiseptic agent on at least the night before the surgery date.[16] A 2015 Cochrane review by Webster and Osborne evaluated seven trials with 10,157 patients that compared bathing with 4% chlorhexidine gluconate with either bar soap or placebo or with no bathing.[67] There was no evidence to support preoperative bathing with chlorhexidine gluconate as a measure to reduce risk of SSI. Another meta-analysis performed by Chlebicki et al. including 16 trials and 17,932 patients yielded similar results.[68] Chlorhexidine gluconate was found to be nonsuperior when compared with soap, placebo, or no shower or bath in reducing the risk of SSI. Considering the results of these two large meta-analyses, there is no support for preoperative bathing with chlorhexidine gluconate and efforts to reduce SSI should focus on interventions with demonstrated efficacy.[68]

Before the first incision, the most commonly used agents for skin antisepsis include alcohol-based solutions, chlorhexidine gluconate, and iodophors such as povidone-iodine. Chlorhexidine works by binding to negatively charged bacterial cell membranes, disrupting them, and precipitating cell contents. Povidone-iodine acts by iodination of cell membrane lipids, and has excellent microbicidal activity against both gram-positive and gram-negative bacteria. The mechanism of isopropyl alcohol is disruption of cell membranes and denaturation of bacterial proteins. Each skin preparation agent has a distinct set of advantages and contraindications, of which the surgical team should be aware. For example, alcohol is an excellent bactericidal agent against gram-positive bacteria; however, when used alone, its benefit is limited by its flammability and lack of residual germicidal activity. Chlorhexidine and povidone-iodine are both very effective in reducing bacterial counts on contact and have excellent activity against skin bacteria. Chlorhexidine has superior duration of activity and has shown a 30% reduced rate of SSI when compared with iodophor-based preparations.[69] Additionally, the iodophors can be inactivated by contact with blood or serum, so the preparation must be allowed to dry to take advantage of its full antibacterial activity. Iodophor-containing agents are also contraindicated in patients with an allergy to iodine and in patients younger than 2 months of age. A further concern with iodophors is that even small concentrations of povidone-iodine (0.5%) are very toxic to fibroblasts and keratinocytes, so it should never be used on open wounds or in postoperative dressings.[35,69]

Skin preparation for head and neck surgery has specific considerations. Alcohol and chlorhexidine should not be used on the face because they can cause conjunctivitis, permanent keratitis, and sensorineural hearing loss.[70] Solutions that are safe to use in the head and neck region are limited to povidone-iodine 7.5% scrub/10% paint (Scrub Care) or chloroxylenol 3% (Techni-Care). Both must be allowed to air dry before incision. When distant sites are also prepped for bone or soft tissue harvest, one may wish to consider a chlorhexidine gluconate–containing solution for the distant preparation site because it has superior length of activity.

Adjunctive strategies that have been advocated to prevent SSIs include use of iodophor-impregnated drapes (Ioban) and microbial skin sealants. Iodophor-impregnated drapes have been shown to reduce wound contamination in the critical care and obstetric literature.[35] They have also been demonstrated to reduce wound contamination in orthopedic surgery but without a concomitant decrease in wound infections.[35] In head and neck surgery, the use of these drapes would not generally be practical except in cases of distant surgical sites, such as in anterior iliac crest graft harvest. In general, however, the use of impregnated occlusive drapes does not seem to reduce the risk of SSI.[35] InteguSeal is a cyanoacrylate microbial sealant that is applied to the skin after preparation is completed with an iodophor or chlorhexidine gluconate solution. On contact with the skin, it forms a barrier that prevents migration of flora onto the incision, and it seals microabrasions on the skin. It has not been associated with any local or systemic toxicity and has activity for several days. However, it is not recommended for use in areas where it may have contact with mucous membranes or with the eyes or on skin with signs of active infection. The evidence on the efficacy of microbial sealants in preventing SSI is mixed.[71,72] Like iodophor-impregnated drapes, it may be considered in preparation of distant surfaces for tissue or bone harvest.

Skin Preparation (Surgical Team)

Skin scrub formulas for the surgical team are similar to those available to prepare the patient. A 2016 Cochrane review aimed to assess the effects of surgical hand antisepsis on preventing SSIs and reducing the number of colony-forming units (CFUs) of bacteria on the hands of the surgical team.[73] This review concluded that there is no definitive evidence to support one type of hand antiseptic over another in reducing risk of SSI. Other investigators have compared chlorhexidine gluconate to povidone-iodine scrubs. Aly and Maibach compared 2-minute scrubbing with chlorhexidine gluconate versus povidone-iodine versus chloroxylenol immediately after scrubbing and at 3 and 6 hours later.[74] Chlorhexidine resulted in significantly reduced bacterial counts compared with both povidone-iodine and chloroxylenol at all measured time points. However, the clinical relevance of this outcome is unclear.[73] Multiple investigators have also studied the efficacy of alcohol rubs, which are non-irritating and tend to have better compliance rates than aqueous scrubs. A 2002 study by Parienti et al. compared hand rubbing with an aqueous alcohol solution to scrubbing with either 4% povidone-iodine or 4% chlorhexidine. The primary endpoint was SSI at 30 days.[75] They found that hand rubbing with the alcohol solution preceded by a nonantiseptic hand wash was not inferior to traditional scrubbing methods with regard to preventing SSI. Furthermore, use of the aqueous alcohol hand rub was better tolerated and had improved compliance by surgical teams compared to traditional scrubbing. In conclusion, chlorhexidine gluconate confers longer antibacterial coverage than povidone-iodine, but aqueous alcohol provides just as effective antibacterial coverage with respect to reducing the risk of SSIs. So, when choosing a method for scrubbing in, aqueous alcohol is fully effective as long as gross contamination has already been removed. However, if one prefers a more traditional method of scrubbing, a combination of alcohol with chlorhexidine gluconate is preferable to chlorhexidine gluconate alone, which is preferable to povidone-iodine.

Temperature Control

Hypothermia is defined as a core body temperature below 36°C (96.8° F). Core body temperature can drop as much as 1.6°C within the first hour of a general anesthetic due to impairment of thermoregulation and exposure to cold temperatures.[76] Perioperative hypothermia has been linked to several complications, including increased blood loss as a result of impaired coagulation, higher incidence of cardiac events, impaired wound healing, longer duration of hospital stay, and elevated risk of SSI.[7,12,15,17,77] Kurz et al. studied a group of 200 patients undergoing colorectal surgery who were randomized to intraoperative hypothermia (34.7 ± 0.6°C) or intraoperative normothermia (36.6 ± 0.5°C) and followed them in a double-blind manner for signs of infection.[78] The study was ended early because of significant results of a 19% wound infection rate in the hypothermia group and a 6% infection rate in the normothermia group. The authors found that lowering core temperature 2°C below normal resulted in a tripling of wound infection rates and prolonged hospital stay by 2.6 days (20%).[78] The hypothermic patients did have a greater transfusion requirement (another effect of hypothermia), but the products transfused were leukocyte depleted, and according to the authors' multivariate regression analysis, the transfusion requirement did not independently contribute to the risk of SSI. It is theorized that hypothermia increases the risk of SSI because it decreases perfusion (and thus oxygenation) and impairs neutrophil function by reducing superoxide radical production.[12,77] Proven methods for maintaining normothermia intraoperatively include the use of warmed intravenous fluids and forced air warmers.[76] Although the anesthesia team will likely take the role of ensuring patient normothermia intraoperatively, it is essential for the surgeon to be aware of the significant impact of maintaining normothermia throughout the perioperative period so as to decrease the risk of SSIs and other complications.

Oxygenation

Researchers hypothesize that perioperative oxygenation with increased fraction of inspired oxygen (Fio_2) reduces risk of SSI. Theoretically, adequate oxygen tension at the wound enhances superoxide production by neutrophils, facilitating bacterial killing. Additionally, adequate oxygen tension is thought to be essential in the development of collagen and epithelium.[12] The purported benefit of perioperative hyperoxia in reducing SSI is controversial. The WHO conducted a meta-analysis of 11 randomized controlled trials analyzing the effect of hyperoxia in reducing SSI. The investigators found that increased perioperative Fio_2 of 80% is beneficial in reducing SSI compared with standard perioperative Fio_2 of 30 to 35% (OR 0.72; 95% CI [0.55, 0.94]). Consequently, the WHO currently recommends that adult patients undergoing general anesthesia with endotracheal intubation receive oxygenation with 80% Fio_2 intraoperatively and in the immediate postoperative period.[17] These findings were in line with two additional meta-analyses on the subject, which reported modest reductions in SSI when perioperative hyperoxia was used.[79,80] In contrast, the PROXI trial, a double-blind randomized clinical trial conducted in 14 Danish hospitals and involving 1400 patients undergoing acute and elective laparotomy between 2006 and 2008, found no significant benefit when comparing administration of 80% Fio_2 versus 30% Fio_2 in reducing the risk of SSI after abdominal surgery (OR 0.94; 95% CI [0.72, 1.22]).[81] In conclusion, perioperative hyperoxia with an Fio_2 2 of 80%, when used in conjunction with other interventions, likely has modest benefit in reducing risk of SSI. Additional research is warranted to determine whether it is beneficial for the head and neck surgery population.

Surgical Technique

Gentle tissue handling, removal of foreign bodies, adequate hemostasis, and debridement of devitalized tissue are technical variables that decrease risk of SSI.[8,82] The use of electrocautery for surgical incisions offers the advantage of decreased operative time and improved hemostasis, two factors that are both implicated in SSIs. Electrocautery is frequently used for tissue dissection and hemostasis in the dermis and deeper layers, but its use for initial skin incisions remains controversial. A 2012 systematic review and meta-analysis evaluated six randomized controlled trials comparing the use of scalpel and electrocautery for skin incisions. The authors found that there was no significant difference in the incidence of SSI between the patient groups. Furthermore, use of electrocautery for skin incision resulted in decreased incision time, less incisional blood loss, and reduced postoperative incisional pain in the electrocautery group.[83] An additional randomized controlled trial by Chau et al. examined 38 patients undergoing bilateral neck incisions. Each side of the neck was randomly assigned to receive skin incision with cold scalpel or electrocautery. No significant difference was appreciated in patient satisfaction or objective measurement of skin incision cosmesis at 6 months postoperatively.[84] Electrocautery is a valuable alternative to scalpel usage for skin incision and appears not to increase risk of poor cosmesis or SSI.

Wound closure technique is also implicated in risk of SSI. When the risk of SSI is low (e.g., wound class 1),

primary closure is favored because of shorter healing times and improved cosmesis. Delayed wound closure 4 to 5 days after injury is recommended for contaminated and infected wounds (class 4) to allow for treatment of the infection with antibiotic therapy, as well as improved tensile strength. No single suture type or closure technique (i.e., interrupted versus continuous) has proven superior in reducing risk of SSI.[82] However, there is moderate evidence to support the use of triclosan-coated antimicrobial sutures. A systematic review evaluating 13 randomized controlled trials and 3568 surgical patients found that the use of triclosan-coated sutures resulted in a lower risk of SSI compared with non–triclosan-coated sutures (fixed effect: RR = 0.734; 95% CI [0.590, 0.913], $P = .005$).[85] The benefit of antimicrobial-coated sutures appears to be independent of suture type and wound contamination classification.[17] Risk of antimicrobial resistance and tissue toxicity is low, further supporting the adoption of triclosan-coated sutures for wound closure. The CDC currently considers the use of triclosan-coated sutures for prevention of SSI a Category II weak recommendation with moderate-quality evidence.[16]

Researchers have also examined the influence of intraoperative drain placement on development of SSI. Drains are typically placed to facilitate removal of fluid, pus, and blood from surgical dead space, because accumulation of these substances can increase the risk of wound complications. It is generally accepted that closed suction drains are preferable to simple conduit drains because there may be retrograde bacteria migration with the use of conduit drains.[15,35] Drains should be used judiciously and removed as soon as clinically indicated because prolonged use has been associated with an increased risk of SSI and possibly higher transfusion requirements.[35,82] The use of drains in head and neck surgery for treatment of infections is indicated. However, in otherwise uninfected cases, the surgeon should carefully consider the necessity of a drain; if a drain is to be placed, a closed suction drain should be used.

Irrigation and Topical Antibiotics

Topical wound irrigation removes debris and decreases bacterial contamination at the surgical site. Sterile saline is the most commonly used irrigant, but formulations including antiseptic and antibiotic solutions are also available. Currently, there is moderate evidence to support the use of aqueous povidone-iodine solutions for incisional irrigation, and strong evidence that opposes the use of topical wound irrigation with antibiotics.[16,17] The WHO conducted a systematic review to investigate whether topical wound irrigation decreases SSI risk. They found that incisional irrigation with saline solution using pulse pressure or administered with force substantially reduced incidence of SSI compared with no irrigation, but acknowledged that the delivery system may be unavailable or cumbersome in low-resource environments. They also conducted a meta-analysis of seven randomized controlled trials comparing irrigation with an aqueous povidone-iodine solution to incisional irrigation with saline solution alone. The evidence demonstrated a significant benefit of irrigation with aqueous povidone-iodine in reducing the incidence of SSI (OR 0.31; 95% CI [0.13, 0.73], $P = .007$). This benefit was mostly attributed to clean and clean-contaminated wound classifications irrigated with povidone-iodine 10% or 0.35%.[17] The CDC also recommends the use of dilute povidone-iodine solutions before wound closure.[16] Other antiseptic irrigation formulas, including chlorhexidine and hydrogen peroxide, have not demonstrated effectiveness in reducing SSI and are potentially harmful.[86] The efficacy of intraoperative incisional irrigation in reducing bacterial contamination may also depend on the method of delivery, which can be classified as high pressure (15 to 35 psi) or low pressure (1 to 15 psi) and can be pulsatile or continuous.[87] Much of the literature concerning high-pressure versus low-pressure irrigation comes from orthopedic surgery. High-pressure pulsatile irrigation appears to be more effective than low-pressure irrigation at debridement of foreign material and bacteria, but results in more tissue damage. High-pressure irrigation also has been linked to an impairment in the immune response and can seed bacteria deeper into tissue or bone.[35,87,88] For this reason, it is recommended to reserve the use of high-pressure irrigation for wounds in which the bacterial contamination is severe enough to warrant the increased risk.[87] In head and neck surgery it is unlikely that one would consider using high-pressure irrigation except potentially when irrigating scalp wounds—in which case the increased risk of bacterial seeding of the skull must be weighed against the benefit of high-pressure irrigation of a heavily contaminated wound. The literature has been equivocal on pulsatile irrigation versus continuous.[87] Furthermore, the optimal volume of irrigation needed to effectively reduce bacterial load has not been determined.[35,87,88]

Topical antibiotics can be administered perioperatively in several forms, including as part of irrigation solutions, powders, ointments, creams, and antibiotic-impregnated beads. The use of antibiotics for wound irrigation has not been demonstrated to reduce incidence of SSI, likely because of insufficient contact time between the agent and its target and low tissue concentrations.[86] The WHO conducted a meta-analysis of five studies that demonstrated no benefit for the use of antibiotic-containing topical irrigation when compared with saline irrigation or no irrigation in reducing risk of SSI (OR 1.16; 95% CI [0.64-2.12], $P = .63$). Furthermore, incorporating antibiotics into topical irrigation formulations can contribute to allergic reactions, tissue irritation, and potentially foster the development of antibiotic resistance.[86] Current evidence also fails to demonstrate that prophylactic use of topical antibiotics prevents the development of SSI. A systematic review by Chen et al. found that transfusion of at least[89] in 2021 evaluated 13 trials comparing the use of topical antibiotics to placebo or other nonantibiotic ingredients in dermatologic, abdominal, orthopedic, spinal, cardiothoracic, and ocular surgery. The delivery method of topical antibiotics varied widely in the studies, including intraoperative vancomycin powder, preoperative

intranasal mupirocin, and postoperative application of antibiotic ointments to the surgical incision. Ten of the included trials were pooled to compare the prophylactic effect of topical antibiotics to no antibiotics in clean postoperative wounds. The authors found that the use of topical antibiotics did not reduce risk of SSI in all populations, including dermatologic surgery (RR 0.89; 95% CI [0.59, 1.32], $P = .56$).[89] Another study highlighted that the moist environment promoted by petroleum-based lubricants may be more beneficial to wound healing than the bactericidal effect of antibiotics.[90] Well-designed randomized controlled prospective studies are needed to better understand the potential role of topical antibiotics and antibiotic irrigation in patients undergoing head and neck surgery. However, based on the evidence available from other surgical specialties, head and neck surgeons should be judicious when recommending topical antibiotics in any patients with clean or clean-contaminated surgical wounds.

Transfusions

When considering blood transfusions, the provider must weigh the risks versus the benefits. A blood transfusion may be required to ensure adequate tissue oxygenation, which is necessary to support the immune system and decrease infection risk. However, blood transfusions themselves stimulate a significant immune response that can also lead to an increased risk of infection, as well as the small risk they pose of transmissible disease and severe transfusion reactions. The mechanisms by which blood transfusions are associated with development of a heightened immune response involve the release of mediators by white blood cells during the storage of blood and the possible downregulation of the recipient's immune system caused by white blood cells in the transfused product.[91] In an effort to mitigate this risk, many U.S. medical centers have incorporated universal leukoreduction of red blood cell stock.[92] The administration of leukocyte-depleted products has been demonstrated to result in a lower risk of infection than products containing white blood cells.[15,93] Studies have demonstrated that the increased risk of sepsis is proportional to the amount of blood transfused as well as to the length of time of blood storage before transfusion.[15,92] Weinberg et al performed a retrospective cohort study of trauma patients who received transfusion of at least 1 unit of leukoreduced blood during the first 24 hours of hospitalization.[92] Patients were stratified based on total number of units transfused, as well as whether they received "young" blood (stored for <14 days) or "old" blood (stored for ≥14 days). Storage life of packed red blood cells is up to 42 days. Weinberg et al. found that transfusion of at least 3 units of "old" blood significantly increased the risk of death compared with at least 3 units of "young" blood.[92] For head and neck surgery, all efforts should be made to reduce intraoperative and perioperative blood loss. Although transfusions should never be withheld from surgical patients as a means to prevent SSI,[16] providers also should be aware of the risk of surgical site, pulmonary, or systemic infection associated with blood products. Every effort should be made to minimize perioperative blood loss, ensure transfused products are leukoreduced, and store transfused blood products for less than 2 weeks.

Conclusions

The prevention of HAIs, including SSIs, requires a targeted and multifaceted approach that involves frequent review and outcomes assessments. Rigorous implementation of guidelines over the last two decades have reduced the incidence of HAIs, but they remain a significant burden to the health care system. SSIs, which comprise an estimated 16% of all HAIs, have well-known risk factors. Evidence-based interventions such as adequate skin preparation, good surgical technique, optimization of nutrition, perioperative glucose control, provision of prophylactic antibiotics, and maintenance of ideal operating room conditions have been shown to reduce risk of SSI. The head and neck surgeon should be able to recognize risk factors in his or her patient population specific to the procedure being performed, and be familiar with implementing these strategies in their own practice.

Acknowledgments

We would like to thank Julie Ann Smith for her contribution to the previous version of this chapter.

References

1. Yokoe DS, Mermel LA, Anderson DJ. A compendium of strategies to prevent healthcare-associated infections in acute care hospitals. *Infect Control Hosp Epidemiol*. 2008;29:S12-S21.

2. Yokoe DS, Anderson DJ, Berenholtz SM. A compendium of strategies to prevent healthcare-associated infections in acute care hospitals: 2014 updates. *Infect Control Hosp Epidemiol*. 2014; 35(8):967-977.

3. Buetti N, Marschall J, Drees M. Strategies to prevent central line-associated bloodstream infections in acute care hospitals: 2022 update. *Infect Control Hosp Epidemiol*. 2022;43(5):553-569.

4. Lessa FC, Mu Y, Bamberg WM, et al. Burden of *Clostridium difficile* infection in the United States. *N Engl J Med*. 2015;372(9):825-834. Available at: https://doi.org/10.1056/NEJMoa1408913.

5. Magill SS, Edwards JR, Bamberg W, et al. Multistate point-prevalence survey of health care-associated infections. *N Engl J Med*. 2014;370(13):1198-1208.

6. Magill SS, O'Leary E, Janelle SJ, et al. Changes in prevalence of health care–associated infections in U.S. hospitals. *N Engl J Med*. 2018;379(18):1732-1744. Available at: https://doi.org/10.1056/NEJMoa1801550.

7. Galway UA, Parker BM, Borkowski RG. Prevention of postoperative surgical site infections. *Int Anesth Clin*. 2009;47(4):37-53.

8. Young P, Khadaroo R. Surgical site infections. *Surg Clin North Am*. 2014;94(6):1245-1264. Available at: https://doi.org/10.1016/j.suc.2014.08.008.

9. Dammling C, Abramowicz S, Kinard B. Current concepts in prophylactic antibiotics in oral and maxillofacial surgery. *Oral Maxillofac Surg Clin North Am*. 2022;34(1):157-167. Available at: https://doi.org/10.1016/j.coms.2021.08.015.

10. Kaye KS, Schmader KE, Sawyer R. Surgical site infection in the elderly population. *Clin Infect Dis*. 2004;39(12):1835-1841. Available at: https://doi.org/10.1086/425744.

11. Kaye KS, Schmit K, Pieper C, et al. The effect of increasing age on the risk of surgical site infection. *J Infect Dis*. 2005;191(7): 1056-1062. Available at: https://doi.org/10.1086/428626.

12. Mauermann WJ, Nemergut EC. The anesthesiologist's role in the prevention of surgical site infections. *Anesthesiology*. 2006; 105(2):413-421.

13. Van den Berghe, Wouters P, Weekers F, et al. Intensive insulin therapy in critically ill patients. *N Engl J Med*. 2001;345.1359-1367.

14. Furnary AP, Zerr KJ, Grunkemeier GL. Continuous intravenous insulin infusion reduces the incidence of deep sternal wound infection in diabetic patients after cardiac surgical procedures. *Ann Thorac Surg*. 1999;67(2):352-360.

15. Alexander JW, Solomkin JS, Edwards MJ. Updated recommendations for control of surgical site infections. *Ann Surg*. 2011; 253:1082-1093.

16. Berríos-Torres SI, Umscheid CA, Bratzler DW, et al. Centers for Disease Control and Prevention guideline for the prevention of surgical site infection, 2017. *JAMA Surg*. 2017;152(8):784-791. Available at: https://doi.org/10.1001/jamasurg.2017.0904.

17. Allegranzi B, Zayed B, Bischoff P, et al. New WHO recommendations on intraoperative and postoperative measures for surgical site infection prevention: an evidence-based global perspective. *Lancet Infect Dis*. 2016;16(12):e288-e303. Available at: https://doi.org/10.1016/S1473-3099(16)30402-9.

18. Shaw P, Saleem T, Gahtan V. Correlation of hemoglobin A1C level with surgical outcomes: can tight perioperative glucose control reduce infection and cardiac events? *Semin Vasc Surg*. 2014;27(3):156-161. Available at: https://doi.org/10.1053/j.semvascsurg.2015.03.002.

19. Blankush JM, Leitman IM, Soleiman A, Tran T. Association between elevated pre-operative glycosylated hemoglobin and post-operative infections after non-emergent surgery. *Ann Med Surg*. 2016;10: 77-82. Available at: https://doi.org/10.1016/j.amsu.2016.07.025.

20. Müller-Richter U, Betz C, Hartmann S, Brands RC. Nutrition management for head and neck cancer patients improves clinical outcome and survival. *Nutr Res*. 2017;48:1-8. Available at: https://doi.org/10.1016/j.nutres.2017.08.007.

21. Wischmeyer PE, Carli F, Evans DC, et al. American Society for Enhanced Recovery and Perioperative Quality Initiative joint consensus statement on nutrition screening and therapy within a surgical enhanced recovery pathway. *Anesth Analg*. 2018;126(6):1883. Available at: https://doi.org/10.1213/ANE.0000000000002743.

22. Talwar B, Donnelly R, Skelly R, Donaldson M. Nutritional management in head and neck cancer: United Kingdom national multidisciplinary guidelines. *J Laryngol Otol*. 2016;130(S2):S32-S40. Available at: https://doi.org/10.1017/S0022215116000402.

23. Son HJ, Roh JL, Choi SH, Nam SY, Kim SY. Nutritional and hematologic markers as predictors of risk of surgical site infection in patients with head and neck cancer undergoing major oncologic surgery. *Head Neck*. 2018;40(3):596-604. Available at: https://doi.org/10.1002/hed.25031.

24. Lee JI, Kwon M, Roh JL, et al. Postoperative hypoalbuminemia as a risk factor for surgical site infection after oral cancer surgery. *Oral Dis*. 2015;21(2):178-184. Available at: https://doi.org/10.1111/odi.12232.

25. Barie PS, Eachempati SR. Surgical site infections. *Surg Clin North Am*. 2005;85(6):1115-1135. Available at: https://doi.org/10.1016/j.suc.2005.09.006.

26. Waisbren E, Rosen H, Bader AM, Lipsitz SR, Rogers SO, Eriksson E. Percent body fat and prediction of surgical site

infection. *J Am Coll Surg.* 2010;210(4):381-389. Available at: https://doi.org/10.1016/j.jamcollsurg.2010.01.004.

27. Wahl TS, Patel FC, Goss LE, Chu DI, Grams J, Morris MS. The obese colorectal surgery patient: surgical site infection and outcomes. *Dis Colon Rectum.* 2018;61(8):938-945. Available at: https://doi.org/10.1097/DCR.0000000000001085.

28. Anderson V, Chaboyer W, Gillespie B. The relationship between obesity and surgical site infections in women undergoing caesarean sections: an integrative review. *Midwifery.* 2013;29(12):1331-1338. Available at: https://doi.org/10.1016/j.midw.2012.12.012.

29. Yuan K, Chen HL. Obesity and surgical site infections risk in orthopedics: a meta-analysis. *Int J Surg.* 2013;11(5):383-388. Available at: https://doi.org/10.1016/j.ijsu.2013.02.018.

30. Pavlovic N, Boland RA, Brady B, et al. Effect of weight-loss diets prior to elective surgery on postoperative outcomes in obesity: a systematic review and meta-analysis. *Clin Obes.* 2021;11(6):e12485. Available at: https://doi.org/10.1111/cob.12485.

31. Sørensen LT. Wound healing and infection in surgery: the clinical impact of smoking and smoking cessation—a systematic review and meta-analysis. *Arch Surg.* 2012;147(4):373-383. Available at: https://doi.org/10.1001/archsurg.2012.5.

32. Mills E, Eyawo O, Lockhart I, Kelly S, Wu P, Ebbert JO. Smoking cessation reduces postoperative complications: a systematic review and meta-analysis. *Am J Med.* 2011;124(2):144-154.e8. Available at: https://doi.org/10.1016/j.amjmed.2010.09.013.

33. Bowater RJ, Stirling SA, Lilford RJ. Is antibiotic prophylaxis in surgery a generally effective intervention? Testing a generic hypothesis over a set of meta-analyses. *Ann Surg.* 2009;249(4):551-556.

34. De Jonge SW, Boldingh QJJ, Koch AH, et al. Timing of preoperative antibiotic prophylaxis and surgical site infection: TAPAS, an observational cohort study. *Ann Surg.* 2021;274(4):e308-e314. Available at: https://doi.org/10.1097/SLA.0000000000003634.

35. Fletcher N, Sofianos D, Berkes MB. Prevention of perioperative infection. *J Bone Joint Surg Am.* 2007;89:1605-1618.

36. Vander Poorten V, Uyttebroek S, Robbins KT, et al. Perioperative antibiotics in clean-contaminated head and neck surgery: a systematic review and meta-analysis. *Adv Ther.* 2020;37(4):1360-1380. Available at: https://doi.org/10.1007/s12325-020-01269-2.

37. Milic T, Raidoo P, Gebauer D. Antibiotic prophylaxis in oral and maxillofacial surgery: a systematic review. *Br J Oral Maxillofac Surg.* 2021;59(6):633-642. Available at: https://doi.org/10.1016/j.bjoms.2020.09.020.

38. Blum IR. Contemporary views on dry socket (alveolar osteitis): a clinical appraisal of standardization, aetiopathogenesis and management—a critical review. *Int J Oral Maxillofac Surg.* 2002;31:309-317.

39. Kolokythas A, Olech E, Miloro M. Alveolar osteitis: a comprehensive review of concepts and controversies. *Int J Dent.* 2010;2010:e249073. Available at: https://doi.org/10.1155/2010/249073.

40. Ren YF, Malmstrom HS. Effectiveness of antibiotic prophylaxis in third molar surgery: a meta-analysis of randomized controlled clinical trials. *J Oral Maxillofac Surg.* 2007;65:1909-1921.

41. Zeitler DL. Prophylactic antibiotics for third molar surgery: a dissenting opinion. *J Oral Maxillofac Surg.* 1995;53:61-64.

42. Piecuch JF, Arzadon J, Lieblich SE. Prophylactic antibiotics for third molar surgery: a supportive opinion. *J Oral Maxillofac Surg.* 1995;53:53-60.

43. Lodi G, Azzi L, Varoni EM, et al. Antibiotics to prevent complications following tooth extractions. *Cochrane Database Syst Rev.* 2021;(2):CD003811. Available at: https://doi.org/10.1002/14651858.CD003811.pub3.

44. Susarla S, Sharaf B, Dodson TB. Do antibiotics reduce the frequency of surgical site infections after impacted mandibular third molar surgery? *Oral Maxillofac Surg Clin North Am.* 2011;23(4):541-546.

45. Halpern LR, Dodson TB. Does prophylactic administration of systemic antibiotics prevent postoperative inflammatory complications after third molar surgery? *J Oral Maxillofac Surg.* 2007;65:177-185.

46. Yanine N, Sabelle N, Vergara-Gárate V, et al. Effect of antibiotic prophylaxis for preventing infectious complications following impacted mandibular third molar surgery: a randomized controlled trial. *Med Oral Patol Oral Cir Bucal.* 2021;26(6):e703-e710. Available at: https://doi.org/10.4317/medoral.24274.

47. Monaco G, Tavernese L, Agostini R, Marchetti C. Evaluation of antibiotic prophylaxis in reducing postoperative infection after mandibular third molar extraction in young patients. *J Oral Maxillofac Surg.* 2009;67(7):1467-1472. Available at: https://doi.org/10.1016/j.joms.2008.12.066.

48. Cho H, Lynham A, Hsu E. Postoperative interventions to reduce inflammatory complications after third molar surgery: review of the current evidence. *Aust Dent J.* 2017;62(4):412-419. Available at: https://doi.org/10.1111/adj.12526.

49. Daly B, Sharif M, Newton T, Jones K, Worthington H. Local Interventions for the management of alveolar osteitis (dry socket). *Cochrane Database Syst Rev.* 2012 Dec 12.

50. Caso A, Hung LK, Beirne OR. Prevention of alveolar osteitis with chlorhexidine: a meta-analytic review. *Oral Surg Oral Med Oral Pathol Oral Radiol Endod.* 2005;99(2):155-159.

51. Davis CM, Gregoire CE, Davis I, Steeves TW. Prevalence of surgical site infections following orthognathic surgery: a double-blind, randomized controlled trial on a 3-day versus 1-day postoperative antibiotic regimen. *J Oral Maxillofac Surg.* 2017;75(4):796-804. Available at: https://doi.org/10.1016/j.joms.2016.09.038.

52. Chow LK, Singh B, Chiu WK. Prevalence of postoperative complications after orthognathic surgery: a 15-year review. *J Oral Maxillofac Surg.* 2007;65:984-992.

53. Zijderveld SA, Smeele LE, Kostense PJ. Preoperative antibiotic prophylaxis in orthognathic surgery: a randomized, double-blind, and placebo-controlled clinical study. *J Oral Maxillofac Surg.* 1999;57:1403-1406.

54. Danda AK, Ravi P. Effectiveness of postoperative antibiotics in orthognathic surgery: a meta-analysis. *J Oral Maxillofac Surg.* 2011;69(10):2650-2656. Available at: https://doi.org/10.1016/j.joms.2011.02.060.

55. Alsharif U, Al-Moraissi E, Alabed S. Systemic antibiotic prophylaxis for preventing infectious complications in maxillofacial trauma surgery. *Cochrane Database Syst Rev.* 2017;(3):CD012603. Available at: https://doi.org/10.1002/14651858.CD012603.

56. Andreasen JO, Jensen SS, Schwartz O. A systematic review of prophylactic antibiotics in the surgical treatment of maxillofacial fractures. *J Oral Maxillofac Surg.* 2006;64:1664-1668.

57. Chole RA, Yee J. Antibiotic prophylaxis for facial fractures: a prospective, randomized clinical trial. *Arch Otolaryngol Head Neck Surg.* 1987;113:1055-1057.

58. Habib AM, Wong AD, Schreiner GC, et al. Postoperative prophylactic antibiotics for facial fractures: a systematic review and meta-analysis. *Laryngoscope.* 2019;129(1):82-95. Available at: https://doi.org/10.1002/lary.27210.

59. Mundinger GS, Borsuk DE, Okhah Z, et al. Antibiotics and facial fractures: evidence-based recommendations compared with experience-based practice. *Craniomaxillofac Trauma Reconstr.* 2015;8(1):64-78. Available at: https://doi.org/10.1055/s-0034-1378187.

60. Michel JC, Amin D, Gelbard RB, Abramowicz S. An evidence-based approach to antibiotic use in maxillofacial trauma. *Oral Surg Oral Med Oral Pathol Oral Radiol.* 2022;134(2):151-158. Available at: https://doi.org/10.1016/j.oooo.2021.12.135.

61. Esposito M, Grusovin MG, Worthington HV. Interventions for replacing missing teeth: antibiotics at dental implant placement to prevent complications. *Cochrane Database Syst Rev.* 2013;(7): CD004152. Available at: https://doi.org/10.1002/14651858. CD004152.pub4.

62. Laskin DM, Dent CD, Morris HF, Ochi S, Olson JW. The influence of preoperative antibiotics on success of endosseous implants at 36 months. *Ann Periodontol.* 2000;5(1):166-174. Available at: https://doi.org/10.1902/annals.2000.5.1.166.

63. Anitua E, Aguirre Anda JJ, Gorosabel A, et al. A multicentre placebo-controlled randomised clinical trial of antibiotic prophylaxis for placement of single dental implants. *Eur J Oral Implantol.* 2009;2:283-292.

64. Tan WC, Ong M, Han J, et al. Effect of systemic antibiotics on clinical and patient-reported outcomes of implant therapy: a multicenter randomized controlled clinical trial. *Clin Oral Implants Res.* 2014;25(2):185-193. Available at: https://doi.org/10.1111/clr.12098.

65. Resnik RR, Misch C. Prophylactic antibiotic regimens in oral implantology: rationale and protocol. *Implant Dent.* 2008;17(2):142. Available at: https://doi.org/10.1097/ID.0b013e3181752b09.

66. Tanner J, Melen K. Preoperative hair removal to reduce surgical site infection. *Cochrane Database Syst Rev.* 2021;8(8):CD004122. Available at: https://doi.org/10.1002/14651858.CD004122.pub5.

67. Webster J, Osborne S. Preoperative bathing or showering with skin antiseptics to prevent surgical site infection. *Cochrane Database Syst Rev.* 2015;(2):CD004985. Available at: https://doi.org/10.1002/14651858.CD004985.pub5.

68. Chlebicki MJ, Safdar N, O'Horo JC. Preoperative chlorhexidine shower or bath for prevention of surgical site infection: a meta-analysis. *Am J Infect Control.* 2013;41:167-173.

69. Privitera GP, Costa AL, Brusaferro S, et al. Skin antisepsis with chlorhexidine versus iodine for the prevention of surgical site infection: a systematic review and meta-analysis. *Am J Infect Control.* 2017;45(2):180-189. Available at: https://doi.org/10.1016/j.ajic.2016.09.017.

70. Bednarek RS, Nassereddin A, Ramsey ML. Skin antiseptics. In: *StatPearls.* Treasure Island, FL: StatPearls; 2023. Available at: http://www.ncbi.nlm.nih.gov/books/NBK507853/.

71. Iyer A, Gilfillan I, Thakur S. Reduction of surgical site infection using a microbial sealant: a randomized trial. *J Thorac Cardiovasc Surg.* 2011;142:438-442.

72. Waldow T, Szlapka M, Hensel J. Skin sealant InteguSeal has no impact on prevention of postoperative mediastinitis after cardiac surgery. *J Hosp Infect.* 2012;81:278-282.

73. Tanner J, Dumville JC, Norman G, Fortnam M. Surgical hand antisepsis to reduce surgical site infection. *Cochrane Database Syst Rev.* 2016;(1):CD004288. Available at: https://doi.org/10.1002/14651858.CD004288.pub3.

74. Aly R, Maibach HI. Comparative antibacterial activity of a 2-minute surgical scrub with chlorhexidine gluconate, povidone-iodine, and chloroxylenol sponge-brushes. *Am J Infect Control.* 1988;16:173-177.

75. Parienti JJ, Thibon P, Heller R. Hand-rubbing with an aqueous alcoholic solution vs traditional surgical hand-scrubbing and 30-day surgical site infection rates: a randomized equivalence study. *JAMA.* 2002;288(2689):722-727.

76. Forbes SS, McLean RF. Review article: the anesthesiologist's role in the prevention of surgical site infections. *Can J Anesth.* 2013;60:176-183.

77. Sessler DI. Complications and treatment of mild hypothermia. *Anesthesiology.* 2001;95:531-543.

78. Kurz A, Sessler DI, Lenhardt R. Perioperative normothermia to reduce the incidence of surgical-wound infection and shorten hospitalization. *N Engl J Med.* 1996;334(19):1209-1215.

79. Qadan M, Akca O, Mahid SS. Perioperative supplemental oxygen therapy and surgical site infection: a meta-analysis of randomized controlled trials. *Arch Surg.* 2009;144:359-366.

80. Hovaguimian F, Lysakowski C, Elia N, Tramèr MR. Effect of intraoperative high inspired oxygen fraction on surgical site infection, postoperative nausea and vomiting, and pulmonary function: systematic review and meta-analysis of randomized controlled trials. *Anesthesiology.* 2013;119(2):303-316. Available at: https://doi.org/10.1097/ALN.0b013e31829aaff4.

81. Meyhoff CS, Wetterslev J, Jorgensen LN, et al. Effect of high perioperative oxygen fraction on surgical site infection and pulmonary complications after abdominal surgery: the PROXI randomized clinical trial. *JAMA.* 2009;302(14):1543-1550. Available at: https://doi.org/10.1001/jama.2009.1452.

82. McHugh SM, Hill ADK, Humphreys H. Intraoperative technique as a factor in the prevention of surgical site infection. *J Hosp Infect.* 2011;78:1-4.

83. Aird LNF, Brown CJ. Systematic review and meta-analysis of electrocautery versus scalpel for surgical skin incisions. *Am J Surg.* 2012;204(2):216-221. Available at: https://doi.org/10.1016/j.amjsurg.2011.09.032.

84. Chau JKM, Dzigielewski P, Mlynarek A, et al. Steel scalpel versus electrocautery blade: comparison of cosmetic and patient satisfaction outcomes of different incision methods. *J Otolaryngol Head Neck Surg.* 2009;38(4):427-433.

85. Edmiston CE, Daoud FC, Leaper D. Is there an evidence-based argument for embracing an antimicrobial (triclosan)-coated suture technology to reduce the risk for surgical-site infections? A meta-analysis. *Surgery.* 2013;154(1):89-100. Available at: https://doi.org/10.1016/j.surg.2013.03.008.

86. Papadakis M. Wound irrigation for preventing surgical site infections. *World J Methodol.* 2021;11(4):222-227. Available at: https://doi.org/10.5662/wjm.v11.i4.222.

87. Barnes S, Spencer M, Graham D. Surgical wound irrigation: a call for evidence-based standardization of practice. *Am J Infect Control.* 2014;42:525-529.

88. Anglen JO. Wound irrigation in musculoskeletal injury. *J Am Orthop Surg.* 2001;9:270-271.

89. Chen PJ, Hua YM, Toh HS, Lee MC. Topical antibiotic prophylaxis for surgical wound infections in clean and clean-contaminated surgery: a systematic review and meta-analysis. *BJS Open.* 2021;5(6):zrab125. Available at: https://doi.org/10.1093/bjsopen/zrab125.

90. Saco M, Howe N, Nathoo R, Cherpelis B. Topical antibiotic prophylaxis for prevention of surgical wound infections from dermatologic procedures: a systematic review and meta-analysis. *J Dermatol Treat.* 2015;26(2):151-158. Available at: https://doi.org/10.3109/09546634.2014.906547.

91. Gunst MA, Minei JP. Transfusion of blood products and nosocomial infection in surgical patients. *Curr Opin Crit Care.* 2007;13:428-432.

92. Weinberg JA, McGwin G, Griffin RL. Age of transfused blood: an independent predictor of mortality despite universal leukoreduction. *J Trauma.* 2008;65:279-284.

93. Friese RS, Sperry JL, Phelan HA. The use of leukoreduced red blood cell products is associated with fewer infectious complications in trauma patients. *Am J Surg.* 2008;196:56-61.

33

Medicolegal Issues Related to Head and Neck Infections

ANTHONY M. SPINA AND JAMES R. HUPP

Patients suffer infections of the head and neck region that are either primary, such as sialadenitis, or occur secondary to an injury. The injury is sometimes part of a surgical intervention or other invasive procedure during which potentially infectious material is introduced into a wound. No matter the cause, infections carry many of the same risks of medicolegal problems as other patient conditions. Patients coming to a clinician for care of a preexisting, existing, or suspected infection bring the possibility of the practitioner being accused of failing to make a timely diagnosis, reaching a misdiagnosis, or providing the wrong treatment. Infections occurring after an invasive procedure run the additional risks of being blamed on negligence in the performance of a procedure or failure to take appropriate steps to prevent infection or mitigate the damage.

To better understand the scope of medicolegal implications of postoperative infections, data were requested from the OMS National Insurance Company (OMSNIC), the leading medical professional liability insurance carrier for oral and maxillofacial surgeons in the United States. The retrospective study evaluated medical malpractice lawsuits against oral and maxillofacial surgeons insured by OMSNIC that closed between January 1, 2018, and December 31, 2022, in which infection after surgery was alleged as an injury. These claims accounted for 14% of all lawsuits closed during this time. Indemnity payments were made in 30% of the infection-related lawsuits, accounting for 15% of all indemnities paid on behalf of OMSNIC policyholders and 14.5% of the total defense costs paid by OMSNIC during this 5-year period; 83% of these allegations were associated with dentoalveolar surgery or dental implant surgery, the most performed oral surgery procedures. From these data, we can conclude that, although a majority of claims do not result in a trial or an indemnity payment, doctors must still defend their care and treatment rendered when faced with litigation—a process that can be stressful and require significant time out of a practice. Although these oral and maxillofacial surgery–specific data are not intended to be representative of the frequency or severity of similar claims made against other providers, risk mitigation strategies can be applied universally.

This chapter discusses how providers can reduce the risk of, and improve the defensibility of, claims related to infections after surgery through the review of common allegations associated with these claims.

Failure to Make a Timely Diagnosis

Clinical signals are usually present that lead one to suspect an infection; however, there may be complicating factors. First, when infection is not high enough or even present on the differential diagnosis list, the clinician may not order needed diagnostic procedures, such as advanced imaging or laboratory tests, early in the patient's workup. Second, even if an infection is included in the differential diagnosis, the causative infectious agent fails to be discovered because of inappropriate or inadequate diagnostic procedures. Third, even when the actual causative agent is identified, an effective drug regimen is not initiated and carried through appropriately.

Osteomyelitis resulting from inappropriate care is a common allegation in this category. The typical case involves a patient who has a localized dull ache that is treated empirically with antibiotics, and the symptoms abate. The patient returns in 2 to 3 weeks complaining of the return of the low-grade discomfort. There is no obvious clinical evidence of infection, and radiographs do not reveal an obvious cause. So again, antibiotics are given empirically. After several weeks, the patient seeks care with a new care provider, who orders a new radiograph that shows bone destruction consistent with osteomyelitis. It typically takes approximately 4 to 5 weeks for an infection to cause sufficient bone decalcification to begin to reveal itself on imaging. Therefore, providers relying solely on an early radiograph may be accused of negligence if the bone infection goes on to produce serious problems.

Clinicians should keep the possibility of an infectious cause of a disease process in mind when conducting an examination of any patient with signs or symptoms of an inflammatory process or when the cause of the patient's problem is not readily apparent. In addition, it is important to remember that an infection can and often does coexist with other disease processes.

Failure to Ensure Appropriate Infection Control

Patients who develop an infection after surgery or other invasive procedure may allege that their infection was the result of a failure to maintain the appropriate degree of sterility or follow infection control guidelines or rules. Patients are observant of their surroundings and are attentive to the actions of the surgeon and staff, such as handwashing, that signify the level of infection control in a practice. If there is a perceived breakdown in infection control practices and an infection occurs, the patient may initiate a claim and report the observation to an attorney. In the case of surgery, the development of a postoperative infection with a pathogen unlikely to be present when proper infection control measures were followed may also trigger medicolegal problems.

In cases in which infections occur after invasive procedures, clinicians may be challenged to prove that all standards related to infection prevention protocols have been met. In any lawsuit arising from the infection, staff members may be deposed, and they will almost always reveal how well the practice's infection guidelines were or were not followed both in the specific case and in general. The health care facility may be required to produce documentation of infection control training procedures and evidence of continuing education for the doctors and staff. Documentation of autoclave maintenance and spore testing to confirm effective sterilization may be requested by plaintiff attorneys.

Therefore, it is critical to place infection control standards and protocols in a facility's operational manuals and require staff training and periodic updates. Sterilization protocols and compliance monitoring should be included. Also, all areas that patients encounter when in the health care facility should be kept clean, including reception areas and restrooms, to set the proper tone of the facility's attention to keeping patients safe.

Failure to Properly Treat

Allegations related to failure to adequately manage an identified or suspected infection include improper and inadequate surgical intervention, ordering the wrong antibiotic, inadequate dosing, improper administration, or wrong duration of treatment. In many circumstances, practitioners use their professional judgment to select the antimicrobials most likely to be effective without first obtaining a specimen for microbiologic testing. However, when an infection worsens and appears to not be responding to the initial treatment, culture and sensitivity testing and perhaps other testing are warranted. In addition, infectious disease specialists can be called on to assist when more complicated or severe infections occur or when an infection appears to be failing to respond to initial treatment.

Failure to Prescribe Antibiotics

A common allegation when a postoperative infection occurs is that preoperative antibiotics were not prescribed. Plaintiff attorneys capitalize on the misconception that preoperative antibiotics should be administered before any invasive procedure. Ironically, attorneys may argue that antibiotics were unnecessarily prescribed when a complication arises related to use of antibiotics. Thus, it becomes imperative that the practitioner documents whether an infection is present before surgery and the indication for antibiotics. Evidence shows that in most cases the removal of the source of infection is the best option, rather than simply prescribing an antibiotic. Many minor localized infections do not need an antibacterial initially; however, if the patient later worsens or the infection persists, an antibiotic can be started.

The practice of prescribing antibiotics before surgery varies among practitioners depending in part on clinicians' training and experience and/or their current institutions' standard practices (often related to geographic location). There are mixed opinions as to the automatic use of antibiotic prophylaxis; no definitive evidence-based studies support prophylactic antibiotics before all surgery as standard of care. This makes it important for practitioners to stay current with respect to scientific studies addressing the efficacy of prophylactic antibiotics. For most hospital-based major surgical procedures, an intravenous antibiotic administered before surgery has become the norm even when no good scientific evidence of its efficacy exists. In addition, the presence of diseases that compromise the immune system's ability to manage pathogens may support the use of prophylactic antibiotics.

Dental providers have a special circumstance surrounding the use of prophylactic antibiotics. This relates to patients with cardiac abnormalities or orthopedic implants. Guidelines published by the American Heart Association, the American Academy of Orthopedic Surgeons, and the American Dental Association address this issue. Therefore, it is imperative for clinicians to stay current with their recommendations because they are subject to change.

Prescribing Unnecessary Antibiotics

Antimicrobial drugs carry the risk of complications similar to those of any other class of pharmaceuticals. Complications from the use of antibiotics include acute hypersensitivity reactions soon after administration. Thus, a detailed history of any previous allergic reactions to drugs or food products must be recorded. In addition, antibiotics may have cross-reactions with other medications, so the clinician should know all the medications a patient is using when an antibiotic is considered. *Clostridioides difficile* infection, if it occurs, can be life-threatening and may be blamed on the injudicious use of antibiotics, although it is usually limited to seriously ill or compromised patients. Informing susceptible patients about this possibility before using an antibiotic and reminding them to immediately report any gastrointestinal disturbances, including bloody diarrhea, allows for early intervention.

Unnecessary overprescribing can occur when several doctors prescribe different antibiotics for the same chronic infection over a period of time. If the patient then has an acute exacerbation, the infecting organism may have become resistant to any antibiotics that were previously effective. Thus, obtaining an accurate medical and medication history is important and, in some cases, conferring with prior-treating doctors when managing a patient's chronic infection may be indicated.

Informed Consent

The informed consent process is integral to any procedure. The opportunity to educate patients about the potential risks of infection and treatment options should occur during the informed consent discussion. When a patient has a reasonable understanding of the procedure, including potential risks such as infection, he or she tends to be much more accepting of a complication if one does occur and will, in general, participate in working toward curing the problem. In addition, a patient with an existing infection should be informed of the possible risks of managing the infection, including those related to medications, procedures, and possible outcomes.

When a patient with an infectious process seeks legal advice, the patient's attorneys will help develop allegations against the doctor. At that moment, the doctor becomes the defendant and in conjunction with the practitioner's legal team, must make every effort to disprove untrue or mischaracterized allegations. The medical record is critical in the defense of a claim. It should be legible, completed in a contemporaneous fashion, and outline the treatment course with adequate detail.

General Recommendations Related to Risk Management

- The best defense against medicolegal claims is to be available, affable, and able.
- If problems occur, communicate with the patient and family, show empathy for the situation, and take the time to explain why the patient is having the problem and the proposed treatment to mitigate any problems.
- Document signs and symptoms before and during the progression of clinical events so that the reasons for your treatment decisions are accurately reflected and recorded.
- Be aware of the financial aspect of care. For example, referring patients to collections for not paying the balance of their bill when they have had a difficult recovery only breeds animosity that may lead to unnecessary litigation.
- All surgical procedures have a risk of infection without any negligence by a provider. The art and science of the profession allows for the use of good judgment in how best to prevent and treat infections. Thorough documentation of decision processes, backed by evidence-based medicine, best serves patients and helps protect practitioners in the event of a malpractice claim.

Illustrative Case Reports

The following case reports illustrate management of dentoalveolar infections against the background of the modern changing bacterial spectrum and in the compromised host (see Chapter 16).

Postextraction Infection

A healthy 24-year-old man underwent extraction of a partially impacted mandibular third molar because of a history of intermittent pain and swelling. Penicillin was prescribed postoperatively for 10 days. Seventeen days after surgery, pain and swelling recurred. Penicillin again was prescribed but had no effect. Surgical drainage of the dentoalveolar abscess was performed, and the culture report revealed the presence of *Acinetobacter calcoaceticus* var. *Iwoffii (Mima polymorpha),* sensitive to ampicillin, gentamicin, and carbenicillin. The infection rapidly resolved.

The causative organism in this patient may have been an oral transient that became an opportunistic invader of the pericoronal culture media, or it may have been a secondary virulent aggressor whose growth was stimulated by penicillin suppression of the normal oral flora. Culture contamination is always a consideration when an unusual organism is encountered, but the response of the infection to the culture-specific antibiotic suggests otherwise.

Pericoronitis in an Immunocompromised Patient

A 26-year-old man was admitted to the hospital for chemotherapy for acute lymphocytic leukemia of 3 months' duration. A previous attempt at chemotherapy had been discontinued because of the development of *Escherichia coli* sepsis and pneumonia.

On the first hospital day the patient reported mandibular pain and submandibular adenopathy was palpable. His temperature was 37.8°C (100°F) and white blood cell count was 1250 cells/mm³, with numerous blast forms present, but platelet counts were well above normal levels. Oral examination revealed pericoronal swelling and tenderness but no erythema or purulence.

Blood cultures were performed and antibiotic therapy was started (tobramycin, 60 mg tid, and ticarcillin, 3 g q4h). By the patient's third hospital day, his temperature was normal and the white blood cell count was 3800 cells/mm³.

Dental radiographs revealed three partially impacted third molars. All three were extracted with the patient under local anesthesia, the wounds were irrigated with bacitracin solution, and the margins were loosely sutured. No further signs of infection were observed, and chemotherapy was reinstituted.

Comments

Patients whose immune systems are compromised or suppressed are at greater risk from odontogenic infection. The lack of erythema and purulence, or even a lack of temperature elevation, is typical of patients with neutropenia who do not demonstrate the classic signs of infection, often until serious generalized sepsis has focused attention on the original site. The patient with leukemia who is receiving chemotherapy has both quantitative and qualitative abnormalities of granulocytes.

The choice of antibiotics for this patient was based on his previous episode of gram-negative sepsis and on the hope of providing the widest possible spectrum of antibacterial activity. The optimal time to perform exodontia for patients with leukemia during remission is when the white blood cell count is above 2000 cells/mm³, and antibiotics, which are considered therapeutic rather than prophylactic, should be used. Some investigators further advocate that impacted teeth should be removed as a prophylactic measure in a patient with leukemia. However, it is difficult to justify subjecting patients who are severely ill or immunocompromised (e.g., leukemia, human immunodeficiency virus infection) to prophylactic surgery when the potential complications of that surgery—the risk of sepsis and the possibility of toxic side effects from high-dose antibiotics—are basically the same as those for an infection in the unextracted third molar. This situation is in contrast to the much better risk-benefit ratio for the extraction of asymptomatic impacted third molars in healthy patients.

The universal extraction of impacted teeth in all compromised hosts has been suggested, but the cost and potential morbidity and mortality suggest otherwise. Careful observation, antibiotic therapy, and selective exodontia seem more prudent in the compromised host.

Canine Space Infection

A 52-year-old man underwent extraction of the maxillary left canine tooth 1 month before the onset of swelling lateral to the nares. Nasal infection had been the diagnosis, and his physician had prescribed penicillin for the swelling.

When the swelling spread to the labial sulcus, the patient could no longer wear his denture and sought a dental consultation. Examination revealed a fluctuant mass lateral to the nares and firm swelling under the upper lip. Dental radiographs revealed a radiolucency in the area of the previously extracted canine root.

With the patient under general anesthesia, an incision into the labial sulcus produced drainage of pus. Blunt dissection superiorly with a small clamp produced greater egress of pus as the lateral nasal abscess (canine space) was entered. The mass collapsed, a drain was placed, and the purulent granulation tissue was curetted from the bony fossa over the canine root.

A culture report later revealed growth of *Citrobacter freundii,* a gram-negative enteric rod. Penicillin therapy was discontinued and further healing was uneventful.

Canine Space Infection

A 29-year-old woman had been examined in numerous hospital clinics because of intermittent swelling and drainage from a fistula "below her eye" (see Figure 16-7). Otolaryngologic, ophthalmologic, and dermatologic examinations had failed to reveal the cause of the lesion, as had radiographs of the sinuses, fungal cultures, chest radiography, and tuberculosis testing. Biopsy of the lesion was scheduled after dental consultation.

Dental examination revealed a carious pulpal exposure of the maxillary canine tooth, and a dental radiograph demonstrated an apical radiolucency at the root tip. Culture of the fistula revealed β-hemolytic streptococci. The tooth was extracted and the fistula promptly closed, terminating the chronic canine space infection.

Buccal Space Infection

A 10-year-old boy had massive swelling of the cheek to the level of the eyelids. Before the onset of the swelling, he had a toothache in a molar tooth, but the commencement of the swelling was associated with diminution of pain. His temperature was 38.3°C (101°F), and the skin of his cheek was warm, tender, and erythematous. The affected tooth was treated by pulpal extirpation, and penicillin therapy was started. Two days later fluctuance was noted in the inferior portion of the cheek, and a percutaneous incision and drainage was performed on an outpatient basis. Ten milliliters of pus was obtained, and a culture later yielded streptococci. Penicillin therapy was continued for 10 days, and the infection resolved. Endodontic filling of the tooth was performed later.

Masticator Space Infection

A 5-year-old girl underwent extraction of an "abscessed" mandibular deciduous molar associated with swelling of the buccal vestibule. Penicillin was prescribed but was never administered by the parent. Sixteen days later the child returned to the hospital with severe trismus, intense pain, brawny erythematous swelling involving the masseteric compartment of the masticator space, and a temperature of 39.2°C (102.6°F) (see Figure 16-11). Radiographs revealed "brushfire" osteomyelitis of the mandible. Her white blood cell count was 16,700 cells/mm³, with 78% polymorphonuclear leukocytes.

Despite intravenous penicillin therapy the swelling and pain intensified and on the third hospital day the girl was taken to the operating room. After blind nasal intubation a curvilinear skin incision was made below the angle of the mandible, and blunt dissection was carried to bone at the mandibular angle. Blunt penetration of the masticator sling resulted in a profuse flow of foul-smelling pus (see Figure 16-12). Specimens for aerobic and anaerobic cultures were obtained and a drain was placed. A Gram stain revealed gram-positive cocci, some in chain formations. Cultures later yielded anaerobic streptococci.

Medical evaluation for defective host defense mechanisms proved fruitless; penicillin therapy was continued orally and parenterally, sequestrectomy was performed later, and after many months the soft tissue and bone infection cleared completely.

Although unusual, this case illustrates masticator space infection and the problems of patient noncompliance. An intraoral incision and drainage might have been technically difficult in a small child and would not have provided dependent drainage. Long-term intraoral purulent flow and the presence of drains might not have been well tolerated. The need for anaerobic and aerobic culturing of deep space infections is also illustrated by this case.

Temporal Space Infection

A 28-year-old male hospital employee underwent forceps extraction of a carious maxillary third molar. Four days later, he noted the onset of trismus, pain, and temporal area headache. By the sixth postextraction day, he had an oral opening of only 12 mm, and examination revealed tender firm swelling in the temporal area just superior to the zygomatic arch. His white blood cell count was 13,950 cells/mm³, and his temperature was 38.8°C (101.8°F).

The patient was admitted to the hospital and underwent percutaneous incision and drainage of the temporal space the next day. A small amount of purulent material was obtained from the superficial temporal pouch, and culture later revealed mixed oral flora. Penicillin was administered, and the infection resolved without further sequelae.

No antibiotic was used at the time of extraction, nor was any antibiotic therapy indicated for extraction of a noninfected maxillary molar. Drainage also could have been accomplished intraorally at the insertion of the temporalis muscle at the mandibular coronoid process. CT scan of the masticator space confirms the diagnosis of infection, *even* if early or occult, and can delineate its extent.

Sublingual Space Infection

A 47-year-old immunosuppressed patient who had received a kidney transplant reported swelling under his tongue. Examination revealed erythematous, firm, tender swelling of the floor of the mouth. Two mandibular incisors were mobile; radiographs revealed diffuse bone loss consistent with periodontitis, and deep gingival pockets were present. His temperature was 38°C (100.4°F).

Penicillin and warm saline solution rinses were prescribed for this ambulatory patient. Two days later, with the patient under outpatient general anesthesia, the teeth were extracted and a mucosal incision parallel to Wharton's duct produced a small amount of purulent drainage from the sublingual space. Culture of specimens revealed streptococci, both aerobic and anaerobic; the infection resolved in 10 days.

Necrotizing Fasciitis

A 63-year-old patient with insulin-dependent diabetes and a history of poorly controlled hyperglycemia was transferred from a rural hospital, where he had been treated with intravenously administered antibiotics for 4 days because of massive swelling of the neck. The infection originally had been localized in the submental area after extraction of a mobile mandibular central incisor.

Examination revealed an obese, febrile man whose neck was swollen and intensely erythematous and tender, with palpable crepitus from the chin to the sternal notch. His white blood cell count was 27,400 cells/mm³, and the fasting blood glucose level was 280 mg/dL. CT scanning revealed gross swelling of the neck associated with profuse gas formation and tissue necrosis.

After fluid resuscitation and intubation, the patient's neck was opened widely and necrotic fascia and muscle were removed. Brown necrotic tissue and fluid, with a fecal odor, extended from the submandibular and submental spaces to the superior mediastinum. After cultures were obtained, multiple drains were placed, small areas of necrotic skin were excised, and intravenous imipenem therapy was started empirically when a Gram stain revealed a mixed flora of gram-positive cocci and gram-negative rods.

Culture later revealed aerobic and anaerobic streptococci and *Fusobacterium* and *Bacteroides* organisms. Healing progressed slowly but uneventfully after hyperglycemia was controlled, and the patient was discharged on the twenty-third hospital day.

In a grossly obese, hyperglycemic patient with insulin-dependent diabetes, periodontal infection is the norm and postextraction infection is commonplace. Whether standard penicillin therapy (or prophylaxis) would have avoided or aborted an infection is debatable. The early concomitant use of metronidazole and clindamycin would have increased the chance of success in this mixed-flora infection.

In this patient a localized submental space infection spread to the submandibular spaces and into the neck, creating a life-threatening necrotizing fasciitis.[1-5]

Submental Space Infection

A 10-year-old child was brought to the emergency department 2 days after a fall from a bicycle. Examination revealed a markedly swollen chin, and imaging revealed a nondisplaced symphyseal fracture and a subcondylar fracture. The central incisors were slightly mobile. Despite rigid fixation and penicillin therapy, the submental area became fluctuant and required incision and drainage, from which streptococci and *Bacteroides* were cultured. After drainage the infection and fracture healed uneventfully.

Antibiotics do not penetrate well into fascial space infections, regardless of the primary source of infection; a scalpel blade often is the therapy of choice. Fractures and surgery may be the cause of space infections.

Ludwig's Angina

A 9-year-old girl in severe respiratory distress was brought to the emergency department by ambulance. Four days earlier a diagnosis of "submaxillary mumps" had been made by the family physician because of unilateral swelling beneath the mandible. Despite progressive swelling, pain, and temperature elevation, only symptomatic therapy was used. A few hours before the patient's hospital admission, the swelling had spread bilaterally and respiratory distress had developed. Examination in the emergency department revealed a cyanotic, semicomatose child with a large firm swelling of the anterior neck. Her tongue was displaced superiorly and posteriorly by wooden-hard erythematous sublingual edema. Laryngoscopy in the emergency department was unsuccessful.

Tracheostomy was attempted but was difficult because of massive edema and displacement of the trachea. The child died within a few minutes while the tracheostomy was being performed, and resuscitation efforts proved fruitless. Postmortem examination confirmed the diagnosis of Ludwig's angina and a deeply carious mandibular molar as its cause.

Submaxillary mumps without parotid involvement is rare, if it exists at all, whereas untreated Ludwig's angina is lethal. Had the association of submandibular swelling with a diseased tooth been noted, the child's death could have been prevented. The rapidly lethal course of the infection, once it had crossed the submandibular midline, illustrates the clear danger of ignoring early signs of this disease. Ludwig's angina leaves little room for misdiagnosis or procrastination, especially in children. Although the overall incidence of Ludwig's angina is decreasing, as is the frequency of mortality, contemporary series of cases reveal that as many as 24% of patients in hospitals with this diagnosis are admitted to the pediatric service. Tonsillitis is a more common cause of deep neck infection in children than is odontogenic infection, and airway compromise is less well tolerated than in adults.

Ludwig's Angina, Sepsis, Disseminated Intravascular Coagulation

A 25-year-old woman, in apparently good health, underwent extraction of a painful, partially impacted third molar tooth in a dental office. No antibiotics were prescribed because there were no obvious clinical signs of infection at the time of surgery.

Low-grade temperature elevation and facial swelling developed during the evening after surgery. By the following day a firm bilateral submandibular swelling, mild trismus, and temperature elevation to 38.2°C (100.8°F) were noted. The patient experienced chills, and the swelling had increased and trismus had intensified later that day. Symptomatic therapy in the form of analgesics and oral rinses was used.

By the morning of the third postoperative day the patient was obtunded and cyanotic. The family physician called to her home was unable to obtain a recordable blood pressure and observed that she was cold, cyanotic, and barely arousable. He noted the presence of purpura and that massive swelling extended from "the jaw to the clavicle."

She was transferred by ambulance to a hospital emergency department and admitted with the diagnosis of Ludwig's angina and septicemia. Laboratory studies at the time of admission revealed visible blood in the urine, red blood cell casts, hemoglobin level of 15.2 g/100 mL, and a white blood cell count of 8300 cells/mm³. Platelets were absent from the peripheral blood smear, and the prothrombin time was markedly prolonged. Because of the presence of shock, acral cyanosis, purpura, thrombocytopenia, and obvious coagulopathy, the diagnosis was modified to disseminated intravascular coagulation secondary to Ludwig's angina of dental origin.

Further laboratory data in the intensive care unit revealed a blood urea nitrogen level of 75 mg/100 mL, platelet count of 39,000/mm³, partial thromboplastin time of 52 seconds, and a moderately decreased fibrinogen level associated with severe depletion of other hemostatic factors. Gram stain of the buffy coat demonstrated large numbers of gram-positive cocci, whereas blood cultures later grew β-hemolytic *Streptococcus* colonies.

Tracheostomy was performed and oxygen administered; fluids, fresh plasma, and blood were infused; penicillin and oxacillin were administered; and heparin therapy was started. Despite all therapy, neck swelling increased, temperature increased to 40.6°C (105°F), urine output decreased, and the blood pressure could be maintained no higher than 90/60 mm Hg with the continuous infusion of vasopressors. A purulent exudate was noted in the oral cavity, and gram-positive cocci were seen on Gram stain.

By the morning of the fourth postoperative day (second hospital day), the shock syndrome and renal failure appeared irreversible and the patient was comatose. The purpura became generalized, and bleeding persisted around the tracheostomy and intravenous catheter sites. Immunoelectrophoresis studies supported the diagnosis of consumption coagulopathy, as did serial coagulation tests.

Assisted respiration and use of plasma, serum albumin, and mannitol infusions were continued. Chest radiography revealed diffuse infiltrates bilaterally, and bloody sputum was obtained from tracheal suctioning. Unremitting

deterioration continued, and late on the fourth postoperative day fatal cardiopulmonary arrest occurred.

Disseminated intravascular coagulation is a well-recognized but fortunately uncommon sequelae of severe infection. It occurs as a result of gram-negative sepsis far more commonly than as a result of streptococcal infection, but severe complications are possible with dental infection. The possible preventive effect of antibiotic use at the time of surgery is purely speculative, inasmuch as the 50 to 70% fatality rate of patients with disseminated intravascular coagulation includes many who were receiving antibiotics at the time of the onset of the consumptive coagulopathy. Generalized sepsis can be the cause of death in Ludwig's angina.

Ludwig's Angina

A 60-year-old woman with a diagnosis of Ludwig's angina and septicemia was admitted to the intensive care unit by a clinician in the hematology section. The patient had a 13-year history of chronic lymphocytic leukemia, which had required chemotherapy only during the last year. She had complained to her dentist about painful swollen gingiva 3 days before admission, and penicillin had been prescribed for the periodontal infection. By the date of admission, her mouth and neck were markedly swollen, airway obstruction was present, and she was in septic shock.

Examination revealed an intubated, obtunded patient with a temperature of 38.3°C (101°F). The tongue was elevated over erythematous indurated sublingual tissue, and the gingivae were edematous and red, especially adjacent to the mandibular incisors. The upper neck was bilaterally swollen and firm. The white blood cell count was 52,000 cells/mm³, consisting exclusively of immature lymphocytes and a few blast forms.

Blood and oral cultures grew *Pseudomonas aeruginosa*. Incision and drainage of the neck was performed, and cultures also revealed *Pseudomonas*. High-dose, intravenous multiple-antibiotic therapy was instituted, but despite a secure airway the patient died of generalized sepsis on the fifth hospital day.

The compromised host is the contemporary patient most at risk from deep fascial space infection, usually from opportunistic organisms. Although the death certificate listed chronic lymphocytic leukemia, septicemia, and Ludwig's angina as causes of death, the initiating factor was gingivitis.

Alternative treatment for Ludwig's angina has been described. Glucocorticoids have been added to antibiotic therapy when the latter did not halt the inexorable progression of the infection. The rationale is to combat the inflammatory edema, with resolution finally accomplished without surgery.[6]

Lateral Pharyngeal and Masticator Space Infection

A 19-year-old man was seen with trismus and dysphagia. Historically, he had multiple episodes of pericoronitis controlled by antibiotics, but he had refused third molar extraction. Examination was difficult because of trismus and pain, but bulging of the lateral pharyngeal wall and soft palate with deviation of the uvula was observed, in addition to tenderness and slight swelling at the mandibular angle. Imaging confirmed the diagnosis of lateral pharyngeal space and masticator space (pterygoid compartment) infection.

After cautious blind nasal intubation, a mucosal incision at the pterygomandibular raphe and an angled skin incision, with deep blunt dissections, released pus from the spaces and relieved the trismus. Mixed oral flora was treated with intravenous penicillin and metronidazole, but persistent pharyngeal swelling and inadequate drainage, confirmed by CT, necessitated second incision and drainage 5 days later, which resolved the infection. The infected tooth was removed.

Medically and legally, a patient must be fully informed of the risks of recurrent pericoronitis. In such situations, the procedure is not elective, but rather is better categorized as urgent.

Dysphagia, like dyspnea, is an alarm in the presence of an odontogenic infection. Anesthesia consultation, prompt imaging, and rapid surgical decompression are necessary.

Failure to respond quickly to incision and drainage, demonstrated by defervescence of fever, lowered white blood cell count, and relief from dysphagia or dyspnea, requires reevaluation by examination and reimaging to determine adequacy of drainage or possible late involvement of other spaces. A second trip to the operating room during the initial hospitalization is medically and legally superior to a later readmission.

Multiple Fascial Space Infections

A 60-year-old man was admitted to the hospital from the emergency department with a diagnosis of multiple space infections and parotitis. Facial swelling had been present for 4 days before admission. His medical history revealed the presence of hepatic cirrhosis and steroid therapy for peripheral neuropathy.

Admission examination demonstrated unilateral facial swelling extending from the temporal region to the angle of the mandible, moderate trismus, bulging of the soft palate, and purulent discharge from Stensen's duct orifice, which was macerated. The mandibular second molar was mobile, and bloody purulent exudate could be expressed from the adjacent gingiva. His temperature was 38.9°C (102°F), and the white blood cell count was 14,850 cells/mm³. Gram stain results suggested streptococci from the gingival purulence and staphylococci from the duct. Specimens for culture were sent to the laboratory, and high-dose intravenous cephalosporin therapy was started. Steroid therapy was reduced gradually and then discontinued during his hospitalization.

Despite treatment, the patient's swelling and pain persisted, and by the second hospital day he reported dysphagia and dyspnea. Soft tissue radiographs revealed narrowing of the upper airway because of expansion of the posterior pharyngeal space.

On the evening of the second hospital day, tracheostomy was performed with the patient under local anesthesia, and general anesthesia was then administered. Drainage of the buccal, masticator, infratemporal, lateral pharyngeal, and retropharyngeal spaces was accomplished intraorally. Profuse purulent flow was obtained and drains were placed. External drainage of the parotid gland was performed by a preauricular approach. Repeat drainage of the temporal spaces was performed on the fourth day; drainage was performed percutaneously because of persistent pain and bulging in the area. Two mandibular molars were extracted. Rapid resolution of the space infections and parotitis followed, but osteomyelitis of the mandible (mixed oral flora) subsequently developed.

Cortisone was a major contributing factor in the rapid and deep spread of this dental infection. The parotitis may have been a result of dehydration or caused by occlusal trauma to the bulging buccal mucosa and duct orifice. It also may have been the result of spread of infection from neighboring spaces. The infection was exacerbated by the antiinflammatory effects of the steroids. This case is a prime example of an overwhelming "minor" infection in a compromised host.

Multiple Fascial Space Infections

A 40-year-old man underwent extraction of an infected third molar, and penicillin was prescribed and taken. However, on the third postextraction day the patient was seen at an emergency department with fever, shaking chills, trismus, and dysphagia. His physician ordered blood cultures and intravenous antibiotics. By the third day of his hospitalization and after two further changes of antibiotics, the patient remained febrile and blood culture revealed *Fusobacterium*. No imaging was performed.

Surgical drainage of the masticator and lateral pterygoid spaces on the fourth hospital day resulted in diminished swelling and defervescence. The patient was discharged the following day taking oral penicillin. Eight days later, he was sent from work back to the emergency department, where he reported chills, headache, and nuchal rigidity. The antibiotic regimen was changed again, but he returned to the emergency department 2 days later semicomatose.

Blood cultures again grew *Fusobacterium* and streptococci, and magnetic resonance imaging revealed a posterior pharyngeal space abscess and an epidural brain abscess near the brainstem. Surgical drainage of both sites and 10 days of intensive intravenous antibiotic therapy resolved all signs of infection, but the patient had severe neurologic deficits, including deafness and hemiparesis. Legal action ensued against the physician, the surgeon, the emergency physician, and the hospital, with a final settlement of almost $2 million.

Fusobacterium, an oral organism, can be virulent, especially when causing generalized sepsis. Patients with positive blood culture results should not be discharged until cultures are sterile or after 10 days of appropriate intravenous antibiotic therapy. Even a lateral plain film might have revealed an incipient posterior pharyngeal space infection. Shaking chills, headache, and neck stiffness should have been strong indicators, especially with the patient's history of recent drainage of a lateral pharyngeal space.

Multiple Fascial Space Infections/Mediastinitis

A 20-year-old student underwent extraction of bilateral painful impacted mandibular third molar teeth in an outpatient facility. His medical history was significant for numerous episodes of staphylococcal pneumonitis and skin infections during childhood. A chronic fungal infection of his nail beds resisted treatment. No antibiotics were used or prescribed at the time of surgery.

Eight days after extraction of the teeth, he was admitted to the hospital because of dyspnea, dysphagia, swelling of the left side of the neck and face, and temperature of 39.7°C (103.4°F). The diagnosis at the time of admission was lateral pharyngeal space abscess, left submandibular space abscess, and left buccal space infection. Dehydration was clinically apparent, and the white blood cell count was 19,700 cells/mm^3 with a marked shift to the left.

Intravenous fluids and clindamycin were administered. On the second hospital day, spontaneous drainage from the buccal space occurred, and gram-stained smears of specimens revealed gram-positive cocci and gram-negative rods. Culturing yielded *Bacteroides* species and peptostreptococci.

Despite extensive antibiotic therapy, his condition worsened, and lateral neck imaging revealed widening of the retropharyngeal space. On the fourth hospital day, he underwent tracheostomy and exploration of the suprahyoid spaces, carotid sheath, lateral pharyngeal spaces, and posterior pharyngeal spaces through submandibular and sternocleidomastoid approaches. Three drains were placed, and mixed aerobic and anaerobic flora was cultured from the heavy purulent fluids suctioned from these spaces.

The patient's condition improved considerably after surgery, with relief of respiratory distress, lowered temperature, and lessened leukocytosis. Blood glucose, B- and T-lymphocyte counts, complement assay, and white blood cell chemotaxis studies were performed and yielded normal findings. Blood cultures yielded *Peptostreptococcus* on two occasions.

On the thirteenth hospital day the patient reported chest pain, his temperature spiked to 40°C (104°F), and radiographs revealed a widened mediastinum and pleural effusions (see Figure 16-22). Thoracentesis produced a cloudy aspirate that yielded *Eikenella corrodens* when cultured. Sputum cultures later yielded *P. aeruginosa;* tobramycin therapy was instituted, and clindamycin was discontinued. On the seventeenth hospital day the mediastinum and a large empyema cavity were drained. Two ribs were resected and drains were inserted.

The patient slowly recovered, but on the twenty-seventh hospital day, swelling of the neck and exacerbation of the fever occurred. His neck was reexplored, a small amount of pus was obtained, and drains were inserted. Cultures revealed *E. corrodens* and peptostreptococci.

All signs of infection resolved, all drains were removed, and the patient was discharged on the fifty-third hospital day. In retrospect, inflammatory markers, such as sedimentation rate and C-reactive protein, might have been used to follow or even predict the course of his disease.

This patient's history was strongly suggestive of compromised host defenses. Although he underwent testing while he had an infection, no defects in the defense system were found, based on contemporary knowledge. Such was the state of the art. His progressive and persistent infectious course may have been related in part to the well-documented failure of clindamycin to destroy *E. corrodens*.

References

1. Zhang WJ, Cai XY, Yang C, et al. Cervical necrotizing fasciitis due to methicillin-resistant *Staphylococcus aureus*: a case report. *Int J Oral Maxillofac Surg.* 2010;39:830.
2. Bahu SJ, Shibuya TY, Meleca RJ, et al. Craniocervical necrotizing fasciitis: an 11-year experience. *Otolaryngol Head Neck Surg.* 2001;125:245.
3. Lin C, Yeh FL, Lin JT, et al. Necrotizing fasciitis of the head and neck: an analysis of 47 cases. *Plast Reconstr Surg.* 2001;107:1684.
4. Umeda M, Minamikawa T, Komatsubara H, et al. Necrotizing fasciitis caused by dental infection: a retrospective analysis of 9 cases and a review of the literature. *Oral Surg Oral Med Oral Pathol Oral Radiol Endod.* 2003;95:283.
5. Whitesides L, Cotto-Cumba C, Myers RA. Cervical necrotizing fasciitis of odontogenic origin: a case report and review of 12 cases. *J Oral Maxillofac Surg.* 2000;58:144.
6. Hutchinson IL, James DR. New treatment of Ludwig's angina. *Br Oral Maxillofac Surg.* 1989;27:83.

Case Reports Related to Osteomyelitis and Osteonecrosis

Infection-Induced Osteomyelitis

A 65-year-old man was referred by his general dentist for the extraction of a symptomatic right mandibular third molar (Figure A-1). The tooth had a communication with the oral cavity and a history of prior episodes of pericoronitis successfully treated with oral antibiotics. The patient was otherwise in good general health, and his list of medications consisted solely of supplemental vitamins. He denied tobacco or alcohol use. The patient underwent an uncomplicated surgical extraction of the third molar and was placed on a 7-day course of amoxicillin. The postoperative course was remarkable for pain and trismus mostly due to muscle spasm.

Panoramic radiographs obtained during postoperative week 1 (Figure A-2) and repeated at postoperative week 4 (Figure A-3) revealed an intact mandible devoid of any obvious signs of osseous pathologic conditions.

At the eighth postoperative week, the patient returned to the clinic with a complaint of a sudden return of right mandibular pain and malocclusion of 3 days' duration. The patient denied any history of trauma and was afebrile. Examination of the mandible was difficult because of trismus and the presence of focal intense pain. Additionally, a small quantity of a purulent exudate was noted at the site of the previous extraction. Culture of the drainage was obtained and submitted to the laboratory for culture and sensitivity studies.

A radiograph obtained on this date revealed a nondisplaced fracture involving the right mandibular angle region (Figure A-4). Radiolucencies consistent with osteolysis, as well as ragged osseous borders and presence of a sequestrum, were noted.

The patient was asked to return to the office the following morning, and under intravenous sedation the wound was explored and repeat culture performed. Additionally, the fracture site was debrided and curettage performed of granulation tissue. Sequestrectomy and saucerization were performed, and specimens were also submitted for biopsy examination to rule out other noninfective pathologic conditions. The patient was then placed in intermaxillary fixation (Figure A-5).

Two days after debridement, the patient reported increased malaise and a decision was made to have the patient admitted for further workup. The patient had a low-grade fever with a slight leukocytosis (13,000 cells/mm^3 consisting of 78% polymorphonuclear leukocytes and 16% bands). Computed tomography (CT) scanning was interpreted as being most consistent with a diagnosis of osteomyelitis of the mandible because of the soft and hard tissue changes present. An infectious disease consult was obtained to assist with the management of the patient. The patient was treated presumptively for osteomyelitis pending the results of the biopsy and the culture and sensitivity studies. He was empirically placed on intravenous broad-spectrum antibacterial coverage. Vancomycin and ampicillin-sulbactam were recommended by the infectious disease consultant and implemented. Rigid fixation was applied to the fracture site on postadmission day 4. The bone biopsy result was consistent with osteomyelitis, and the culture revealed mixed oral flora. The patient was placed on a 4-week course of intravenous penicillin followed by a 3-month regimen of amoxicillin-clavulanate. The patient tolerated the antibiotic course and had a full recovery from the infection. The pathologic fracture of the mandible fully healed without sequelae. He has been symptom-free for 12 months since the initial presentation.

Radiation-Induced Osteonecrosis

A 58-year-old man was referred by his general dentist for the evaluation of a nonhealing fistulous tract involving the anterior mandibular vestibule. The patient had presented to his general dentist about 6 weeks prior with a complaint of slight swelling and pain involving the anterior mandibular region. The patient wears a mandibular overdenture supported by dental implants. The patient's general dentist had prescribed at least three 1-week courses of antibiotics; each course 1 week apart (two 1-week courses of amoxicillin and a 1-week course of clindamycin). The patient had been responsive to these regimens while on the antibiotics, but would have recurrences of the infection on discontinuation. The patient's medical history was significant for irradiation to the upper neck for an isolated enlarged right neck lymph node that had been found positive for squamous cell carcinoma with no known primary lesion. He had received a total radiation dose of 6000 cGy 1 year before the onset of his signs and

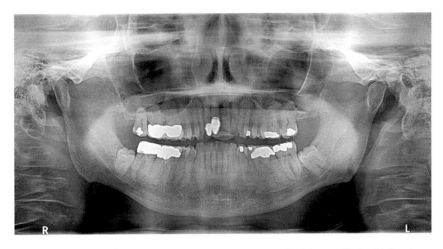

• **Figure A-1** Pretreatment radiograph showing symptomatic right mandibular third molar.

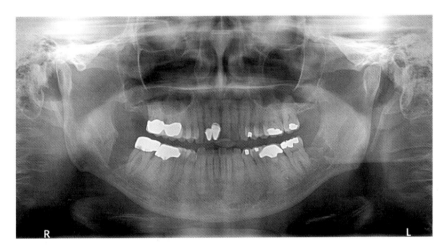

• **Figure A-2** Radiograph 1 week after surgery shows the mandible intact and devoid of signs of an osseous pathologic condition.

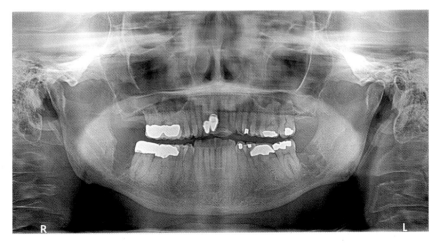

• **Figure A-3** Radiograph 4 weeks after surgery shows the mandible intact and devoid of signs of an osseous pathologic condition.

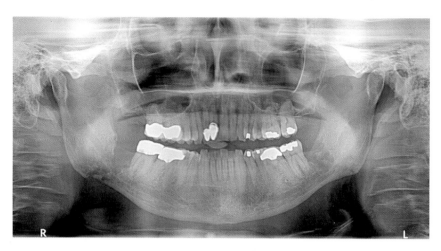

• **Figure A-4** Radiograph 8 weeks after surgery shows a nondisplaced fracture involving the right mandibular angle, radiolucencies consistent with osteolysis, ragged osseous borders, and the presence of a sequestrum.

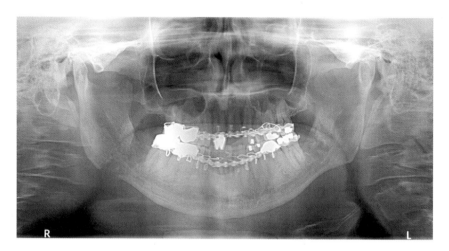

• **Figure A-5** Radiograph showing intermaxillary fixation.

symptoms. Review of radiotherapy documents confirmed that the mandible was in the field of radiation. Of note, the implants had been placed 2 years before the discovery of his neck mass. He reported a 30-pack-year smoking history. On the initial presentation, the patient was afebrile and had gingival erythema and slight fullness in the mandibular vestibule. There was a small fistulous tract opening with scant purulence. The left dental implant was mobile; however, the right dental implant appeared stable (Figure A-6).

A panoramic radiograph revealed areas of radiolucency and irregular osseous borders involving the anterior mandibular region (see Figure A-6). The exudate was swabbed for culture and sensitivity studies. The patient was asked to return in a week for a follow-up appointment, and given the history of irradiation to his mandible, he was referred to a wound center for evaluation and to receive hyperbaric oxygen (HBO) therapy.

The patient returned 5 days later with increased swelling and pain and the new finding of an orocutaneous fistula in the submental region. Additionally, the right implant appeared mobile (Figure A-7).

A decision was made to perform incision and drainage, perform repeat culture of the wound, remove the mobile implants, debride, and remove any necrotic free-floating bone and submit for biopsy (Figure A-8).

The patient was referred to an infectious disease specialist and was empirically placed on amoxicillin-clavulanate. The culture results were positive for mixed oral flora. The biopsy results confirmed osteomyelitis with colonies of actinomyces. A diagnosis of spontaneous osteoradionecrosis of the mandible secondary to denture trauma and subsequent superinfection with actinomyces was made.

The patient received 30 dives of HBO per the Marx Protocol and was placed on amoxicillin for 6 months. The patient had a full recovery, with no recurrences of the infection 18 months after the initial presentation (Figure A-9).

Drug-Induced Osteonecrosis

An 85-year-old woman presented for the extraction of a symptomatic mandibular right second molar (Figure A-10). The patient stated that the tooth had become symptomatic

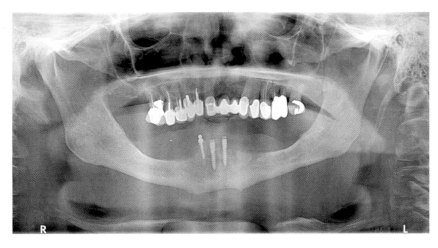

• **Figure A-6** Pretreatment radiograph showing radiolucency and irregular osseous borders involving the anterior mandibular region.

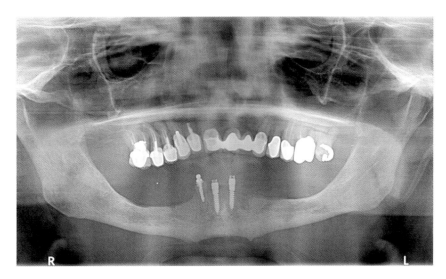

• **Figure A-7** Five days after the initial presentation, radiograph shows an orocutaneous fistula in the submental region; the right implant now appears mobile.

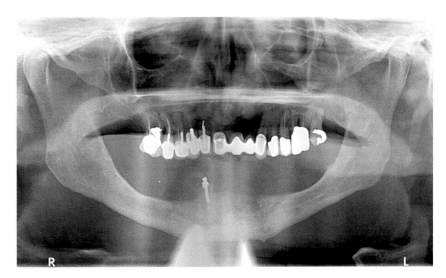

• **Figure A-8** Post-treatment radiograph. Treatment included incision and drainage, repeat culture of the wound, removal of the mobile implants, debridement, and removal of necrotic free-floating bone.

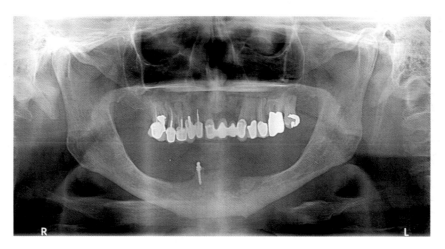

• **Figure A-9** Radiograph 18 months after the initial presentation. The patient fully recovered.

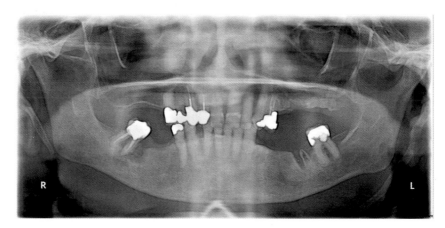

• **Figure A-10** Pretreatment radiograph showing symptomatic mandibular right second molar.

1 week earlier. The patient's medical history was significant for being on alendronate for 5 years for osteoporosis; however, her physician had discontinued the bisphosphonate 1 year earlier. The patient was also on etanercept for rheumatoid arthritis. On examination, the patient had gingival fullness with no purulent exudate and the tooth was very sensitive to palpation. Given the presence of symptoms, the tooth was extracted atraumatically and the patient was placed on amoxicillin and chlorhexidine rinses.

A follow-up appointment a week later revealed a normally healing socket with small amounts of granulation tissue, but no exudate. The patient also reported a slight paresthesia in the area of distribution of the right inferior alveolar nerve. The patient returned to the clinic 2 weeks later with the new onset of an orocutaneous fistula in the right submandibular region. Exposure of alveolar bone measuring 5 mm was noted at the extraction site. Panoramic radiography revealed extension of the radiolucency within the mandible compared with the baseline (Figure A-11). The presence of irregular osseous borders could also be appreciated. The drainage was

swabbed for culture and sensitivity, and amoxicillin was prescribed. The patient was referred to an infectious disease specialist. The culture results confirmed polymicrobial cause, including presence of actinomyces. Given the patient's history, a diagnosis of drug-induced osteonecrosis of the mandible with superinfection with actinomyces was made. The patient was placed on intravenous penicillin G for 8 weeks, followed by a 4-month course of amoxicillin.

The orocutaneous fistula did not completely resolve until the third month. The antibiotic therapy was discontinued by the infectious disease specialist after a total of 6 months. One month later, the patient returned with the recurrence of an orocutaneous fistula at the same site. A decision was made to maintain the patient on the amoxicillin regimen indefinitely as a suppressive modality. Exposed bone at the extraction site persisted for over 18 months. Over 24 months after the initial presentation, while still on amoxicillin, the patient is asymptomatic, the exposed bone is no longer present, and there has been no recurrence of the orocutaneous fistula (Figure A-12).

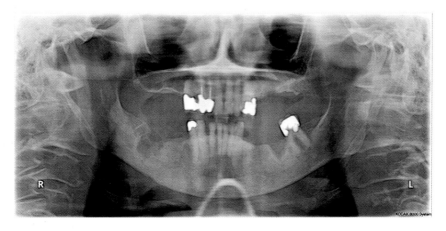

• **Figure A-11** Two weeks after tooth removal. Radiograph shows extension of the radiolucency within the mandible compared with the baseline.

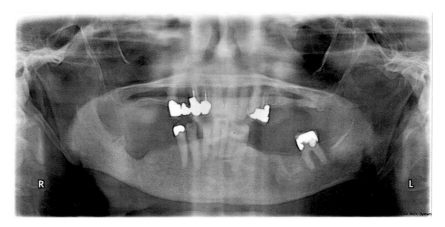

• **Figure A-12** Radiograph 24 months after the initial presentation. The patient is asymptomatic.

Index

Page numbers followed by *b* indicate boxes, *f* indicate illustrations, and *t* indicate tables.